Illustrated Manual of Nursing Techniques

Illustrated Manual of

Third Edition

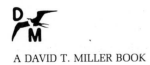

A DAVID T. MILLER BOOK

**J. B. Lippincott
Company**
Philadelphia

London
Mexico City
New York
St. Louis
São Paulo
Sydney

Sponsoring Editor: David T. Miller/
  Joyce Mkitarian
Manuscript Editor: Mary K. Smith
Indexer: Deana Fowler
Art Director: Tracy Baldwin
Design Coordinator: Anne O'Donnell

Designer: Arlene Putterman
Production Supervisor: Kathleen P. Dunn
Production Assistant: Susan Hess
Compositor: Circle Graphics
Printer/Binder: The Murray Printing Company

Library of Congress Cataloging in Publication Data

King, Eunice M.
    Illustrated manual of nursing techniques.

    King's name appeared first on the t.p. in earlier eds.
    "A David T. Miller book."
    Bibliography: p.
    Includes index.
    1. Nursing—Handbooks, manuals, etc.   I. Wieck, Lynn.
II. Dyer, Marilyn.   III. Title. [DNLM: 1. Nursing—
outlines.   WY 18 K51i]
RT51.K54   1986   610.73   85-24097
ISBN 0-397-54521-5

The authors and publisher have exerted every effort to ensure that drug selection and dosage set
forth in this text are in accord with current recommendations and practice at the time of publication.
However, in view of ongoing research, changes in government regulations, and the constant flow of
information relating to drug therapy and drug reactions, the reader is urged to check the package
insert for each drug for any change in indications and dosage and for added warnings and
precautions. This is particularly important when the recommended agent is a new or infrequently
employed drug.

Techniques 26, 27, 28, 29, 30, 49, 59, 60, 61, 69 contain illustrations from the Lippincott Learning
System, units Application of Heat and Cold, Asepsis, Bedmaking, Care of the Mouth, Care of the
Skin, Wound Care; copyright J. B. Lippincott Company. Techniques 22, 31, 33, 39, 42, 51, 80 contain
illustrations from the Lippincott Learning System, units Anatomical Terminology, Joint Classification
and Range of Motion, Bowel Elimination, Urine Elimination; copyright Regents of the University of
Wisconsin/Milwaukee and J. B. Lippincott Company. Technique 67 contains illustrations from the
Lippincott Learning System, units Oral Medication, Parenteral Medication; copyright Regents of the
University of Wisconsin/Milwaukee.

Nursing Tech

Lynn Wieck, R.N., M.S.

Adjunct Faculty, West Texas State University
Assistant Director of Nursing Service,
Nursing Quality Assurance Chairperson,
Northwest Texas Hospital, Amarillo, Texas

Eunice M. King, R.N.,

Administrator of Medical Staff Services and F
Northwest Texas Hospital, Amarillo, Texas

Marilyn Dyer, R.N., M.

Assistant Dean,
West Texas State University School of Nursin

To my husband, Steve, for his patience,
and our sons, Joey, Scott, and Doug,
for their perseverance
L.W.

To my daughters Janet and Kathy,
who have encouraged and inspired me
in my professional endeavors
E.K.

To Mindi, Cheri, Mark, Keith, Trent, and Brooke,
who enjoy having a nurse for a mother
M.L.D.

Preface

In preparing this third edition of *Illustrated Manual of Nursing Techniques*, we have attempted to reflect the changing roles of the nurse and the client in today's evolving health care system. Acknowledging the partnership shared by client and nurse and the growing emphasis on client and family participation in care, we have focused on assessment and education as an integral part of every technique. The client's right to know and responsibility for self permeate each procedure described in this book. The role of the family as provider, supporter, and consumer of health is a unique and dominant factor.

Consumer awareness and involvement are a welcome trend in the health care field. Cognizant of the Orem Self-Care Model, we have attempted to help the nurse and nursing student to identify the client's self-care deficits and potentials. With an understanding not only of how to perform the particular technique, but also why, we feel that the nurse will gain confidence and the consumer will receive competent care.

Responses from users of previous editions have indicated consistently that this manual provides a vital how-to aspect to the theoretical and analytic textbooks used in teaching and practice. Its aim is to present comprehensive coverage in a concise manner that will complement medical–surgical, pediatric, and obstetric texts. For this edition, each technique has been thoroughly revised and updated, and the nursing intervention sections now follow an action/rationale format. New features include technique-specific discussions of *quality assurance*, *infection control*, and *discharge planning*. In addition, the inclusion of an *anatomy and physiology* segment for each technique, along with attention to relevant *pathophysiological aspects*, gives the reader a sound basis for nursing diagnosis and competent performance. *Technique checklists* provide structured performance criteria and a convenient self-assessment tool. Techniques are organized by the steps in the nursing process, according to the following outline:

Overview
  Definition
  Rationale
  Terminology
Assessment
  Pertinent anatomy and physiology
  Pathophysiological concepts
  Assessment of the client
Plan
  Nursing objectives
  Client preparation
  Equipment
Implementation and interventions
  Procedural aspects: Action and rationale
  Special modifications
  Communicative aspects
    Observations
    Charting

Discharge planning aspects
  Client and family education
  Referrals
Evaluation
  Quality assurance
  Infection control
  Technique checklist

We wish to thank our colleagues in nursing service and nursing education who have collaborated with us to make this book a reality. We particularly wish to thank those clinical experts who took the time to read and review each technique to make sure that each was accurate, readable, and current: Tedi Beckett, R.N., M.S.N., medical–surgical techniques; Christy Blake, R.N., M.S.N., pediatric techniques; Shirley Brock, R.N., B.S.N., obstetric techniques; Kitty Padgett, R.N., B.S.N., obstetric techniques; Mary Jo Arend, R.N., B.S.N., neonatal techniques; Linda Gast, R.N., B.S.N., critical care techniques; and Debbie Davenport, R.N., M.S.N., C.C.R.N., critical care techniques. Special thanks is due to Ona Goad Baker, R.N., B.S.N., President of the Texas Association of Infection Control Nurses for her valuable input in regard to infection control considerations.

For the improved quality of the art and photography, we wish to thank Ann Kime, artist and illustrator; Robert Bradshaw, photographer; Sandy Hutchens, R.N., B.S.N., obstetrical photography; and Tracy Baldwin of J. B. Lippincott Company for her valuable advice and feedback.

Sincere appreciation goes to Joyce Mkitarian of J. B. Lippincott Company, whose editorial assistance was invaluable, and to David T. Miller of J. B. Lippincott, for his continued support and friendship, we owe our thanks.

Lynn Wieck, R.N., M.S.N.
Eunice M. King, R.N., M.ED., F.A.A.N.
Marilyn Dyer, R.N., M.S.N.

Contents

Unit One

Techniques for Diagnostic Studies

Unit Two

Techniques for Adult Clients

Unit Three

Techniques for Pediatric Clients

Unit Four

Techniques for Obstetric Clients

Unit Five

Techniques for Neonatal Clients

Appendixes

The Nursing Process in the Presentation of the Nursing Techniques

Nursing continues to undergo dynamic change. These changes are the result of the fluid society in which we live and the many internal and external pressures that are exerted on the health care milieu. An important aspect of modern health care delivery is provision of individualized care to an interacting member of society. The provision of care based on the unique needs of the person is embodied in the nursing process, which ensures that care will be systematic, scientific, deliberate, and individualized.

The components of the nursing process: assessment, planning, implementation, and evaluation, are the basis for the provision of comprehensive nursing care geared to help the client to reach the greatest potential of self-care. Basic to the nursing process is an understanding of the goals and components of each technique. To that end, each technique is prefaced with a short definition, the rationale relating why the technique is performed, and pertinent terminology used in the technique. Fortified with this introductory material, the nurse will move easily into the dynamics of the nursing process.

Assessment Phase

The assessment phase involves a process that requires the ability to make decisions and judgments. These judgments are based on data collected by the nurse about the state of the client's health. Data collection is accomplished by methods such as observation, physical examination, and the interviewing process. This information is then organized and analyzed so that the nurse can arrive at a diagnosis of the client's nursing problems and begin the planning stage for resolution.

The nurse must bring to the assessment phase a basic understanding of the situation, how it evolved, and what may be anticipated. Hence, in this book the assessment phase includes a basis of the anatomy and physiology pertinent to the technique, an introduction to the pathophysiology that is occurring, and a guide to client assessment that includes client, family, and environmental considerations.

Planning Phase

The planning phase is a guide for the nursing care actions of the nurse. Based on the assessment, the nurse can assist in setting priorities and identifying objectives in conjunction with the client and family. Specific nursing actions for the achievement of objectives, as well as educational deficits of the client and family, can be identified. Expected outcomes can be stated in the form of a written plan that adds clarity and provides cohesiveness for the team of client, family and nurse.

The nursing objectives specific to each technique are clearly stated. Because carefully written objectives are important in establishing goal direction, the objectives reflect the goals of both the client and the nursing care provider, arising from the mutual interest in promoting self-help from the client. Self-help begins with preparing the client for the technique. Preparation steps, both physical and psychological, are included for each procedure. The therapeutic client–nurse relationship, which begins with identification and addressing the preparatory needs, is essential to the proper implementation of each technique. Another aspect of planning is the provision of essential equipment. Needed equipment is identified in each technique.

Implementation Phase

The implementation phase is the action phase of the nursing process. During this phase, client and family responses to the nursing actions will be identified. Priority is given to assisting the client to gain independence and confidence in providing for self-needs. For every action, a rationale is given to assist the nurse in understanding not only what to do, but why. The rationale aspect adds a dimension of understanding that is necessary for the nurse to make an informed decision about the progress of care.

Integral to the implementation of nursing interventions is an understanding that there are exceptions to every rule. A section within each appropriate technique handles special modifications relating to those exceptions. Although these sections cannot be all-inclusive, the most common exceptions are addressed.

The communicative aspects include observations and documentation. Observation as an element of nursing intervention can help the nurse identify the client's and family's responses to the care. When the nurse reviews the objectives for the technique, responses indicative of change emerge. Effective documentation is an essential component of health care communication. This book offers standardized examples of charting for specific techniques. To acknowledge the vast divergence in charting styles and methodology, from check lists to computerized records, the emphasis in this manual is on charting observations made during the implementation of the nursing technique.

Discharge planning is a vital part of the nursing intervention phase. This process actually begins in the assessment phase, when information is obtained regarding how this client will be assisted to as much independence as possible within the physical, emotional, and environmental confines present. The emphasis in discharge planning is on client and family education. Knowledge deficits are identified, and information is supplied according to individual needs. Some clients will need more information and will respond to different teaching styles than others. This book provides the essential elements for the client's knowledge base. It is up to the nurse to identify each client's deficits and provide the information to fill those gaps in a meaningful way.

Evaluation Phase

The fourth step in the nursing process is the evaluation phase. Although this step takes place throughout the entire process in the form of assessment and reassessment, it is organized and finalized in this final section of each technique. Assurance of quality nursing care is the right of every client. The Quality Assurance section emphasizes those ways in which hospitals and individual nurses can make sure that quality care was given. The focus of quality care assessment by the Joint Commission for the Accreditation of Hospitals is on documentation. This book takes that approach as well. Documentation of nurs-. ing assessments, anticipated and unanticipated problems and their resolutions, and nursing actions and client responses all fall within the Quality Assurance framework.

One aspect of quality care is the assurance that each client will be protected from hospital-acquired infections and will receive the education needed to prevent self-infection after discharge. Because prevention of infection is such a priority, a separate section of each technique involves identification of recommended infection control measures.

The technique checklist at the end of each procedure provides the final vehicle for comprehensive evaluation. It provides a synopsis of the important features of the technique to serve as a reminder for discharge planning activities and as a reaffirmation that quality care was given.

The nursing process works because it is flexible enough to allow nurses to meet the individualized needs of every client, yet structured enough to prevent omission of vital care aspects. A client living up to the fullness of his or her health potential is the goal; the nursing process is the means.

Nursing the Older Person

The over-65 age group is said to be the fastest growing segment of the U.S. population. This phenomenon, which has been called the "greying of America," has great implications for the health care industry. By the year 2020, the elderly may constitute one fifth of the total population. Adequate health care for the elderly, the senescent, and the senile will require special knowledge and skills on the part of the health care professionals. The emergence of the geriatric nurse practitioner and the addition of geriatric components to nursing school curricula are evidence that nursing is recognizing that care of the elderly client requires a unique body of knowledge.

Past attitudes toward aging, which emphasized maintenance of the status quo and a custodial existence to death, will no longer suffice. In recognition that the elderly also have rights to self-determination, new emphasis is now being given to exploring the potential of the elderly and dealing with each person's right to independence and self-care individually. Degeneration in many elderly persons can be reversible. The rights of the elderly to both ends of the hierarchy of needs is being recognized. Not only do the elderly deserve shelter and nourishment, but they deserve and are seeking socialization and self-actualization. Work patterns are changing to keep pace with the demands of an aging work force; so too will the health care industry be molded into the form needed for quality care of the elderly.

The dynamics of aging have been the focus of considerable study and research in recent years. The common denominator that has evolved is only that there is no common denominator. The elderly are a diverse group of people, with individual needs and desires. The responsibility of nursing administrators, practitioners, educators, and students addressing the aging population is to recognize their differences while accepting their common, special needs.

The Aging Population

The causes of aging are multidimensional, encompassing physiological, psychological, social, and cultural factors. Literature available in the area identifies some of the general characteristics as follows:

1. Susceptibility to stress increases. This is a critical area; authorities generally agree that stress can cause illness and that vulnerability to stress-induced diseases increases with old age.

2. Loss is more prevalent among the elderly, who often and inevitably experience drastic life changes, such as loss of spouse, lifelong friends, job, or home.

3. Many older adults suffer from low self-esteem because of cultural neglect.

4. Loneliness has been identified as the most common mental health problem.

5. Chronological age is not a valid indicator of aging. Individual differences are great, and a total assessment of each person is needed to determine the degree of aging and the physiological, sociological, and psychological changes that have occurred.

6. The elderly are not a homogeneous group. Each person is unique in background, current health status, needs, goals, and reactions.

7. Change is gradual; persons age at vastly different rates.

8. Elderly people generally have been stereotyped as hostile, inflexible, senile, prejudiced, and "set in their ways." Although some elderly persons may fit this image, many do not whereas some younger persons do.

9. A small percentage of the elderly are in institutions (fewer than 5%); for many, old age is a satisfying time of life with only minor physical or mental impairment.

10. Old age is not synonymous with disease, yet age increases susceptibility to disease, and disease tends to intensify the aging process.

11. A major need of the elderly is the desire to be involved and not isolated or neglected. Noninvolvement usually leads to rapid mental and physical deterioration.

12. Personality is a key factor in the person's response and adjustment to the aging process.

13. Activity is important, and new avenues should be developed; when lifelong activities must be given up, satisfactory substitutes should be found.

14. A major cause of emotional disorders in the elderly is the loss of self-esteem and a lowered social status.

Common Physical Changes

The physical changes that occur with aging vary markedly among different persons, and they may appear at varying points along the life-span continuum. Some of the commonly found changes are: weight loss, progressive structural decline of the body, greying of the hair, tooth loss, hearing and visual deterioration, and wrinkling and discoloration of the skin.

Diseases commonly found in the elderly are osteoporosis, atherosclerosis, cardiovascular disease, stroke, cancer, severe or mild organic brain disease, arthritis, arteriosclerosis, rheumatoid arthritis, and diabetes mellitus.

A major problem in physical illness is that elderly clients may not report their physical symptoms and may resort to uniformed self-treatment. Many physical diseases impair mental ability. Drug tolerance varies in older persons and must be monitored closely. For example, antihypertensive drugs can decrease the cerebral blood flow, diuretics may affect the electrolyte balance, and digitalis may cause adverse reactions in the central nervous system.

Common Emotional Changes

Attitudes in caring for the elderly are vital. Aging is not necessarily accompanied by a decline in mental abilities. In fact, much can be done to reverse mental dysfunction by the way the elderly person is treated. When an older person faces loss of memory, anxiety is a common reaction. This may predispose the older adult to physical and psychological manifestations. Multiple losses, such as those of status, income, home, spouse, friends, or self-image, often intensify the mental stress.

The most prevalent functional disorders found in elderly persons are depression, paranoid states, and late-life schizophrenia. Depression, which is widespread, is characterized by feelings of helplessness and sadness, poor self-image, lack of interest, and emotional withdrawal. Physical symptoms are fatigue, constipation, sleep disturbances, and loss of appetite.

Nursing Implications

An important part of nursing responsibility to the elderly is to assist in maintenance of independence. The older client should be encouraged to take part in or assist as much as possible with self-care. Conservation of physical strength is important, but should not be used as an excuse for disenfranchisement of the older person's rights to self-determination and independence.

A basic need of the elderly is the need to talk to someone. The nurse should allot time to spend with the elderly client, encouraging verbalization and expression of feelings. All nursing measures and treatment should be explained thoroughly, allowing time for questions and frank, honest answers.

Isolation and loneliness can result in depression, loss of purpose, loss of willpower, and physical and mental deterioration. The older person should be encouraged to visit with other clients, participate in recreational and social activities, read, watch television, and participate in arts, crafts, or other activities that are a means of achievement and satisfaction for the client.

The needs of the elderly are much more than day-to-day physical needs; aging persons have deep needs for security, dignity, self-esteem, independence, and respect. The whole person must be understood. The nurse's awareness of the special needs of the elderly is as important as it is for any other age group.

Psychosocial Aspects of Nursing Care

Psychosocial aspects in the care of clients include all of the intrapersonal and interpersonal processes that stimulate and modify behavior. Illness very often alters a person's usual behavior pattern, as well as the ability to cope with new and sometimes unpleasant situations. It is the nurse's responsibility to assist the client in adjusting to evolving situations, and at the same time to assist in retaining a sense of self-worth.

The format of this book is focused on clients and families, not on procedures or diseases. The core of the nursing process is the client–nurse relationship. Florence Nightingale, in her *Notes on Nursing* (1859), referred to the behavioral aspects of illness and the effect of the body on the mind. The inclusion of the behavioral sciences in nursing is not a new concept.

Concern for Individual Needs

Procedures should never be viewed as "routine"; rather, nursing intervention should be approached as an individual process concerned with the total needs of the client. Within this framework, therapeutic procedures become an integral part of total care. It is the responsibility of the nurse to strive continuously to increase knowledge and understanding of human needs and their relationship to the preservation of the person's psychosocial and physiological equilibrium. A broad view of the psychosocial aspects of human behavior is presented in this introduction; content specific to nursing technique is included in each chapter.

The Need for Security

One basic human need is to feel safe, comfortable, and accepted in any possible situation. Confrontation with an illness at home or admission to a hospital are situations that can cause fear and anxiety. As humans, we fear the unknown and the idea that our role in the family may change or that we may lose our identity and become a case or number instead of a person. The ways in which the health care provider responds to these fears and worries will greatly influence the client's experience during illness.

The Need for Knowledge and Reassurance

The best method to allay fear of the unknown is adequate explanation. This builds trust and security, promotes comfort and safety, and greatly enhances interpersonal relationships. Explanation of physical care procedures also advances the client–nurse relationship by establishing trust and two-way communication. Allowing the client to ask questions and express feelings provides security and comfort in an unfamiliar environment.

A person who is fearful will react with increased anxiety if caretakers show doubt or lack of concern. The nurse must maintain a calm attitude and convey competence through actions and demeanor. The close client–nurse association allows the nurse a unique opportunity to enhance security and comfort.

Self-esteem and Self-image

In addition to being a fear-provoking experience, illness represents a threat to a person's self-esteem and self-image. Plunged into an unfamiliar state of dependency, the client may be unable to meet even the most basic human needs. The nurse should emphasize the positive aspects of treatment and expected therapeutic results to combat negative feelings on the part of the client. Performance of tasks carefully and confidently creates an attitude of acceptance. Of extreme importance in enhancing self-esteem is concern for the client's privacy and modesty. The need for adequate use of screening and draping cannot be overemphasized.

Opportunities to encourage independence should be sought and used. If the client is allowed to participate in care, feelings of helplessness and dependence are decreased. Cooperation may also be enhanced if the client is allowed to follow established behavior patterns within the limitations of the hospital setting. The nurse must be aware of physical restrictions and assist the client to remain within them. If the client understands the reason for the restrictions, cooperation may be enhanced. Knowledge of limits may give the client a sense of security and increases self-esteem by knowing that others care; however, the client still retains autonomy and the right to self-determination.

Relieving Anxiety

Tension and anxiety may increase one's perception of pain. Measures that can be taken to relieve the anxiety level and possibly reduce the amount of pain perception include two-way communication, explanations, and reassurance. Hospitalized clients may have unexpected emotional reactions to their conditions. Emotions may be controlled by diversionary techniques such as backrubs, reading, television, and crafts. Inclusion of the client's family in therapy and teaching will enrich the therapeutic atmosphere and aid in acceptance and compliance with prescribed therapy.

Fear of disfigurement or bodily injury is a persistent problem, especially if the client will undergo surgery. Clients should be prepared in advance if there is a possibility of alteration to body image from treatment, surgery, or medication. Perception of body image is developed from childhood and usually is firmly established. Adjustments to changes in body image evolve slowly. The nurse should avoid unnecessary or premature demands for adjustment.

Fear of illness or death is also an emotion that must be faced on entry to a hospital. Many people at this time come face to face with the reality of their own mortality. Societal attitudes about illness and death may guide behavior. The nurse should allow the client to verbalize feelings about illness and death and provide honest answers to questions. Acceptance as a valued member of society, without regard to physical condition, is an important need of every client. The way in which a person perceives a situation usually is related to past experiences with the same or similar situations. A past unpleasant experience with illness may prompt the client to seek additional explanation and reassurance.

Aesthetic Needs

Americans place high values on both beauty and cleanliness. Each client should be clean and comfortable. Attention to personal hygiene is a part of every client's hospital day. This is based on the premise that if the client feels fresh and clean, outlook and feelings will be more positive. Each person is an individual, and one of the most personal and valued possessions is self-image. Nurses owe it to their clients to help them to leave the hospital with self-images intact.

Environmental Needs

People tend to evaluate and modify their environments constantly to protect themselves against potential danger. The nurse can aid in this process by removing unpleasant stimuli, such as bright lights, sudden noises, or temperature extremes. Concern for the client's safety also may be shown by such simple actions as raising siderails or offering adequate instructions.

The Need for Value As a Person

A hospitalized client is sensitive to verbal and nonverbal communications; difficulties arise when inconsistencies are noted. When the nurse expresses concern about the client, this concern may be manifested by a gentle touch or attentive listening. Before a client can practice self-acceptance, the feeling of acceptance by others must be present.

Health Teaching

The nurse has many opportunities for health teaching in the hospital setting. Motivation is a prerequisite to learning; hence, the client must be able to see some correlation between what the nurse is saying and the self. The client has learned when health problems, actions, and outcomes are internalized. The client's educational and intellectual levels also affect the ability to understand. The nurse should assess the client's level of understanding and knowledge and should gear explanations appropriately.

Psychosocial Resources

If a person is to receive adequate medical and nursing care, the area of psychosocial functioning must receive attention. In treating the "whole" person, nurses will draw on knowledge and skills from the social sciences, sociology, psychology, and anthropology. It is the hope of the authors that nurses will use the unlimited reference materials available in this area, and that the application of principles from the social sciences will be a major objective in planning care.

Unit One

Techniques for Diagnostic Studies

1 Barium Enema

Overview

Definition

X-ray visualization of the large intestine after rectal instillation of contrast medium

Rationale

Reveal the presence of polyps, tumors and other lesions of the lower bowel. Determine the site of pathology in the lower bowel.

Terminology

Colonoscopy: Direct visualization of the rectum and colon by means of a flexible hollow instrument with glass fibers to provide light from an external source

Fluoroscopy: Use of a fluorescent screen to visualize shadows in the body cavities

Hemorrhoid: A dilated blood vessel internally or externally located in the colon, rectal or anal region

Impaction: Retention of hard, dried stool in the rectum and colon

Peristalsis: The wavelike movement of the intestinal tract that is responsible for the onward movement of intestinal contents

Polyp: A growth with a pedicle, commonly found in a vascular area such as the rectum

Assessment

Pertinent Anatomy and Physiology

See Appendix I: *anus, intestine (large), rectum, sigmoid colon.*

Pathophysiological Concepts

1. A common symptom of abnormalities of the bowel is diarrhea. Large-volume diarrhea results from an increase in the water content of the stool, and small-volume diarrhea from an increase in the peristaltic action of the bowel. Small-volume diarrhea usually is characterized by cramping, as well as by frequent, explosive stools. This form of diarrhea often is associated with intrinsic disease of the colon, such as ulcerative colitis.

2. Another common symptom of pathology of the bowel is impaction. Fecal impaction stimulates secretion of mucus in the portion of the bowel proximal to the blockage, which results in watery, diarrhealike stools as the body attempts to evacuate the mass.

3. Cancer may occur in any part of the colon, but it is found most commonly in the rectum. Usually cancer of the colon and rectum are present for a long time before producing any symptoms. Bleeding is a highly significant symptom of colorectal cancer. Other symptoms are changes in bowel habits and a sense of urgency or incomplete emptying of the bowel. Pain is often the last symptom.

Assessment of the Client

1. Assess the general condition of the client to ascertain tolerance of the preparation regimen for a barium enema. If the client is already in a weakened condition, it may be necessary to space the cleansing enemas farther apart to allow adequate time to rest.

2. Ascertain the client's perception of the reason for the diagnostic study. Determine if malignancy is suspected. The reason motivating the client to have the test will greatly affect cooperation during the procedure and reaction to the results.

Plan

Nursing Objectives

Provide adequate information about the examination to allay fear and anxiety.

Cleanse the colon thoroughly of fecal matter.

Client Preparation

1. Thoroughly explain the bowel preparation procedure, as well as the examination procedure itself. Assure the client that the barium is insoluble and is not absorbed by nor is it toxic to the body.

2. Thoroughly and completely cleanse the bowel so that adequate visualization may be accomplished. A liquid supper and a strong laxative, such as castor oil, may be given to the client the evening before the x-ray. An enema at bedtime may also be ordered (see Technique #51, Enema and Rectal Tube). The client will usually be NPO at midnight to reduce the possibility of nausea or fecal accumulation. On the morning of the examination, the client may receive enemas until the return is clear, signifying that no fecal matter remains in the bowel to interfere with the x-ray.

3. For the client having the lower gastrointestinal tract examinations done on an outpatient basis, commercial kits are available which eliminate the necessity of numerous enemas. Preparations which may accompany the use of such kits include forced clear fluids, no enemas, and a rectal suppository early in the morning of the test day.

3. If colonoscopy is to be done, it is usually done before the barium enema as the barium may obscure the visualization. The preparation for colonoscopy may require high volumes of an electrolyte-complete, oral bowel evacuation preparation (such as Colyte). Enemas are not necessary; however, food and fluids are withheld from midnight.

Equipment

Enema Setup

Specific bowel preparation package

Implementation and Interventions

Procedural Aspects

ACTION	*RATIONALE*
1. For soft tissues to be visualized, barium sulfate is used to fill the organs and cause them to cast an outline shadow on the film (Fig. 1-1 shows a normal colon).	X-rays are a form of radiant energy that penetrate according to the density of the tissue. Barium sulfate is a fine, white, odorless, tasteless bulky powder, insoluble in water and impermeable to the x-ray beam. The barium coats the lining of the bowel.
2. In the x-ray department, the client lies on the left side on the x-ray table. The physician inserts a balloon-tipped tube into the rectum, which is inflated to prevent backflow of barium. The barium is allowed to run into the large intestine. The client may be asked to roll to the supine position and then to the right side so that the	The portion of the bowel immediately proximal to the rectum is the ascending colon, which is located along the left side of the body. With the client on the left side, the barium flows by the natural force of gravity into the left colon.

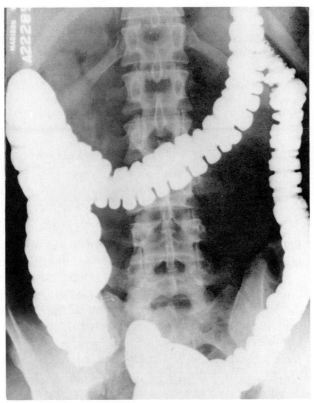

Figure 1.1

ACTION

    barium is more generally dispersed.

3. Adequate cleansing of the colon is essential so that the contour of the colon (including cecum and appendix) is clearly visible.

4. Films are made with the barium in place and after it has been evacuated. The peristaltic activity of each portion of the bowel also can be observed.

5. Occasionally, air may be used to inflate the bowel.

RATIONALE

Fecal material in the bowel will appear as a dense shadow on the film and will obscure the position of other anatomically significant structures.

The natural tendency of the full bowel is to evacuate the contents. This peristaltic activity can be seen on the radiologic examination, and adequacy of elimination capacity can be evaluated.

Inflation of the bowel allows the outline to be illuminated better, which enhances the visualization of polyps and small tumors.

Special Modifications

1. Administer enemas with care to clients with conditions such as ulcerative colitis. Assess any bleeding carefully and report if the amount appears excessive. Suppositories may be used for bowel cleansing in clients with known rectal disease.

In certain inflammatory diseases of the colon, any irritation of the colon may initiate bleeding.

ACTION	*RATIONALE*
2. If resistance to insertion of the enema tube is encountered, do not force it into the rectum. Notify the physician of inability to insert the tube.	Some bowel disturbances may be due to tumor growth in the lower rectal area. These may impede the passing of the enema tubing.

Communicative Aspects

OBSERVATIONS

1. Observe the client carefully during the bowel cleansing procedure for signs of fatigue and hemorrhage.

2. Check any rectal bleeding carefully and report it to the physician. Laxatives, suppositories, and enemas can irritate hemorrhoids and cause minor rectal bleeding.

3. Observe for electrolyte imbalances due to repeated enemas and withholding of fluids. Watch for altered vital signs and mental confusion or disorientation.

4. After the x-ray examination, ask the client to report the next bowel movement so that the nurse can verify that the barium is passing satisfactorily. If it is not, additional measures (e.g., laxatives, suppositories, or forcing fluids) may be necessary to avoid impaction.

CHARTING

DATE/TIME	OBSERVATIONS	SIGNATURE
5/23 0730	Enemas until clear in preparation for barium enema. Cleansing enemas given (4×). Last enema returned clear. Encouraged to rest until time for x-ray. No rectal bleeding noted.	C. Allen RN

Discharge Planning Aspects

CLIENT AND FAMILY EDUCATION

1. Some colon conditions may be improved by a change in the diet that eliminates foods high in fiber and roughage. Calling attention to the types of low-fiber foods served in the hospital will acclimate the client and family to dietary modifications that might be made after discharge. On the other hand, some colon discomfort actually may be decreased by high-fiber diets. Once the cause of the client's problems has been established, arrange for dietary counseling so that future dietary changes may be incorporated into the client's life-style after discharge.

2. Caution the client about the need to expel all of the barium after the x-ray examination. It should be understood that failure to evacuate the barium could lead to impaction. Stress the importance of fluids in aiding the elimination process.

3. Offer sound guidance and practical information about exercise and activity, and guidelines for judicious use of over-the-counter medications for relief of minor gastrointestinal disturbances. Help the client develop a positive, flexible attitude about elimination patterns.

4. If a malignancy is found, surgical intervention may be necessary. The client and family will need support and reassurance. If a colostomy is to be done, begin early with a positive attitude preparing the client and family for care at home. Stress and dwell on the things that the client will be able to do rather than limitations. A positive attitude at the earliest stages of diagnosis and treatment will greatly enhance the client's adjustment to any alterations in lifestyle.

REFERRALS

If a cancerous process is discovered, the client and family may benefit from the support available from the American Cancer Society.

Evaluation

Quality Assurance

The documentation should reflect the nature of the results of the preparation procedure as well as the client's response to these results. Record the number of preparatory enemas, the appearance of the return, and the client's condition before and after the procedure. Document the evacuation of the barium or instructions to the client and family regarding passage of barium after discharge from the hospital.

Infection Control

Thorough handwashing before and after the administration of an enema cannot be stressed enough. Likewise, encourage the client to engage in thorough handwashing after each bowel movement and enema evacuation. Transfer of microorganisms from the colon is greatly reduced by proper handwashing. Equipment that is used for consecutive clients must be thoroughly cleaned and disinfected after each use.

Technique Checklist

	YES	NO
Client given explanation of barium enema procedure before beginning preparations	_____	_____
Laxative or suppository given	_____	_____
Medication _____		
Amt. _____		
Enemas until clear (no. given _____)	_____	_____
Clear fluids forced	_____	_____
NPO at midnight	_____	_____
Adequate visualization accomplished	_____	_____
Evacuation of barium before discharge	_____	_____
Instructions on diet before discharge	_____	_____
Instructions regarding medications before discharge	_____	_____
Proper eliminatory habits explained to client and family	_____	_____

2   Blood Samples, Arterial and Venous

Overview

Definition

Removal of a small amount of blood from an artery, vein, or capillary for laboratory analysis

Rationale

Determine the normal constituents of the blood by analysis of a blood specimen.
Analyze blood gases to determine the effectiveness of ventilation.
Assess the blood to detect the presence of foreign substances.

Terminology

Antecubital area: The area at the internal aspect of the elbow on the forearm

Brachial artery: The artery located in the antecubital area of the arm

Coagulation: Clotting or solidifying of blood from a liquid state into a semisolid mass

Femoral artery: The artery located in the groin

Peripheral resistance: The resistance, which maintains adequate blood pressure, offered by arterioles to the flow of blood

Radial artery: The artery located at the internal aspect of the wrist

Thrombus: A clot, formed from constituents of blood, in a blood vessel or one of the cavities of the heart

Venipuncture: Puncture of a vein for the purpose of obtaining a blood sample or administering a substance intravenously.

Assessment

Pertinent Anatomy and Physiology

See Appendix I: *blood, blood vessels.*

Pathophysiological Concepts

1. Veins used repeatedly for venipuncture may become knotted or inflamed. Such damage can cause a vasoconstrictive reflex; this can lead to thrombus formation owing to prolonged slowing of the blood.
2. Certain conditions can lead to hemorrhage. These include thrombocytopenia (a decrease in the number of circulating platelets), impaired platelet function, and hemophilia. Platelets are involved in the formation of the sticky plug that stems the flow of blood from leaking vessels. In hemophilia, which is an inherited lack of plasma clotting factor needed to initiate clot formation, there is a prolonged coagulation time and a tendency toward bleeding in the skin, muscles, and joints. Clients who have been undergoing anticoagulant therapy also may experience abnormal bleeding tendencies. Obtaining blood specimens from these clients should be done cautiously to avoid hemorrhage.

Assessment of the Client

1. Assess the knowledge level of the client about pretest requirements, the procedure itself, the reason the blood analysis is being done, and the possibility of complications.
2. Assess the client's overall physical condition. Question the client about pre-

vious problems with clotting and about familial conditions such as frequent bruising, difficulty stopping bleeding, or known cases of hemophilia.

Plan

Nursing Objectives

Minimize trauma at the puncture site.

Allay nervousness by reassurance and assistance of the client as needed.

Preserve the specimen appropriately.

Assure that the client is aware of pretest and post-test requirements (e.g., fasting, positioning, and activity).

Client Preparation

1. Before beginning, carefully explain how the procedure is to be done and why it is necessary. Emphasize that although the amount of blood removed may seem excessive, in reality it is a very small amount. Explain that the body is continually manufacturing new blood even when none is lost, and that the amount taken for the specimen will not cause any physical effects or problems.

2. Inform the client that the blood specimen(s) may be drawn very early in the morning. Blood drawn before a person has eaten breakfast is usually more chemically uniform and offers a closer indication of the true status of the vascular system.

3. The client should know that there may be a momentary deep throbbing pain when the artery is punctured.

4. The specimen should not be taken from the arm in which an intravenous infusion is in place because the specimen may be diluted and therefore not indicative of the true composition of the blood.

5. The client should be in a reclining or semireclining position. Comfort is important in decreasing anxiety. Some people faint at the sight of blood, so precautions must be taken to avoid falls and anxiety.

6. Ulnar circulation must be present before radial artery puncture is attempted. Check this by compressing the radial artery tightly while the client makes a fist. While maintaining compression of the radial artery, instruct the client to relax the hand, which should return to normal color if adequate ulnar circulation is present.

Equipment

VENIPUNCTURE

1. Tourniquet
2. Alcohol sponge or topical cleanser
3. Needle (usually 20-, 21-, or 23-gauge)
4. Cotton ball and tape
5. Syringe or vacuum container
6. Labels for specimens
7. Requisition form for tests to be done

ARTERIAL PUNCTURE

1. 5-ml or 10-ml syringe (preferably glass)
2. Heparin (1,000 U/ml)
3. 20-gauge needle
4. Blood gas syringe cap (metal or cork)
5. Alcohol sponge
6. Cup of ice
7. Labels for specimens
8. Requisition form for tests to be done

Implementation and Interventions

Procedural Aspects

	ACTION	*RATIONALE*

Venipuncture

1. Be familiar with the state laws governing the removal of blood from living persons.

   Laws regarding who can legally do venipuncture vary among states.

2. Thorough handwashing is essential before withdrawing blood samples.

   Handwashing decreases the chance of cross-contamination.

3. Apply the tourniquet tightly several inches above the site of intended venipuncture. The arm should be in a dependent position. Common sites for venipuncture are the cubital, basilic, and cephalic veins of the arm (Fig. 2-1).

   Withdrawal of blood by venipuncture depends on differences of pressure. Blood in the vein comes under greater than normal pressure by the damming action of the tourniquet and by the dependent position of the arm, at a level lower than that of the trunk.

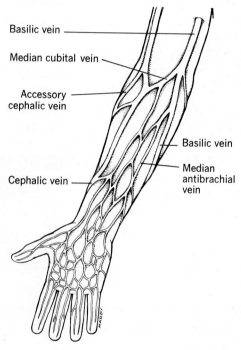

Basilic vein

Median cubital vein

Accessory cephalic vein

Basilic vein

Median antibrachial vein

Cephalic vein

Figure 2.1

4. Cleanse the venipuncture site thoroughly with a circular motion using the alcohol sponge. Venipuncture for blood culture and sensitivity requires additional measures (See Technique No. 6, Cultures).

   Microorganisms normally found on the skin may be pathogenic if allowed to enter the bloodstream.

5. Locate the vein by sight (bluish appearance) or by feel (a firm, rubbery rebound sensation). Pumping the fist may help distend the vein in the upper extremity.

   The vein of choice is usually located in the antecubital area. Activity in the area will increase blood supply to that area.

ACTION	*RATIONALE*
6. Assure that the needle is large enough to withdraw the blood easily, usually at least a 23-gauge needle, and preferably a 20- or 21-gauge.	Use of too small a needle results in hemolysis of the blood as it is withdrawn and inaccurate test findings.
7. Hold the skin taut. Hold the needle with the syringe attached at a 45° angle with the bevel up. When the needle enters the vein, venous return is visible immediately in the syringe. Obtain the specimen by gently drawing back on the plunger of the syringe. It may be necessary to release the tourniquet if the blood flow diminishes.	Tautness of the skin helps prevent rolling or movement of the vein. The pressure needed to pierce the skin is sufficient to force the needle into the vein. Negative pressure will cause the blood to enter the syringe.
8. When using a vacuum container, insert the external needle on the adapter into the vein. Once venous return is visible, the vacuum container is pushed down onto the needle and the tube fills with blood. If more than one tube is needed, the first tube may be replaced with a second without removing the needle from the vein (Fig. 2-2).	The vacuum inside the container creates enough negative pressure to withdraw the blood from the vein.

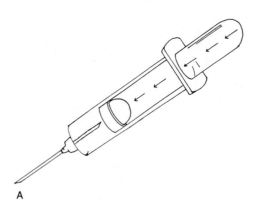

A

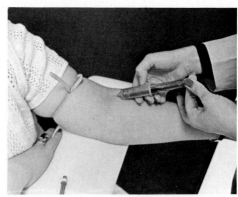

B

Figure 2.2 A and B

9. After venipuncture, release the tourniquet and remove the needle. A dry cotton ball should be held firmly on the venipuncture site for several minutes. An adhesive strip may prevent oozing.	Stemming the flow of blood will allow time for a clot to form.
10. Transport the specimen to the laboratory in an expeditious manner. Label every specimen and ensure that the correct requisition is attached.	Delays may compromise results. Avoid errors by labeling properly.

ACTION

Arterial Puncture

1. Determine the site of arterial puncture at any artery in which the pulse is easily palpable, usually radial, brachial, or femoral (Figs. 2-3, 2-4). Before the radial artery is punctured, ensure that there is an adequate ulnar pulse (see Client Preparation, above).

RATIONALE

Direct puncture of an artery may be done for a variety of reasons. The most common is to ascertain the effectiveness of ventilation by study of blood gases. A blood sample from any of these arteries will indicate clearly the adequacy of gaseous exchange occurring in the cardiopulmonary system.

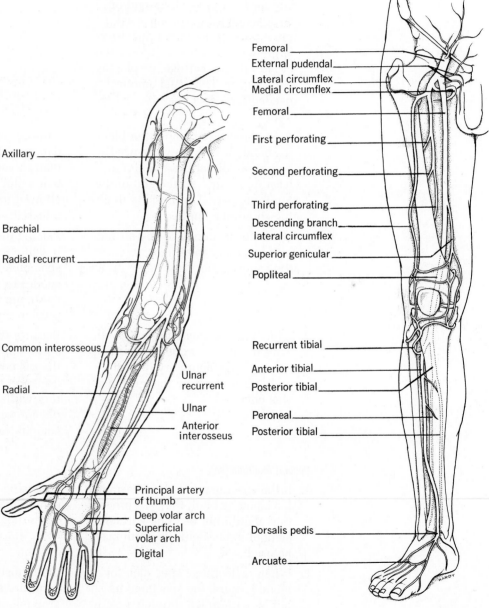

Figure 2.3

Axillary

Brachial

Radial recurrent

Common interosseous

Radial

Ulnar recurrent

Ulnar

Anterior interosseus

Principal artery of thumb

Deep volar arch

Superficial volar arch

Digital

Femoral

External pudendal

Lateral circumflex

Medial circumflex

Femoral

First perforating

Second perforating

Third perforating

Descending branch lateral circumflex

Superior genicular

Popliteal

Recurrent tibial

Anterior tibial

Posterior tibial

Peroneal

Posterior tibial

Dorsalis pedis

Arcuate

Figure 2.4

2. Use a glass syringe to obtain the arterial specimen.

Gases can permeate the walls of a plastic syringe and cause inaccurate test results.

ACTION

RATIONALE

3. Lubricate the syringe with 0.5 ml of heparin. After the barrel has been coated, discard the remainder of the heparin.

Heparin is an anticoagulant and will help to prevent the specimen from clotting.

4. Cleanse the area with an alcohol sponge. Palpate the artery with the middle and index fingers of the free hand. When the pulsation is felt, insert the needle at a 90° angle between the two fingers into the artery. The wrist may be anchored on the surface near the puncture site for finer control. Extend or hyperextend the extremity as much as possible. Once the artery is pierced, pressure will force the blood into the syringe, displacing the plunger. The usual amount needed for a specimen is 2 ml to 4 ml.

Cleansing reduces the chance of introducing microorganisms into the bloodstream. Because arterial pressure is greater than the venous pressure, vascular pressure usually is sufficient to cause the syringe to fill.

5. After the desired amount of blood is obtained, withdraw the needle and apply direct pressure for at least 5 minutes. At the end of the 5-minute period, a pressure dressing should be applied.

Arterial pressure is so great that the danger of hemorrhage is more acute than in venipuncture. It is essential that a clot of sufficient strength be allowed to form before pressure is released.

6. Clear the specimen of any air bubbles by gently rotating it; replace the cap and place specimen on ice.

Placing the specimen on ice will keep it stable for several hours; whereas a specimen left at room temperature is good only for about 10 minutes. The specimen must be handled gently to prevent destruction of red blood cells.

7. Label the specimen correctly and send it with the appropriate requisition to the laboratory immediately. Note the time the specimen was obtained.

Because the study of the arterial specimen includes measurement of the gas components, it is essential to transport the specimen to the laboratory while the gas composition is stable and representative of the actual state of the client's blood.

Special Modifications

1. If the specimen is to be measured for blood alcohol, the skin preparation should not be done with an alcohol swab. Benzalkonium may be used.

Cleansing the skin with alcohol may contaminate the results.

2. When collecting a specimen for a blood culture, the specimen must not be withdrawn through a catheter, such as a subclavian IV. Transport the specimen for culture to the laboratory immediately and call the attention of the lab personnel to the fact that it is for culture.

Care must be taken not to contaminate a culture specimen. Organisms start growing quickly, so that the specimen must be handled in an efficient manner to ensure correct results.

ACTION	*RATIONALE*
3. Arterial blood samples may be withdrawn through an arterial line. Arterial lines should be handled only by nurses with critical care experience and expertise.	Because of the great potential for contamination or complications, a thorough knowledge of arterial monitoring is essential in dealing with arterial specimens and lines.
4. Capillary specimens may be used to determine hemoglobin, glucose, and blood type. The tip of the middle or ring finger is cleansed with alcohol, and the end is punctured with a sterile object. "Milking" the finger by grasping it at the base and applying pressure in a progressive manner toward the tip will produce several drops of blood, which are allowed to run by gravity into a pipette tube for testing.	Applying pressure over the length of the finger from the base to the tip will cause accumulation and pooling of blood, making the specimen easier to collect.
5. The client should not be receiving any oxygen, positive pressure breathing (PPB) treatments, or other ventilatory assistance when blood gas specimens are drawn, unless the purpose of the test is to measure the effectiveness of the assisting apparatus. If oxygen is in use, note the amount of liters per minute the client is receiving on the requisition.	Alterations in aeration will change the amount of oxygen and carbon dioxide in the blood. If the laboratory knows how much oxygen the client is receiving, they can provide a more accurate interpretation of the results.

Communicative Aspects

OBSERVATIONS

1. Observe the site of arterial puncture or venipuncture for signs of oozing or leaking into tissue. Small hematomas are common, but excessive bleeding may indicate a clotting deficit.

2. Observe the reaction of the client to the puncture, including comments and nonverbal communication.

CHARTING

DATE/TIME	OBSERVATIONS	SIGNATURE
2/20 1800	Arterial puncture of radial artery for blood gas analysis. Adequate ulnar collateral circulation present. Iced specimen to laboratory stat. Pressure to radial artery for 7 min. ———————————————————————	F. White RN

Discharge Planning Aspects

CLIENT AND FAMILY EDUCATION

1. Tell the family and client that arterial and venous puncture may cause slight discoloration of the skin; however, large areas of discoloration or continued oozing from the puncture site may indicate problems. These should be reported to the nurse.

2. Alert the client and family that abnormal bruising or bleeding may indicate problems with the normal clotting mechanism of the blood. This is usually a reversible condition if diagnosed early enough. Any abnormal bleeding or bruising should be reported to the physician.

3. Inform the client and family to check the site for inflammation, heat, or continued oozing, which would indicate that the site had not sealed properly.

Evaluation

Quality Assurance

Documentation should reflect the reason for obtaining the blood specimen, the site used, and any complications noted. The client's reaction to the procedure and explanations offered should also be documented. Note the type of skin preparation utilized. Findings of the blood analyses should be present on the chart. Document efforts to reinforce or clarify the interpretation of results to the client and family.

Infection Control

1. Adequate cleansing of the puncture site will decrease the chance of introducing microorganisms into the vascular system. Exercise care when inserting the needle between the fingers during arterial puncture. The needle must not come in contact with the nurse's fingers.

2. Some pathogenic microorganisms may be carried in the blood. For the protection of laboratory personnel, specimens obtained from persons with communicable diseases should be labeled legibly and prominently, stating the type of isolation precautions required.

3. Accidental needle puncture is a common mechanism of transmission of certain blood-borne diseases to healthcare personnel (especially hepatitis B). Such accidents frequently occur when one is attempting to recap or destroy the needle. Carefully dispose of all needles used in obtaining blood specimens according to hospital procedure. Attention to safety precautions and common sense will help to ensure that accidents are prevented. If needle puncture occurs, immediate attention should be given to the accident according to hospital policy.

Technique Checklist

	YES	NO
Test ordered by physician on chart	_____	_____
Client understands why test is to be done	_____	_____
Pretest preparations completed	_____	_____
Fasting _____		
Medication _____		
Removal of ventilatory aids _____		
Adequate amount of blood withdrawn	_____	_____
Specimen uncontaminated	_____	_____
Complications present		
Hematoma		
Bleeding		
Site Infection		
Other _____		
Procedure carried out in adequate time frame	_____	_____
Time specimen drawn _____		
Time specimen to lab _____		
Time results obtained _____		
Test results in normal range	_____	_____
If not, physician notified:	_____	_____
Date _____		
Time _____		

3   Bone Marrow Aspiration

Overview

Definition

Puncture and withdrawal of marrow from thin, flat bones, e.g., sternum, spinous process of vertebra, iliac crest. It is also called a *sternal puncture* or *bone tap*.

Rationale

Determine the presence of blood dyscrasias.

Assess the progression of serious blood diseases such as leukemia.

Determine the level of immunity.

Terminology

Dyscrasia: Abnormality of the blood

Marrow: The soft tissue, occupying most bone cavities, which is involved in the formation of blood cells

Osteomyelitis: Inflammation of the bone marrow

Periosteum: The outer layer of the bone

Assessment

Pertinent Anatomy and Physiology

1. See Appendix I: *bone marrow.*
2. With the exception of the joints, bones are completely covered with a dense fibrous membrane called the periosteum. Periosteum is important in the early growth of bones as well as in the nourishment of bone tissue.

Pathophysiological Concepts

1. Pernicious anemia and leukemia are diseases specific to the blood that result in abnormal formation of certain cells. These cells are concentrated in the marrow of the bones.
2. The bone may become infected. The resulting inflammation of the bone and its marrow is called osteomyelitis. Because of the difficulty in reaching the offending organism in the bone, these infections are very difficult to control and often become chronic.
3. If the client has been receiving chemotherapeutic agents for the treatment of cancerous conditions, watch for suppression of bone marrow function and of blood cell formation. These drug effects, leading to anemia, leukopenia, and thrombocytopenia, place such clients at particular risk for developing serious infections.

Assessment of the Client

1. Assess the physical condition of the client. Aspiration of marrow is a painful procedure and may necessitate a period of bedrest after completion. It is also important to have baseline measurements before the procedure so that signs of infection and complications can be seen and corrected early. Assess the client's ability to maintain the necessary position during the procedure.
2. Assess the ability of the client to understand why this procedure is necessary. Bone marrow aspiration may be repeated at intervals during chemotherapy or other selected treatment regimen to ascertain progress. The client should be assessed each time the procedure is done to determine knowledge

deficits and emotional response. Fears, anxieties, and depression tend to intensify with each subsequent bone marrow aspiration procedure.

3. Determine whether the client has any allergies, especially if a local anesthetic or a topical antiseptic is to be used. If iodine is to be used to prepare the skin, assess prior sensitivity to iodine or allergies to shellfish and other iodine preparations.

4. Assess the client during the procedure for signs of pallor, diaphoresis, or syncope, all of which are usually a result of the pain.

5. Assess the client for pain, bleeding, and signs of shock following the procedure.

6. Advise the client that localized tenderness and discomfort over the puncture site is to be expected for 48 to 72 hours.

Plan

Nursing Objectives

Allay the client's fear and nervousness regarding the procedure.

Prevent complications after the puncture.

Support the client during the procedure.

Transfer properly labeled specimen to the laboratory promptly.

Maintain the mental and physical comfort of the client.

Client Preparation

1. The client will need a great deal of reassurance and explanation because the procedure itself is uncomfortable and fear of the results may be overwhelming. A complete explanation should be offered before the puncture is done. A surgical consent form should be signed by the client or legal guardian if required by hospital procedure.

2. Withholding food and fluids is unnecessary. The client may be given a sedative, tranquilizer, or pain medication before bone marrow aspiration is begun, however.

3. A 3- 5-minute scrub may be required before bone marrow aspiration. The skin preparation of the client may include use of a broad-spectrum antiseptic, such as an iodine-containing solution. Preparation should be done in a circular motion, moving outward from the potential puncture site.

Equipment

Cotton balls or gauze swabs

Antiseptic cleaning solution

Sterile gloves

Bone marrow puncture tray containing syringe, bone marrow needles with stylets, additional sterile swabs, and drapes

Glass slides with covers, test tubes, and labels

Syringe, needle, and local anesthetic

Adhesive bandage or tape for pressure dressing

Implementation and Interventions

Procedural Aspects

ACTION

1. In addition to a complete explanation before the procedure is begun, an ongoing explanation during the procedure with continuing reassurance may be necessary.

RATIONALE

An understanding of what is happening will help reduce stress and anxiety.

ACTION

2. Position the client according to the site from which the specimen will be obtained. Specimens may be withdrawn from the sternum, ilium, or vertebrae (Fig. 3-1). If the sternum is to be used, position the client in the back-lying position flat in bed (Fig. 3-2). If the ilium is used, position the client sitting on the side of the bed and leaning forward supported by the nurse or overbed table (Fig. 3-3). The client may also lie in bed on the unaffected side. For vertebral puncture, place the client in the side-lying position with knees drawn up to the chest. (Fig. 3-4)

RATIONALE

Positioning should allow optimal visualization of the site with consideration given to the comfort and safety of the client.

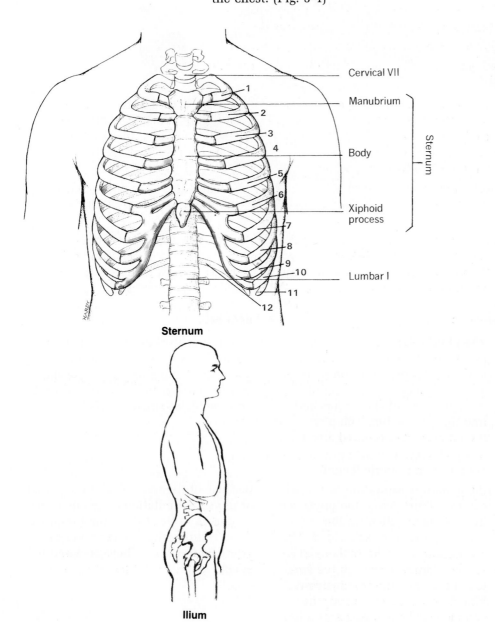

Sternum

Ilium

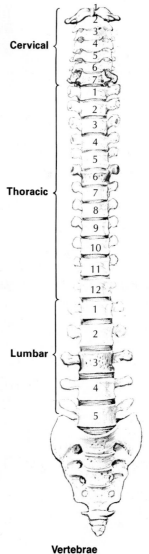

Vertebrae

Figure 3.1

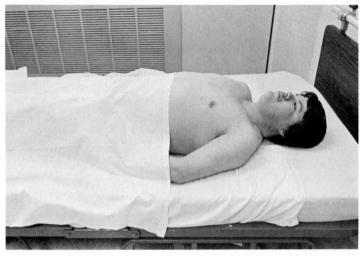

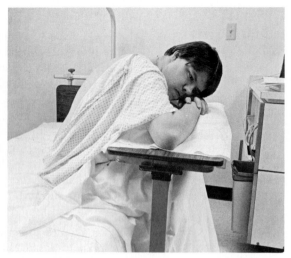

Figure 3.2

Figure 3.3

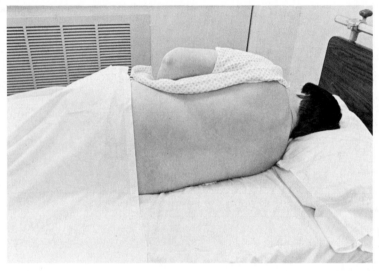

Figure 3.4

ACTION	RATIONALE
3. The physician will then clean the puncture site thoroughly with a topical antiseptic solution. A local anesthetic may also be administered through all skin layers and into the periosteum. The physician then drapes the prepared area with sterile drapes. The procedure is done utilizing sterile technique.	The unbroken skin offers a natural barrier to pathogenic organisms. Microorganisms present on the skin may be pathogenic when introduced into the blood-stream or tissues.
4. Bone marrow aspiration is a medical procedure. Assist the physician by holding the client in the desired position or as needed. The bone marrow needle with stylet in place is inserted through the cortex of the bone into the marrow. The stylet is then removed, the syringe is attached, and aspiration	Because of the tension of the situation or physical limitations, the client may be unable to lie still during the procedure. Holding the client promotes safety and may also have a reassuring effect.

ACTION	*RATIONALE*
is accomplished. The actual aspiration may cause a brief moment of intense pain.	
5. The physician will place the marrow on sterile slides, which are then covered and sent directly to the lab. Proper labeling of each slide is essential. The physician may place the specimen in a test tube, which also must be labeled properly. Laboratory personnel may be present for the biopsy to make the smears and transport the specimens to the lab.	The uncontaminated slides must be received in the lab immediately. Labeling will prevent accidental confusion of results.
6. Apply pressure to the puncture site for 5 to 10 minute. If there is any indication of bleeding or oozing, apply a pressure dressing and watch it carefully. If no oozing is apparent after pressure has been applied, place an adhesive strip to the site and observe it frequently for signs of complications	Hemorrhage is always a possibility after invasion of the marrow. It is essential that the puncture site seal completely before pressure is released.

Special Modifications

Infants and young children must be adequately restrained during this procedure. (See Technique No. 111, Restraints for Pediatric Clients)	Due to the pain involved, compliance of small children cannot be expected; therefore, physical restraint is necessary.

Communicative Aspects

OBSERVATIONS

1. Observe the puncture site carefully for oozing of blood.
2. There is a slight chance of hemorrhage after marrow aspiration. Check vital signs every 15 minutes for 2 hours; significant changes warrant immediate attention.

CHARTING

DATE/TIME	OBSERVATIONS	SIGNATURE
4/6 1115	Bone marrow puncture of sternum done. Seemed relaxed throughout procedure. Intense pain reported during the needle insertion, but no discomfort stated now. Pressure applied to the site for 7 minutes after aspiration. No bleeding noted. Specimen to lab ——————————————	P. Dillon RN

Discharge Planning Aspects

CLIENT AND FAMILY EDUCATION

1. The client and family should understand why it is necessary to do this procedure and what the expected results are. In preparing the client for the procedure, explain that there may be pain when the actual specimen is withdrawn. There may be a crunching sound when the needle penetrates the periosteum into the soft, spongy bone layer. This is expected and is not dangerous. Tell the client and family that the entire procedure takes about 15 to 30 minutes. The client then may have to remain in bed for a period ordered by the physician (usually 4 to 12 hours depending on physical condition and complications). Bedrest usually is advised after vertebral puncture but not after sternal or iliac puncture.

2. Interpret the physician's explanation of the test results, if necessary, to allay anxiety and stress.

Evaluation

Quality Assurance

Documentation should reflect the client's condition before, during, and after the procedure. Hospital policy should provide for an adequate method of transporting specimens to the laboratory in an safe and expedient manner. Documentation should reflect that the nurse was aware of the possible side-effects of this procedure and took precautions to avoid them.

Infection Control

1. Meticulous handwashing is essential before bone marrow aspiration. Some institutions require a surgical scrub. The threat of cross-contamination is great, and the immunosuppressed client is already in a compromised state.

2. The most common causes of infections in the immunosuppressed client are the client's own microorganisms; therefore, it is essential to perform an adequate skin preparation to prevent introducing such organisms during the invasive procedure.

3. A variety of infection control techniques may be deemed appropriate to reduce the quantity of pathogenic organisms to which the client is exposed. These may involve special attire and environmental measures (such as positive air-flow rooms). Careful attention to handwashing prior to client contact remains the single most important measure to prevent infection in the immunosuppressed individual.

Technique Checklist

	YES	NO
Consent form signed	_____	_____
Client understands why procedure is to be performed	_____	_____
Sedative or tranquilizer given	_____	_____
Medication _____		
Time given _____		
Careful handwashing by health personnel	_____	_____
Equipment assembled before procedure	_____	_____
Thorough skin preparation done	_____	_____
Bone marrow puncture accomplished	_____	_____
Number of attempts _____		
Client was able to remain still during procedure	_____	_____
Client required medication for pain	_____	_____
Specimens labeled	_____	_____
Specimens		
Time obtained _____		
Time taken to lab _____		
Pressure applied for site for _____ min	_____	_____
Adhesive strip applied	_____	_____
Vital signs checked q15min	_____	_____
Complications		
Bleeding	_____	_____
Oozing	_____	_____
Vital signs unstable	_____	_____
Client understands the results of the test	_____	_____

4   Bronchoscopy, Assisting With

Overview

Definition

Direct visualization of the trachea and bronchial tree by means of a rigid or flexible tube called a bronchoscope

Rationale

Visualize the tracheobronchial tree for diagnostic purposes.

Obtain a tissue specimen.

Remove a foreign body.

Terminology

Bronchi: The major branches of the respiratory tract leading from the trachea to the lungs

Bronchioles: The smaller subdivisions of the bronchi

Bronchoscope: A rigid, hollow metal instrument that is passed into the upper portions of the bronchi to visualize the respiratory tract (Fig. 4-1)

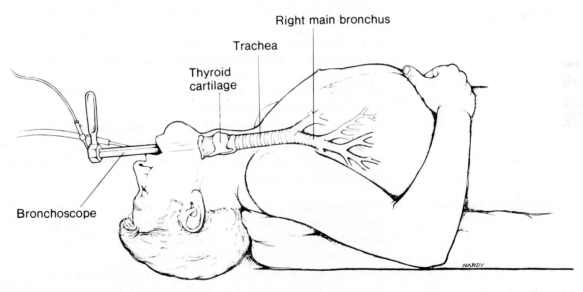

Figure 4.1

Fiberoptic bronchoscope: A flexible instrument of smaller diameter than the metal bronchoscope used for visualization of the respiratory tract (Fig. 4-2)

Tracheobronchial tree: The trachea, bronchi, and bronchial tubes

Assessment

Pertinent Anatomy and Physiology

Appendix I: *bronchial tree, trachea.*

Pathophysiological Concepts

1. Because of the irregular size and shape of the right bronchus, foreign bodies are more likely to lodge in this area.

35

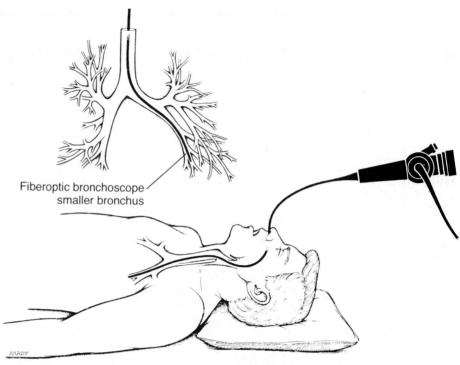

Fiberoptic bronchoscope
smaller bronchus

HARDY

Figure 4.2

2. Collection of fluid in the bronchial passages subsequent to bronchitis causes interference with normal inspiration and expiration. The fluid may be expelled by coughing. Localized pathologic dilatation of larger bronchi as a result of bronchiectasis compromises the normal elastic action of the bronchi, resulting in recurrent infection with excessive production of purulent sputum. When the lung tissue loses its elasticity because of permanent scarring, such as in pulmonary emphysema, lung capacity diminishes because the inspired air cannot be pushed out of the lungs.

3. Lung cancer is a leading cause of death among men, and a steadily increasing cause among women who smoke. Metastatic cancer of the lung is a fairly common condition that is often visible if located in the bronchial tree or if it infringes on the bronchi.

Assessment of the Client

1. Assess the client's respiratory capacity before the bronchoscopic examination. Some discomfort and swelling of the throat is possible after bronchoscopy; therefore, it is important to ascertain whether the client is suffering from respiratory impairment before the procedure.

2. Ascertain the client's understanding and acceptance of the need for the bronchoscopic examination. This procedure sometimes is performed with the client under local anesthesia. The client must understand how to comply with the physician for ease of tube insertion and visualization of the bronchial area. If the client has reservations about the procedure or is overly anxious, notify the physician so that the client's ability and willingness to cooperate during the procedure can be assessed adequately.

3. Assess the state of dental health of the client. Note the presence of partial or total dentures. It is especially important to note the presence of any loose teeth that might become dislodged during bronchoscopic examination.

Plan

Nursing Objectives

Assist the physician by promoting maximum efficiency and minimal time expenditure.

Prepare the client adequately to ensure compliance and comfort during the procedure.

Beware of and observe continually for adverse reactions or complications.

Client Preparation

1. Thoroughly explain the need for cooperation to the client before the procedure. Compliance and relaxation on the part of the client will facilitate the passage of the bronchoscope greatly and will enhance the success of the procedure. Many clients fear that they will be unable to breathe with the scope in place. Give instructions and demonstrate breathing through the nose with the mouth open. Ask the client to demonstrate this technique. Offer reassurance that breathing will not be inhibited during the examination.

2. Withhold food and drink for several hours before the bronchoscopic examination. The mucous lining of the respiratory tract will be stimulated to secrete additional mucus with the insertion of a foreign body, such as a bronchoscope. Limiting fluids and administering a mucus-inhibiting agent may decrease the amount of mucus secretion and the danger of vomiting.

3. Either local or general anesthetic may be used. If local anesthetic is chosen, the client should understand that application of the anesthetic will be uncomfortable because it may stimulate the gag reflex. Local anesthetic is administered by spray, swab, or drip-through cannula.

4. Remove dentures or partial plates. Provide mouth care before the examination so that the client will feel refreshed.

Equipment

Bronchoscopic setup from surgery

Anesthetic agent

Syringe and cannula or swabs (local anesthetic)

Suction pump and tubing

Suction catheters or aspirating tubes

Specimen container, biopsy forceps

Tissues

Emesis basin

Lubricating jelly

Basin with sterile saline solution

Sterile slides with cover (for smear)

Implementation and Interventions

Procedural Aspects

ACTION	RATIONALE
1. The bronchoscopic examination may be done in the surgical suite or on the unit. It may be done with the patient under either local or general anesthesia. If the client is awake, dim the lights and place a towel over the client's eyes.	Dimmed lights provide an environment conducive to optimal visualization of the tracheobronchial tree. A towel over the eyes may help the client relax and remain calm.
2. Withhold food and fluids by mouth for several hours after the procedure until the gag reflex returns. A feeling of swelling of the tongue and throat may follow application of the anesthetic. This is a false sensation, as is the feel-	The local anesthetic inhibits the gag reflex. It also creates a sensation of fullness in the throat. When explaining to the client, use the analogy of the feelings in the mouth after one has dental work under local anesthesia.

ACTION	RATIONALE
ing of the inability to swallow. Reassure the client that these sensations are normal and that actually there is little or no swelling present. Suctioning will eliminate the drooling that results from the client's not swallowing.	
3. Remain with the client during the procedure and offer reassurance and reminders to relax and breathe normally through the nose.	Relaxation of the neck muscles and breathing normally will facilitate the procedure. The more the client relaxes, the less pressure will be felt.

Special Modifications

Children are usually placed under general anesthesia for bronchoscopic examination.	Due to the discomfort and potential for injury if the child moves, general anesthesia is considered practical for children.

Communicative Aspects

OBSERVATIONS

1. Although the local anesthetic creates a sensation of swelling in the tongue and throat, this is usually a false sensation. However, swelling is a complication that may occur after bronchoscopy. Because the client cannot assess the actual amount of swelling adequately, observe the throat at frequent intervals (q15min for several hours) until sensation returns to the anesthetized area.

2. Severe complications may follow bronchoscopy. For this reason, the client must be observed carefully for respiratory distress (may indicate laryngeal edema) and for frank bleeding (indicating hemorrhage). Signs of laryngeal edema include dyspnea, cyanosis, and restlessness.

3. If a foreign body is removed, listen to all lung lobes to ensure that all are clear and trauma is not evidenced by abnormal breath sounds.

CHARTING

DATE/TIME	OBSERVATIONS	SIGNATURE
1/12 1000	Returned to room following bronchoscopy. Swallow reflex diminished. Placed on right side to facilitate drainage of saliva. Slight blood-tinged mucus from coughing. B/P 110/88, P 90, R 20, T 97.8°. Daughter remaining in room, states she understands complications to watch for and will call if help is needed.	F. White RN

Discharge Planning Aspects

CLIENT AND FAMILY EDUCATION

1. Teach the client to use tissues to catch expectoration so that the presence of blood can be noted, as well as for sanitation purposes. Teach the client to dispose of tissues in a receptacle or paper bag near the bedside.

2. The client and family should be told to report any blood in the mucus. A small amount is expected, but frank bleeding indicates a serious complication.

3. The client may have a sore throat for several days and should avoid further irritation (caused by smoking, coughing, or excessive talking) as much as possible.

REFERRALS

If an abnormality or disease of the respiratory tract is discovered, referral to the American Lung Association may be appropriate.

Evaluation

Quality Assurance

Documentation should include teaching done before and after the procedure. Make frequent notation of the aftereffects of the procedure with emphasis on continued monitoring of respiratory sufficiency and blood in the mucus.

Infection Control

1. Bronchoscopy is accomplished under aseptic conditions.
2. Before and after the procedure, remind the client that covering the mouth when coughing and expectorating into a tissue will help to prevent the spread of airborne microorganisms. Provide a bag at the bedside for the disposal of such waste.

Technique Checklist

	YES	NO
Consent form signed	_____	_____
Client understands why the procedure is to be done	_____	_____
Food and fluids withheld for _____ hours	_____	_____
All equipment assembled before beginning of procedure	_____	_____
Specimen obtained	_____	_____
Time obtained _____		
Time to lab _____		
Client observed for respiratory distress for _____ hours	_____	_____
Dyspnea	_____	_____
Cyanosis	_____	_____
Restlessness	_____	_____
Client observed for blood in sputum for _____ hours	_____	_____
Other complications		
Coughing	_____	_____
Sore throat	_____	_____
Vomiting	_____	_____
Other _____	_____	_____

5 Cholangiogram and Cholecystogram

Overview

Definition

X-ray visualization of the gallbladder (cholecystogram, Fig. 5-1) or the entire biliary tree (cholangiogram) after the ingestion of radiopaque dye or by nuclear scan or sonogram.

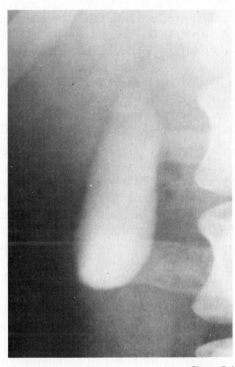

Figure 5.1

Rationale

Determine the presence of stones or other pathology blocking the bile duct.

Differentiate between biliary pain and pain originating because of gastric, abdominal or coronary pathology.

Terminology

Biliary: Having to do with the bile system

Cholecystectomy: Surgical removal of the gallbladder

Duodenum: The first portion of the small intestine, lying between the pylorus of the stomach and the jejunum; this segment is crucial to digestion because many of the digestive enzymes, including bile, are secreted into this section.

Nuclear scan: Radiologic study of an organ (in this case the biliary system) after the intravenous injection of radioactive isotopes to allow visualization of contour and assessment of function

Sonogram: A scan of a body part in which the density of organs contrasted against a body fluid (in this case, the bile in the biliary system) creates outlines on a monitor or on a film

> **T-tube:** A T-shaped tube that is inserted into the common bile duct and sutured into the wound after cholecystectomy; provides a mechanism for the drainage of bile into a collection bag

Assessment

Pertinent Anatomy and Physiology

1. See Appendix I: *biliary system, gallbladder.*
2. The common bile duct is the connecting tubule between the liver and the gallbladder for the transport of bile into the duodenum. The common duct descends and passes behind the pancreas and enters the descending duodenum. Sphinctures regulate the flow of bile into the duodenum. When the sphincture controlling the flow of bile into the common duct is closed, the bile moves back into the gallbladder, where it is stored.

Pathophysiological Concepts

1. Cholelithiasis (gallstones) can occur in the gallbladder and in the common bile duct. These stones are due to precipitation of substances contained in bile, mainly cholesterol and bilirubin. The majority of biliary calculi are composed of cholesterol. Three factors contribute to this formation: a) abnormalities in the composition of bile, b) stasis of bile, and c) inflammation of the gallbladder. Biliary stones cause problems when they obstruct bile flow. Small stones (not greater than 8 mm in diameter) may pass into the common duct, producing symptoms of indigestion and biliary colic. Larger stones may obstruct flow of bile with jaundice resulting. Some biliary stones are translucent and may not show up on radiologic examination.
2. Cholecystitis is an acute or chronic inflammation of the gallbladder. Acute cholecystitis almost always is associated with complete or partial obstruction of bile flow. The gallbladder usually is distended markedly. Bacterial infections may arise, and ischemia may result in gangrene of the gallbladder. Chronic cholecystitis may be due to spasms or stenosis of the common bile duct. Symptoms for both chronic and acute cholecystitis include pain in the right upper quadrant of the abdomen radiating to the right scapular area, intolerance of fatty foods, belching, and other signs of discomfort. The partial obstruction of bile flow may result in cholelithiasis.

Assessment of the Client

1. Assess the physical condition of the client. If the client is in a weakened state, provide the opportunity for as much uninterrupted rest as possible the evening and night before. Ascertain baseline vital signs.
2. Take a complete history of the client's allergies. This is essential because the oral dye contains iodine, a substance to which many people are sensitive. Assess any allergies to shellfish or iodine preparations.
3. Assess the bowel status of the client. If the bowel is full, the fecal material may distort adequate x-ray visualization of the biliary system.

Plan

Nursing Objectives

Contribute to the production of an adequate x-ray film on which sound diagnostic judgment may rely.

Allay the client's fear and anxiety.

Prevent allergic complications.

Client Preparation

1. Inform the client that there is no pain involved in radiologic examinations and that the exposure to radiation is very minimal. The entire procedure usually takes about 30 to 45 minutes; however, subsequent later films may be necessary.
2. The client may receive fatty meals for a few days before the test. Bile emulsi-

fies fat; therefore, the increased intake of fat will cause the gallbladder to empty before the test. The meal on the evening before the cholangiogram is usually low in fat.

3. An x-ray is a form of radiant energy that penetrates according to the density of tissue. The stomach and bowel should be empty so they will not interfere with the biliary x-ray. Food may be withheld for 12 hours before the test, and a laxative, enema, or both may be ordered to precede the x-ray study.

  Cholecystogram: For x-ray visualization of the gallbladder, the dye is taken orally. Administer the dye tablets the evening before the test. After the oral tablets are ingested, the dye takes about 13 hours to reach the liver, where it is excreted in the bile and passes through the gallbladder, making both the ducts and gallbladder radiopaque.

  Cholangiogram: Visualization of the biliary system usually is accomplished by a nuclear scan. Radioactive isotopes are injected intravenously, usually in the brachial vein. At 15-minute intervals, films are taken to show function of the biliary system.

  Sonogram: A sonogram may be performed to provide a graphic picture of how the biliary system is functioning and to locate possible pathology. The client usually will be NPO for at least 8 hours before the test.

Equipment

1. Oral dye tablets
2. Enema setup (see Technique No. 5, Enema and Rectal Tube)
3. Hospital gown
4. Wheelchair or stretcher for transport

Implementation and Interventions

Procedural Aspects

ACTION	RATIONALE
1. Ensure that the client has been prepared thoroughly and correctly for the x-ray before being transported to the radiology department. If the client is fatigued or feeling ill, transport should be by stretcher; otherwise a wheelchair is used.	If the client is not prepared, it will be a needless expense to do the examination. The client should be transported to the radiology department in a safe and expedient manner that will conserve energy and prevent additional fatigue.
2. When the client returns to the unit, ensure that all of the films are complete before offering food or liquids.	The initial x-ray and subsequent films may take several hours to complete. Sometime the client may be returned to the unit to await further films and should not be fed until all of the films are complete.
3. After completion of the x-ray examination, a regular diet usually is resumed. If the client is hungry, provide a snack.	The client may have been NPO for a long period. Provide nourishment as soon as possible.

Special Modifications

After cholecystectomy, a T-tube may be left in place for a short time to allow for the drainage of bile. Dye may be inserted through the T-tube in an effort to ascertain if more stones are present.	The T-tube provides for the direct drainage of bile. Insertion of dye through the tube allows immediate visualization of the portion of the biliary system below the T-tube.

Communicative Aspects

OBSERVATIONS

1. Reactions to the contrast medium range from no reaction to nausea, vomiting, hives, or anaphylactic shock. The nurse should observe the client carefully for any signs of an allergic reaction.

2. Note the client's condition before and after the x-ray to ascertain the amount of fatigue. Plan to minimize further fatigue.

CHARTING

DATE/TIME	OBSERVATIONS	SIGNATURE
1/5 0945	Cholangiogram completed. No nausea, vomiting, or signs of allergy noted. Alert and requesting food. Informed that x-ray results will be available by 1500 hr	K. Hicks RN

Discharge Planning Aspects

CLIENT AND FAMILY EDUCATION

1. Tell the client and family that there are a variety of ways to administer the dye for visualization of the biliary system. The dye may be administered orally or through the T-tube. T-tube cholangiogram often is done after chole-cystecomy to determine the status of the remaining portion of the biliary system.

2. If visualization is not achieved the first time, the test often is repeated. If the biliary system is not visualized the second time, pathology is considered and surgical intervention may be required. Explain to the client that the examination may have to be repeated.

3. If the diagnosis is a chronic condition, dietary modifications may need to be made. Dietary counseling for fat-free meals should be given before discharge.

4. Explain the signs and symptoms of an acute biliary attack to the client who has never experienced this phenonomen. This situation dictates that immediate attention be sought to relieve the pain and determine the proper treatment. Signs of an acute attack are spasmodic pains in the midepigastric region of the abdomen, which later are noticeable in the right upper quadrant. Often the pain is referred to the right scapula or interscapular area. Tenderness and muscle guarding over the area of the gallbladder may be present, with fever and leukocytosis. Nausea and vomiting also may be present.

Evaluation

Quality Assurance

Document preparations for the x-rays and the client's reaction to the procedure. Of particular importance is addressing the problem of allergies in relation to the use of dye. The chart should reflect an order for the test. A report of the results also should be on the chart within a reasonable length of time. Explanations of the results and an appraisal of the client and family's understanding should be noted. Follow-up treatment and counselling (such as dietary) should be documented.

Infection Control

Adhere to hospital policy regarding transport of hospitalized clients to minimize cross-infection from unit to unit. If viral hepatitis is included in the differential diagnosis, enteric as well as blood–body fluid precautions should be observed in all departments. The radiology department must be informed in advance in order to arrange for special precautions in this area. The client is transported according to specified isolation policy.

Technique Checklist

	YES	NO
Explanation of test to client	_____	_____
Allergies checked		
Iodine	_____	_____
Shellfish	_____	_____
Other _____	_____	_____
Preparatory laxative _____	_____	_____
Time given _____		
Preparatory enema	_____	_____
Oral dye tablets (taken at 5-min intervals with 4–6 oz of water the evening before the test)	_____	_____
Fasting from midnight the evening before the test	_____	_____
Client taken to x-ray by		
Wheelchair	_____	_____
Stretcher	_____	_____
Nourishment offered after completion of x-ray	_____	_____
Client understands the results of the x-ray	_____	_____

6   Cultures

Overview

Definition

Obtaining a specimen for laboratory study to determine the presence and specific type of microorganism

Rationale

Determine the presence of pathogenic microorganisms.

Identify the specific microorganism in determining drug sensitivity and methods of treatment.

Terminology

Aerobe: An organism that requires oxygen to survive

Anaerobe: An organism that can live in an environment without oxygen

Contaminated: Containing pathogenic microorganisms

Infection: A disease process produced by pathogens

Microorganism: A microscopic living body that may or may not be capable of producing disease

Pathogen: A microorganism that causes disease

Assessment

Pertinent Anatomy and Physiology

See Appendix I: *skin.*

Pathophysiological Concepts

1. The types of microorganisms that cause infection are

   Bacteria: Microorganisms that are responsible for most of the infections in humans. They are single-celled organisms that are described according to their shape (rod, sphere, cone), staining technique (Gram's stain or acid-fast stain), oxygen requirements (anaerobe or aerobe), and by the presence of spores or capsules (spore-forming).

   Protozoa: One-celled animals that are much larger than bacteria and are usually harmless to humans, although they are implicated in diseases such as malaria.

   Fungi: Single-cell (yeast) and multicell (mold) forms that are actually plants. They produce conditions such as ringworm and monilia.

   Rickettsiae: Microorganisms that are intracellular; that is they live within the cells of living tissue. They are larger than viruses but smaller than bacteria. They are transported largely by rodents and ticks and may produce such conditions as Rocky Mountain spotted fever.

   Viruses: Extremely small microorganisms or fragments of DNA that live and grow within the cells of the host's living tissue. Viruses remain a mystery and seem to be controlled best by vaccinations.

2. Certain environmental conditions favor the growth of microorganisms. All microorganisms require moisture, as well as some type of nourishment, to live. Most microorganisms require organic food for growth. The environment temperature is also a vital concern. Temperatures over 77°C (170°F) and un-

der 0°C (32°F) will inhibit the growth of most bacteria, although these temperatures may not be bactericidal. The acidity and alkalinity of the environment also has an effect on the growth of microorganisms.

Assessment of the Client

1. Assess the health history of the client in relation to infectious processes. Determine the frequency of infections and manifestations. Ask the client about past problems with boils, slow-healing wounds, and any pus-forming condition.

2. Assess the apparent area of microbial infestation of the client in determining where to culture. Areas of drainage, especially when pus is present, may indicate infection.

3. Assess the familiarity of the client with the culturing procedure. If the client has never had a throat culture, the procedure may seem frightening. If the client has had a yearly Pap smear for many years, a vaginal culture may not seem intimidating.

Plan

Nursing Objectives

Obtain the culture efficiently without undue discomfort for the client.

Obtain and transport the specimen in such a way that contamination is avoided.

Interpret the results to the client in understandable terms.

Initiate the isolation techniques appropriate for the results of the culture.

Client Preparation

1. Explain the culture technique to the client. Relate why the culture must be done, what is expected from the results, and how the client can participate effectively.

2. Remove any dressings or coverings from the area to be cultured. If infectious processes are suspected, handle the dressings as if they were contaminated.

Equipment

Sterile swabs

Sterile culture tube for transporting the swab

Sterile culture container with tight-fitting lid

Blood agar plate for certain equipment culture

Implementation and Interventions

Procedural Aspects

ACTION	RATIONALE
Swab Technique	
1. To culture the mucous membranes or a draining wound, use sterile swabs. If there is danger of the hands coming in contact with infective materials, wear sterile gloves. Remove the swab from the package and place the cotton end into the area that is suspected of being infected. If it is a wound, obtain the specimen from the draining portion of the wound (Fig. 6-1). Do not touch the skin. If more swabs are used to take specimens from various areas around the wound, label each swab container with the location from	Microorganisms flourish in the warm, moist environment of the mucous membranes or a wound on the skin. A specimen of the cells on the outer layer of mucous membranes will yield a sample of the microorganisms present throughout the area. This is also true of wound drainage. Do not touch the skin around the wound to prevent contamination of the wound.

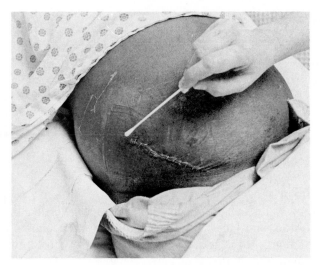

Figure 6.1

ACTION

which it came. The culture of an abscess should contain a specimen of the fluid from within the abscess.

2. If the nose or throat is cultured, place the swab well into the orifice and rub it along the side with a rotating motion. The usual area of culture of the throat is the tonsil area or the back of the throat below the uvula (Fig. 6-2). Ask the client to say "ahhh" when obtaining a throat culture.

RATIONALE

The most common site of infection is around the tonsils and below the palate. Saying "ahhh" relaxes the throat muscles and decreases the gag reflex.

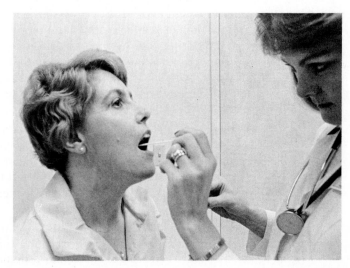

Figure 6.2

3. The rotating action is used for a vaginal culture; however, the swab should be labeled whether it came from the external opening of the

Different tests may be ordered for specimens from different locations. It is necessary to be able to tell which specimen came from which location.

ACTION	**RATIONALE**
vagina, the vaginal wall, or the cervix during vaginal examination with a speculum.	
4. To obtain a specimen of drainage from an orifice (e.g., urethra, vagina, nose, or ear), place the swab so that a maximum amount of drainage is absorbed. Take care that the swab does not touch the skin, however.	Touching the skin or mucous membrane may contaminate the swab and render the specimen results invalid.
5. Place the swab in a sterile container and label with the client's name and the source of the specimen (Fig. 6-3).	Sterile surroundings prevent the specimen from being contaminated with foreign microorganisms.

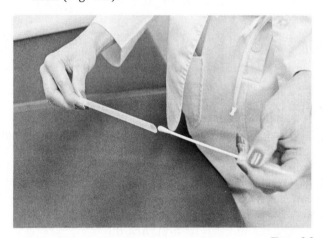

Figure 6.3

Sputum Specimen

1. Ask the client to cough and bring up sputum from the chest and throat. Provide a sterile sputum cup for the client to expectorate the sputum. Also, provide tissues for the client to use in covering the mouth to prevent the spread of disease.	A sterile container will prevent contamination of the specimen with extraneous material. *Sputum* is an accumulation of the bronchi and trachea that is peculiar to disease conditions. Be sure the client does not expectorate saliva, the liquid secretion of the salivary glands in the mouth.
2. If the client is suspected of having a communicable disease, place the sputum container in an impenetrable bag and label.	This prevents accidental contamination of laboratory personnel, who can use special techniques for retrieving the specimen they know is contaminated.
3. Assist the client to engage in handwashing after sputum specimen collection.	This not only helps prevent the spread of infection but also provides a good role model for the client who should be encouraged to wash hands after any contact with potentially infected secretions.

Blood Specimen

1. Prepare the skin with an iodine preparation if the client has no	The skin must be cleansed of any microorganisms that may contaminate

ACTION

allergies to iodine. If so, use alcohol swabs. Withdraw 5 ml of blood from a vein which does not have an intravenous infusion. Remove the needle used for venipuncture and place a sterile needle on the syringe. Swab the top of two blood culture bottles and inject 2½ ml of blood into each one, using a new sterile needle for each injection. In 15 minutes, a second specimen may be taken by percutaneous stick. The skin is prepared as before and the specimen is again placed into two different containers.

2. Use direct pressure to prevent the leakage or oozing of blood after penetrating the skin barrier.

Urine Specimen

The urine specimen for culture may be obtained by clean catch, catheterization, or aspiration from an indwelling catheter. (Refer to Technique No. 22, Urine Examinations.) Place the specimen in a sterile container and transport to the laboratory at once.

Stool Specimen

1. Obtain the specimen by allowing the client to have a bowel movement in a clean bedpan. With a sterile tongue depressor, place a small amount of the stool (about 1 tbsp) in a sterile container. Be careful not to contaminate the sides of the container. Place the lid on securely and label the container with the client's name and the contents. Transport the specimen to the laboratory at once. If there is a delay, the specimen should be kept in a cold refrigerator. If the stool is liquid and soaks into the linen or diaper, saturate a sterile swab with the fecal material and place it in a sterile swab container.

2. If the client has been receiving antibiotics or sulfonamides, note this on the requisition.

All Cultures

1. Transport the culture specimen to the laboratory at once.

RATIONALE

the specimen. The needle that has accomplished venipuncture is contaminated and must be changed before injecting the specimen into the specimen containers. This is also the rationale for each change of the needle, to prevent contamination of the blood specimen.

Once the wound is closed, the danger of pathogen entry is reduced.

The goal for urine culture specimen is to provide a sterile specimen for testing.

Cold will inhibit the growth of extraneous microorganisms and will allow a more accurate reflection of the stool flora. The container and tongue blade should be sterile to prevent contaminating the specimen.

Antibiotics and sulfonamides may produce false-negative results from cultures.

If the culture is allowed to sit in the container for an extended period, the

ACTION	RATIONALE
	results may be compromised by the growth of extraneous microorganisms.
2. Use careful handwashing technique after collection of any specimen for culture.	Handwashing will prevent spread of infection by cross-contamination.

Special Modifications

Children

When obtaining specimens from children, be sure that adequate assistance is available to restrain the child so that injury does not occur. Before obtaining the specimen, explain to the parents and to the child as appropriate for the age and level of understanding.	Obtaining nose and throat specimens is an unpleasant procedure for the client. The child must be restrained properly so that accidental trauma to the delicate mucous membranes is avoided.

Contaminated Equipment

1. Use the swab technique for suspected colonization of large pieces of equipment or those that cannot be taken safely to the laboratory.	Some equipment is stationary. If it is not practical to move the equipment or if the equipment is not disposable, use the swab technique.
2. For a suspected contaminated venous catheter, remove the catheter from the client, being careful not to touch it. Hold the catheter over a blood agar plate and with sterile scissors, cut off the last 1½ inches of the catheter. Let the cut portion fall onto the blood agar plate. With a sterile swab, roll the catheter across the surface of the agar. Replace the cover and label and transport to the laboratory immediately. Do follow-up care for the venipuncture site.	Touching the catheter might contaminate it with extraneous material and render the culture unreliable as to causative organism. Rolling the catheter spreads out the organisms and enhances the chance that they will grow successfully.

Communicative Aspects

OBSERVATIONS

1. Observe the condition of the area from which the specimen is taken. Note the presence of abnormalities as well as any specific symptoms described by the client.
2. Observe the condition of the wound from which the specimen is taken. Note the amount and color of drainage. Determine the progress of healing and note symptoms that prompted the culture.
3. Note the appearance of vaginal or urethral discharge. Normal discharge is whitish or clear, nonpurulent, does not contain blood, and is usually minimal in amount.

CHARTING

DATE/TIME	OBSERVATIONS	SIGNATURE
2/5 0730	Throat and nasal specimens obtained using sterile technique for culture. To lab stat. Small amount of gagging but no problems obtaining specimens. Continues to express discomfort from sore throat. ———————	F. White RN

**Discharge Planning
Aspects**

**CLIENT AND FAMILY
EDUCATION**

1. Explain to the client and family how the specimens will be taken, why they are necessary, and what the results should provide. Answer any questions.

2. If the parents of small children wish to assist in restraining during specimen collection, be sure that they understand exactly what will occur. Allow them the option of being absent during the procedure. It is often difficult for parents to deal with procedures that cause discomfort to their children.

Evaluation

Quality Assurance

The hospital infection control policies should address specific situations in which cultures are to be done to prevent the spread of infection in the hospital and to protect the clients and staff. Documentation should include signs and symptoms that indicated the need to take a culture initially. The appearance of the area and the drainage, if appropriate, should be noted. The actual culturing procedure should be described in relation to area cultured, type of culturing media or equipment, disposition of specimens, and any problems noted. Results of the culture and sensitivity, if ordered, should be on the chart within a reasonable time.

Infection Control

1. The basic premise for culturing is control of infection. Any time an area is suspected of being infected or colonized in the preinfective stage, it should be cultured.

2. Because cultures are done to discover the presence and type of microorganisms, care must be taken not to transmit the infective material to other persons. Using sterile technique and proper labeling of specimens should help protect laboratory personnel.

3. Sterile gloves should be worn to do culturing. All equipment and containers should be sterile. These efforts will help to minimize the chance of contaminating the specimen.

Technique Checklist

	YES	NO
Procedure explained to client and family	_____	_____
Type of specimen		
Swab _____		
Sputum _____		
Blood _____		
Equipment _____		
Exact location of specimen collection _____		
Specimen to laboratory immediately	_____	_____
Labeled	_____	_____
Bagged	_____	_____
Specimen to lab _____ (date)		
Results on chart _____ (date)	_____	_____

7

Electrocardiogram (ECG, EKG)

Overview

Definition

A recording of the electrical impulses produced by the heart (Fig. 7-1)

Bedside ECG: an ECG done at the client's bedside or anywhere the client may lie in the supine position; used for assessment of usual cardiac activity

Stress test: an ECG done during and after controlled exercise, usually on a treadmill-type machine; used for cardiac assessment during periods of stress and exertion

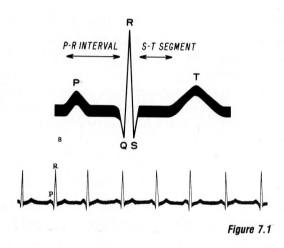

Figure 7.1

Rationale

Provide grounds for the diagnosis of cardiac arrhythmias, arteriosclerotic heart disease, cardiac enlargement, electrolyte abnormalities, and myocardial infarction.

Assess the status of a client in a life-threatening situation as a basis for medical or nursing action.

Provide a visual image of the heart rhythms.

Terminology

Atrium (pl. atria): The upper chamber of each half of the heart

Atrioventricular (AV) node: The area of the heart through which the electrical impulse travels before initiating ventricular contraction; located between the atria and the ventricles

P wave: The first graphic wave of the electrocardiograph (ECG) caused by contraction of the atria

Q,R,S, and T waves: The second series of waves on an ECG, related to contraction of the ventricles

Sinoatrial (SA) node; normal pacemaker: The area where the electrical impulse stimulating a heartbeat begins; located in the superior aspect of the right atrium

Ventricle: The lower chamber of each half of the heart that propels blood into the arteries

Assessment

Pertinent Anatomy and Physiology

See Appendix I: *heart*.

Pathophysiological Concepts

1. The heart muscle is unique in its ability to generate its own electrical impulse independently of the nervous system. Disorders of the heartbeat arise as a result of disturbances in the generation and conduction of impulses in the heart. There are many causes of altered cardiac rhythms, including congenital defects, degenerative changes, ischemia, myocardial infarction, electrolyte imbalances, and drug ingestion. Arrhythmias are not necessarily pathologic but may occur in the healthy heart.

2. Any pathologic process that disturbs the electrical activity of the heart will produce characteristic changes in one or more of the wave deflections on the ECG. The electrical charge may not originate at all, may originate in an abnormal site, or may go astray of its intended destination. All of these occurrences result in alterations of the client's normal cardiac function. Diagnosis of conduction defects and cardiac arrhythmias is usually made on the basis of the ECG tracing.

Assessment of the Client

1. Assess the client's baseline vital signs for later comparisons.

2. Assess the knowledge level of the client about the ECG procedure. If the client has not had ECGs previously, a thorough explanation of what will happen may help relieve anxiety.

3. Assess the physical condition of the client to determine limitations, such as impaired ambulation, dizziness, nausea and vomiting, and respiratory problems that might interfere with the client's ability to perform the exercise required for the stress test.

Plan

Nursing Objectives

Assist the client to a position of comfort and provide privacy.

Ensure the client's cooperation and decrease anxiety by thorough explanations.

Ensure the client's safety by continuous monitoring during the stress test.

Client Preparation

BEDSIDE ECG

1. Explain that there is no pain associated with the bedside ECG itself. The client must lie still during the actual test, which takes about 10 to 15 minutes.

2. There is little actual physical preparation. A sedative may be ordered before the ECG. If so, be aware that the sedation may have an effect on the ECG results. Remove restrictive clothing so that the client's wrists, ankles, and chest are accessible.

3. Explain that a conductive paste will be applied to the areas of attachment of the electrodes (leads), which will measure the client's electrocardiographic reading. This paste facilitates the reception and recording of the electrical impulses. Leads with a prepared nonsticky gel are also available. These are neater and more pleasant to the client than those that use the electrode paste.

STRESS TEST

1. Reinforce that the exercise during the stress test will be supervised closely and will not be beyond the level of the client's endurance. The exercise usually consists of walking at progressive speeds on a treadmill-type device. The device may be set for the desired speed and degree of incline. Blood pressure will be taken before the test begins and at regular intervals (usually q3min). The ECG tracing will be recorded during the entire test.

2. If the stress test is done near mealtime, it is advisable to withhold the meal until after the test so the client will not become nauseated during exercising.

Equipment   ECG machine
             Treadmill

Implementation and Interventions

Procedural Aspects

ACTION	RATIONALE

ACTION

1. For a bedside ECG, have the client lying down in a relaxed and comfortable position. The ECG technician may apply a conductive paste to each lead or may use leads prepared with a gellike material. The technician will place leads on the client's ankles and wrists and will move one lead progressively across the client's chest (Fig. 7-2). Reassure the client throughout the procedure.

RATIONALE

The metal leads applied to the skin conduct a current to an instrument, which makes a graphic tracing of the activity. The gel or paste maximizes the ability of the machine to depict electrical impulses accurately.

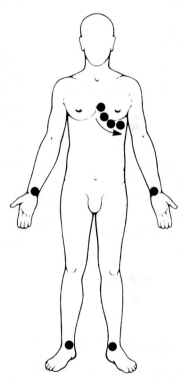

Figure 7.2

2. The stress test involves a period of exercise during which the client is supervised and monitored closely. Amount of time and degree of difficulty on the treadmill are specified for each person of a certain height and age. Monitor tracings will be available throughout the test; graphic tracings will be made at specified intervals.

Because the client may be at risk from symptoms or previous cardiopathy, extreme fatigue must be avoided. It may be desirable to ascertain function under extreme conditions, however. Often this is the only time pathology is seen. Because of the chance of serious complications from the strain on the heart muscle, constant monitoring is essential.

Communicative Aspects

OBSERVATIONS

1. Observe the client closely during the exercise phase of the stress test to ensure that exercise itself does not precipitate a cardiac emergency
2. Observe the client for compliance with the test. Movement during the ECG will cause extraneous lines on the tracing.
3. Observe for a regular ECG tracing.

CHARTING

DATE/TIME	OBSERVATIONS	SIGNATURE
3/9 1400	ECG done at bedside. Relaxed and tolerated procedure very well. Seems to understand the need for repeat ECG in the morning and does not appear anxious.	F. White RN

Discharge Planning Aspects

CLIENT AND FAMILY EDUCATION

1. Excitation waves produced from the heart muscle cells are recorded as electrical phenomena. This activity is detected on the skin surface because body fluids are an excellent conductor of electricity. Electrodes placed on the skin surface record voltage and intervals of electrical activity over time. Emphasize that there is no danger of electrical shock. The machine measures the naturally occurring electrical impulses emanating from within the client and does not transmit electricity to the client.
2. The client and family should understand that subsequent ECGs may be needed to provide comparisons and determine the effectiveness of treatment or the extent of heart damage. The performance of repeated ECGs during the course of recovery is expected and should not be construed as a setback or sign of additional problems.
3. If cardiac abnormality is found, the client and family will need help adjusting to and coping with this condition as part of their everyday lives. Close family members must be familiar with the technique for cardiopulmonary resuscitation (CPR). This should be approached in a matter-of-fact, routine way so that the family will not be alarmed and feel that the situation is worse than they have been led to believe. Knowledge of CPR can save lives, and this is the point that should be stressed.

REFERRALS

The American Heart Association has been very active in research and public awareness of cardiac-related problems and prevention. The client and family may be able to find support groups and additional information through referral to this organization.

Evaluation

Quality Assurance

Documentation should reflect the baseline vital signs and subsequent measurements, especially if the ECG procedure involved physical exertion. The symptoms that resulted in the need for the ECG should be noted. Document the client's reaction to the ECG and any complications.

Infection Control

1. Health care providers must wash their hands thoroughly between clients.
2. All equipment in contact with the client should be cleaned with a disinfectant after each use to minimize the risk of cross-infection.

Technique Checklist

	YES	NO
Test ordered on chart	_____	_____
Client understands why test is being done and what will happen during test	_____	_____

	YES	NO
Sedative given	_____	_____
Drug _____		
Time given _____		
Meal withheld	_____	_____
Baseline vital signs		
Pulse _____		
Respiration _____		
Blood pressure		
Lying _____		
Sitting _____		
Standing _____		
Complications after ECG		
Pain _____		
Nausea	_____	_____
Vomiting	_____	_____
Shortness of breath	_____	_____
Other _____	_____	_____
(Additional for stress test)		
Amount of time client was able to exercise	_____	_____
Complications of exercise	_____	_____
Client and family understand the reason for the stress test	_____	_____
Client and family understand the results of the test	_____	_____

8 Electroencephalogram (EEG)

Overview

Definition

A graphic record of the electrical activity passing through the surface of the brain

Rationale

Detect and determine the location of abnormal electrical activity in the brain, which may indicate such conditions as epilepsy, tumors, or brain damage.

Assess the presence or absence of electrical activity in determining brain death.

Assessment

Pertinent Anatomy and Physiology

1. The averge adult human brain weighs about 1400 g (3 lbs) and is the largest and most complex mass of nervous tissue in the body. It is housed in the cranial cavity and reaches full growth by the 18th to 20th year of life. The primary divisions of the brain are the forebrain, midbrain, and hindbrain. Within these divisions are ventricles which are concerned with the formation and the circulation of cerebrospinal fluid.
2. The ability to transmit nerve impulses is a highly developed property of nerve tissue. The records of the brain waves are really records of electrical changes in the brain.

Pathophysiological Concepts

1. A *seizure* is a spontaneous, uncontrolled, paroxysmal, transitory discharge from the cortical centers in the brain causing symptoms based on the location of the involved area. Seizure activity may be initiated by abnormal cells within the brain caused by a change in the permeability of membranes. Symptoms can include bizarre muscle movements, strange sensations and perceptions, and loss of consciousness. A seizure is not a disease, but is a symptom of underlying pathology.
2. Nerve impulses are propelled through the body over an intricate network of nervous tissue to and from the brain. There are various disorders of the brain that may disturb the normal conduction pattern. These include malignancy, epilepsy, and trauma.

Assessment of the Client

1. Assess baseline vital and neurologic signs on admission and at various intervals during hospitalization. Periodic assessments are essential to determine the extent and progress of pathology as evidenced by neurologic changes.
2. Assess the knowledge level of the client about EEG procedure. The EEG is a noninvasive procedure. However, anything concerning the brain may have a frightening connotation for the client. Determine if the client has any preconceived notions about the test or any fears or anxiety about undergoing electroencephalographic examination. The entire test may take about 45 minutes to 2 hours.

Plan

Nursing Objectives

Prepare the client adequately by a thorough explanation to reduce anxiety about the test.

Elaborate on the physician's interpretation of the test results if the client does not understand.

Maintain the client's safety if seizures occur.

Client Preparation

1. Provide a thorough explanation of the need for and procedure of the EEG. Make sure that the client understands that there is no danger of electrical shock from the electrodes.

2. The client should avoid the consumption of stimulants (coffee, cola, etc) and depressants (alcohol) before the EEG. Smoking is not allowed before the test. The client is not NPO for an EEG because the resulting hypoglycemia may alter the test results. Medications that may be withheld unless specified otherwise by the physician are tranquilizing, sedative, or hypnotic drugs.

3. Before the test, shampoo the client's hair and scalp. Do not use any hair preparations after the shampoo.

4. If the physician orders a sleep-deprivation EEG, the client should not sleep during the 12 hours preceding the test. The EEG is often done early in the morning after the client has been kept awake all night.

Equipment

EEG machine and electrodes

Conductive paste or jelly

Implementation and Interventions

Procedural Aspects

ACTION

1. Assist the EEG technician as needed. The client is usually lying down or reclining during the EEG. Electrodes are placed at various intervals over the scalp by means of a sticky conductive paste (Fig. 8-1).

RATIONALE

With the client at rest, brain waves will not be distorted by extraneous activities. The conduction paste maximizes ability of the machine to accurately depict the electrical impulses.

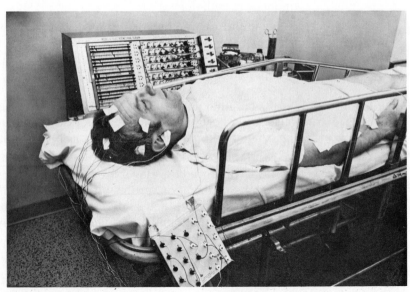

Figure 8.1 (Courtesy of Roche Laboratories)

ACTION	RATIONALE
2. Tracings are taken over a period during which the client is relaxed or asleep. The client may be asked to hyperventilate, do simple mental activities, or take certain medications.	It is desirable to measure electrical impulses of the brain while at rest. Simple activities may help to determine the presence of pathology.
3. Assist the client in shampooing the hair after the EEG is finished. If the client is comatose, thoroughly cleanse the scalp and hair.	The electrode paste is sticky and will cause discomfort if not removed as soon as possible.

Special Modifications

In the comatose client, the absence of brain activity on the EEG signifies "brain death" and is used in various medicolegal decisions depending on the laws of the state.	The American Medical Association (AMA) and the American Bar Association (ABA) support the concept of "irreversible cessation of all functions of the entire brain, including the brain stem" as a part of the criteria for death.

Communicative Aspects

OBSERVATIONS

1. Hyperventilation, the use of external stimulants (such as a strobe light), and sleep deprivation may induce a grand mal seizure in the epileptic client. Because measurement of brain conductivity during seizure is desirable, however, this is not considered a great hazard. The important consideration is to protect the client from injury should a seizure occur.
2. Observe the client for willingness and ability to follow instructions.

CHARTING

DATE/TIME	OBSERVATIONS	SIGNATURE
6/19 0745	To Radiology for sleep-deprivation EEG. Has remained awake with some difficulty since 2100 last night. Up in hall most of the night. States he has no reservations about the test. No coffee or cigarettes this night. ————————	G. Ivers RN

Discharge Planning Aspects

CLIENT AND FAMILY EDUCATION

1. Instruct the family and client about the signs of impending seizure (aura) if the client is diagnosed as epileptic.
2. Management of the epileptic as a functioning participant in modern society should emphasized. Unfortunately, the stigma attached to seizure still lingers in some segments of society. If this is the first experience with the reality of epilepsy for the client, a matter-of-fact, accepting attitude on the part of the nurse can do much to serve as a model for the family to emulate. Emphasizing what the client *can* do rather than what the client *cannot* do is very important.

REFERRALS

If the client has a head injury, there are many support groups for families of this type client across the nation. There are also clubs and groups for those who have suffered from stroke or for the families of stroke victims. The National Epilepsy Foundation may provide help and support for the newly diagnosed epileptic client and family.

Evaluation

Quality Assurance

1. Documentation should reflect a complete neurologic assessment with baseline vital and neurologic signs. Also reflected should be the underlying symptoms that prompted the client to seek attention in the first place. Ongoing evidence of neurologic assessment is important. Documentation of seizures should include any precipitating events, description by the client of feelings before the seizure, duration and description of the seizure, and any aftereffects.

2. Some states include the absence of brain waves in their definition of death. This definition usually is based on the assumption that the coma is irreversible and that responsiveness and respirations are absent. Consult the particular state law for the legal definition of death.

Infection Control

Whenever equipment is used consecutively for different clients, it is essential to decrease the possibility of cross-infection by cleaning and disinfecting the equipment after each use. The nurse and technician must also wash their hands thoroughly after each procedure and before contact with the next client.

Technique Checklist

	YES	NO
Is there an order for the EEG?	_____	_____
Explanation to client and family	_____	_____
Medications withheld	_____	_____
For _____ hours		
Sleep deprivation	_____	_____
From _____ to _____		
Abnormalities found	_____	_____
Client understands test results	_____	_____

9 Endoscopy of the Upper Gastrointestinal Tract

Overview

Definition

Endoscopy is the direct visual examination of certain natural openings or cavities by means of a hollow, lighted instrument. Types include

Duodenoscopy: Direct visualization of the duodenum by means of a flexible endoscope

Esophagoscopy: Direct visualization of the esophagus by means of a flexible endoscope

Gastroscopy: Direct visualization of the stomach by means of a flexible endoscope

Jejunoscopy: Direct visualization of the jejunum by means of a flexible endoscope

Rationale

Determine the presence of pathology or abnormalities in the upper gastrointestinal (GI) tract (e.g., tumors or ulcers).

Assess the motility and thickness of the gastric wall.

Determine the presence of right atrial enlargement that usually impinges on the esophagus.

Assess the presence and severity of esophageal varices.

Obtain a tissue biopsy.

Remove a foreign body.

Terminology

Adhesions: The abnormal joining of organs or structures by the formation of fibrous bands

Anorexia: Loss of appetite

Dysphagia: Difficulty swallowing

Eructation: Raising of gas from the stomach (belching)

Flatulence: Excessive gas in the stomach and intestines

Incarcerated: Confined; constricted

Intussusception: The slipping of one part of the intestine into the part just below it

Obstruction: Blocking of a structure, preventing normal function

Peritonitis: Inflammation of the peritoneum, the membranous coat lining the abdominal cavity

Stricture: Narrowing of the lumen (opening or channel) of a tube, duct, or hollow organ

Ulcer: An open lesion of the skin or mucous membrane

Urticaria: An inflammatory condition characterized by the eruption of wheals and severe itching (hives)

Assessment

Pertinent Anatomy and Physiology

See Appendix I: *esophagus, stomach, intestine (small)*.

Pathophysiological Concepts

1. Pathology of the esophagus may manifest itself in dysphagia. If it is due to narrowing of the esophagus because of tumor encroachment or lesions, it may be detected by endoscopic visualization. Esophageal diverticulum is an outpouching of the esophageal wall caused by a weakness in the muscle layer.

2. Other disorders that may be visualized by endoscopy include gastric and peptic ulcers, inflammatory bowel disease, diverticulitis, appendicitis, and cancer.

3. Intestinal obstruction may be due to incarcerated hernia; foreign bodies; stricture from an ulcer, peritonitis, or tumor; knotting or twisting of the intestine (volvulus); intussusception, or telescoping of one part of the intestine into another part; or adhesions. Intestinal obstruction is very serious and warrants immediate attention.

4. Esophageal varices are dilatations of the esophageal veins and capillaries. They arise with persistent obstruction of blood flow through the portal vein, resulting in diversion of blood flow to the other venous channels, such as the gastric and esophageal veins. Esophageal veins are relatively small and inelastic and are subject to rupture. The final outcome of varices is often massive and fatal hemorrhage.

Assessment of the Client

1. Assess the physical condition of the client. Assess the described symptoms in relation to gastric pain and problems. Determine baseline vital signs to monitor the progress of symptoms. The client may be weak and debilitated from episodes of vomiting or from an inability to digest or absorb food. Baseline vital signs may be useful in determining the degree of fatigue as the diagnostic screening progresses. Because the procedure may cause slight trauma to the throat, resulting in soreness, dysphagia, and slight bleeding, it is important to assess the presence of these symptoms before the examination.

2. Assess the client's dental condition. Note the presence of dentures or partial plates. It is particularly important to note the presence of loose teeth, which may become dislodged during the procedure.

3. Assess the amount of understanding the client exhibits regarding the endoscopic examination. It is essential that the client understand what will occur without becoming alarmed or frightened.

Plan

Nursing Objectives

Prepare the client adequately and ensure maximum compliance during the procedure.

Monitor the client during and after the procedure to detect early signs of complications.

Client Preparation

1. Endoscopy often is performed with the patient having been given a local anesthetic. A thorough explanation of what to expect and what will be expected of the client may enhance cooperation (Fig. 9-1). Because endoscopy is an invasive procedure, consult the hospital procedure manual to determine if a consent form is necessary.

2. Glands of the mucous membranes lining the GI tract normally produce secretions. When irritated, these glands secrete increased amounts, which may interfere with the endoscopic examination. For this reason, a mucus-inhibiting agent may be administered. Because fluid is essential to the formation of these secretions, restrict fluids before the examination. This also decreases

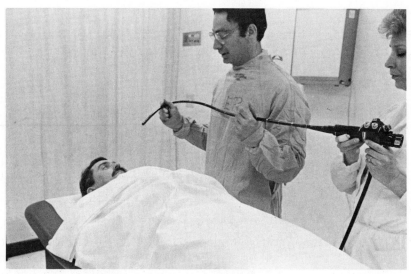

Figure 9.1

the possibility of vomiting and aspiration. If the endoscopic examination is done as an emergency measure, aspiration of gastric contents usually will be done first.

3. Because passage of an endoscope may induce vomiting if the stomach is full and gastric contents may obscure visualization, it is usually desirable to empty the contents of the stomach by gastric aspiration or to have the client NPO for 12 hours before the examination.

4. Suppression of the gag reflex is necessary before passage of the endoscope. This is accomplished by general or by local anesthesia. If local anesthesia is selected, tell the client that there will be stimulation of the gag reflex during application but that this will pass.

5. Remove dentures and partial plates and give mouth care before the examination.

Equipment

Endoscope of appropriate size (setup is usually available in surgery or in the central supply area of the hospital)

Suction pump and tubing

Topical anesthetic setup (including the anesthetic agent, syringe and cannula, and swabs)

Specimen container or slides and covers

Basin with sterile saline solution

Emesis basin

Tissues

Implementation and Interventions

Procedural Aspects

ACTION	RATIONALE
1. Dim the lights in the examination room, and place a towel over the client's eyes before the endoscopic procedure.	Endoscopy depends on illumination of the cavity by an adjacent light source. Maximum visualization is achieved in subdued lighting. The cloth will shield the client from viewing what is happening and perhaps decrease anxiety.
2. The physician applies the topical anesthetic and waits for a short	Several minutes are required for the topical anesthesia to take effect. Con-

ACTION	RATIONALE
time before passing the endoscope. Reassure the client during this interim period. Turn the client onto the left side during insertion (Fig. 9-2). Instruct the client to swallow as the tube is passed. Speak in low, unhurried tones. The client will be awake during the procedure; offer support throughout the entire time.	tinual reassurance in a calm, confident voice will help the client remain calm and follow the physician's directions as the tube is passed. Swallowing facilitates tube passage by normal peristaltic activity. Because the stomach lies toward the left of the body, turning the client to the left allows gravity to aid the natural movement of the tube into the stomach.

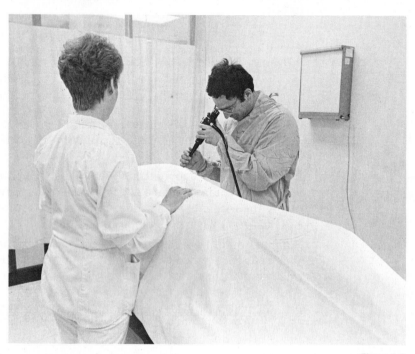

Figure 9.2

3. A brief, cramping sensation may be experienced when the endoscope is passed into the stomach and again when air is pumped into the stomach to inflate it for optimal visualization. Reassure the client that this is expected and is no cause for alarm.	Distention of the stomach causes reflex discomfort, resulting in a cramping sensation.
4. After endoscopy, allow the client time to rest. No foods or fluids are given until the gag reflex is restored completely.	When a bolus of food enters the pharynx, it is grasped by the constrictor muscles and propelled into the esophagus. When these muscles are anesthetized temporarily, the food may remain in the pharynx and cause choking and aspiration of food particles.

Special Modifications

Slight pain may be experienced if a tissue biopsy is taken. Inform the cli-	The trauma of tube insertion, as well as the bleeding edges left after biopsy,

ACTION	*RATIONALE*
ent to expect some bloody sputum if the biopsy is high in the esophagus. The stool and emesis must be observed carefully after biopsy to detect abnormal bleeding.	may result in a small amount of bleeding that will show up in the sputum. Large amounts of bleeding are indicative of hemorrhage, a serious emergency.

Communicative Aspects

OBSERVATIONS

1. Note the client's ability to relax and comply with the tube insertion.
2. Frequently monitor vital signs after GI endoscopy to ensure early detection of any complications. Elevated temperature may indicate rupture of the esophagus. Appropriate monitoring may be every 30 minutes for 3 hours. Observe for such complications as vomiting, bleeding, inability to swallow, excessive salivation, or intense pain. Observe for the return of the gag reflex by noting the client's ability to swallow saliva. The gag reflex may be assessed by opening the client's mouth and holding down the tongue with a tongue blade. Stimulate the gag reflex by touching the back of the client's pharynx on each side with an applicator stick. Watch for any long-lasting, previously unnoted dysphagia.

CHARTING

DATE/TIME	OBSERVATIONS	SIGNATURE
5/6 1015	Gastroscopy done in OR. Returned to Room 650. Gag reflex present, able to swallow with only slight sore throat. States no pain and is requesting liquids. B/P 120/78, P 84, R 16, T 98.2°.	F. White RN

Discharge Planning Aspects

CLIENT AND FAMILY EDUCATION

1. The client should be told to report any sharp chest pains or stomach pains after the procedure. The client and family should understand that it will be several hours before the gag reflex returns, and no food or water may be consumed until the reflex is completely normal.
2. A sore throat is not unusual after endoscopy of the GI tract, owing to tracheal irritation by passage of the tube. The client should report any bleeding in the sputum or continued inability to swallow, however.
3. Inform the client that increased flatulence or eructation are expected after endoscopy if air has been pumped into the stomach to enhance visualization.

REFERRALS

If a carcinogenic lesion is found, referral to the American Cancer Society may be appropriate.

Evaluation

Quality Assurance

Documentation should include education of the client in regard to preparation before the examination, as well as complications to expect after. Baseline vital signs and post-treatment vital signs must be reflected for an adequate time to ensure that the nurse knew which complications were possible and took precautions to see that none occurred or that they were reported to the physician promptly. The client's tolerance of the procedure and understanding of the findings should be documented. Note the presence or absence of bleeding. In addition, note the time of the return of the gag reflex and its proximity to the next meal consumed by the client.

Infection Control

Although the GI tract is not sterile, use of rigid medical asepsis helps minimize the likelihood of transferring organisms from one body site to another, or from the surrounding environment to the client. Sterilization or manufacturer-approved high-level disinfection of the endoscope after every use is critical in reducing cross-infection. Handwashing after the procedure is also necessary to ensure that microorganisms are not transmitted to the nurse, technician, or other persons.

Technique Checklist

	YES	NO
Consent form signed	_____	_____
Client understood what would happen during endoscopy	_____	_____
Food and fluids withheld for _____ hr	_____	_____
All equipment assembled before beginning of procedure	_____	_____
Specimen or biopsy obtained	_____	_____

Time obtained _____

Time to lab _____

| Client observed for complications for _____ hours | _____ | _____ |

Dysphagia _____

Coughing _____

Bloody sputum _____

Vomiting _____

Pain in chest or stomach _____

| Pathology found | _____ | _____ |
| Client and family understand the nature and ramifications of the findings of the endoscopic examination. | _____ | _____ |

10   Gastric Analysis

Overview

Definition

Aspiration of the stomach contents through a nasogastric tube for laboratory study

Rationale

Determine the presence or absence of acid in the stomach.

Determine the presence of gastric carcinoma.

Assess the need for or results of gastric or duodenal surgery.

Screen the client for pernicious anemia, gastric bleeding, tuberculosis, and drugs in the stomach.

Terminology

Analogue: Similar to in function but differing in structure

Anorexia: Loss of appetite

Chyme: Food that has been mixed with gastric juice

Dysphagia: Difficulty swallowing

Eructation: Raising of gas from the stomach (belching)

Flatulence: Excessive gas in the stomach and intestines

Pernicious anemia: A severe form of blood disease marked by a progressive decrease in red blood cells, muscular weakness, and gastrointestinal (GI) and neural disturbances

Ulcer: An open lesion of the skin or mucous membrane

Urticaria: An inflammatory condition characterized by the eruption of wheals and severe itching (hives)

Assessment

Pertinent Anatomy and Physiology

1. See Appendix I: *esophagus, intestine (small), stomach.*
2. Gastric juice is the highly acid secretion produced by glands in the mucosa of the stomach. Secretion occurs in three phases: the *cephalic* stage, which is stimulated by the sight, smell, taste, or thought of food; the *gastric* phase, which occurs because of the presence of food in the stomach; and the *intestinal* phase, during which gastric juice continues to be secreted as long as chyme is present in the duodenum.

Pathophysiological Concepts

1. Hydrochloric acid is normally present in the stomach to aid in digestion. If no acid is present, the client is said to have *achlorhydria,* a finding in pernicious anemia. Less than the normal amount of acid is called *hyposecretion* and occurs in cancer of the stomach. If there is an unusually high content of acid, the condition is called *hyperacidity* or *hypersecretion.* This last finding may be associated with ulcer formation.
2. Signs and symptoms of GI tract disorders often include anorexia, nausea, vomiting, and GI bleeding. Bleeding may be either in the vomitus or feces.

Assessment of the Client

1. Assess the client's physical condition, with emphasis on gastric symptoms.

2. Do a complete allergy assessment because some substances used to stimulate gastric secretion can cause allergic reaction in sensitive persons. Note any past allergic manifestations including asthma, dermatitis, urticaria, and hay fever.

3. Assess the client's familiarity with the procedure for obtaining gastric secretions for analysis. If the client has never undergone nasogastric intubation, assess anxiety level to determine how detailed to make the explanation.

Plan

Nursing Objectives

Allay the fear and anxiety of the client by adequate preparation.

Offer reassurance during the course of the procedure.

Protect the client from allergic reaction.

Client Preparation

1. Tell the client in advance of the procedure what is going to take place. Because of the duration and the unpleasant aspects of gastric analysis, foreknowledge may enhance cooperation and tolerance by the client.

2. Prior to the gastric aspiration, insert a nasogastric tube (Fig. 10-1). (See Technique No. 57, Gastric intubation.)

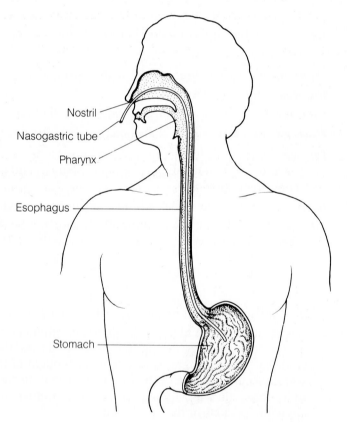

Figure 10.1

3. Ensure that the stomach is empty by having the client fast for 10 to 12 hours before the test. Eliminate any stimulants that might increase gastric secretion; these include smoking, chewing gum, and the consumption of any food or liquids.

Equipment

Gastric intubation equipment

Specified amount of stimulant (histamine, caffeine, betazole, alcohol)

Aspiration syringe

Specimen containers and labels

Sterile saline solution

Implementation and Interventions

Procedural Aspects

ACTION

Determine the method ordered by the physician for obtaining gastric secretions for analysis. Withhold food and fluids before the gastric analysis.

RATIONALE

The primary concern is prevention of allergic complications due to certain stimulants. Food and fluids in the stomach will stimulate secretions before the test and will render the quantitative analyses invalid.

Twelve-hour Secretion Test

Pass the nasogastric tube in the evening, rinse the stomach with saline solution, and drain the stomach. Discard the gastric juice collected in the first 15 minutes. Aspirate the nasogastric tube periodically during the next 12 hours and save all contents. Flush the tube periodically with sterile saline solution. Aspirate all contents at the end of the test before removing the tube.

Because of the duration of the test, it usually is performed at night to minimize discomfort from having the tube in place for so long and withholding of food and fluids. The client also may rest between aspirations. Amount of secretion is an important part of the analysis, so that it is necessary to record how much saline is used to rinse the tube.

Histamine Test

Histamine is a strong gastric stimulant that can cause severe allergic reactions. An alternative is the use of betazole HCl (Histalog), the side-effects of which are milder. If histamine is used, inject 0.1 ml intradermally to test for allergy. If a wheal appears that is greater than 10 mm across, the test result is positive and its use is contraindicated. Histamine is not used in clients with a history of asthma, urticaria, or other allergies. If no contraindication is present, pass the nasogastric tube and aspirate gastric contents. Histamine 0.01 mg/kg body weight or Histalog 0.05 mg/kg body weight is injected intramuscularly. Aspirate gastric content at 15 to 20 minute intervals for the prescribed time, usually one hour. Note the quantity and send the specimen to the lab.

Histalog is an analogue of histamine and is less likely to cause a reaction. A sensitivity test offers an opportunity to assess allergies without endangering the client with anaphylactic shock. These potent stimulants cause enough gastric secretion to determine adequacy of gastric function.

Caffeine

Insert the nasogastric tube and aspirate gastric contents. Insert a solution of 0.5 g caffeine sodium benzoate in 200 ml water through the tube at the

Caffeine is a gastric stimulant. Quantity as well as quality of contents will be analyzed for diagnostic purposes.

ACTION	*RATIONALE*
prescribed time. Aspirate gastric contents in 30 minutes and every 10 minutes for 2 hours.	

Communicative Aspects

OBSERVATIONS

1. When histamine is used, observe the client carefully for the following side-effects: flushing of the face, headache, hypotension, dizziness, pain at injection site, and nausea.

2. Observe the amount of gastric secretions.

3. Note the appearance of gastric secretions. If the return is yellowish green (indicating bile), the position of the tube may be in question (*i.e.*, it may be in the duodenum). Small streaks of blood may indicate slight trauma during insertion of the tube. Frank red bleeding indicates a medical emergency; notify the physician at once.

CHARTING

DATE/TIME	OBSERVATIONS	SIGNATURE
4/12 2230	Histalog gastric analysis begun. No reaction noted to skin test. Procedure explained to Mr. J and wife, who state understanding of why the test is to be done and what will occur. Nasogastric tube inserted and gastric content (60 ml) discarded. Histalog given IM. Resting quietly at this time. ————————	G. Ivers RN

Discharge Planning Aspects

CLIENT AND FAMILY EDUCATION

1. Before the gastric analysis, warn the client and family about the signs of allergic reaction, which should be reported at once.

2. If the client is suspected of or found to have an ulcer, dietary counseling about the effects of certain foods on stimulation of the gastric juices should be arranged.

3. The reasons for frequent disturbance of the client to withdraw gastric contents should be explained. This is especially important if the client will be awakened frequently during the night.

Evaluation

Quality Assurance

Documentation should include education of the client in regard to preparation before the examination. Evidence of a thorough assessment of allergic history should be present. The amount of gastric content and its appearance should be noted, as well as the client's tolerance of the procedure.

Infection Control

The gastric contents specimen must be handled aseptically in collection and transport to the laboratory. Contamination with exogenous organisms could lead to erroneous laboratory results. Thorough handwashing before and after performing gastric aspiration will reduce the chance of transmitting infection.

Technique Checklist

	YES	NO
Order for the test on chart	_____	_____
Test explained to client	_____	_____
Food and fluids withheld for _____ hr	_____	_____
Equipment assembled before test	_____	_____
Allergy assessment on chart	_____	_____
Nasogastric tube inserted at _____		

	YES	NO
Stimulant given _____	_____	_____
Time _____		
Original gastric aspiration discarded	_____	_____
Specimen gathered at intervals of _____		
Test completed at _____		
Total amount of specimen _____		
Specimen to lab at _____		
Complications _____	_____	_____
Nasogastric tube removed at _____		
Client and family understand test results	_____	_____

11   **Gastrointestinal X-Ray Studies**

Overview

Definition

Radiologic study of the gastrointestinal (GI) tract after consumption of a radi-opaque substance, also called or including esophagography, barium swallow, upper GI series, and small bowel examination. (The normal stomach and duodenum are shown in Fig. 11-1.)

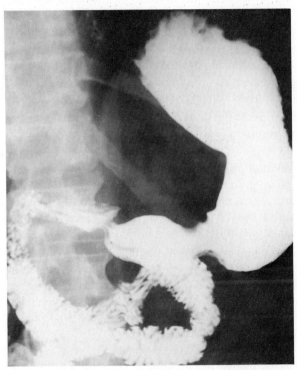

Figure 11.1

Rationale

Determine the presence of pathology or abnormalities in the GI tract (e.g., tumors or ulcers).

Assess the motility and thickness of the gastric wall.

Determine the presence or absence of right atrial enlargement, which usually will impinge on the esophagus.

Assess the presence and severity of esophageal varices.

Terminology

Adhesions: The abnormal joining of organs or structures by the formation of fibrous bands

Anorexia: Loss of appetite

Diverticulitis: Inflammation of a pouch in the intestine

Dysphagia: Difficulty swallowing

Eructation: Raising of gas from the stomach; belching

Flatulence: Excessive gas in the stomach and intestines

Incarcerated: Confined; constricted

Intussusception: The slipping of one part of the intestine into the part just below it

Obstruction: Blocking of a structure, which prevents normal function

Peritonitis: Inflammation of the peritoneum, the membranous coat lining the abdominal cavity

Stricture: Narrowing of the lumen (opening or channel) of a tube, duct or hollow organ

Ulcer: An open lesion of the skin or mucous membrane

Assessment

Pertinent Anatomy and Physiology

See Appendix I in the back of the book: *esophagus, intestine (small), stomach.*

Pathophysiological Concepts

1. Signs and symptoms of GI tract disorders are anorexia, nausea, vomiting, abdominal distention, constipation, decreased or increased bowel sounds, and GI bleeding. Bleeding may be either in the vomitus or feces.

2. Pathology of the esophagus may manifest itself in dysphagia. If it is due to narrowing of the esophagus because of tumor encroachment or lesions, it may be detected by radiologic visualization. *Esophageal diverticulum* is an outpouching of the esophageal wall caused by a weakness in the muscle layer.

3. Other disorders that may be visualized by x-ray study include gastric and peptic ulcers, inflammatory bowel disease, diverticulitis, appendicitis, and cancer.

4. Intestinal obstruction may be due to incarcerated hernia; foreign bodies; stricture from an ulcer, peritonitis, or tumor; knotting or twisting of the intestine (volvulus); intussusception, or telescoping of one part of the intestine into another part; or adhesions. Intestinal obstruction is very serious and warrants immediate attention.

5. *Esophageal varices* are dilatations of the esophageal veins and capillaries. They arise with persistent obstruction of blood flow through the portal vein, resulting in diversion of blood flow to the other venous channels, such as the gastric and esophageal veins. Esophageal veins are relatively small and inelastic and are subject to rupture. The final outcome in this instance often is massive and fatal hemorrhage.

Assessment of the Client

1. Assess the symptoms described by the client in relation to gastric pain and problems. Determine baseline vital signs to monitor the progress of symptoms.

2. Assess the dietary habits and knowledge of the client and family. Determine amount and duration of alcohol consumption. Determine if the client is aware of the basic food groups and assess current eating patterns in relation to the symptoms. Define knowledge deficits and assess the teaching strategy that seems most likely to succeed with this client.

3. Assess the amount of familiarity and experience the client has had with radiologic examinations. Determine the amount of teaching necessary to reassure the client and to enhance the chances of compliance with the preparation and completion of the x-ray studies.

Plan

Nursing Objectives

Explain the procedure thoroughly to the client.

Ensure that proper preparation takes place for maximum results.

Client Preparation

1. Explain to the client what will occur during the x-ray examination and why the study is necessary. Tell the client that follow-up films may be taken as

the barium progresses through the GI tract. This may require several hours, and anxiety may be reduced if the client anticipates the lengthy time requirements.

2. No physical preparation is necessary except withholding food and fluids for 12 hours before the test. If prior barium studies have been done, it may be necessary to administer one or more enemas to evacuate the barium in the GI tract so that it will not interfere with the progressive visualization of the upper GI tract.

3. Instruct the client not to smoke or chew gum because these activities stimulate the secretion of gastric juices, a state that is undesirable preceding barium studies.

Equipment	Hospital gown
	Wheelchair or stretcher for transport

Implementation and Interventions

Procedural Aspects

ACTION	RATIONALE
1. To visualize the soft tissues, barium sulfate is used to fill the organs and cause them to cast an outline shadow on the film.	X-rays are a form of radiant energy that penetrate according to the density of the tissue. Barium sulfate is a fine, white, odorless, tasteless, bulky powder, insoluble in water and impermeable to the x-ray beam.
2. In GI studies, the client swallows the "barium milkshake," and the progress of the barium through the GI tract is visualized on the x-ray film.	The barium is flavored to disguise the chalky taste; however, little can be done to disguise it completely. Peristalsis carries the barium through the GI tract; its adequacy can be determined on radiologic examination.
3. Explain that the client will be asked to stand against a tilting table in the upright position. After the initial swallow, the client will be secured to the table and tilted at various angles to ensure maximum visualization of all areas. As the barium travels the length of the GI tract, x-ray films will be taken. The client may be asked to swallow air to add additional contrast. Pressure may be applied manually or by using a dome-shaped projection on the x-ray machine. This may be slightly uncomfortable. The client may be returned to the room to await follow-up films. Films may be taken as late as 24 hours after the barium swallow.	Tilting the table allows the barium to infiltrate the GI tract by means of gravitational pull. Pressure may be applied to ensure spreading of the barium throughout the GI system. It can take several hours to complete the x-ray study.
4. Films are made with the barium in place and after it has been evacuated. The peristaltic activity of each portion of the bowel can also be observed.	The natural tendency of the GI tract is to evacuate its contents. This peristaltic activity can be seen on the radiologic examination, and the adequacy of eliminatory capacity can be evaluated.

Communicative Aspects

OBSERVATIONS

1. Signs and symptoms of GI tract disorders are anorexia, nausea, vomiting, abdominal distention, constipation, decreased or increased bowel sounds, and GI bleeding. Bleeding may be either in the vomitus or feces.
2. Observe the stools for the next few days to verify the passage of the barium.

CHARTING

DATE/TIME	OBSERVATIONS	SIGNATURE
8/2 0930	Returned to room after GI series. Remains NPO. To return to Radiology in 1 hr for follow-up films. States no problems or discomfort at this time. ——	G. Ivers RN

Discharge Planning Aspects

CLIENT AND FAMILY EDUCATION

1. Inform the client and family that there will be a long wait during the x-ray procedure as the barium progresses through the GI tract. Advise the client to take along some reading material or a craft to help pass the time.
2. After the x-ray examination, ask the client to report the next bowel movement so that the nurse can verify that the barium is passing satisfactorily. If it is not, additional measures may be necessary. Inform the client that chalky stools may occur for several days after the examination. A laxative, increased intake of high-fiber foods (if not contraindicated by findings of the x-ray studies), and large amounts of fluid may help pass the barium easily.
3. Caution the client about expelling all of the barium after the x-ray examination. It should be understood that failure to evacuate the barium could lead to impaction. Stress the importance of fluids in aiding the elimination process.
4. Offer sound guidance and practical information about exercise and activity, and guidelines for judicious use of over-the-counter medications for relief of minor GI disturbances. Also, help the client to develop a positive, flexible attitude about elimination patterns.
5. If the client swallowed significant amounts of air during the procedure, eructation and increased flatulence will occur until the excess air is eliminated.

Evaluation

Quality Assurance

Documentation should reflect the symptomatology that prompted the examination. The baseline vital signs should be recorded, as well as vital signs after the examination. The nurse should document frequent monitoring of pulse and blood pressure if the suspected diagnosis involves a pathologic condition that may predispose hemorrhage (e.g., ulcer and esophageal varices). The client's response to the examination should be noted, as well as when the barium was evacuated. The presence of the first normal stool after barium studies is significant.

Infection Control

If the preparation involves administration of enemas, the nurse must be sure to engage in thorough handwashing both before and after the procedure. Special attire and other measures are required for the client with an infectious process.

Technique Checklist

	YES	NO
Examination ordered on chart	_____	_____
Client understood why the test was ordered and what would occur during the examination	_____	_____
Preparations complete		
Enema(s) × _____	_____	_____
NPO at midnight	_____	_____
Transported safely to X-ray dept.	_____	_____
X-ray procedure successfully completed	_____	_____
Client and family understand what the results of the x-ray signify	_____	_____

12   Glucose and Acetone Testing

Overview

Definition

Diagnostic testing to assess the status of the client's diabetic condition

Rationale

Determine the presence of glucose in the blood and urine.

Determine the presence of ketone bodies (acetone) in the system.

Provide a guideline on which to assess the client's need for insulin.

Terminology

Anorexia: Loss of appetite

Glycosuria: The presence of an abnormal amount of glucose in the urine

Ketosis: Accumulation in the body of ketone bodies

Reagent: A substance involved in a chemical reaction—often to detect the presence of another substance

Assessment

Pertinent Anatomy and Physiology

1. Metabolism allows for the continuous release of energy. Anabolism is the phase of storage and synthesis of cell constituents which requires energy. Catabolism involves the breakdown of complex molecules into substances that can be used in the production of energy. Carbohydrates, fats, and proteins are transformed into adenosine triphosphate (ATP), which is the energy source of all body cells.

2. Glucose is broken down into carbon dioxide and water. Its entry into the blood is regulated by the liver, which stores and synthesizes glucose. When blood sugar is increased, the liver removes glucose from the blood, converts it into glycogen, and stores it in the liver and muscle tissues for future use. When the blood sugar drops, the liver releases its stored glucose.

3. About three fourths of body solids are proteins that are essential for the formation of all body structures. Amino acids are the building blocks of proteins.

4. Insulin is the hormone that is released in response to an increase in blood sugar levels. The actions of insulin are currently being researched. It is believed to be involved in glucose storage, prevention of fat breakdown, and increasing protein synthesis. Insulin is produced by the pancreatic cells in the islets of Langerhans. It is secreted by the beta cells directly into the liver, where it is either used or degraded.

Pathophysiological Concepts

1. *Diabetes mellitus* is an insulin deficiency state that interferes with carbohydrate, protein, and fat metabolism. The uncontrolled diabetic is unable to transport glucose into fat and muscle cells. This results in an increased breakdown of fat and protein. Diabetes is accompanied by a predisposition to vascular changes. There are two types of diabetes: type I and type II. Type I diabetes (formerly called juvenile diabetes) occurs in clients who manufacture little or no insulin. It usually develops in younger persons and requires

daily injections of insulin as well as regulated diet and exercise. Type II diabetes is the noninsulin-dependent condition, which usually occurs in persons over 40 years of age. The pancreas does produce insulin, and treatment mainly is centered on diet and exercise regulation. Factors that contribute to the development of diabetes include heredity, obesity, pregnancy, physical or emotional stress, and aging.

2. Determination of the urine glucose level is interpreted as a "reflection" of the actual blood glucose level. Optimal analysis of the diabetic status is ascertained from actual testing of the serum level of glucose. This is considered the preferred method of insulin regulation. A variety of reagent strips and equipment such as self blood glucose meters enable the diabetic to monitor actual serum glucose level with a finger stick in a minimal amount of time.

3. *Renal threshold* is the level at which the blood spills excess glucose into the urine. If the threshold is higher or lower than normal, the results of the urine testing will be misleading. Renal thresholds tend to become higher as people age. The normal renal threshold for most people up to about age 50 is 160 mg to 180 mg of glucose per 100 ml of blood.

4. *Hypoglycemia* (often called insulin reaction or insulin shock) occurs when the blood sugar level falls below 50 mg per 100 ml of blood. It is characterized by sudden onset and rapid progression. Symptoms include headache, altered behavior, anxiety, hunger, sweating, cool and clammy skin, coma, and convulsions. The most effective treatment of an insulin reaction is the immediate ingestion of a concentrated carbohydrate source (e.g., sugar, candy, or orange juice). If the client is comatose, glucagon may be given intravenously, intramuscularly, or subcutaneously.

5. *Diabetic ketoacidosis* occurs when ketone production by the liver exceeds utilization and excretion. The body compensates for the inadequacy of the insulin supply by increasing the blood sugar levels in the muscles. The muscles cannot use this oversupply of glucose without insulin, however. The liver, in response, forms acidic substances called ketone bodies to supply the needed additional energy to the muscles. The resulting condition, called ketosis, leads the liver to lose further glycogen. When the blood sugar level reaches 150 to 200 mg/100 ml, the kidney cannot absorb all of the filtered glucose, and glycosuria results. The onset of ketoacidosis is slower and the recovery more prolonged than in insulin reaction. Symptoms include a characteristic fruity smell on the breath, an increase in the rate and depth of respirations (Kussmaul breathing), anorexia, nausea and vomiting, excessive urination and thirst, weakness, fatigue, abdominal pain, blurred vision, lethargy, stupor and coma. Treatment involves returning the pH of the blood to normal levels by the administration of insulin and intravenous electrolyte replacement.

Assessment of the Client

1. Assess the client for signs and symptoms of diabetic complications. Do a complete diabetic history of the patient on admission, including the onset of the condition and the client's familiarity with the diabetic condition. Initial assessment should include vital sign assessment, measurement of weight, and glucose and acetone determination on both the blood and urine.

2. Assess the knowledge level of the client and family regarding the diabetic condition. Determine knowledge deficits and the willingness and ability of the client and family to learn about the treatment of diabetes. Assess the receptivity of the family and client to the restrictions and modifications which may be necessary. This is important in determining which approach teaching efforts should take.

Plan

Nursing Objectives

Perform the tests correctly.

Ensure the stability and freshness of the reagent tablets or equipment.

Report and take immediate actions when tests indicate glucose and acetone levels above normal.

Teach the client and family to perform the tests.

Client Preparation

1. To perform these tests, a blood or urine specimen is necessary. The blood test is performed with a drop of blood obtained from a finger stick. Have the client wash both hands thoroughly with soap and water. To gain greater compliance from the client, explain why the test is being done and the significance of the results in determining the status of the diabetic condition. Because these tests may be done frequently during the day, the cooperation and understanding of the client are especially significant.

2. Provide the client with sufficient liquids to ensure adequate hydration if urine specimens are to be used to monitor the diabetic condition. Fluids should be of the noncaloric type or should be figured into the overall calorie count for the day.

Equipment

Soap and water to cleanse hands

Clean specimen receptacle for urine testing

Reagent materials

Test tube and dropper for Clinitest and Acetest

Blood glucose meter and reagent strips

Implementation and Interventions

Procedural Aspects

ACTION	RATIONALE
1. During the initial period of beginning self-glucose monitoring, the client may check the serum glucose level four times a day, that is, before each meal and at bedtime. After several days, a glucose profile of the client is done, and it may be possible to measure the serum glucose accurately by intermittent analysis such as before breakfast one day, before lunch the next day, and so forth. Check the glucose level as ordered by the physician. The ultimate goal is to allow the client to assume the responsibility for the testing so that testing will be done more frequently during illness, unusual stress, or if any type of reaction should occur.	Because the testing requires a finger stick, client compliance may be enhanced if the need for sticks is kept to a minimum. Because glucose monitoring assesses actual serum glucose levels, it is possible to determine adequacy of treatment and need for adjustments. Determining the usual levels of glucose will allow the client some flexibility in monitoring.

ACTION

RATIONALE

2. Urine testing for glucose and acetone may be done to determine the success of current treatment modalities. Because urine reflects the status of the body at a time several hours before the time at which the urine specimen is obtained, the tests do not necessarily reflect the current amount of glucose in the client's blood. Tell the client to check the urine for ketones whenever blood sugar levels are running high (>240 mg) and whenever symptoms or illness are present.

Urine testing may be ordered to complement serum glucose monitoring. Ketones in the blood are important indicators that the client is at risk for ketoacidosis. This should not be neglected when the client is doing self-monitoring of serum glucose.

3. A variety of equipment and materials are commercially available for use in diabetic monitoring

The type of monitoring device(s) may depend on the stability of the client's condition, availability of equipment, motivation of the client, and economic status.

Glucose Reagent Strips:

These strips are available for use with a portable meter or alone. Cleanse the client's finger with soap and water. Stick the tip of the finger (Fig. 12-1) with the sterile lancet (puncture device) that accompanies the kit (Fig. 12-2). "Milk" the finger (Fig. 12-3). Blot away the first drop of blood and place the second directly on the strip. Follow the manufacturer's instructions regarding the remainder of the test. Some strips are simply blotted, some must be washed and then blotted. Compare the strip with the accompanying color chart.

The second drop of blood is used for analysis because of the possibility of body fluids diluting the first drop. Comparison with a color chart provides a semiquantitative estimation of serum glucose levels. For quantitative results the strips should be read with a glucose scan meter.

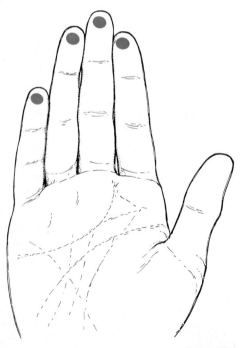

Figure 12.1

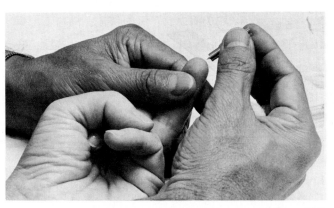

Figure 12.2

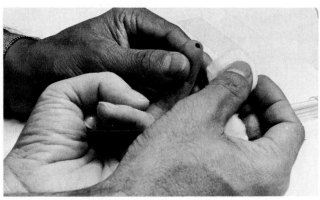

Figure 12.3

ACTION

Serum Glucose Meters:

The meter is a self-contained box that may be as small as a pocket calculator. A drop of the client's blood is placed on the accompanying strip. After a short time has elapsed (usually 1 min), the strip is placed into a slot on the meter. The meter gives a digital readout of the status of the client's serum glucose.

Urine Reagent Methods:

Clinitest (5-drop method):
Have the client void into a clean container. Hold the dropper vertically and fill it with urine. Place 5 drops of the urine into the test tube. Rinse the dropper and add 10 drops of water to the urine in the test tube. Drop one Clinitest tablet into the tube and observe the reaction taking place. Do not touch the bottom of the test tube or shake it during the reaction or for 15 seconds after the reaction concludes. If no pass-through reaction occurs, gently shake the tube and compare the results with the color scale accompanying the Clinitest set.

Clinitest (2-drop method):
Have the client void into a clean container. Hold the dropper vertically and fill it with urine. Place 2 drops of the urine in a test tube. Rinse the dropper and add 10 drops of water to the tube. Drop one Clinitest tablet into the test tube. Do not shake the test tube during the reaction or for 15 seconds after completion. Compare the resulting color with the chart accompanying the Clinitest set to determine the approximate percentage of glucose in the urine.

RATIONALE

Meters are calibrated and give a measurement of the client's blood glucose level at the time the drop of blood is removed.

Careful observation of the reaction is essential because a pass-through color change can occur for a high glucose level. If the solution passes through orange and dark greenish-brown, it indicates a level of 4+ (or urine sugar >2%) and is recorded as such. Clinitest reaction is a chemical reaction that generates heat; the bottom of the test tube gets very hot when the tablet boils in the presence of urine and water.

See rationale for the 5-drop method above.

ACTION	RATIONALE
Reagent Strips Method: Diastix (glucose), Testape (glucose), and Ketostix (acetone) are strips permeated with reagent. Dip the strip into undiluted urine and compare the result with the color chart which accompanies that particular strip. Keto-Diastix is a combined ketone–glucose reagent strip and is used in the same way as those previously mentioned.	The strips undergo a chemical reaction on urine contact. The resulting color determines levels of the particular substance being measured.
Tablet Testing Method: Acetest tablets are useful in detecting acetone bodies in the urine. Place a tablet on a clean paper towel and place 1 drop of urine directly on top of the tablet. Compare the results with the accompanying color chart.	The tablet undergoes chemical reaction upon contacting urine. The resulting color is used to determine the level of acetone in the urine.
4. Rinse all equipment thoroughly after use and return it to its proper place.	In addition to maintaining a clean, germ-free environment, it is essential to set a good example for care of the testing equipment so that the client will understand proper care after discharge.

Special Modifications

1. If the condition is particularly unstable, it may be necessary to do serum glucose determinations more often than once or four times a day. The client eventually should learn when it is necessary to test and when it would be safe to go for longer periods without performing glucose testing. Generally, testing more frequently is warranted during periods of illness, high stress, or when symptoms of insulin reaction or ketoacidosis are present.	When the body is under unusual stress from illness, metabolism is altered. Diabetic status may change and should be monitored carefully.

Communicative Aspects

OBSERVATIONS

1. Note the level of comprehension and motivation of the client in regard to glucose testing. Observe the client demonstrating the method of testing ordered by the physician and note any knowledge or physical deficiencies that must be addressed before discharge.

2. Careful observation of the chemical reaction during Clinitest is important in detecting pass-through color changes.

3. Note any problems in obtaining the specimens.

4. Observe the client for the following signs of diabetic problems which warrant immediate attention:

   Insulin Reaction: sweating, pallor, tremor, hunger, altered behavior, anxiety, tachycardia, palpitation, headache, confusion, slurred speech, incoordination, double vision, drowsiness, convulsions, and coma.

Diabetic Ketoacidosis: thirst, anorexia, nausea, vomiting, abdominal pain, headache, blurred vision, drowsiness, weakness, shortness of breath or an increase in the rate and depth of respirations, air hunger, fruity-smelling breath, excessive urination, lethargy, stupor, and coma.

CHARTING

DATE/TIME	OBSERVATIONS	SIGNATURE
2/10 1330	Taught finger-stick technique to obtain specimen for glucose determination. Comparison with table explained and demonstrated. Glucose within normal range. Expressed no hesitation about doing the testing herself this evening. States that she understands the diet instructions and insulin administration technique. Expressed anticipation of getting back to her family. ————	F. White RN

Discharge Planning Aspects

CLIENT AND FAMILY EDUCATION

1. The major goals of diabetic management are to avoid the symptoms of uncontrolled diabetes and to avoid or delay diabetic complications. This is accomplished largely by keeping glucose levels at or near normal levels and keeping blood fat and cholesterol levels low. An organized and comprehensive teaching program is essential for the diabetic client and family.

2. If the client will be checking the urine at home, teach the procedure to the client and family members. There are several products available for glucose monitoring. Emphasize that the color scales that accompany each product are not interchangeable.

REFERRALS

The American Diabetes Association is very active in screening procedures and in the assistance of active diabetics. In addition, the A.D.A. supplies a large assortment of reading material to help the diabetic remain current on the latest advancements in diabetic research and management. Some insurance companies cover certain diabetic testing equipment, such as glucose meters, on health insurance coverage. Advise the client to consult the insurance company to determine if assistance with purchase of equipment is possible.

Evaluation

Quality Assurance

Documentation should include aspects of client teaching in addition to the results of glucose and acetone determinations made in the hospital. The response of the client and likelihood of compliance with diabetic restrictions after discharge should be addressed. Evidence should be apparent in the chart that the nurse(s) knew and understood the symptoms of diabetic crises, that precautions were taken to minimize the risk of complications, and that the client and family are familiar with the symptoms and management before discharge.

Infection Control

Infections are a common concern for the diabetic. Infections that may occur are soft-tissue infections, osteomyelitis, urinary tract infections and pyelonephritis, candidal infections of the skin and mucous surfaces, and tuberculosis. Vascular impairment may hinder the body's defense mechanisms in the production of an adequate inflammatory response to effect adequate healing. Sensory deficits may cause the diabetic person to ignore a minor trauma, which then becomes an infection. It is essential that diabetics engage in meticulous skin care and that extreme caution be exercised in avoiding cross-infection during hospitalization. Maintenance of sterile technique during finger-stick procedures must be stressed.

Technique Checklist

	YES	NO
Assessment of diabetic history	————	————
Glucose and acetone determination techniques taught to client	————	————
Method used:		
Serum glucose strips	————	————
Serum glucose meter	————	————
Urine glucose monitoring	————	————
Urine acetone monitoring	————	————
Glucose and acetone test results kept on an accessible record during hospitalization	————	————
Client (and family) demonstrated an understanding of how, when, and why to do the diabetic monitoring.	————	————
Diabetic complications ———————————————		

13   Intravenous Pyelogram (IVP)

Overview

Definition

An x-ray study of the kidneys and ureters by means of an injected dye

Rationale

Determine abnormalities in the outline of the urinary tract signifying pathology.
Assess the level of kidney functioning.
Assess the efficiency of bladder emptying.

Assessment

Pertinent Anatomy and Physiology

See Appendix I: *bladder, kidneys, ureters.*

Pathophysiological Concepts

1. Congenital defects of the kidneys are a fairly common occurrence. These defects include absence of one kidney, fusion of the kidneys (horseshoe kidney), polycystic kidney, hypoplasia (abnormally small kidneys), and dysplasia (abnormal differentiation of the renal structures during the embryonic period) of the kidneys.

2. Urinary obstruction may result from congenital defects, stones, pregnancy, benign prostatic hypertrophy, infection, and certain neurological disorders. Obstruction results in a greater chance of infection and stone formation, as a result of urine pooling. Permanent damage to the kidney may occur.

3. Kidney stones (renal calculi) may form in the pelves of the kidneys, causing pain and hematuria. Stones that escape from the kidney into the ureter may cause excruciating pain (renal colic) as they move toward the urinary bladder. The usual cause of stones is an increased concentration of the constituents that make up the stones causing precipitation and crystallization. The four types of stones are calcium stones, magnesium ammonium phosphate stones, uric acid stones, and cystine stones.

Assessment of the Client

1. Completely assess the client's allergy history before the injection of the iodine dye used in IVP. Allergies of any kind should be noted, especially allergies to shellfish and iodine preparations.

2. Assess the client's knowledge of the reason for and expected outcome of the test. Assess anxiety level and determine the appropriate teaching strategies.

3. Determine if the client has had any barium studies in the past several days (e.g., GI series or barium enema). The presence of barium in the system may obscure the IVP.

Plan

Nursing Objectives

1. Protect the client from the threat of allergic reaction.
2. Prepare the client adequately to ensure maximum visualization.

Client Preparation

1. An x-ray is a form of radiant energy that penetrates according to the density of tissue. For this reason, the stomach and bowel should be empty so that

they will not interfere with the x-ray visualization of the kidneys, ureters, and bladder, which lie in proximity. Food and fluids may be withheld for 12 hours preceding the test. A laxative, enema, or both may be used to ensure that the bowel is empty in preparation for this x-ray examination.

2. Barium in the gastrointestinal (GI) tract will obscure the urinary tract. If the client has undergone barium studies recently, a period of about 2 days should elapse before urologic studies are begun.

Equipment

Hospital gown

Wheelchair or stretcher for transport

Implementation and Interventions

Procedural Aspects

ACTION	**RATIONALE**
1. Transport the client safely to the radiology department by stretcher or in a wheelchair as tolerated. The client will be placed on an x-ray table. An initial x-ray film of the kidneys, ureters, and bladder is usually performed. A test dose of the dye may be given intradermally to ensure that the client is not allergic to it. If no symptoms occur, the iodine-based dye is then injected by venipuncture. A warm, flushing feeling and an unpleasant taste sensation in the mouth often accompany injection, but these effects are short-lived. X-rays are taken at designated intervals. A post-voiding film may be taken when the IVP is completed. The entire study takes about 1 hour.	An initial x-ray of the urinary system may be of value for comparison with subsequent films. A post-voiding x-ray will help to determine the efficiency of the bladder emptying.
2. After the x-ray examination, provide the client with a quiet environment for rest and recuperation. Force fluids and offer nourishment unless contraindicated.	Fluids help flush the dye from the client's system. Food will help to counteract the effects of dehydration and fasting.

Communicative Aspects

OBSERVATIONS

1. Observe the client for any indication of an allergic reaction to the iodine dye.
2. Note the effect of laxatives or enemas to determine if the colon has been emptied adequately.

CHARTING

DATE/TIME	OBSERVATIONS	SIGNATURE
7/4 0700	To x-ray for IVP per wheelchair. States no history of allergies. Has used iodine topically without problems. Good results from enema prep. States no further right flank pain.	F. White RN

Discharge Planning Aspects

CLIENT AND FAMILY EDUCATION

1. Stress the role of adequate hydration in the prevention of urinary stones and urinary infection.

2. Emphasize the inherent safety of x-ray techniques, especially if the client voices any concern about radiation.

REFERRALS

If abnormalities are found, the National Kidney Foundation may be able to offer services or assistance to the client and family.

Evaluation

Quality Assurance

Document preparatory measures taken to ensure that extraneous matter would not obscure the x-ray. Show evidence that the nurse recognized the problem of barium and fecal matter in the bowel and took steps to rectify the situation. Document the steps taken to ensure that no allergic reaction occurred.

Infection Control

1. Cystitis, or infection of the bladder, is a common infection, especially in women. Stress to all female clients the importance of cleansing the female genitalia from front to back to avoid transporting bacteria from the rectum and vagina to the urinary meatus. Pyelitis is an infection of the renal pelvis that may follow infection of the bladder. Infection may spread along the mucous membrane of the ureters from the bladder.

2. Equipment used for consecutive clients should be cleaned between uses. This includes wheelchairs, which should either be cleaned with a disinfectant after use or covered by a sheet that is changed between clients. Outbreaks of infection that have been associated with a variety of urinary tract diagnostic measures may be reduced by rigid attention to cleansing procedure and handwashing before and after procedures.

Technique Checklist

	YES	NO
Order for IVP on chart	_____	_____
Test explained to client	_____	_____
Allergy assessment completed	_____	_____
Adequate preparation before exam		
Laxative _____		
Enema (number) _____		
NPO at midnight	_____	_____
X-ray completed satisfactorily	_____	_____
Renal pathology found	_____	_____
Client understands x-ray findings	_____	_____

14   Lumbar Puncture

Overview

Definition

Insertion of a needle into the lumbar subarachnoid space for the purpose of examining and withdrawing cerebrospinal fluid for diagnostic study or spinal anesthesia. Lumbar puncture is also called *spinal tap.*

Rationale

Determine the presence of infection, hemorrhage, increased intracranial pressure (IIP), and other pathology.

Facilitate determining the cause of headaches, numbness in the legs and arms, and other neurologic symptoms.

Administer spinal anesthetic.

Inject dyes or gases for the purpose of diagnostic x-ray examination of the spine.

Relieve pressure by removal of a small amount of cerebrospinal fluid.

Terminology

Cisternal puncture: Insertion of the needle into the cisterna magna just below the occipital bone in the back of the neck

Hydrocephalus: Increased accumulation of cerebrospinal fluid within the ventricles of the brain

Lumbar spine: The five vertebrae below the thoracic spine

Manometer: The graduated tube through which fluid flows to determine the pressure of the spinal fluid

Myelogram: Radiologic study of the spinal column using a radiopaque medium

Pneumoencephalogram: Radiologic study of the subarachnoid area of the brain, accomplished by injecting gas into the space

Queckenstedt test: Compression on one or both of the jugular veins for 10 seconds during lumbar puncture; this should cause a rapid rise in pressure of the cerebrospinal fluid of healthy persons. The rise in pressure quickly subsides when pressure on the neck is released. When there is a block in the spinal canal, the pressure of the spinal fluid is scarcely affected by this test. This test is contraindicated in the presence of intracranial disease, (*i.e.,* hemorrhage or IIP).

Thoracic spine: The twelve vertebrae below the cervical spine

Assessment

Pertinent Anatomy and Physiology

1. See Appendix I: *vertebral column.*
2. The cerebrospinal fluid is a clear, colorless fluid that fills the ventricles of the brain and the subarachnoid spaces around the brain and spinal cord. Some of the constituents are water, sodium chloride, potassium, glucose, traces of protein, and a few white blood cells. Although about 500 ml of cerebrospinal fluid is secreted each day, the total volume in the spinal canal and ventricular system is only about 150 ml. The fluid is completely replaced about three times a day.

3. The spinal cord begins at the level of the foramen magnum in the brain and extends downward through the vertebral canal to the level of the disk between the first and second lumbar vertebrae. The spinal cord is an elongated, cylindrical mass of nervous tissue consisting of 31 segments, each of which gives rise to a pair of spinal nerves. The cord is covered and protected by three membranes called meninges. The dura mater is the outermost. The space between the walls of the vertebral canal and the dura mater is the epidural space. The next layer of the meninges is the arachnoid membrane and the innermost layer is the pia mater. The subarachnoid space is a relatively roomy area between the arachnoid and the pia mater. It is filled with the cerebrospinal fluid. (Fig. 14-1)

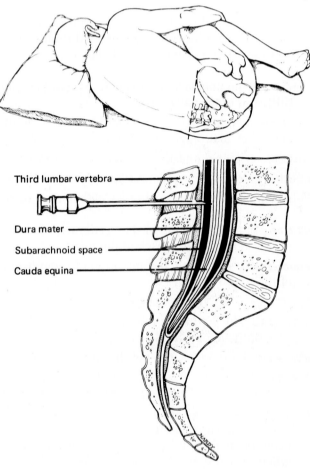

Third lumbar vertebra

Dura mater

Subarachnoid space

Cauda equina

Figure 14.1

Pathophysiological Concepts

1. The rigid structure of the skull prevents its expansion when the intracranial pressure increases. The normal intracranial pressure is 60 to 180 mm of water. Causes of increased pressure are impaired production, circulation, or absorption of the cerebrospinal fluid and edema from brain tumor, stroke, or injury. When intracranial pressure increases, destruction of brain tissue is possible, as well as internal hydrocephalus. A progression or worsening of increased pressure can be detected by changes in the level of consciousness, pupil size and reaction, vital signs, and motor function. Another danger is the withdrawal of too much fluid during lumbar puncture. Sudden decompression may result in spontaneous protrusion of the edematous brain into the vertebral column, resulting in death.

2. Infections in the central nervous system (CNS) are classified according to the structure involved: meninges—meningitis; brain parenchyma—encephalitis;

spinal cord—myelitis; both brain and spinal cord—encephalomyelitis. Pathogens generally enter the CNS by the bloodstream, crossing the blood–brain barrier in a systemic disease, or by direct invasion through skull fracture or bullet hole, or from contamination during surgery or lumbar puncture.

3. The presence of blood in the cerebrospinal fluid is an indication of trauma or hemorrhage in the CNS. The cerebrospinal fluid will be pinkish. Immediate action is indicated because blood is not a normal constituent of the cerebrospinal fluid.

4. Headache is a universal phenomenon, the cause of which is not really known. Some headaches may be the result of tension or muscle contraction. Migraine headaches may be due to changes in blood flow and oxygen availability. Headache is a symptom of some types of CNS disorders.

Assessment of the Client

1. Assess the baseline vital and neurologic signs for later comparison. Assess the client's neurologic condition also, including the presence and description of headaches.

2. Assess the client's allergy history if a dye is to be injected for x-ray studies. Determine if the client has any allergy to topical or local anesthetic or a known or suspected sensitivity to shellfish, iodine, and other contrast media.

3. Assess the physical agility of the client in relation to ability to curve the torso to facilitate the insertion of the needle between the vertebrae. Assess respiratory capacity as breathing will be hindered somewhat while in the position required for successful lumbar puncture. If the client is obese, separation of vertebrae may be more difficult.

Plan

Nursing Objectives

Prevent contamination and the possibility of infection.

Minimize the chance of postlumbar-puncture headache.

Allay the anxiety and enhance cooperation by providing a thorough explanation.

Secure the client to ensure immobility during lumbar puncture.

Transport the labeled specimen to the laboratory in an expeditious manner.

Client Preparation

1. Offer a thorough explanation including a description of the spine and spinal cord. Many clients are afraid that they will be paralyzed by needle insertion into the spinal cord. Emphasize that the cord descends to the level of the first or second lumbar vertebra, where it ends. The spinal needle is inserted well below the area of the spinal cord, usually at the level of the third and fourth vertebrae. There are many nerve endings in this area, and the needle may encounter one of these. The client should be reassured that no permanent damage will result, but the physician should be notified if a sharp pain is felt in the legs or groin area. Explain positioning so that the client will be prepared in advance. Check hospital procedure to determine if a consent form should be signed.

2. Minimize, but do not ignore, the possibility of postspinal headaches. Many people will have been exposed to other people who will have greatly exaggerated the likelihood, the duration, and the severity of these headaches. A positive attitude may do a great deal to prevent the "spinal headache." Headaches may occur, however, although the exact cause is uncertain. Some feel that the headache may be caused by leaking of the cerebrospinal fluid, which reduces the fluid's cushioning effect on the brain. When the brain then settles to the base of the skull as the client assumes the erect position, pain results from pressure on the nerves. The likelihood of headache can be reduced if the client remains flat in bed for 12 to 24 hours after the lumbar puncture.

3. Because the client will remain in bed for an extended period after the lumbar puncture, complete emptying of the bladder should precede invasive procedures of the spinal column.

Equipment

Spinal tap tray containing syringes and needles for local anesthetic, spinal needle, drapes, specimen tubes and stoppers, gauze sponges, forceps, and cups for antiseptics

Sterile gloves

Manometer with three-way stopcock

Local anesthetic

Topical anesthetic

Sterile adhesive strip bandage

Labels for specimens

Low pillow

Hospital gown (back-opening)

Implementation and Interventions

Procedural Aspects

ACTION	RATIONALE
1. Hyperextend the spine by asking the client to assume the side-lying position with knees drawn upward onto the abdomen and with the chin displaced onto the chest. Assist in maintaining this position by placing one arm on the back of the client's neck and the other behind the client's knees (Fig. 14-2). Other positions for lumbar puncture include having the client sit on the side of the bed leaning forward on an overbed table or against the nurse. This is often used for spinal anesthesia; however, the pressure readings in this position are inaccurate (Fig. 14-3).	Proper positioning allows maximum separation of the third and fourth lumbar vertebrae and optimizes the insertion of the needle. Sitting on the bedside causes pressure to be altered due to the gravitational pull on the fluid. This pull is, however, desirable when spinal anesthesia is administered because it causes the initial flow to be downward allowing more control of the area to be anesthetized.

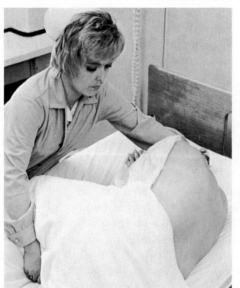

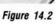

Figure 14.2

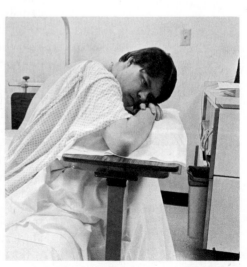

Figure 14.3

ACTION

2. Careful disinfection of the skin is essential. The site of the puncture also is draped to provide a sterile field. A local anesthetic may be administered and allowed to take effect before the actual lumbar puncture is performed.

3. Reassure the client during the procedure. Encourage normal breathing and relaxation. Assist the client to lie still.

4. After the physician inserts the spinal needle into the subarachnoid space, the manometer is attached. The fluid is allowed to flow freely into the manometer until it stops. The level at which the fluid stops indicates the spinal pressure. Specimens of the fluid are then placed in test tubes for subsequent laboratory analysis. The stopcock is turned, and the fluid is allowed to run or drip out into the tubes naturally. Because the rate of flow varies and may be slow, the client must be reassured if the procedure seems to be uncomfortably long. Three specimens are usually obtained. The sequence of the specimens must be noted, for example, #1, #2, and #3 and marked on the labels. Also, the requisitions must be marked to indicate which tests are to be done on which specimen. Send the specimens and requisitions to the laboratory immediately.

5. A Queckenstedt test may be done while the manometer is still in place if the initial pressure was normal. Apply digital (finger) pressure to both jugular veins.

6. After specimen collection is completed, the physician will remove the needle. Apply direct pressure to the puncture site for a short time (3–5 min). Apply a sterile ahesive strip and place the client flat in bed. Ask the client to remain flat for the specified time, usually 12 to 24 hours. Some physicians allow a small pillow. Turning from side to side may be allowed.

RATIONALE

The normal microorganisms present on the skin may become pathogenic when introduced into the spinal column. Penetration of the body's natural defense barrier, the skin, may predispose to such conditions as meningitis and encephalitis.

Movement, coughing, tenseness of muscles, and breathholding will alter the client's cerebrospinal fluid pressure.

A total of 10 ml of fluid usually is collected, with 2 ml to 3 ml in each tube. The measurement of the spinal fluid pressure is based on the displacement of the mercury by the spinal fluid. It is measured at its highest peak.

The normal response is an increase in the pressure of the cerebrospinal fluid. This test is contraindicated if IIP is present because permanent brain damage may result.

Prevent seepage of the cerebrospinal fluid from the puncture site by allowing the site to seal itself by applying a small pressure dressing in the form of an adhesive strip. Every effort should be made to prevent postspinal headache.

ACTION

RATIONALE

Special Modifications

1. A lumbar puncture usually is not performed on a client with head trauma or IIP. The CT (computerized tomography) scan usually is considered the diagnostic method of choice to determine intracranial bleeding.

2. Restraining a child for lumbar puncture is accomplished by holding the child across the front of the nurse securely with one arm restraining the legs at the knees and the other restraining the upper portion of the child's body (Fig. 14-4).

Computerized tomography (CT) scan is a type of examination in which several beams of x-ray are passed through the portion of the body to be examined at different angles. Variations in density are recorded graphically.

The child must be securely restrained to ensure that the needle is not dislodged.

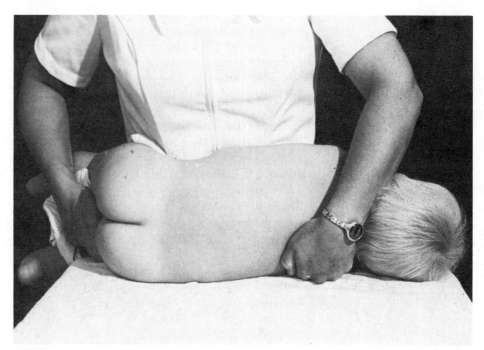

Figure 14.4

3. After spinal anesthetic is administered, place the client flat on the table and lower the head of the table. Progression of anesthesia is assessed by pin pricks on the client's legs and lower abdomen. When the desired height of anesthesia is reached, the table is leveled or the head slightly elevated, and surgical preparation begins.

The natural pull of gravity is used to disperse the anesthetic to the desired level in the spinal column.

Communicative Aspects

OBSERVATIONS

1. Note the color and appearance of the spinal fluid. Blood-tinged fluid may indicate a subarachnoid hemorrhage, and cloudiness may indicate infection.

2. The pressure of the cerebrospinal fluid should be noted, as well as the length of time necessary for the fluid specimens to be taken. Pressures over 200 mm H_2O are considered abnormal.

3. A Queckenstedt's test may be done before removal of the spinal needle. Note the pressure variations and the length of time necessary for the pressure to normalize.

4. Assess the client's response to the procedure. Note symptoms such as pallor; faintness; changes in vital and neurological signs; changes in level of consciousness; headache; swelling, bleeding, or seepage at puncture site; and numbness, tingling, or pain radiating down the legs. Vital signs and neurologic signs must be monitored frequently during the next 24 hours (q15min for 2 hr, then q2hr).

5. Observe the client for adequate hydration including output of urine. Immobility and inability to retain fluids because of nausea may inhibit urination.

CHARTING

DATE/TIME	OBSERVATIONS	SIGNATURE
4/9 1100	Lumbar puncture done by Dr. K. Needle insertion accomplished with difficulty. Pressure 100 mm H_2O. Fluid appears red-tinged—specimens labeled consecutively and sent to lab stat. Remains flat in bed without pillow. Site sealed with sterile adhesive strip, no signs of leakage. States severe headache. Dr. K notified. B/P 110/80, P 74, R 22, T 99.4°F (orally). Wife in attendance.	P. Dillon RN

Discharge Planning Aspects

CLIENT AND FAMILY EDUCATION

1. Inform the client of what to expect during the procedure. There will be slight discomfort when the local anesthetic is administered. When the spinal needle is inserted, there will be some pressure. Ask the client to inform the physician of any feelings of pain. Reinforce to the client that it is important to remain still throughout the procedure.

2. Discuss the subject of postspinal headaches in a matter-of-fact way, so that the client does not become alarmed if this phenomenon should occur. A positive attitude may greatly reduce the chances of a headache occurring, however.

3. If spinal anesthesia is administered, the client must understand that feeling in the lower portion of the body will be regained in several hours. Usually, no headache occurs.

Evaluation

Quality Assurance

Documentation should include the educational preparation of the client as well as assessment of allergies. The amount of spinal fluid removed and the pressure readings are important. The response of the client to the procedure must be noted. The written documentation should reflect the follow-up care rendered to prevent complications after lumbar puncture. It should also reflect that the nurse was aware of the possible complications and took measures to avoid them.

Infection Control

1. Rigid sterile technique must be observed during the lumbar puncture procedure to prevent introduction of exogenous organisms into the CNS. Proper skin preparation, maintenance of the sterile field, and traffic control are key measures to reduce infection risk to the client.

2. Care must be exercised in handling and transporting the cerebrospinal fluid specimens because the fluid may contain pathogenic organisms. Be sure that the specimens are marked clearly as to origin and note if any infectious process is suspected.

3. Any dressing placed over the puncture site should be sterile to help to prevent the threat of infection. Because the CNS is particularly at risk for infection, the lumbar puncture site must be observed frequently to ensure that no leakage is occurring.

4. Reusable equipment from the procedure should be bagged and marked contaminated if there is any suspicion of infection. Caution must be taken to protect personnel such as transport clerks and supply personnel (who clean used equipment) from the chance of accidental exposure to contamination. Special attention must be given to the handling of used needles. Disposable supplies should also be appropriately bagged and marked before discarding.

Technique Checklist

	YES	NO
Order for lumbar puncture on the chart	_____	_____
Operative permit signed (if hospital policy)	_____	_____
Client understood procedure	_____	_____
Client was able to comply with instructions during the procedure	_____	_____
Cerebrospinal fluid specimen obtained	_____	_____
Cerebrospinal fluid pressure _____		
Queckenstedt's test performed	_____	_____
Positive _____		
Negative _____		
Lumbar puncture completed at _____		
Labeled specimens to lab at _____		
Client flat in bed for _____ hr	_____	_____
Postspinal headache	_____	_____
Leakage of fluid from puncture site	_____	_____
Any complications _____		
_____		
Client and family understand the results	_____	_____

15   Mammography

Overview

Definition

X-ray visualization of the breasts

Rationale

Determine the presence of tumors of the breasts.
Determine whether breast tumors are malignant.

Terminology

Fibrocystic breast disease: The formation of fibrous tumors that have undergone cystic degeneration or that have accumulated fluid in the interspaces

Galactorrhea: The continuation of lactation after the cessation of nursing

Mastitis: Inflammation of the breast

Assessment

Pertinent Anatomy and Physiology

See Appendix I: *breast, skin.*

Pathophysiological Concepts

1. Breast tissue is never static; it is constantly responding to changes in hormonal, nutritional, psychological, and environmental stimuli, all of which cause continual cellular changes. Benign conditions of the breast are nonprogressive and include mastitis, galactorrhea, and fibrocystic disease.

2. Cancer of the breast is one of the leading causes of death among women in the United States. It may present as a mass, a puckered area, nipple retraction, or an unusual discharge. Menopause and aging cause significant structural changes in the breast, such as atrophy and loss of muscle tone. Women most at risk for breast cancer are menopausal, those who have had their first baby after age 34, those with a family history of breast cancer, those who have been exposed to radiation or carcinogenic agents, and those who work at a high-stress job and eat a diet high in fat and red meat.

Assessment of the Client

1. Assess the anxiety level of the client. Determine the reason for the client's seeking medical attention.

2. Assess the client's family history in relation to breast cancer and other high-risk factors, including the age of the client at the birth of her first baby and exposure to carcinogens and radiation. Determine the client's stress level and usual dietary habits.

Plan

Nursing Objectives

Reduce the client's anxiety about possible breast malignancy.
Establish a sound diagnostic base on which to base further action, if needed.

Client Preparation

1. A client facing mammography has usually had some basis for suspicion of breast malignancy, such as an unexplained lump or family history of breast cancer. This suspicion may produce a great deal of anxiety as the client faces the procedure. Offer reasonable reassurance about the procedure

2. Offer an explanation of how the procedure is done and the fact that no pain is involved. A small amount of discomfort may be experienced if the breasts must be compressed against the radiology film holder for clearer films.

Equipment

In the x-ray department

Implementation and Interventions

Procedural Aspects

ACTION	*RATIONALE*
The client will be asked to remove all clothing above the waist. X-ray films are taken in the standing, sitting, and lying positions. The breasts are placed one at a time on the film holder and compressed to ensure even density throughout.	An x-ray is a form of radiant energy that penetrates according to the density of tissue. Clothing bulk or metal fasteners will distort the x-ray film.

Communicative Aspects

OBSERVATIONS

1. All female clients should be examined for lumps or irregularities in their breasts during the admission physical assessment.
2. The client should be observed for undue anxiety about the examination.

CHARTING

DATE/TIME	OBSERVATIONS	SIGNATURE
3/7 1030	To X-ray for mammography. Examination explained in detail. Seemed less nervous after explanation.	F. White RN

Discharge Planning Aspects

CLIENT AND FAMILY EDUCATION

1. The client and her female family members should be taught how to do breast self-examination. They should be encouraged to do this every month, preferably 5 to 7 days after the menstrual period ends, when the breasts are soft and pliable. In postmenopausal women, examinations should be done on a set date each month.
2. Men develop breast cancer at a much lower rate than women. Nevertheless, men at risk should be taught to do breast self-examination and should do so in a regular and consistent manner. Men at risk are older, widowed or divorced, and may have a history of estrogen use or endocrine imbalance. Men with a family history of breast cancer, a history of orchitis, cirrhosis, orchiectomy, transsexuality, or Klinefelter's syndrome are also at risk.
3. The need for an annual Pap smear for clients considered at risk should also be discussed as a form of cancer detection and prevention.

REFERRALS

The American Cancer Society has booklets explaining self-examination of the breast (SEB), which are free and readily available. If a malignancy is found, the American Cancer society also may assist by furnishing supplies, such as dressings. There are also local groups, such as "Reach for Recovery," who will assist by counseling and visiting the client should a malignant tumor be found. These agencies usually seek the permission of the attending physician before visiting.

Evaluation

Quality Assurance

Documentation should include an assessment of the history of the current problem, family tendency toward malignancy, and the status of the client's emotional adjustment. Note preparation of the client for the examination. The results of the mammogram should be reflected, as well as the client's understanding and acceptance of the results.

Infection Control

All equipment used on consecutive clients should be cleaned between each use. In addition, the nurse and other health care workers should wash their hands thoroughly between clients.

Technique Checklist

	YES	NO
Client and family understood what was involved in the examination before going for x-ray	_____	_____
X-ray successfully completed	_____	_____
Results explained to and understood by client and family	_____	_____
Self-examination of breasts taught to client and family	_____	_____

Follow-up treatment needed

Surgery _____

Chemotherapy _____

Radiation _____

Other _____

16 Myelogram

Overview

Definition

X-ray visualization of the subarachnoid space around the spinal column by injection of dye (Fig. 16-1 shows a normal myelogram.)

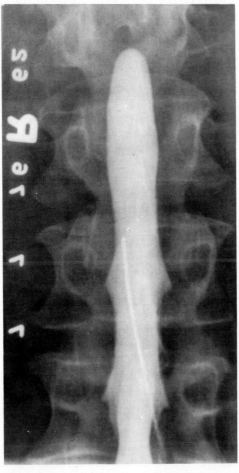

Figure 16.1
(Courtesy of H. Revollo, M.D. Photograph by D. Atkinson)

Rationale

Determine the reason for unexplained numbness of legs and arms.

Rule out pathology of the spinal column (e.g., cysts, herniated discs, or tumors).

Determine the cause of headaches.

Terminology

Cervical spine: The first seven vertebrae

Cisternal puncture: Insertion of a needle into the cisterna magna just below the occipital bone in the back of the neck

Lumbar puncture: Insertion of a needle into the subarachnoid space in the area of the third and fourth lumbar vertebrae

Lumbar spine: The five vertebrae below the thoracic vertebrae

Thoracic spine: The twelve vertebrae below the cervical spine

Assessment

Pertinent Anatomy and Physiology

1. See Appendix I: *vertebral column.*
2. The cerebrospinal fluid is a clear, colorless fluid that fills the ventricles of the brain and the subarachnoid spaces around the brain and spinal cord.
3. The spinal cord begins at the level of the foramen magnum in the brain and extends downward through the vertebral canal to the level of the disk between the first and second lumbar vertebrae. The spinal cord is an elongated, cylindrical mass of nervous tissue consisting of 31 segments, each of which gives rise to a pair of spinal nerves. The cord is covered and protected by three membranes called meninges. The dura mater is the outermost. The space between the walls of the vertebral canal and the dura mater is the epidural space. The next layer of the meninges is the arachnoid membrane, and the innermost layer is the pia mater. The subarachnoid space is a relatively roomy area between the arachnoid and the pia mater. It is filled with the cerebrospinal fluid.
4. Major weight-bearing is accomplished through the column of vertebral bodies, and flexibility of the vertebral column is provided by cartilaginous disks that lie between each two vertebrae. A firm, gelatinous structure called the nucleus pulposus gives substance to the disk, which is held in place by a strong, ventral ligament and a weaker dorsal ligament.

Pathophysiological Concepts

1. If the dorsal ligament, which supports the vertebral column, becomes weakened, the nucleus pulposus can be squeezed out of place resulting in the condition called a slipped disk.
2. Headache is a universal phenomenon, the cause of which is not really known. Some headaches may be the result of tension or muscle contraction. Migraine headaches may be due to changes in blood flow and oxygen availability. Headache is a symptom of some types of central nervous system (CNS) disorders.

Assessment of the Client

1. Assess allergy history, with special attention to sensitivity to shellfish, iodine, and other contrast media.
2. Assess baseline vital and neurologic signs. Determine baseline motor and sensory functions as well.
3. Assess the knowledge level of the client. The myelogram is very uncomfortable. Determine the client's anxiety level and past experience with x-ray procedures to decide which teaching strategy will be most effective.

Plan

Nursing Objectives

Allay the anxiety and enhance the cooperation of the client by a thorough explanation.

Minimize unpleasant side-effects.

Client Preparation

1. Offer a thorough explanation. Lumbar or cisternal puncture is performed (Technique No. 14, Lumbar Puncture). A small amount of cerebrospinal fluid is removed, and a radiopaque dye is injected. The client is then strapped to a movable table, which is tilted to various angles to provide complete visuali-

zation. X-ray films are taken at intervals. After the films are taken, the table is tilted so that the contrast medium collects at the puncture site, where it is withdrawn. Removal of the contrast medium on completion of the x-ray examination may cause some pain in the legs and other areas. Alerting the client before this sensation is experienced may reduce the chances of alarm and fright if and when the pain occurs. The entire procedure may take several hours.

2. If ordered, consider giving the client a relaxant or tranquilizer as well as an antiemetic before the myelogram. Withhold food and fluids for 4 to 6 hours before the test unless the physician orders otherwise.

3. Because the client will remain in bed for a time after myelogram, complete emptying of the bladder should precede the diagnostic test.

Equipment

Hospital gown
Stretcher for transport
Emesis basin
Low pillow

Implementation and Interventions

Procedural Aspects

ACTION

1. Lumbar puncture and myelogram are done in the radiology area. Transport the client by stretcher (Fig. 16-2).

RATIONALE

Even though the client may feel like going to radiology in a wheelchair, transport after myelogram will require the client to remain in the supine position and will require transportation by stretcher

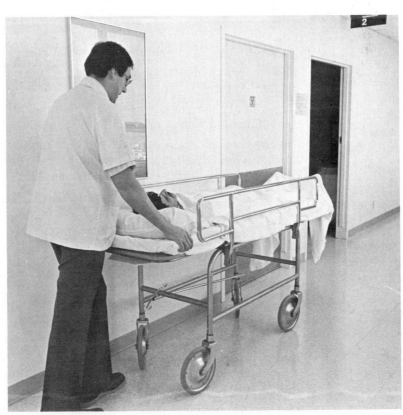

Figure 16.2

ACTION	*RATIONALE*
2. After returning from the radiology department, the client is treated as a postlumbar puncture client. Lying flat in bed for the specified period may help to reduce the chance of headache. Offer the client a small pillow for comfort, if allowed. Check the client at frequent intervals and provide an emesis basin if needed. Force fluids as soon as nausea subsides	Lying flat reduces the risk of headache and nausea. Nausea is a common side-effect of myelogram. Fluids will help to counteract the effects of fasting and nausea as soon as the client is able to take them.

Special Modifications

1. The needle may have to be manipulated somewhat in an effort to remove all of the dye. Manipulation of the needle in the spinal column may cause irritation of the surrounding nerves, resulting in some pain, numbness, and tingling in nearby anatomical structures.	Failure to remove all of the contrast medium may cause inflammation of the subarachnoid space.
2. Use of the computerized tomography (CT) scanner may yield a satisfactory film of the spine so that myelogram is not necessary. The client has to be prepared for myelogram in case the CT scan films are inconclusive, however.	Computerized tomography (CT) scan is a type of x-ray in which several beams of x-ray are passed through portion of the body to be examined at different angles. Variations in density are recorded graphically.

Communicative Aspects

OBSERVATIONS

1. Observe the client closely for any signs of allergy to the contrast medium.
2. Observe for side-effects such as headache, nausea, back pain, and stiff neck. Be alert for fever.
3. Observe the client for adequate hydration including output of urine. The immobility and nausea may inhibit urination.
4. Check neurologic signs and vital signs on return from the radiology department and periodically for the next 24 hours (q15min for 1–2 hr, then q2hr). Observe for any postlumbar puncture complications.

CHARTING

DATE/TIME	OBSERVATIONS	SIGNATURE
3/5 1020	Returned from Radiology after myelogram. Lying flat in bed with small pillow. Expresses some feelings of nausea and slight headache. Antiemetic given. B/P 112/68, P 64, R 16, T 97.2°F. Pupils equal and reactive, grip in both hands equal and strong. Resting at this time. ——————————	F. White RN

Discharge Planning Aspects

CLIENT AND FAMILY EDUCATION

1. Inform the family and client that the procedure will take from 45 minutes to 2 hours. Be sure that they know why the procedure is necessary and what the results are expected to show.
2. Prepare the client and family for the postmyelogram period so they will not think that the client's weakened condition is an indication that the general

condition is worsened, but will realize that this is the normal recuperation process.

3. If back pain is the symptom that prompted the client to seek medical attention, demonstrate proper body mechanics and lifting techniques before the client is discharged.

Evaluation

Quality Assurance

Documentation should include a physical and neurologic assessment before and after the myelogram. Document the client's reaction to the test and any side-effects that arose. Documentation should reflect that the nurse knew what complications could arise and the precautions taken to prevent them or the actions taken to alleviate them. Baseline and periodic assessment of vital signs should be in evidence.

Infection Control

The dressing placed over the puncture site should be sterile to help to prevent the threat of infection. Because the CNS is particularly at risk for infection, the lumbar puncture site must be observed frequently to ensure that no leakage is occurring that might predispose to infection.

Technique Checklist

	YES	NO
Order for myelogram on the chart	_____	_____
Client and family understood procedure	_____	_____
To Radiology at _____		
Myelogram completed at _____		
Client flat in bed for _____ hours	_____	_____
Nausea	_____	_____
Postspinal headache	_____	_____
Leakage of fluid from puncture site	_____	_____
Any complications _____		
_____		
Client and family understand the results	_____	_____

17 Ophthalmoscopic Examination

Overview

Definition

Examination of the interior of the eye using a lighted instrument

Rationale

Examine the inner structures of the eye to determine abnormalities.

Locate the presence of pathology in the eye.

Terminology

Nystagmus: Constant involuntary movement of the eyeball

Strabismus: An eye disorder that occurs when the optic axes cannot be directed to the same object; squint

Assessment

Pertinent Anatomy and Physiology

See Appendix I: *eye (external), eye (internal).*

Pathophysiological Concepts

1. A *cataract* is an opacity of the lens or its capsule. Light rays cannot pass through the lens to reach the retina. The lens must be removed and corrective lenses used to see clearly. The cataract is often visible on gross examination of the eye and also on ophthalmoscopic examination.

2. Pathologic conditions such as hypertension and diabetes mellitus are accompanied by typical changes in the retinal vessels. A rise in the intracranial pressure, as occurs in the case of a brain tumor, may obstruct the flow of blood away from the eyeball through the central vein, causing a reddening and swelling of the optic disks (papilledema). If the intraocular pressure rises, such as happens in glaucoma, the disk becomes cup-shaped as it is pushed backward (cupped disk). Loss of vitreous, the jellylike substance that fills the space posterior to the lens and supports the retina, is a serious complication of eye surgery that may result in detached retina.

Assessment of the Client

1. Ophthalmoscopic examination of the eye is a basic part of the general physical assessment of any client. Determine if the client has ever had this type of examination previously.

2. Assess general physical condition and health history. Note especially the presence of diabetes, complaints of cloudy vision (especially in the older client), sensitivity to light, headaches, and reports of trauma to or pain in the eye.

Plan

Nursing Objectives

Examine thoroughly the inner portion of the eye.

Minimize the possibility of trauma to the eye and surrounding structure.

Establish a basis for sound scientific investigation of physiological abnormalities.

Client Preparation

1. Explain what will happen during ophthalmoscopic examination, stressing the proximity of the nurse to the client. Because the ophthalmoscope is held so

closely to the client's eye, sudden movement could traumatize the delicate eye tissue. Elicit the client's cooperation in remaining still before beginning eye examination.

2. If the eye is excessively teary, a thin crust may form around the eyelids. This debris may interfere with optimal visualization and may cause some discomfort for the client. Gently wash the eye with a soft, moist cloth to remove excess debris.

Equipment

Ophthalmoscope

Extra batteries

Soft cloth for cleansing

Implementation and Interventions

Procedural Aspects

ACTION

1. Ophthalmoscopic examination is one method of accurately assessing the client's health status. Observing signs and symptoms of pathology are important functions of the nurse. Be accurate in reporting and recording findings.

2. Dim the room lights and turn the scope on. Direct the client's vision to a distant object in front and slightly to the peripheral side of the eye being examined.

3. To examine the client's right eye, hold the scope in front of your right eye with whichever hand feels most comfortable. Place the scope at "eyelash distance," or at the point of brushing the client's eyelashes. Place the free hand on the client's forehead to help ascertain proximity to the client. Repeat the same procedure for the left eye using the left eye for visualization (Fig. 17-1).

RATIONALE

Observation is fundamental to all scientific investigation. Comparison with baseline data is only as good as the accuracy of the original data.

A dim environment allows maximum visualization of the internal eye with the artificial light source. Fixing the vision on one object will minimize the amount of involuntary movement of the eye during the examination.

Because of the proximity, the examiner should strive to avoid actual contact with the client, which might elicit an involuntary movement.

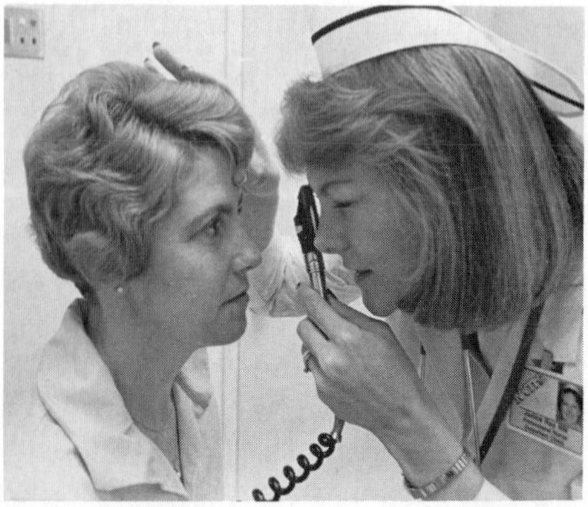

Figure 17.1

ACTION

RATIONALE

4. Direct the ophthalmoscope beam onto the client's eye. A red glow will indicate the point of focus for the examination of the inner aspect. The fundus should be visible. Look for the macula, the optic disk, the condition of the vessels, and the general color and condition of the inner eye (Fig. 17-2).

Visualization of all of the landmarks of the eye is very difficult without continuous practice. Strive to view the vessels and note abnormalities such as bulging pockets, feathering at endings, and red hemorrhagic areas.

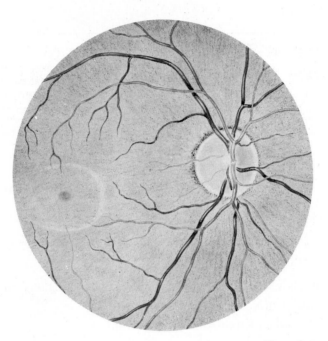

Figure 17.2

5. Examine the eye thoroughly; however, do not extend the length of the examination unnecessarily.

The closeness of the examiner and the ophthalmoscope may cause anxiety in the client. Terminate the examination as quickly as possible. Offer reassurance to the client that the procedure is safe and will last only a few minutes.

Special Modifications

If the examiner wears glasses, it is best to remove them during the examination.

The ophthalmoscope has a dial that may be turned for optimal focus.

Communicative Aspects

OBSERVATIONS

1. Observe for undesirable conditions of the outer eye and surrounding parts:

   Eyelids: Closure, drooping, swelling, or cysts

   Conjunctiva: Inflammation, blood

   Lacrimal ducts: No tears or excessive tears

   Cornea: Cloudiness, excessive sensitivity

   Sclera: Thinning, bulging, cysts, inflammation

Anterior chamber: Abnormal contents such as blood or pus

Iris: Difference in color, notching, congestion, or infiltration

Pupil: Inequality, dilation, or constriction

Extraocular muscles: Strabismus, crossed eyes, or nystagmus

2. Observe the condition of the interior eye:

Retina

Optic nerve

Optic disk

Blood vessels

Macula

CHARTING

DATE/TIME	OBSERVATIONS	SIGNATURE
6/9 0945	Continues excessive tearing of both eyes. Ophthalmoscopic exam of the right and left eyes. No visual abnormalities of the outer eyes except continuous tearing. Retinal vessels appear to be normal. Optic disk sighted, appears normal. Dr. J. notified of tearing. ———————————————	K. Wells RN, FNP

Discharge Planning Aspects

CLIENT AND FAMILY EDUCATION

1. Provide the client information about proper eye care and the importance of yearly checkups if any problems are found.

2. Diabetic and hypertensive clients are particularly vulnerable to pathology of the eyes. Clients diagnosed as diabetic should be encouraged to have frequent ophthalmoscopic examinations.

REFERRALS

Clients with chronic eye damage may get assistance from the following agencies:

Office of Vocation Rehabilitation

American Foundation for the Blind

Braille Institute of America

National Society for the Prevention of Blindness

Evaluation

Quality Assurance

Documentation should reflect the condition of the eye as seen through the ophthalmoscope. The nurse should document that the physical condition was assessed and show evidence of an understanding of the possible visual complications arising from the physical condition of the client.

Infection Control

Eye infections are fairly common and many are readily transmissible. Care must be taken not to touch the client with the ophthalmoscope. After examination, the ophthalmoscope should be wiped clean with a disinfectant. Health care personnel should engage in thorough handwashing between clients.

Technique Checklist

	YES	NO
Procedure explained to client	———	———
Client cooperated during examination	———	———
Interior of eye seen clearly	———	———
Pathology found ————————————	———	———

18   Otoscopic Examination

Overview

Definition

Visual examination of the ear using a lighted instrument

Rationale

Determine the condition and the presence of pathology in the external auditory canal.

Instill medications in the ear.

Clean the ear and remove wax accumulation or foreign bodies.

Terminology

Mastoid process: The portion of the temporal bone lying behind the pinna

Pinna: The external ear (auricle)

Tympanic membrane: Membrane separating the external auditory canal from the middle ear

Assessment

Pertinent Anatomy and Physiology

See Appendix I: *ear (external), ear (internal).*

Pathophysiological Concepts

1. The ceruminous glands lining the auditory canal secrete a waxy substance called cerumen. Excessive amounts of this wax may block the ear canal and exert pressure on the tympanic membrane. This pressure causes earache and may result in temporary deafness.

2. The mucous membrane that lines the middle ear is continuous with that of the pharynx. Thus it is possible for infection to travel along the mucous membrane from the nose or the throat to the middle ear (otitis media). When pus forms in the middle ear, the tympanic membrane may have to be lanced. Having the patient chew gum may help to remove the pus by way of the eustachian tube.

Assessment of the Client

1. Otoscopic examination of the ear is a basic part of the general physical assessment of any client. Determine if the client has ever had an otoscopic examination. Determine the health habits of the client in relation to ear care. Decide if knowledge deficits are present and the best strategy to improve them.

2. Assess the condition of the external ear. There should be no redness, abrasions, foreign bodies, or discharge. Assess the consistency and amount of earwax.

3. Assess the condition of the middle ear.

4. Assess the hearing competency of the client. Stand behind the client and speak softly. Assess whether the client may be suffering from a hearing deficit. Hearing screening may be advisable if the client seems to have suffered hearing loss.

5. Assess any history of problems with hearing such as ear infections, "broken" ear drums, tubes in the ears, surgery on the ears or inner mechanisms, use of hearing aids, or irrigation to remove ear wax.

Plan

Nursing Objectives

Protect the integrity of the lining of the external auditory canal.

Allay the anxieties of the client.

Obtain the client's cooperation in remaining still during otoscopic examination.

Client Preparation

1. Offer a thorough explanation of what will occur during the examination. Emphasize the necessity of the client's remaining still while the otoscope is in the ear.

2. Ear treatments often cause anxiety because the sound produced is exaggerated because of the closeness to the inner ear. Decrease the client's anxiety with gentleness and efficiency. Have all of the equipment gathered before beginning and ensure that the light on the otoscope is working.

3. If medication is to be instilled or wax removed by irrigation, place the client lying on the unaffected side.

Equipment

Otoscope with assorted sizes of specula

Extra batteries

Irrigation syringe or bulb syringe and irrigation solution

Basin

Otic medication

Cotton ball

Soft cloth

Implementation and Interventions

Procedural Aspects

ACTION

1. Cleanse the external ear with a soft cloth to remove any drainage (Fig. 18-1).

RATIONALE

A cotton-tipped applicator should not be used because this type device may cause damage and infection if used generally at home and particularly

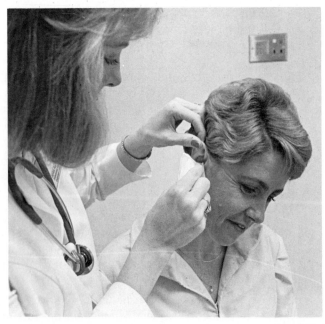

Figure 18.1

ACTION

RATIONALE

with small children. The nurse should use this opportunity to set a good example and warn the client never to place anything sharp or small into the ear.

2. Place a rounded speculum on the end of the otoscope. Use the largest speculum that will comfortably fit into the external auditory canal. Check to see that the light is working.

The larger the speculum, the better the visualization. The speculum should not cause pain or discomfort when being inserted, however.

3. Insert the speculum just inside the external opening. In adults, the pinna should be pulled greatly upward and backward. To visualize the entire canal, tilt the otoscope and change body position accordingly. The client should remain immobile (Fig. 18-2).

Pulling the ear and inserting the speculum along normal curves of the canal will minimize discomfort and the chance of trauma. If the client remains motionless, unintentional trauma is less likely.

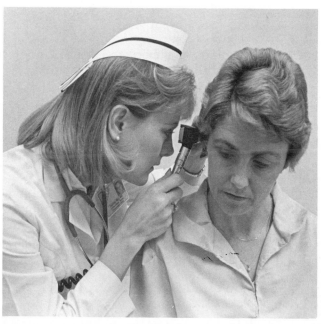

Figure 18.2

Special Considerations

1. Minor treatments may be administered through the speculum. Instillation of medication may be accomplished with or without the otoscope. To instill otic drops, straighten the client's ear canal by gently pulling upward and backward. Instill the correct number of drops, which have been warmed. Warming may take place by hold-

Gently pulling the ear up and back allows the drops to flow straight down the canal. If the medication is too hot, it may injure delicate mucous membranes. The lining of the auditory canal is very delicate. Nothing should ever be pushed forcefully into the canal. The pinna should never be pulled forcefully in any direction as this action is sufficient to injure the

ACTION	*RATIONALE*
ing the bottle in the hand for a few minutes or by placing it in warm water. Be sure that the medication is not hot. Have the client remain in the side-lying position for about 5 minutes. Insert a small cotton ball gently into the meatus of the auditory canal for 15 minutes. Do not force the cottonball into the canal.	lining of the ear canal.
2. Irrigation of the external auditory canal may be done to remove wax accumulation or a foreign object. Flush the ear with warm fluid such as sterile saline or whatever is ordered by the physician. Allow the fluid to return by turning the client over and placing the affected ear downward over a basin or towel.	Allowing the natural pull of gravity to return the fluid from the ear decreases the chance of traumatizing delicate membranes by suction.

Communicative Aspects

OBSERVATIONS

1. Observe the pinna for abnormalities, fistulas, infection, boils, ulcers, or rash. Check the condition of the mastoid by pulling the pinna forward. Swelling or extreme tenderness may signify mastoiditis.

2. Inspect the external auditory canal for occlusion, redness, swelling, drainage, foreign body, or tumors.

3. The tympanic membrane has a dull, bluish or pearly gray, translucent appearance. It is stretched across and continuous with the auditory canal. Observe for any abnormalities.

4. If the ear is being flushed to remove wax or a foreign body, observe the return closely to determine whether the procedure was successful. Describe the return and the client's tolerance of the procedure.

5. Observe the compliance of the client with the procedure. Note any tenderness or signs of extreme anxiety.

CHARTING

DATE/TIME	OBSERVATIONS	SIGNATURE
7/2 0845	States right ear hurts and "feels like there is something in it." Otoscopic examination done. No evidence of foreign objects, however, the external canal is reddened. Slight clear discharge from right ear. Dr. J. notified.———	L. Collins RN

Discharge Planning Aspects

CLIENT AND FAMILY EDUCATION

1. Emphasize the importance of keeping sharp objects out of the ears. This is especially important for the parents of small children who might be tempted to clean their child's ears with a cotton-tipped swab. Cleaning the pinna with a soft cloth is usually adequate to maintain proper hygiene. Caution the client and family against rubbing vigorously or pulling the pinna roughly because these actions can cause ear damage.

2. Foreign objects in the ear should be removed only by qualified health care personnel.

3. Ear wax serves the purpose of protecting the inner ear from infectious organisms. Its sticky substance traps foreign particles that enter the ear. The wax is constantly moving toward the outside thus removing potentially hazardous particles. Cerumen, or ear wax, serves a vital purpose and should never be removed by cotton swabs. Some persons have dry earwax, which does not move and easily becomes impacted. This dry earwax must be softened regularly with an oil and may require irrigation.

4. Direct the client and family to chew gum and drink large amounts of fluid if they feel fluid building up in the middle ear.

REFERRALS

Persons with severe hearing impairment may be referred to the American Society for the Hard of Hearing.

Evaluation

Quality Assurance

Documentation should reflect that the nurse knew and adhered to the proper method of viewing the internal ear through an otoscope. Note measures taken to ensure that no cross-contamination occurred. The appearance of the internal ear should be reflected as well as the tolerance of the client to the procedure. If medication was instilled, documentation should show that the nurse knew and understood the desired action of the medication as well as the side-effects. Irrigation procedures should be documented, including reason and results as well as the tolerance of the client. Note teaching about proper ear care.

Infection Control

1. Nose and throat infections may travel to the ear, causing infection there. These infections warrant close attention because they may spread to the mastoid air cells that lie in proximity to the venous sinuses and the meninges of the brain.

2. Careful handwashing must be carried out before and after the otoscopic examination.

3. Specula must be scrupulously cleaned and disinfected after use. Because of the unusual shape of this equipment, care must be taken to remove all wax.

Technique Checklist

	YES	NO
Procedure explained to client	_____	_____
Examination completed without complications	_____	_____
Pathology found	_____	_____
Otic medication administered	_____	_____
Name _____		
Amount _____		
Which ear _____		
Irrigation completed	_____	_____
Reason _____		
Results _____		
Order on chart	_____	_____
Client tolerated procedure well	_____	_____
Proper ear care taught to client and family	_____	_____

19   Proctoscopic Examination

Overview

Definition

Direct visualization of the distal end of the large intestine by use of a lighted, tubular instrument (Fig. 19-1)

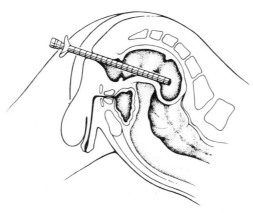

Figure 19.1

Rationale

Reveal the presence of polyps, tumors, and other lesions of the lower bowel.

Determine the site of pathology.

Provide a means to cauterize to stop rectal bleeding.

Provide a method of obtaining a rectal biopsy.

Remove rectal polyps.

Terminology

Anoscopy: Visualization of the anus

Endoscopy: Inspection of cavities using an illuminated rigid or flexible tube

Eructation: Raising of gas from the stomach (belching)

Flatulence: Excessive gas in the stomach and intestines

Hemorrhoid: A dilated blood vessel in the anal region

Impaction: Retention of hard, dried stool in the rectum and colon

Polyp: A growth with a pedicle commonly found in a vascular area such as the rectum

Sigmoidoscopy: Visualization of the sigmoid colon

Assessment

Pertinent Anatomy and Physiology

See Appendix I: *anus, intestine (large), rectum, sigmoid colon.*

Pathophysiological Concepts

1. A common symptom of abnormalities of the bowel is diarrhea. Large-volume diarrhea results from an increase in the water content of the stool, and small-volume diarrhea from an increase in the peristaltic action of the bowel.

Small-volume diarrhea is usually characterized by cramping and frequent, explosive stools. This form of diarrhea often is associated with intrinsic disease of the colon, such as ulcerative colitis.

2. Another common symptom of pathology of the bowel is impaction. Fecal impaction stimulates secretion in the portion of the bowel proximal to the blockage. This results in watery, diarrhealike stools as the body attempts to evacuate the mass.

3. Other symptoms of bowel problems are abdominal discomfort, hypoactive or hyperactive bowel sounds, and blood in the stool.

4. Cancer may occur in any part of the colon, but it is found most frequently in the rectum. Usually, cancers of the colon and rectum are present for a long time before producing any symptoms. Bleeding is a highly significant symptom of colorectal cancer. Other symptoms are changes in bowel habits and a sense of urgency or incomplete emptying of the bowel. Pain is the last symptom.

5. There are a variety of conditions that are detectable by proctoscopy. Rectal veins may become dilated and tortuous; this condition is called hemorrhoids. Most diverticula (sacs or pouches in the wall of a canal or organ) occur in the sigmoid colon.

Assessment of the Client

1. Assess the general condition of the client to ascertain the ability to tolerate the preparation regime for proctoscopy. If the client is already in a weakened condition, it may be necessary to space the cleansing enemas farther apart to allow adequate time to rest between.

2. Ascertain the client's perception of why the diagnostic study is being done. Determine if a malignancy is suspected. The reason motivating the client to have the test will affect cooperation greatly during the procedure and reaction to the results.

3. Assess the physical condition of the client in relation to agility if the procedure will be done in the knee–chest position in bed. If a proctoscopic table is used, the client will be tilted forward with the head lower than the rest of the body. Assess respiratory adequacy because ventilation may be compromised in this unaccustomed position.

Plan

Nursing Objectives

Provide adequate information about the examination to allay fear and anxiety.

Prepare the bowel adequately to ensure maximum visualization results.

Ensure that all equipment is in proper working order before beginning the procedure.

Client Preparation

1. Thoroughly explain the bowel prepartion procedure as well as the examination procedure itself. If the client is to assume the knee–chest position in bed for the examination, show the client how to gain maximum comfort while in this position by resting the weight on the legs and chest, not the hands and elbows. The client may be asked to assume the knee-chest position while in the side-lying position if particularly weak and debilitated. Most hospitals have a special proctoscopic table that breaks in the middle and tilts to allow the client to be adequately supported and maximally positioned (Fig. 19-2).

2. Thoroughly cleanse the bowel so that adequate visualization may be accomplished. A light supper and a strong laxative (e.g., castor oil) usually are given to the client the evening before the x-ray. To reduce the possibility of nausea or fecal accumulation, the client may be NPO for several hours before the examination. On the morning of the examination, the client may receive enemas until the return is clear, signifying that no fecal matter remains in

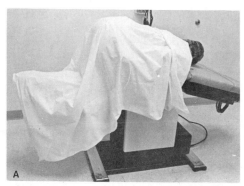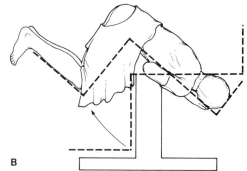

Figure 19.2A and B.

the bowel to interfere with the procedure (see Technique No. 51, Enema and Rectal Tube).

Equipment

Enema setup

Appropriate endoscope

Suction tips and machine

Rectal biopsy forceps and specimen container

Sheet for drape

Lubricating jelly

Rectal swabs

Implementation and Interventions

Procedural Aspects

ACTION	RATIONALE

1. Place the client in one of the following positions:
  a. in bed on the left side with the right leg flexed;
  b. on the chest and knees with the buttocks in the air;
  c. in the knee-chest position side-lying in bed;
  d. on a proctoscopic table.
	Positioning for optimal visualization will help to reduce the amount of time the client has to remain in the strained position.

2. Continually reassure the client throughout the examination. Drape the client with a special sheet with a hole in the center for tube insertion or with a folded sheet.	Avoid embarrassing the client and protect privacy throughout the procedure.
3. Provide lubricating jelly to coat the endoscope. Talk to the client during the procedure. Offer frequent reminders to take slow, deep breaths. Offer praise and reassurance.	Lubrication will reduce friction, which is the force opposing motion between two contacting surfaces. Slow, deep breaths will enhance relaxation of the anal sphincter and will facilitate scope insertion.
4. The examiner may use rectal swabs or suction tip if debris is present in the rectum. Inflation of the lower colon by means of a bulb attached to the scope may cause a cramping sensation. Remind the client to take slow, deep breaths.	The rectum is composed of muscular folds. Forcing air inside will provide visualization between these folds. It may also stimulate peristalsis which will cause a full, cramping sensation. Relaxation will decrease discomfort.

Procedural Aspects

ACTION	*RATIONALE*
5. For biopsy, the forceps are inserted through the scope and a small piece of tissue is removed. This may be painful. Place the biopsy in a prepared container that has an appropriate preservative and is clearly labeled with the client's name and the location from which the biopsy came.	The biopsy must be adequately preserved and transported to the laboratory as quickly as possible.
6. After the scope is removed, clean the lubricating jelly from the client's buttocks. If the client has been in a position of having the head lower than the body, slowly raise the client's head to an even plane with the body and allow a few minutes to stabilize before raising to the upright position. When feelings of dizziness and fainting have passed, place the client in a wheelchair for return to the hospital room.	Nerve impulses in the inner ear are sensitive to the pull of gravity. This abnormal position in which the client has been placed may have upset the sense of balance and may cause some dizziness and nausea. Allow time for the sense of balance to be restored by not hurrying the client.
7. Ensure that all equipment is either cleaned thoroughly or disposed of properly.	Fecal material contains bacteria that may be harmful if transmitted.

Special Modifications

1. Administer enemas with care to clients with conditions such as uclerative colitis. Assess any bleeding carefully and report if the amount appears excessive.	In certain inflammatory diseases of the colon, any irritation of the colon may initiate bleeding.
2. If resistance to insertion of the enema tube is encountered, never forcefully push it into the rectum.	Some bowel disturbances may be related to tumor growth in the lower rectal area. These growths can impede the passing of the enema tubing.

Communicative Aspects

OBSERVATIONS

1. Observe the client carefully during the bowel cleansing procedure for signs of fatigue or hemorrhage.

2. Check any rectal bleeding carefully and report it to the physician. Laxatives and enemas can irritate hemorrhoids and cause minor rectal bleeding.

3. Observe the client's tolerance of the procedure. Note sweating, shortness of breath, dizziness, pain, and any other problems.

4. Observe the client after the procedure for recovery from the unnatural positioning on the proctoscopic table. Note the presence and appearance of stools to detect any rectal bleeding. Observe the rectal area for bleeding or trauma.

CHARTING

DATE/TIME	OBSERVATIONS	SIGNATURE
12/2 1015	Proctoscopy done in treatment area. Tolerated procedure well. Slight abdominal cramping. Biopsy taken and sent to lab. Assured nurses that he will save stool for inspection. Before proctoscopic exam B/P 114/60, P 68, R 16. After proctoscopic exam B/P 132/72, P 78, R 20. No dizziness. ———————	C. Allen RN

Discharge Planning Aspects

CLIENT AND FAMILY EDUCATION

1. Inform the client that a sense of fullness, as well as increased flatulence and eructation, may occur because of the instillation of air into the colon for better visualization.

2. Some colon conditions may be improved by a change in the diet that eliminates foods high in fiber and roughage. Call attention to the types of low-fiber foods served in the hospital to acclimate the client and family to dietary modifications that may be made after discharge. On the other hand, some colon discomfort actually may be decreased by high-fiber diets. Once the cause of the client's problems has been established, arrange for dietary counseling so that future dietary changes may be incorporated into the client's life-style after discharge.

3. Offer sound guidance and practical information about exercise and activity, and guidelines for judicious use of over-the-counter medications for relief of minor gastrointestinal (GI) disturbances. Help the client to develop a positive, flexible attitude about elimination patterns.

4. If a malignancy is found, surgical intervention may be necessary. The client and family will need support and reassurance. If a colostomy is to be done, begin early with a positive attitude preparing the client and family for care at home. Stress and dwell on the client's capabilities rather than limitations. A positive attitude at the earliest stages of diagnosis and treatment will greatly enhance the client's adjustment to any alterations in life-style.

REFERRALS

If a cancerous process is discovered, the client and family may benefit from the support available from the American Cancer Society.

Evaluation

Quality Assurance

The documentation should reflect the nature of the results of the enema preparations as well as the client's response to them. Record the number of preparatory enemas, the appearance of the return, and the client's condition before and after the procedure. Document the response of the client to the proctoscopic examination. Note all follow-up care and show evidence that the nurse anticipated possible side-effects and took measures to avoid or rectify them.

Infection Control

Thorough handwashing before and after the administration of an enema cannot be stressed enough. Likewise, encourage the client to engage in thorough handwashing after each bowel movement and enema evacuation. Transfer of microorganisms from the colon is greatly reduced by proper handwashing. Equipment that is used for consecutive clients must be cleaned and disinfected thoroughly after each use.

Technique Checklist

	YES	NO
Procedure explained to client	_____	_____
Light meal evening before proctoscopy	_____	_____
Laxative or suppository	_____	_____
Castor oil given (amt. _____)	_____	_____
Other _____	_____	_____
Enemas until clear (no. given _____)	_____	_____
Equipment gathered before procedure and in proper working order	_____	_____

	YES	NO
Position for proctoscopy		
On right side of bed _____		
Knee–chest _____		
Proctoscopy table _____		
Difficulty inserting proctoscope	_____	_____
Complications after proctoscopy		
Nausea/vomiting _____		
Dizziness _____		
Faintness _____		_____
Bleeding _____		
Cramping _____		
Pathology found	_____	_____
Instructions on diet before discharge	_____	_____
Instructions of medications before discharge	_____	_____

20   Residual Urine, Measurement of

Overview

Definition   Determination of the amount of urine left in the bladder after urination

Rationale   Ascertain the adequacy of the bladder's emptying mechanism.

Assess the possibility of enlarged prostate.

Terminology   ***Catheterization:*** Insertion of a tube directly into the bladder to obtain a sterile urine specimen

Benign Prostatic Hypertrophy (BPH): An enlargement of the prostate gland, often associated with advancing age

Urinary calculus: An abnormal concentration of mineral salts adhering to form a "stone" somewhere in the urinary system

Assessment

Pertinent Anatomy and Physiology   See Appendix I: *bladder, kidneys, ureters, urethra, urination.*

Pathophysiological Concepts   The male urethra is completely surrounded by the prostate gland. When this gland begins to enlarge, as it commonly does in elderly men, it compresses the prostatic urethra and interferes with the flow of urine. Another condition that may interfere with the ability to empty the bladder is *stricture,* or narrowing of the urethra as a result of adhesions. *Urinary obstruction* may result from congenital defects, stones, pregnancy, infection, and certain neurologic disorders. Obstruction causes a greater chance of infection and stone formation as a result of pooling of urine. Permanent damage to the kidney may occur.

Assessment of the Client
1. Assess the recent physical history of the client in relation to urinary problems. Note symptoms of urinary retention such as incontinency, inability to start the urine stream, and urgency.
2. Assess the dietary habits of the client, especially in regard to amount and types of fluids usually ingested.
3. Assess the client's knowledge of the reasons for and expected outcomes of the procedure. Assess the client's previous experience with catheterization. Assess the anxiety level of the client and family to determine appropriate teaching strategies.

Plan

Nursing Objectives   Empty the client's bladder completely.

Measure the amount of residual urine to assess emptying capability.

Client Preparation
1. Explain to the client why the catheterization must be done and why the bladder must be emptied voluntarily first.

129

2. Refer to Technique No. 39, Catheterization, Urethral, for further preparation steps.

Equipment

Catheterization equipment (see Technique No. 39, Catheterization, Urethral)

Graduated cylinder for measurement

Bedpan, urinal, or commode container

Implementation and Interventions

Procedural Aspects

ACTION	RATIONALE
1. Instruct the client to void into a container. Immediately afterward, perform urethral catheterization and completely drain the bladder.	The amount of urine left in the bladder after voluntary emptying is called residual urine.
2. Measure the urine from the voided specimen and the amount of urine from the catheterized specimen. Record both amounts.	Ability of the bladder to empty is of valuable diagnostic significance. Measuring both specimens provides a basis for comparison.

Communicative Aspects

OBSERVATIONS

1. Note and record the amount of residual urine. Also note and record the amount of voided urine.

2. Observe the appearance and color of the urine.

3. Note any difficulty in voiding.

CHARTING

DATE/TIME	OBSERVATIONS	SIGNATURE
5/23 1430	Voided 350 ml of dark urine. Catheterized for residual urine with return of 175 ml of dark urine. No discomfort at this time. States no problems voiding; has been catheterized previously.	C. Blake RN

Discharge Planning Aspects

CLIENT AND FAMILY EDUCATION

1. Stress the importance of adequate fluid intake.

2. Urge male clients over the age of 60 years to report any feelings of incomplete emptying and difficulty starting the urinary stream to their physicians. These are symptoms of benign prostatic hypertrophy.

3. Stress the importance of voiding as soon as the sensation appears. Voiding should be frequent and complete. Persons who ignore or postpone emptying the bladder when the need arises invite damage to the bladder musculature.

Evaluation

Quality Assurance

Document the amount of voided urine and the amount of residual urine. Document assessment of the symptoms of urinary retention in the client. The chart should reflect the teaching done for the client and family in relation to preventing further retention of urine. If surgical intervention was necessary, documentation should reflect diagnostic support for the decision to operate.

Infection Control

1. Urinary catheterization is a procedure that places the client at great risk of infection. Scrupulous adherence to sterile technique is absolutely essential. The microorganisms normally found on the skin and perineum may become

pathogenic when introduced into the urinary system. Careful handwashing should precede and follow catheterization.

2. Stasis of the urine in the bladder after failure to empty completely provides an excellent medium for the growth of bacteria. Incomplete emptying of the bladder often results in infection.

Technique Checklist

	YES	NO
Order for procedure on chart	_____	_____
Procedure explained to client	_____	_____
Amount of urine voided _____		
Amount of urine from catheterization _____		
Physician notified of results	_____	_____
Cause of incomplete emptying found	_____	_____
Cause of incomplete emptying corrected	_____	_____
Client and family understand what caused retention and how to prevent it in the future	_____	_____

Specific Gravity of Urine, Measurement of

Overview

Definition

Measurement of the ratio the weight of a given volume of urine bears to the weight of the same volume of water

Rationale

Test the ability of the kidneys to dilute and concentrate urine.

Evaluate the extent of kidney damage.

Evaluate glandular efficiency, such as ADH secretion by the pituitary gland.

Terminology

Urinometer: An instrument that contains a mercury bulb attached to a stem with a graduated scale indicating a range of concentration from 1.000 to 1.040

Assessment

Pertinent Anatomy and Physiology

1. See Appendix I: *kidneys*.
2. *Urine* is a watery solution of nitrogenous waste and inorganic salts that is removed from the plasma and eliminated by the kidneys. The color is usually amber. The specific gravity is usually between 1.016 and 1.020, but may vary from 1.002 to 1.040 in normal kidneys, according to whether the urine is very dilute or very concentrated.

Pathophysiological Concepts

1. In the normal person, the kidneys are able to vary the specific gravity of the urine from 1.002 to 1.040. Lack of the ability to concentrate the urine is one of the earliest signs of kidney damage. Normally, the specific gravity of urine is responsive to the water and electrolyte situation in the body. Profuse perspiration with decreased intake produces a high specific gravity. High fluid intake with no excessive loss lowers the specific gravity. Damaged kidneys cannot adjust to these extremes; and regardless of the degree of hydration, the specific gravity remains constant, usually between 1.010 and 1.015.
2. Reabsorption of water by the kidney is regulated by the antidiuretic hormone (ADH), which is synthesized in the hypothalamus. A rise in ADH levels causes increased reabsorption of water from the kidneys. ADH levels are controlled by the volume and osmolar changes in the extracellular fluids. Stress situations such as pain, trauma, surgery, and some anesthetics and analgesics cause an increase in release of ADH. Diabetes insipidus occurs because of a failure of the kidneys to respond normally to ADH concentrations. In a large number of cases, diabetes insipidus is related to tumors or lesions of the pituitary body. Temporary diabetes insipidus may follow surgery or trauma to the pituitary gland. Large quantities of urine are excreted (up to 15 liters/day), and excessive thirst is present. If the person can balance the fluid loss by intake of fluid, the problems are less critical. Problems develop when the person is unconscious or otherwise unable to take in adequate fluids. Serum osmolality increases with subsequent dehydration of tissue.

Assessment of the Client

1. Assess the physical appearance of the urine to determine if other abnormalities such as blood may be present.
2. Assess the knowledge level of the client and/or family about why the testing is being done and what is being determined. Assess the anxiety level of the family. If the client is unconscious or in critical condition, provide information to the family. Determine amount of information to share by the willingness and ability of the family to seek and accept information.

Plan

Nursing Objectives

Allay client apprehension about diagnostic testing.

Obtain an adequate amount of urine to ensure accurate test results.

Carry out the specific gravity testing in a capable manner.

Client Preparation

1. If the test is being done to determine the ability of the kidneys to dilute and concentrate urine, the client may be dehydrated before one specimen and overhydrated before the second specimen.
2. Offer an explanation of why the test is being done and the amount of urine needed, in order to gain greater client cooperation.

Equipment

Urine specimen collection container

Graduated container holding at least 150 ml

Urinometer

Implementation and Interventions

Procedural Aspects

ACTION	RATIONALE
1. At least 20 ml of urine is needed to test specific gravity. Place the urine in a graduated container and lower the urinometer gently into the urine. The specific gravity is the level of the urine on the graduated scale when the urinometer is still. It is read 00, 01, 02, etc., through 10, 20, 30, etc. These are interpreted as 00 (1.000), 01 (1.001), 10 (1.010), 20 (1.020), etc., as measured against the specific gravity of distilled water (1.000) (Fig. 21-1).	The principle upon which this measurement is based is displacement. The more concentrated the urine, the more the urinometer will be displaced upward, and the higher will be the specific gravity.
2. After the test is completed, all equipment should be thoroughly rinsed and stored properly. Reassurance should be offered if the client expresses concern over the frequency or results of the diagnostic testing.	Neatness adds to the client's and family's confidence in the nurse as they see evidence that everything is under control.

Communicative Aspects

OBSERVATIONS

1. Note the color, odor, and appearance of the urine when the specimen is obtained.
2. Observe the client's degree of apprehension regarding diagnostic testing.

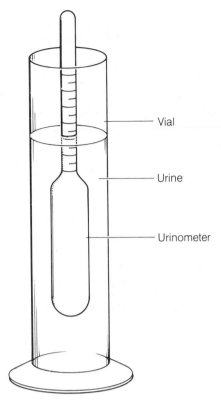

Vial

Urine

Urinometer

Figure 21.1

	DATE/TIME	OBSERVATIONS	SIGNATURE
CHARTING	9/1 1100	150 ml urine obtained for testing. Color yellow, clear with no foul odor. Specific gravity of urine is 1.015. ——————————————————	G. Ivers RN

Discharge Planning Aspects

CLIENT AND FAMILY EDUCATION

1. Explain the importance of adequate fluid intake in ensuring proper kidney function. Adequate hydration is also important in preventing kidney stones and urinary infection. Adults should consume from 4 to 6 glasses of water daily unless fluids are restricted because of physical condition.

2. Relate to the client and family the purpose of the specific gravity determinations and interpretation of the results, if they indicate an interest and desire to know.

Evaluation

Quality Assurance

Documentation should reflect the times and readings of the specific gravity determinations. In addition, the nurse should indicate an awareness of the potential causes and complications of abnormally high and abnormally low specific gravity determination. Actions taken to rectify abnormal specific gravity readings should be documented.

Infection Control

1. Equipment for specific gravity measurement should be assigned for use on a single client or should be thoroughly disinfected after each use.

2. Outbreaks of infection have been associated with a variety of urine testing/ measuring equipment. Rigid attention to handwashing after such procedures is essential to prevent infection of other clients.

Technique Checklist

	YES	NO
Specific gravity determinations done at prescribed or indicated intervals	_____	_____
Explanation of test given to client and/or family	_____	_____
Abnormal values reported to physician	_____	_____
Equipment maintained in a neat and clean manner	_____	_____

22   Urine Examinations

Overview

Definition

An analysis of the constituents of urine

Rationale

Assess the functional effectiveness of the urinary system.

Determine the presence of pathology.

Terminology

Catheterized specimen: A sterile urine specimen obtained by insertion of a tube directly into the bladder

Clean-catch specimen (midstream): A voided specimen caught in a sterile container after cleansing the meatus and voiding a small amount prior to catching the specimen

Random specimen: Urine collected under clean conditions for laboratory study

Timed specimen: Urine collected for a specified period of time, usually 12 to 24 hours

Urinalysis: Analysis of the urine to obtain a description of color and degree of cloudiness, pH, specific gravity, and presence of protein or glucose, and a microscopic examination of the sediment

Assessment

Pertinent Anatomy and Physiology

See Appendix I: *bladder, kidneys, ureters, urethra, urination.*

Pathophysiological Concepts

1. The time when the urine specimen is collected has a great bearing on the results of the diagnostic tests. Early morning specimens are often desirable for urinalysis because the specimen is more concentrated because of decreased fluid intake during the hours immediately preceding collection. Tests for certain metabolic disorders may require a specimen collected after a meal. Abnormal constituents of urine include blood, pus, albumin, glucose, and ketone bodies.

2. Urinary tract infection is a frequent form of infection. These infections range from bacteria in the urine to cystitis (infection of the bladder) and pyelonephritis (infection of the kidney). Cystitis is especially common in women because of the shortness of the urethra and the proximity of the vagina and rectum, which provide microorganisms with easy access to the urinary system.

3. Reabsorption of water by the kidney is regulated by the antidiuretic hormone (ADH), which is synthesized in the hypothalamus. A rise in ADH levels causes increased reabsorption of water from the kidneys. ADH levels are controlled by volume and osmolar changes in the extracellular fluids. Stress situations, such as pain, trauma, surgery, and some anesthetics and analgesics, cause an increase in ADH release. Diabetes insipidus occurs because of a failure of the kidneys to respond normally to ADH concentrations. A large number of cases of diabetes insipidus are related to tumors or lesions of the pitu-

itary body. Temporary diabetes insipidus can follow surgery or trauma to the pituitary gland. Large quantities of urine are excreted (up to 15 liters a day), and excessive thirst is present. If the person can balance the fluid loss by intake of fluid, the problems are less critical. Problems develop when the person is unconscious or otherwise unable to take in adequate fluids. Serum osmolality increases, with subsequent dehydration of tissues.

Assessment of the Client

1. Assess the recent physical history of the client in relation to urinary problems. Note symptoms of urinary problems such as incontinence, inability to start the urine stream, pain and burning during urination, and urgency.

2. Assess the dietary habits of the client, especially in regard to amount and types of fluids usually ingested.

Plan

Nursing Objectives

Assist the client to overcome the embarrassment sometimes associated with urine elimination.

Collect an adequate amount of urine under clean or sterile conditions.

For timed specimens, collect all of the urine excreted during the specified time period.

Client Preparation

1. The voluntary process of voiding can be inhibited by feelings of fear, excitement, pressure, and embarrassment. Give the client adequate time and privacy to produce the desired specimen.

2. Give precise instructions on the method of specimen collection prior to the actual request for the specimen so that the client will have time to adjust accordingly and produce the desired results.

3. If the specimen is to be gathered over a specified period of time, explain to the client that *all* of the urine must be saved and relate the exact length of time involved.

Equipment

RANDOM SPECIMEN

Clean urinal, bedpan, or commode container
Specimen container

CATHETERIZED SPECIMEN

See Technique #39, Catheterization, Uretheral.

CLEAN-CATCH SPECIMEN

Cotton balls and cleansing solution
Sterile specimen container

TIMED SPECIMEN

Urinal, bedpan, or commode container
Large specimen container with appropriate preservative
Ice (if indicated)

Implementation and Interventions

Procedural Aspects

ACTION

1. For a random specimen, ask the client to void into a clean receptacle (usually a bedpan, urinal, or commode container). Pour a small amount of the specimen (usually about 30 ml to 50 ml) into a labeled specimen container. Send

RATIONALE

This is the usual method of obtaining a specimen for routine urinalysis. If the urine is allowed to remain on the unit for an extended time before being transported to the laboratory, its usefulness as a diagnostic tool is compromised.

ACTION

the labeled specimen to the laboratory with a requisition as soon as possible. Discard the remainder of the specimen and rinse the receptacle thoroughly.

2. For specifics about obtaining a catheterized specimen, see Technique #39. Once the catheterized specimen has been placed in the container, care must be taken not to contaminate it when replacing the lid. The container should be labeled and sent to the laboratory at once, especially if the specimen is for culture. A labeled requisition should accompany the specimen.

3. In obtaining the clean-catch specimen, careful instructions must be given so that the specimen is not accidentally contaminated. The cap of the sterile container is removed and replaced with the finger-tips on the outside edge to avoid touching the sterile portion (Fig. 22-1). Instruct the client to place the cap top side down on the table when voiding.

Women: Clean the vulva with an accepted cleansing solution from front to back (Fig. 22-2). Separate the labia and have the client pass a small amount of urine, which is not saved (Fig. 22-3). Then, have the client void directly into the sterile specimen container (Fig. 22-4).

RATIONALE

Delay in taking the specimen to the laboratory increases the risk of contamination and distorted results.

Voiding a small amount prior to saving a specimen allows flushing of the urethra of any contaminants that might be located near the meatus or in the urethra itself.

Women should always clean from front to back to avoid contaminating the urinary meatus with fecal or vaginal flora.

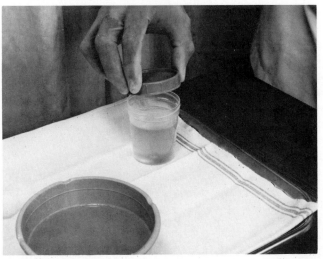

Figure 22.1

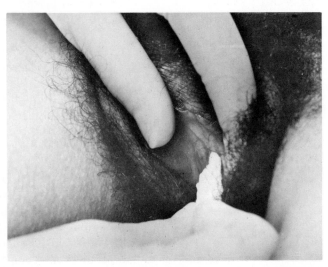

Figure 22.2

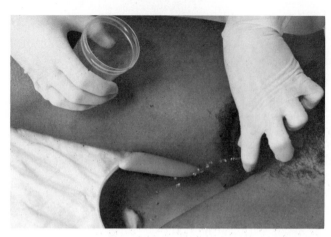

Figure 22.3

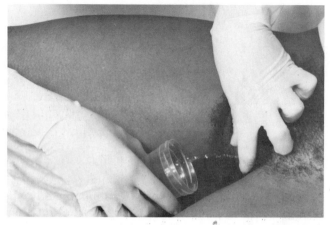

Figure 22.4

ACTION	RATIONALE
Men: Clean the meatus and surrounding area with a cotton ball and cleansing solution (Fig. 22-5). Have the client pass a small amount of urine, which is not saved (Fig. 22-6). Then, have the client void directly into the sterile specimen container (Fig. 22-7). If no cleansing solution is available, soap and water are adequate. If an iodine preparation is used for cleansing, care must be taken to rinse off the iodine thoroughly with water before taking the specimen.	The meatus is cleansed in a circular motion from the meatus outward so microorganisms are carried away from the opening into the urinary tract. Iodine in the specimen will skew the results of the test.
4. For a timed specimen, collect all of the urine for the exact time specified. Explain to the client that all of the urine must be saved. A bottle from the laboratory, containing a preservative, should be labeled and placed in a convenient place where it will not be accidentally spilled. The specimen should be kept cold during collection, either in a refrigerator or in a basin of ice. Place an appropriate sign in the client's bathroom to alert nursing personnel and family members that a timed specimen collection is in progress. To begin the collection, ask the client to void an initial specimen, which is then discarded. *All* urine voided thereafter is saved and poured into the collection container. At the time the collection is scheduled to end, the client voids, and this specimen is also saved in the container. Take the bottle to the laboratory.	The initial specimen is discarded because it represents urine that has been produced earlier in the day. The specimen should contain all of the urine produced within the specified time; this includes the final specimen, which is collected before the container is taken to the laboratory. Extra precautions to alert everyone of the urine collection measures will help ensure accuracy and efficiency.

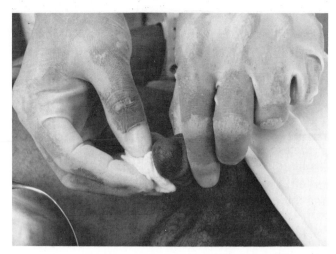

Figure 22.5

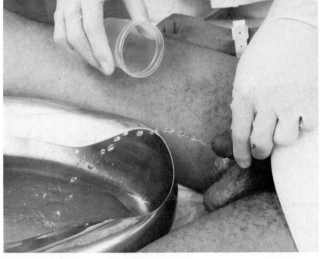

Figure 22.6

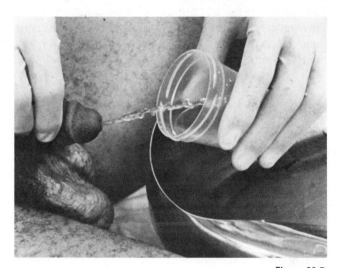

Figure 22.7

Communicative Aspects

OBSERVATIONS

1. Note the color and appearance of the urine.

2. Note any dififculty in voiding.

3. Note the approximate amount of urine.

CHARTING

DATE/TIME	OBSERVATIONS	SIGNATURE
12/4 0600	24-hour urine secimen collection begun. Container for urine placed on ice in bathroom. Initial specimen of 240 ml discarded. Complete instructions given to Mr. J and wife to save all urine. Instructed to call the nurse after each voiding. Expresses willingness to follow directions. ————	P. Dillon RN

Discharge and Planning Aspects

CLIENT AND FAMILY EDUCATION

1. Explain carefully how to obtain the urine specimen. Offer specific explanations about clean-catch specimens, with emphasis on the need to cleanse and flush the urethra by voiding a small amount before catching the specimen in the container.

2. For a timed specimen, involve the entire family in efforts to save all of the urine. If everyone knows that the test is being done, no one will accidentally throw away a specimen. Use written as well as verbal instructions to alert everyone to the fact that the urine is to be saved.

3. This is an excellent time to emphasize to female clients the importance of cleansing their genitalia from front to back. The urinary meatus lies in close proximity to the vagina and rectum, both of which contain normal flora that is very pathogenic should it be introduced into the urinary system. Cleansing from front to back greatly reduces the chance of contamination. Stress that all women, young and old, should adhere to this procedure.

4. Relate to the client and family the purpose of the urine examinations and assist them in understanding the results.

Evaluation

Quality Assurance

Documentation should reflect what type of specimen was obtained and what the ordered test was. Any problems in obtaining the specimen should be reflected. The results of the test should be a permanent part of the client's hospital record. The record should reflect the times of urine collection and whether the specimen was kept on ice or in the refrigerator. Teaching efforts and actions taken to rectify abnormal results should be documented.

Infection Control

1. Cystitis, infection of the bladder, is common, especially in females. Stress to all female clients the importance of cleansing the genitalia from front to back to avoid transporting bacteria from the rectum and vagina to the urinary meatus. Pyelitis, a more serious infection of the renal pelvis, may follow urinary infection. Health-care personnel should wash their hands after assisting with specimen collection and after transporting the specimen to the laboratory. Likewise, the client's hands should be washed after participation in specimen collection.

2. If a clean-catch specimen is collected, the client should be carefully taught how to cleanse the urethral area to prevent contamination.

3. If the urine specimen is from a client with an infectious process requiring infection-control precautions for body fluids, label the specimen clearly with the type of precautions necessary and adhere to all appropriate precautionary measures (see Technique #66, Isolation Precautions).

Technique Checklist

	YES	NO
Procedure explained to client	_____	_____
Uncontaminated specimen obtained	_____	_____
Timed specimen	_____	_____
Initial specimen discarded	_____	_____
Time parameters of collection from _____ to _____		
Specimen to laboratory at _____		
Test results are on the chart	_____	_____
Client and family understand the test results and implications	_____	_____

Unit Two

Techniques
for
Adult
Clients

---

23 Abdominal Thrust (Heimlich Maneuver)

Overview

Definition

The manual technique used to dislodge foreign bodies or food from the airway by forcing the diaphragm upward to cause the residual air in the lungs to be forcefully exhaled, thereby dislodging the object occluding the airway

Rationale

Dislodge foreign bodies or food from the airway.

Establish and clear the airway.

Terminology

Anoxia: Lack of oxygen

Residual air: Air remaining in the lungs after normal expiration

Xiphoid process: The lower 1 to 2 inches of the sternum in the midchest region

Assessment

Pertinent Anatomy and Physiology

1. See Appendix I: *bronchial tree, lungs.*
2. The thorax is a cone-shaped bony cage, narrow at the top and broad at the bottom. Twelve pair of ribs form the outer perimeter of the cage, which encloses the heart and lungs. The ribs are slender, curved, and fairly flexible. Some of the ribs join the sternum by means of the costal cartilage, allowing flexibility of the rib cage during breathing.
3. The diaphragm is the sheet of 2 muscles that forms the floor of the thorax. When the muscle fibers of the diaphragm contract, the central portion is pulled downward, and the thoracic cavity is enlarged, allowing inspiration. The dome of the diaphragm is constantly changing. Upon sudden compression of the abdominal area directly below the sternum, the diaphragm spontaneously contracts, forcefully pushing air from the lungs through the trachea. Each side is innervated and moves separately.

Pathophysiological Concepts

1. Aeration of the tissues in the body depends on transport of oxygen through the circulatory system. The carbon dioxide removed from the tissues is transported to the lungs, where it is exchanged for oxygen in the alveoli. Oxygen is continuously supplied to the alveoli by inspiration of atmospheric air. If the supply of air is obstructed, the amount of oxygen in the lungs is quickly depleted. Oxygen is then unavailable for functioning of vital organs, such as the brain, and anoxia leads to unconsciousness and death.
2. Pulmonary arrest is usually preceded by a short period of shallow breathing. The client's breathing becomes increasingly labored, cyanosis and flushing occur, and the client becomes agitated because of feelings of suffocation. Unconsciousness, coma, and cardiac arrest follow.

Assessment of the Client

1. Assess the client to determine if choking is actually occurring. The universal sign for choking is placing a hand on the throat. Assess the client's color. Ask the client to place a hand on the throat if choking is occurring.
2. Assess the size and position of the client to determine how to deliver the ab-

dominal thrusts effectively. If the client is too large to encircle with the arms, place the client on the floor and deliver the thrusts from the floor. Quickly assess the position of the client so that if falling occurs, further injury from hitting sharp or dangerous objects may be prevented.

Plan

Nursing Objectives

Ascertain from the client's gestures and appearance whether choking is indeed taking place.

Perform the abdominal thrust maneuver in a proper and efficient manner.

Prevent complications associated with choking and with the abdominal thrust maneuver.

Observe and record the client's condition after the technique has been completed.

Client Preparation

Since choking is a sudden and unplanned condition, there is usually no time or necessity for client preparation. The procedure may be done with the client standing or lying.

Implementation and Interventions

Procedural Aspects

ACTION	RATIONALE
1. Act quickly to ascertain if the client is choking. If so, initiate the abdominal thrust immediately.	Prolonged deprivation of oxygen to the brain will lead to death.
2. If the victim is standing, assume a position directly behind the client and place both arms around the client's waist. Make a fist with one hand and place the other hand over the fist. Position the hands halfway between the xiphoid process and umbilicus, with the thumb side against the client's abdomen. Press the fist into the client's abdomem with a quick upward thrust. The client's head, arms, and upper torso will probably fall forward. Repeat the thrusts until the object is dislodged. (Figs. 23-1, 23-2).	The goal of the technique is to force the diaphragm upward, increasing the pressure of the air in the tracheobronchial tree and forcing the obstructing object from the airway.

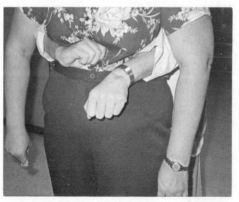

Figure 23.1

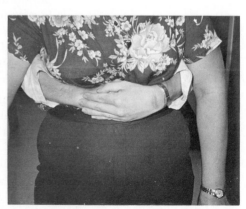

Figure 23.2

ACTION

RATIONALE

3. If the victim is lying down, place the victim in the supine position. Kneel beside the client's hips. Place the heel of one hand over the area between the xiphoid process and the umbilicus. Place the other hand over the first and press the heel of the first hand firmly upward with a quick thrust (Fig. 23-3). Repeat until the object is dislodged. If the client vomits, turn the head to one side.

The firm thrust against the epigastric region forces exhalation of air through the airway, which may dislodge the obstruction. Aspiration of vomitus must be prevented.

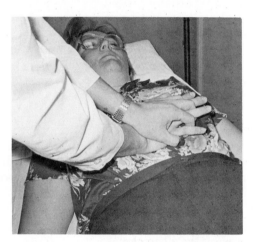

Figure 23.3

4. Remove the obstructing object from the client's mouth. Turn the client's head to one side and spread the jaws open. Remove dentures if they are obstructing actions. Bending the index finger into the form of a hook, attempt to snare and remove the object from the client's throat or mouth. After the object has been removed, continue to clear the client's mouth of any debris, such as vomitus, blood, or saliva, using several fingers in a scooping motion.

If foreign objects are not removed from the client's mouth, they may fall back into the throat and again cause airway obstruction. Liquids may be aspirated into the lungs.

Special Modifications

Infants and Toddlers

1. With the child seated on the nurse's lap, lower the child's head to a position below the trunk while maintaining a firm grip on the child. Deliver 4 rapid back blows between the shoulder blade while the head is supported with a hand around the jaw and chest (Fig. 23-4). If the object is not dis-

Using the abdominal thrust causes too much compression, which might cause internal injury to the small child. If the child with partial airway occlusion is turned upside down, the foreign body may become lodged against the underside of vocal cords causing complete obstruction.

ACTION	*RATIONALE*

lodged, place the child supine across the nurse's lap with the head lower than the trunk. Supporting the child's head and neck with one hand, use the other to deliver 4 chest thrusts in the same manner as chest compressions are done for the infant (*i.e.*, place the tips of the index and middle fingers at midsternum level to depress the chest ½ to 1 inch). Do not turn the child upside down if the airway is only partially obstructed (some air is moving in and out of the lungs).

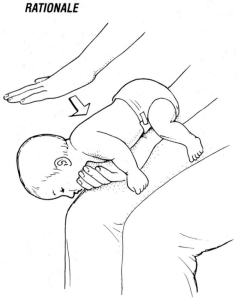

Figure 23.4

Young and School-aged Children

2. The child is draped over the thighs of the kneeling nurse. Keep the child's head lower than the trunk. Deliver 4 back blows with greater force than that used on an infant (Fig. 23-5). The child is then placed supine on the floor, and 4 chest thrusts are delivered in the same manner as chest compression for the young child (*i.e.*, using the heel of one hand, compress the chest 1 to ½ inches at the midsternum area).

Abdominal thrusts are not used with small children because of the danger of trauma to the delicate abdominal organs.

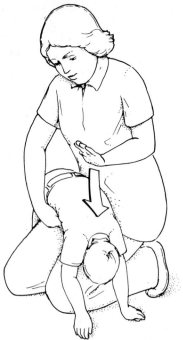

Figure 23.5

ACTION	*RATIONALE*
3. For the pregnant woman or those who are very obese, the chest thrust is used. Stand behind the victim and place both arms under the victim's axillae to encircle the chest. Grasp one fist with the other hand and place the thumb side on the middle of the sternum. Press with quick backward thrusts.	Chest thrusts are easier to accomplish in some cases. If the rescuer's arms will not go around the victim's waist, the abdominal thrust will not be effective unless the victim is lying down and the abdominal thrust is accomplished in this manner.

Communicative Aspects

OBSERVATIONS

1. Observe the client for signs of inadequate oxygenation after the object has been removed. These signs may be dyspnea, restlessness, and cyanosis, which may be from failure to completely dislodge the object or swelling of the throat due to trauma of the obstruction.

2. Observe the respiratory sufficiency of the client after removal of the foreign object. Auscultate breath sounds. Assess rate and depth of respirations.

3. Observe for trauma to the throat and mouth during digital removal of the foreign object.

CHARTING

DATE/TIME	OBSERVATIONS	SIGNATURE
4/13 1215	Found choking while lying in bed after lunch. Abdominal thrusts × 3 administered to epigastric area with heel of hand. Small bone dislodged. No vomiting. No apparent trauma to throat. Resting quietly at this time. B/P 136/76, P 82, R 18. Dr. J notified.	P. Dillon RN

Discharge Planning Aspects

CLIENT AND FAMILY EDUCATION

1. The abdominal thrust maneuver should be taught to all parents of small children. In addition, it is a valuable tool for everyone. The technique may be demonstrated to the client and family after the crisis is over if they express an interest and willingness to learn.

2. Inform the client and family about signs of complications following trauma to the throat. Ask the client to notify the nurse of any feelings of fullness in the throat, difficulty breathing or swallowing, or pain.

Evaluation

Quality Assurance

Document the signs and symptoms that preceded administration of the abdominal thrust. Document any signs that might have indicated that the client was choking. Note the number of thrusts and the outcome of the procedure. The notes should reflect any complications, such as vomiting or bleeding. Assess and record the client's condition after successfully dislodging the obstruction. Include vital signs, physical appearance of the client, and appearance of the mouth and throat. Identify the obstruction, if possible, and describe its size. Reflect any teaching done about administration of the abdominal thrust procedure.

Technique Checklist

	YES	NO
Signs and symptoms of choking documented on chart	_____	_____
Number of thrusts _____		
Client standing		
Client supine		
Patent airway restored	_____	_____
Trauma to throat	_____	_____
Complications		
Bleeding	_____	_____
Emesis	_____	_____
Client and family taught abdominal thrust technique	_____	_____

24   Admission of the Adult Client

Overview

Definition

The incorporation and implementation of a series of activities that occurs when the client enters the hospital

Rationale

Provide basic, pertinent information to the client.

Obtain baseline information from the client.

Create a comfortable environment in which the client feels welcome and secure.

Initiate discharge planning objectives and rehabilitation potential.

Assessment

Pertinent Anatomy and Physiology

Homeostasis is the dynamic, steady state that exists in the internal environment of the body. Illness has been described as an alteration in this steady state. Homeostasis serves its most important function in providing a reference point for understanding pathologic changes that have occurred in the body. Baseline parameters help determine the extent of disturbance to the homeostasis state of the person.

Pathophysiological Concepts

Stress has been defined as a dynamic state within the body occurring in response to a demand for adaptation. Adaptation to stress involves cooperation among mental and physical activities. The three processes involved in the interaction of person and environment are perception (an awareness of objects), analysis (breaking down the whole into its parts), and reaction (the body's response to stimulation). These tools are used by a client in adapting to the stress of the hospital experience. Every disease has some element of stress, and adapting to the stress is an important part of the client's reaction to illness.

Assessment of the Client

1. Admission is the proper time for the nurse's physical assessment of the client. The initial assessment includes the immediate appraisal of the client's physical, mental, and emotional status. Follow this with an in-depth assessment of the general condition, the health history, and any other information that will augment the development of nursing goals. Assess the history and severity of any allergies. Do a systems review, noting problems in addition to those responsible for the client's hospitalization. (See Technique No. 75, Physical Assessment of the Adult Client.)

2. Begin the assessment of the client with an analysis of the presenting problem. Relieve major discomfort and allay initial anxiety as much as possible. Elicit as much information as can reasonably be expected from the client and the family at this particular stage of hospitalization. A well-grounded assessment takes note of information from a variety of sources, such as the client, family, referral forms, and past records.

3. A brief review of the major complaint and presenting symptoms will be an indicator of the depth of the initial assessment. Certain information is essential: known or suspected allergies; onset, duration, and location of present problem; major health problems in the past; and the name of a person to call

in case of emergency. If the client is in no acute distress, elicit information about the complete health history and ancillary problems and initiate mutual discharge-planning goals.

4. A review of systems will establish a sound baseline from which to judge future findings. Ascertain baseline measurements of temperature, pulse rate, respiratory rate, and blood pressure for every newly admitted client. Measure and record height and weight if possible.

Plan

Nursing Objectives

Make the client and family feel welcome and facilitate their adjustment to the hospital.

Observe the client's condition and reactions.

Institute primary diagnostic measures.

Maintain the individuality of the person being admitted.

Client Preparation

1. Greet the client and family in a courteous manner. Orient them to their surroundings and answer any immediate questions they may have.

2. Offer to the client and family courteous explanations of hospital regulations concerning valuables, visiting hours, televisions, telephones, and any other items that might ease their apprehension and increase their comfort. Also explain hospital routines (e.g., meals, shift changes, physicians' rounds). Knowing what to expect reduces unnecessary fear and apprehension, enabling the client to concentrate energy on adjusting to the hospital experience. Impart all information at the time of admission in the context of its importance to the client.

Equipment

Stethoscope and sphygmomanometer

Watch capable of measuring seconds

Hospital gown or personal bed clothing

Portable scale

Labeled bedpan and urinal, if needed

Admission kit (wash basin, emesis basin, lotion, and tissues)

Electric or regular thermometer

Admission record

Implementation and Interventions

Procedural Aspects

ACTION	RATIONALE
1. Take vital signs immediately.	Anxiety often causes increases in blood pressure and pulse rates. Retake the vital signs after the client has rested 1 hour.
2. Take temperature, pulse respiration, and blood pressure. Record weight and height as actually measured or, if necessary, as stated by the client or family.	Vital signs are indicators of the client's general condition. Physical-care procedures also serve a secondary purpose of establishing positive interpersonal relationships between the client and family and the hospital staff.
3. Obtain appropriate specimens, such as blood and urine, at this time.	Delays in obtaining specimens may result in delayed treatment and longer hospitalization.

ACTION

RATIONALE

4. Place an identification card on the bed and label personal equipment. Allergies should be noted prominently on the chart and on the client's identification band. Attach an identification band securely to the client's body in some manner (Fig. 24-1).

Adequate identification can help prevent errors and cross-contamination.

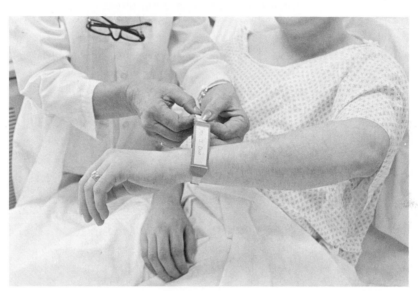

Figure 24.1

5. Make the client comfortable and secure with the call signal left in a convenient place. Send valuables and personal clothing home with the family. If the client brought any medications from home, this should be noted, and the information should be passed on to the physician. Adhere to the specific hospital policy on the proper handling of medications from home.

Unfamiliar surroundings and a sense of isolation can create stress for the newly admitted client. The ability to obtain assistance quickly is of paramount importance to hospitalized persons.

6. Initiate the nursing care plan on admission. Involve the client and family in the identification of goals and the initiation of the care plan.

Early initiation of the care plan gives a sense of purpose and organization to the activities that will occur during the rest of the hospital stay.

7. Notify the physician of the admission of the client as soon as possible. Orders already on the chart should be noted and initiated as soon as possible.

Orders should be started in an expedient manner to ease the client's discomfort and anxiety.

Modifications for Special Situations

1. In emergency situations, the usual explanations may have to be postponed until the client's condition has been stabilized. However, it is

High-stress situations are particularly difficult when no information is available. Keeping the family informed may defuse anxiety and promote ad-

Procedural Aspects	*ACTION*	*RATIONALE*
	imperative to keep the family informed and to give them information about hospital routines as soon as they are emotionally able to assimilate it.	justment to the hospital environment.
	2. When the client is hospitalized for a 1-day stay or day-surgery procedure, take extra precautions to measure accurately baseline physiological parameters.	Accurate measurement of baseline vital signs is especially important because of the brevity of the client's stay and the resulting scarcity of data should complications arise.

Communicative Aspects

OBSERVATIONS

1. Include the client and family in all admission explanations. Written instructions may be available for them.

2. Convey confidence and security by answering questions readily and cometely.

CHARTING

1. Record the time, date, and mode of admission.

2. Record pertinent observations such as general appearance and facial expression, location and type of pain, rashes, bruises, abrasions, drug and food sensitivities, complaints, medication brought by the client, clothing, valuables, specimens obtained, name of physician, and time physician was notified of admission.

3. Sign the admitting entry on the chart.

DATE/TIME	OBSERVATIONS	SIGNATURE
2/14 0900	Admitted to Room 214 via wheelchair from the Emergency Room. States nausea since yesterday evening, some vomiting, and severe pain in the right, lower quadrant of abdomen. CBC and UA done. Operative permit for appendectomy signed by client. Clothes and wristwatch given to husband. States she is allergic to Demerol and tomatoes. States she has not been in the hospital since her last child was born 6 years ago. Appears apprehensive. Seems more at ease after being interviewed by head nurse. B/P 142/80, P 68, R 14, T 98.4°, HT 66 in, WT 132 lb. ———————————	F. White RN
0910	Dr. A notified of admission. ———————————	F. White RN

4. Computerized admission forms may facilitate the recording of baseline admitting data. Check the accuracy of input carefully before it is added to the computer memory.

5. Client classification is a method of categorizing clients according to the amount of care they require. It is an effort to use more efficiently the number and level of nursing staff available. After the initial assessment by a professional nurse, classify the client according to the estimated amount of care that will be required. This classification is flexible and is subject to change as the client's condition changes. (Since different hospitals use different classification systems, consult the hospital procedure manual for specifics about classification systems.)

Discharge Planning Aspects

CLIENT AND FAMILY EDUCATION

1. Begin discharge planning during the initial admitting procedure. The goal of health promotion is to return the client to the optimal level of function. Assess health potential during admission and reflect goals in the care plan that are specific to the client retaining maximal health potential after discharge.

2. A positive attitude about the client's ability to regain health and the nurses' abilities to offer the expertise needed can get the hospitalization off to an optimal start. This optimism can be of great comfort to the client and family as they face a time when they are unsure of what will happen and are relatively helpless to control events.

3. Explain visiting hours, dining facilities' locations and hours, and parking accommodations and answer any questions about the hospital situation.

4. Tell the client and family as early as possible of the approximate time of and pertinent details about surgical and diagnostic procedures.

Evaluation

Quality Assurance

Charts should be audited periodically to ensure that all pertinent admitting information is being obtained. If the sensorium of the newly admitted client is in doubt, take appropriate precautions such as raising the siderails or requesting a family member to remain in attendance. Document in the chart all safety precautions taken.

Infection Control

1. Use proper handwashing techniques after admitting the client to help reduce the chance of cross-contaminating other clients.

2. Proper labeling of each client's equipment will help reduce the chance of using it for someone else and thereby spreading infection.

Technique Checklist

The following checklist offers the nurse a convenient method of making sure that all items are explained to the client during the admission process. This checklist will enable the nurse to return when circumstances are different and include those items omitted during the initial interview. In addition, see the physical assessment checklist in Technique No. 75, Physical Examination of the Adult.

ADMISSION CHECKLIST

Place your initials in the blank when the item has been discussed with the client and/or family. Make narrative comments in the Nurses' Notes:

BEDSIDE ENVIRONMENT

_____ Nurse call signal

_____ Telephone

_____ Television

_____ Bad controls

_____ Siderails

_____ Heating/cooling devices

_____ Lighting

_____ Apparel

HOSPITAL ENVIRONMENT

_____ Visiting hours

_____ Valuables

_____ Meals

_____ Shift change

_____ Physicians' rounds

_____ Public-address system

_____ Cafeteria services for family and guests

25   Ambulation, Assisting With

Overview

Definition

The act of walking, with or without assistance, in an attempt to regain normal activity

Rationale

Build up the physical stamina of the client in preparation for surgery or treatment.

Offer a diversion from hospital routine.

Facilitate wound healing and return of homeostasis.

Prevent complications, such as pneumonia and contracture.

Contribute to the rehabilitation potential of the client.

Assessment

Pertinent Anatomy and Physiology

1. See Appendix I: *skeletal muscles, skeletal system.*
2. The chief muscles involved in ambulation are those of the legs and thighs. For the client who must use assistance devices to ambulate, the upper limb muscles are used to a great extent to hold the cane, crutches, or walker or to grasp the handrails. The normal walking pace for adults is 70–100 steps per minute. Elderly people may have a slower pace.

Pathophysiological Concepts

1. Muscle tone is often reduced when one is in poor health, particularly if prolonged bed rest is necessary. Early ambulation of hospital clients markedly reduces this hazard. With inactivity, muscles decrease in size and strength. When clients are immobilized and unable to exercise, their muscles become weak and atrophied.
2. Changes in the joint result when the surrounding tissue is immobilized. When muscle movement decreases, the connective tissue in the joints, tendons, and ligaments becomes thickened and fibrotic. Chronic flexion or hyperextension of the joints can cause permanent contracture. Hyperextension results in pain and discomfort for the client and abnormal stress and strain on the surrounding ligaments and tendons of the joint.
3. A *spasm* is a sudden involuntary contraction of a skeletal muscle. If persistent, it is called a *cramp*. When the spasm is characterized by alternate contraction and relaxation, it is called a *clonus*. Spasmodic contractions are accompanied by pain.

Assessment of the Client

1. Assess the client for dizziness or faintness upon arising to the vertical position, preferably while sitting on the side of the bed. Assess the client's sense of balance, and note any signs of weakness or fatigue. Assess the presence and severity of pain in determining the best time to ambulate.
2. Assess the client's postoperative progress in relation to wound healing and pain in the incision site. Assess the site for proper closure and adequate tension before undertaking ambulation.
3. Assess the client's posture for alignment during ambulation. The well-aligned posture is with head erect, vertebral column straight, toes and kneecaps

pointing forward, and elbows slightly flexed. Include in this assessment the normal gait of the client in relation to physical body structure.

4. Assess the range of mobility while the client is still in bed. Continue the mobility assessment with the client sitting on the side of the bed and then, standing beside the bed. From this assessment, the amount of assistance that will be needed with ambulation can be determined.

Plan

Nursing Objectives

Promote feelings of mental, emotional and physical well-being in the client.

Maintain an environment conducive to client safety.

Assist with ambulation as dictated by the client's condition and progress.

Offer explanations and reassurance to allay anxieties about ambulation.

Teach the client and family optimal ambulatory techniques and proper posture.

Client Preparation

1. After prolonged immobility, it may be necessary to strengthen and tone the muscles used in ambulation prior to undertaking the first steps. A program of muscle tone exercises should concentrate on the quadriceps femoris, which is responsible for extension of the leg and flexion of the thigh. To strengthen these muscles, ask the client to tense the muscle by drawing the kneecap upward and inward, pushing the back of the knee against the bed, and raising the heel off of the bed surface. This tension is held for three counts and relaxed for two counts. Repeat this tension and relaxation only to the point of tiring, never to the point of actual fatigue. This exercise may be done several times an hour during the day.

2. Before beginning the ambulation process, the client should be told exactly what will happen, what will be expected, and what limitations, if any, will be placed on participation (e.g., no weight bearing on right leg or no extension of affected limb).

3. Assemble all pertinent equipment prior to beginning the procedure to reduce delays and avoid overtiring the client unnecessarily.

4. Older clients, especially those who have suffered cerebral vascular accident or Parkinson's disease, may benefit from passive range-of-motion exercises to warm up the muscles and pathways.

5. Adjust the ambulation schedule so that the client does not walk immediately after eating. A large portion of the available blood supply will be diverted from the muscles to assist in digestion.

Equipment

Belt (around client's waist for support)

Robe

Nonskid slippers

Implementation and Interventions

Procedural Aspects

ACTION	RATIONALE
1. Begin ambulation as soon after surgery or treatment as possible. Clients in the hospital for diagnostic tests and examinations should be encouraged to ambulate to preserve their muscle tone and sense of well-being. If activity limitations have been imposed by the physician, the client should fully understand the extend of these limitations and the reasons for them.	Ambulation helps restore a sense of equilibrium and enhances self-confidence.

ACTION	RATIONALE
2. During the initial attempts to ambulate after surgery or severe debilitating illness, two attendants should accompany the client. Prevention of injury (from falls, for example) and complications (such as wound dehiscence) should be kept uppermost in mind. A belt may be placed around the client's waist for guidance and support by the attendant. However, if the client has an abdominal incision, a belt is not practical, and an attendant should be on each side during the first several ambulation attempts. Place slippers on the client's feet. It may benefit the client to have pain medication 30 minutes before getting up to ambulate to reduce discomfort and anxiety.	Muscle tone deteriorates after prolonged inactivity. During initial ambulation attempts, the client may overestimate capabilities. Adequate assistance must be available during the first ambulation attempts to make sure that no problems arise. Slippers will help prevent falls and infection.
3. Place the bed in the lowest position with the head raised; have the client sit on the side of the bed and gain a sense of equilibrium. Do not attempt ambulation until the client is stable, with no feelings of dizziness or nausea. Tell the client not to look down during ambulation, but to assume as near normal posture as possible. Begin slowly and deliberately at first (Fig. 25-1).	Prolonged bed rest distorts the sense of balance because of the action of gravity on the fluid in the inner ear. It takes a few seconds for stability and equilibrium to return upon rising. Standing erect encourages deep breathing and lessens the possibility of wound complications. It also contributes to a sense of balance and well-being.

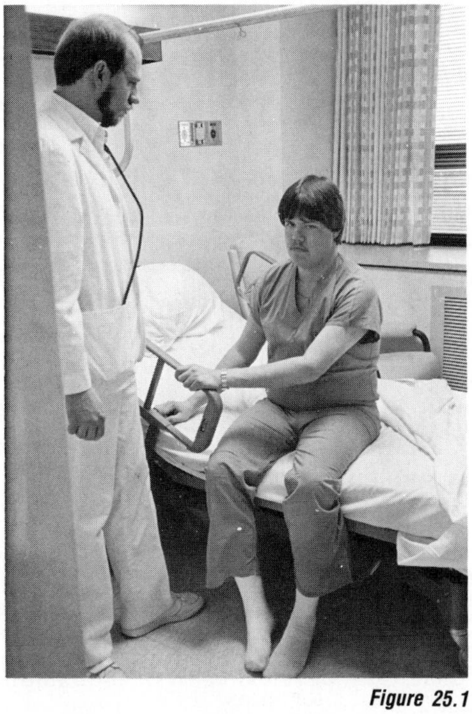

Figure 25.1

ACTION	RATIONALE

Two Attendants

4. With one attendant on each side of the client, each places one hand under the client's axilla and the other on the forearm (Fig. 25-2). Use the hands for support, guidance, and reassurance.

Two attendants provide a more secure feeling for the client, as well as ensuring greater safety during the first ambulation attempts after lengthy bed rest.

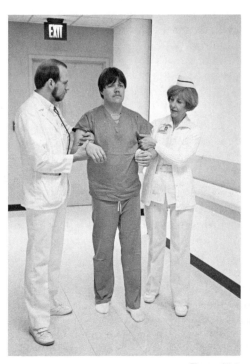

Figure 25.2

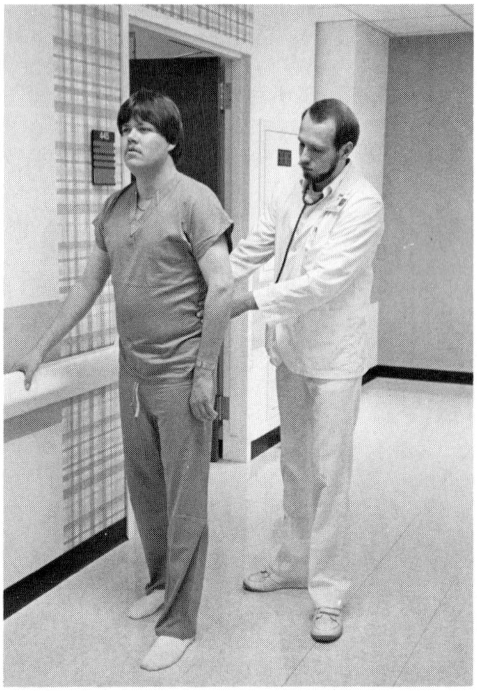

Figure 25.3

One Attendant

5. Stand behind the client, who is standing next to or near the bed. Place both hands on the client's waist to provide support (Fig. 25-3). If the client has a pronounced weakness on one side, stand on the affected side to add support and stability.

Standing behind the client helps to maintain the center of gravity. It allows the client to stand erect and not lean to one side in a dependent position against the nurse. When standing on the weak side, the nurse allows the client to compensate for the weakness and may prevent falls.

6. Leave the bed in the low position after completion of ambulation.

It is unsafe to leave a client in a bed in the high position.

7. Encourage the client to deep breathe after walking.

Deep breathing helps replenish the oxygen supplies used by the skeletal muscles.

Special Modifications

Special equipment, such as catheters and chest tubes, need not restrict ambulation. Consult the physician's orders about ambulation. Carry the

The benefits of ambulation by far outweigh the slight inconvenience of ambulating with drainage bags and tubes.

ACTION	**RATIONALE**
urinary drain bag during ambulation. Always keep the bag at a level below the client's bladder. Nasogastric tubes may be clamped, if allowed, and secured to the client's gown with a pin to prevent pulling and discomfort. Chest tubes may be placed on rollers, and ambulation can occur with the suction still in operation. See the appropriate techniques for ambulation with other specialized equipment, such as crutches or walkers.	

Communicative Aspects

OBSERVATIONS

1. Observe carefully for readiness to ambulate prior to getting the client up. Do not hurry the client; if dizziness or nausea occurs, wait a few minutes before beginning.

2. After ambulation, observe dressings for more profuse drainage and tubes for changes in the amount and appearance of drainage.

3. Observe carefully during ambulation for signs of fatigue and return the client to bed when signs of tiring become evident.

CHARTING

DATE/TIME	OBSERVATIONS	SIGNATURE
7/1 1050	B/P 110/64, R 14, P 76	F. White RN
1100	Amb. to door and back. No nausea or dizziness. Wearing nonskid slippers and safety belt. Some incisional discomfort. Suture integrity maintained, small amount of serosanguineous drainage on dressing. B/P 124/70, R 22, P 82. Resting at this time.	F. White RN

Discharge Planning Aspects

CLIENT AND FAMILY EDUCATION

1. Stress the positive benefits of early ambulation, including prevention of pneumonia, earlier return to normal activities, and promotion of wound healing. Assure the client that ambulation will not injure the suture line or operative area.

2. Emphasize the need to stand erect even though the sutures may pull and some discomfort may be present. Walking in a slumped position inhibits breathing and contributes to complications.

3. Tell the client that momentary dizziness may occur upon arising, but it should pass quickly. Notify the client that some pulling sensation in the operative area may also be noticed, but it is normal and not an indication of wound breakdown.

4. Stress the importance of correctly estimating capabilities. Some clients begin to feel better and try to undertake activities that exceed their stamina. *Moderation* is a key word in ambulation therapy.

5. If the client will require assistance in ambulation after discharge, the family should be taught proper body mechanics, transfer terchniques, and safety precautions.

REFERRALS

If continued assistance and teaching will be needed after discharge, or if the client has unusual difficulties in ambulation, refer the client to a physical therapist. A physician's concurrence is usually required for this action.

Evaluation

Quality Assurance

Documentation should include the condition of the client prior to and after ambulation. Comparison between the two should be made with emphasis on changes in vital signs and amount and location of pain. Duration, length, and any assistive devices used during ambulation should be noted. The appearance of the wound, dressings, and drainage should be documented, as well as any unusual occurrences. Documentation should reflect safety precautions taken to ensure the client's well-being.

Infection Control

1. When ambulating the client with an indwelling catheter, always keep the drainage apparatus below the level of the bladder. If the drain bag is elevated above this level, the natural pull of gravity will allow the urine in the tubing to flow back into the bladder. Since the tubing is no longer considered sterile once it is used, the chance of contaminating the bladder is great. The risk of infection is increased if urine is allowed to flow back into the bladder.

2. Handwashing before and after procedures is an excellent method of preventing the spread of infections.

3. Have the client wear slippers to decrease the chance of contacting infectious agents with the bare feet during ambulation.

Technique Checklist

	YES	NO
Order on chart for ambulation	_____	_____
Procedure explained to client	_____	_____
Problems encountered upon arising:		
Nausea _____		
Dizziness _____		
Fainting _____		
Pain _____		
Safety precautions taken:		
Two attendants	_____	_____
Belt around waist	_____	_____
Slippers	_____	_____
Client ambulated successfully		
Duration _____		
Distance _____		
Appearance of wound checked before ambulation	_____	_____
Appearance of wound checked after ambulation	_____	_____
Tubing clamped during ambulation		
Catheter _____		
Nasogastric tube _____		
Other _____		
Ambulation procedure demonstrated to family if appropriate	_____	_____
Bed left in low position after walk	_____	_____

26 Backrub

Overview

Definition
The massaging of an individual's back as a therapeutic and comfort measure

Rationale
Stimulate circulation and thus increase blood supply to the area.
Observe the skin for signs of impaired circulation or breakdown (pressure sore).
Relieve tension and promote relaxation.
Convey personal concern for the client.

Terminology
Effleurage: Deep or superficial stroking in massage

Petrissage: A kneading movement in massage

Pressure sore (decubitus ulcer): Gangrene of the skin due to pressure; also known as a bed sore (See Technique No. 78, Pressure Sores, Prevention and Treatment.)

Tapotement: Percussion in massage

Assessment

Pertinent Anatomy and Physiology

1. See Appendix I: *skin, vertebral column.*
2. The blood supply to the skin is important in the regulation of temperature and nourishment of the tissue cells.
3. The motion of the backrub maneuver on the skin releases endorphins from the brain. These endogenous peptides have an opiatelike action on the body.

Pathophysiological Concepts

1. The two layers of the skin are firmly cemented together. However, excessive rubbing of the skin may cause the two layers to become forcibly separated, allowing interstitial fluid to accumulate in the area. This is called a *blister*.
2. Interference with the normal blood supply to the skin will cause death of cells and result in areas of ulceration. Decubitus ulcers may occur when pressure is extended over a long period against one area of the skin. Those areas of the body particularly susceptible to ulceration are areas over the bony prominences, including the spine and rib cage.

Assessment of the Client

1. Assess the client's ability to tolerate this procedure while in the prone position. If the client cannot lie face down because of difficulty in breathing or abdominal pathology, a modified backrub may be done. The client may be positioned in the side-lying position or sitting on the side of the bed leaning forward on the bedside table.
2. Assess the client's skin during the backrub for whitish or reddened pressure areas that do not disappear after a few minutes of rubbing. Determine the presence of any broken or raw areas caused by friction from rubbing against the sheet.
3. Assess the body structure of the client to determine the type of stroke to be used and the amount of pressure to be applied during the backrub to prevent trauma and make the stroke effective. Tapotement should not be used on an

emaciated client. More pressure will have to be applied to the obese or muscular person when using effleurage in order to affect more than just the superficial layer of the skin.

Plan

Nursing Objectives

Make sure that the client has been made as comfortable as possible, especially at bedtime.

Prevent skin breakdown for the client who must spend the majority of time in bed or is unable to change position easily or often.

Open and improve lines of communication between the client and the nurse.

Client Preparation

1. An important reason for administering a backrub is to relieve tension and promote relaxation, especially at bedtime. Therefore, the nurse should make sure that the client is comfortable prior to beginning. General hygiene measures undertaken prior to bedtime, including emptying the bladder, should be completed before the backrub. Bed linen should be wrinkle-free, and the lights lowered appropriately.

2. Determine if the client has any preference for the type of lotion to be used. Also, check to see if the physician has ordered any special type of lotion for the client's skin.

Equipment

Lotion, powder, or alcohol
Towel

Implementation and Interventions

Procedural Aspects

ACTION	RATIONALE
1. Provide the backrub at the times best suited to the client's wishes and the purpose of the procedure, unless it is specifically ordered by the physician at certain times. If the purpose is to stimulate circulation to all areas of the back, the best times might be in the morning after the bath and at other times during the day when the client has been lying in bed for an extended period. If the purpose is to promote rest and relaxation, the optimal times might be at bedtime and after injection of pain medication.	Relaxation promotes rest and sleep. A backrub may alleviate discomfort, tension, and anxiety. The rubbing motion increases circulation and will help nourish pressure areas and prevent decubitus ulcers.
2. Apply lotion or powder to the client's back. Warm the lotion in the hand prior to placing it on the skin. Apply the lotion with firm, long strokes, beginning at the base of the spine and proceeding upward to the shoulders and downward to the buttocks.	Lotion or powder reduces the friction between the nurse's hands and the client's back. Cold lotion may stimulate a shocking sensation, which is not conducive to relaxation.
3. Determine which type of effect is desired so that the proper technique can be used: for a sedative effect, use long, slow stroking motions such as effleurage; for a	Long, slow strokes produce relaxation, while short, firm strokes are stimulating.

ACTION	RATIONALE

stimulating effect, use firm, rapid strokes such as petrissage and tapotement.

4. Strokes should begin near the spine and rotate outward to include the entire back (Figs. 26-1 to 26-5). The thumb and first three

The duration of the backrub should be long enough to provide the desired effect, but not so long as to tire or irritate the client.

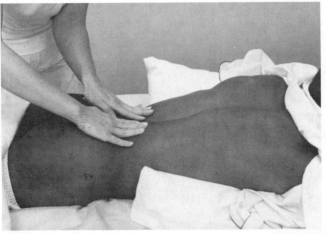

Figure 26.1

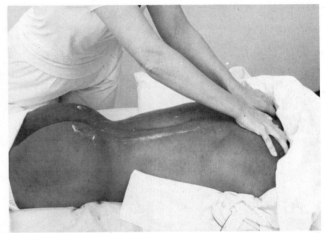

Figure 26.2

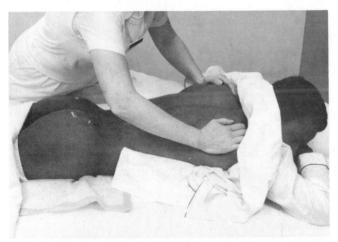

Figure 26.3

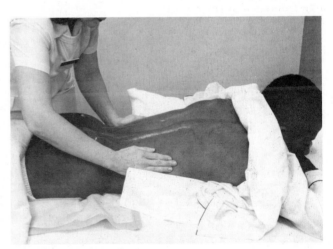

Figure 26.4

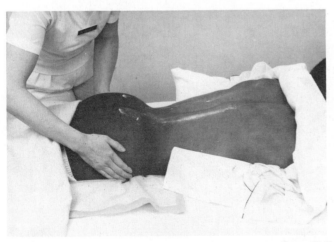

Figure 26.5

ACTION	RATIONALE

fingers of one hand may rub the nape of the neck. The entire process should be continued for 3 to 5 minutes.

5. Give special attention to the bony prominences (Fig. 26-6). This is particularly important if the client is immobile or has reddened or irritated areas on the back.

Pressure on the skin is exaggerated over the bony areas of the back. Rubbing these areas stimulates circulation and aids nourishment of the tissue.

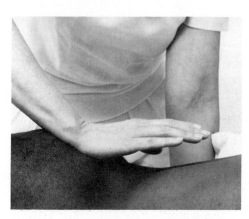

Figure 26.6

6. Leave the client properly positioned. Wipe away all excess lotion.

Comfort will facilitate sleep.

Special Modifications

If the client has a condition that prevents lying in the prone position, the benefits of a backrub need not be denied. Position the client in the side-lying position, sitting up in bed or on the side of the bed leaning forward slightly on the bedside table. Be certain that the client is adequately supported to prevent falls. Rub the back and bony prominences as in a regular backrub being careful to avoid excess pressure (Figs. 26-7, 26-8).

The positive therapeutic benefits of the backrub make the extra effort worthwhile and present a challenge to the creativity and innovation of the professional nurse.

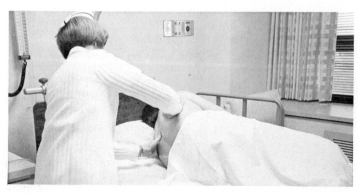

Figure 26.7

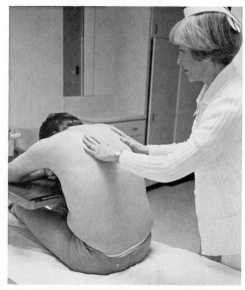

Figure 26.8

Communicative Aspects

OBSERVATIONS

1. Record the reaction of the client to the backrub.

2. Note the appearance of the back, particularly any areas of discoloration or skin breakdown. Note any abnormal findings or responses. Observe for any changes in pressure areas.

CHARTING

DATE/TIME	OBSERVATIONS	SIGNATURE
12/9 2100	Backrub given to prepare for sleep. Skin over back appears pink and intact with no pressure areas. Range-of-motion exercises preceded backrub, with full dexterity of all but right arm and right leg. Weakness in these areas seems to be improving.	P. Dillon RN

Discharge Planning Aspects

CLIENT AND FAMILY EDUCATION

1. Teach the family the proper backrub technique if the client will be confined to bed at home. Explain to them and to the client the purpose of the backrub in the prevention of decubiti. If the client is to be bedridden for an extended time, stress the importance of meticulous skin care, including frequent back-rubs and position changes.

2. Explain to the client the purpose of the backrub (sedation, prevention of pressure, relaxation). Explain that there will be some pressure during the back-rub; however, if the pressure becomes excessive, the client should report it so that the technique can be adjusted appropriately.

Evaluation

Quality Assurance

The nurse should reflect in the documentation an awareness of the possible complications of prolonged bed rest and the measures taken to prevent them. The technique used for the backrub should be reflected, as well as the rationale for this selection. The appearance of the client's back and reaction to the procedure should be documented. If complications resulting from bed rest and inhibited circulation do occur, treatments and procedures aimed at reversing them should be noted.

Infection Control

1. The skin is the natural protective barrier of the body. As long as it is intact, the chances of infection are minimized. The nurse should be careful not to scratch or otherwise traumatize the skin during backrub. Remove rings and shorten long fingernails before giving back care.

2. Decubitus ulcer is a gangrenous process characterized by localized decaying and sloughing of skin. This dead tissue is an excellent medium for the growth and proliferation of infectious agents. The decubitus must be cleaned and cared for frequently (see Technique No. 78, Pressure Sore, Prevention and Treatment).

3. Meticulous handwashing before and after the backrub should be carried out to avoid the chance of cross-infection between clients.

Technique Checklist

	YES	NO
Procedure explained to client	_____	_____
Friction-reducing agent used	_____	_____

    Lotion _____

    Powder/cornstarch _____

    Medicated lotion ordered by physician _____

Desired effect of backrub

    Sedation _____

    Stimulation _____

    Healing _____

	YES	NO
Was skin breakdown prevented?	_____	_____
Were the lines of communication opened and maintained?	_____	_____
Family taught the proper technique for backrub	_____	_____

27 Bandaging

Overview

Definition

The application of a continuous strip of woven material to a body part. Types of bandages are as follows:

Ace: A commercially prepared bandage of woven elastic material capable of giving strong support

Gauze: A soft, porous, woven, light-weight cotton, which molds easily to body parts and is used frequently to retain dressings

Kling/Kerlix: A woven, porous gauze that stretches and molds to body contours and is self-adhesive.

Rationale

Limit motion of the affected part.

Secure a dressing.

Secure splints.

Provide support.

Apply pressure.

Secure traction apparatus.

Aid the return of venous circulation from the extremities to the heart.

Terminology

Distal: Farthest from the midline of the body

Proximal: Nearest the point of attachment

Assessment

Pertinent Anatomy and Physiology

See Appendix I: *skeletal muscles, skeletal system, skin.*

Pathophysiological Concepts

1. *Muscle tone* refers to a normal state of vigor or tension that is common to all healthy muscle. It involves a sustained mild contraction of some muscle fibers, along with relaxation of others; this gives the muscle firmness and supportive potential. Muscle tone is often reduced when one is in poor health, especially if prolonged bed rest is necessary. Improper application of bandages can promote the formation of *contractures*, or abnormal positioning of the joints due to fibrous growth and shortening or lengthening of the involved muscles.

2. Young skin is extensible and elastic, but as one grows older, certain changes occur. The skin becomes thinner, there are fewer elastic fibers, and fat disappears from the lower tissue, resulting in wrinkling. The blood supply to the skin is important in the regulation of body temperature and the nourishment of tissue cells. Interference with the blood supply to the skin will cause death of cells and result in areas of ulceration.

Assessment of the Client

1. Assess the bandages to ascertain the degree of mobility possible and the adequacy of blood supply to the dependent part.

2. Assess the adequacy of the bandaging technique in achieving the desired effect.

3. Assess the emotional and physical condition of the client in relation to ability to cooperate with and accept the necessary course of treatment.

Plan

Nursing Objectives

Allay fear and anxiety.

Promote physical comfort.

Maintain body alignment.

Make sure that the bandage accomplishes its intended purpose (e.g., support or immobilization).

Prevent contact of two skin areas by applying appropriate padding.

Protect bony prominences by applying appropriate padding.

Prevent venous stasis.

Client Preparation

1. Microorganisms flourish in warm, moist, contaminated areas. Wounds should be aseptically prepared before bandaging (see Technique No. 49, Dressings, Surgical). In addition, prolonged heat and moisture on the skin may cause epithelial cells to deteriorate. A bandage should be applied only over a clean, dry area. It should not be excessively thick or extensive, since this promotes an overly warm environment. Porous materials allow air to circulate more thoroughly.

2. Complete assembly of equipment prior to initiating the procedure will reduce the risk of tiring the client because of delays.

Equipment

Specified bandage

Medications, dressings, equiment as ordered

Tape (for some types of bandages)

Pins, clips (for some types of bandges)

Implementation and Interventions

Procedural Aspects

ACTION	*RATIONALE*
1. Place the part to be bandaged in a normal functioning position.	Placing the part in the position of normal function helps to prevent deformities and discomfort. It also enhances the circulation to the involved part.
2. Apply appropriate padding to separate adjacent skin areas and protect bony prominences (Fig. 27-1).	Friction and pressure can cause mechanical trauma to the skin.

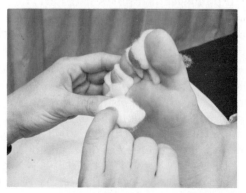

Figure 27.1

Procedural Aspects

ACTION

3. Apply the bandages from distal to proximal parts.

4. When applying the bandage, take care to ensure even distribution of pressure throughout. Securing the end of the bandage helps maintain even pressure along the entire length of the bandage. Secure with tape or clips.

5. If possible, leave a small area at the end of the bandaged extremity exposed, such as a toe or finger. This is not practical when the area is actually involved in the healing process, such as the stump of an amputated part (Fig. 27-2).

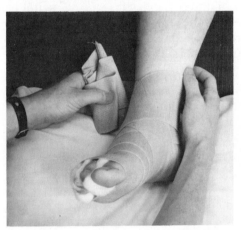

Figure 27.2

6. Basic bandage patterns:

   Circular: Each round of bandage slightly overlaps the entire previous round, thus creating a bandage that is the width of the material itself (Figs. 27-3 to 27-6).

RATIONALE

Application of the bandage toward the midline of the body encourages return of venous flow to the heart.

Uneven pressure can interfere with blood circulation and cell nourishment and slow the healing process. Secure application prevents the bandage from moving when the client moves, causing friction that may result in skin abrasions and chafing.

Direct visualization of an affected limb is desirable in order to check the adequacy of circulation.

A circular bandage is used primarily for anchoring a bandage where it begins and terminates.

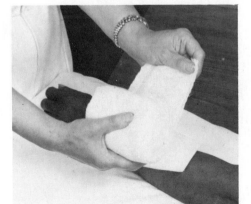

Figure 27.3

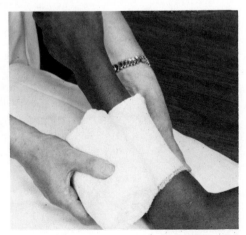

Figure 27.4

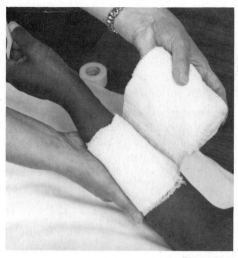

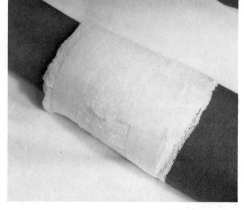

Figure 27.6

Figure 27.5

ACTION

Spiral: Each round of bandage slightly overlaps the previous round to create a progression up the limb (Figs. 27-7 to 27-10).

RATIONALE

A spiral bandage is useful for a cylindrical body part, such as the finger, wrist, or trunk.

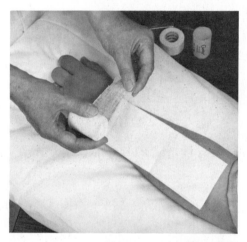

Figure 27.7

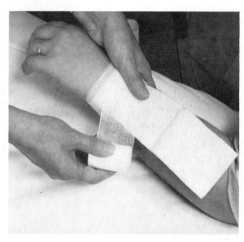

Figure 27.8

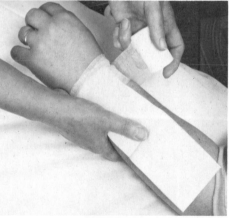

Figure 27.9

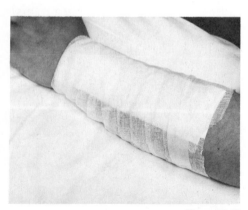

Figure 27.10

ACTION	**RATIONALE**
Spiral reverse: The bandage is anchored by several rounds of spiral. Then, with each round, the top of the bandage is turned under. (Figs. 27-11 to 27-14).	A spiral reverse bandage is used for bandaging a cone-shaped body part, such as the thigh, leg, or forearm.

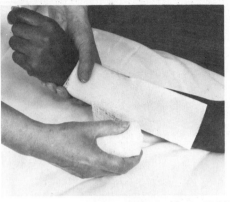

Figure 27.11

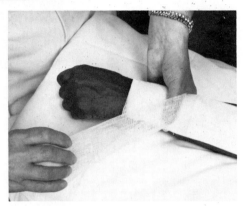

Figure 27.12

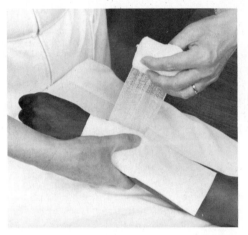

Figure 27.13

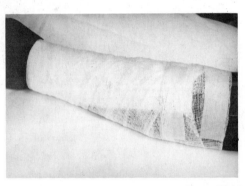

Figure 27.14

Figure 8: A figure 8 bandage is used for joints. It is anchored by several rounds of spiral below the joint. A round is then made above the joint and alternately below and above until the entire joint is covered (Figs. 27-15 to 27-18).	A figure 8 bandage provides a snug fit and is therefore used for immobilization around joints such as the knee, elbow, ankle, and wrist.

ACTION

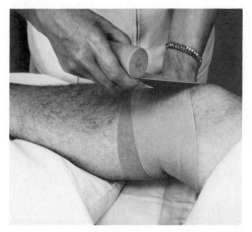

Figure 27.15

RATIONALE

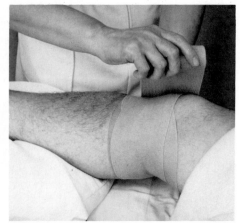

Figure 27.16

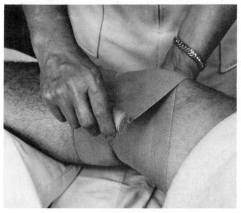

Figure 27.17

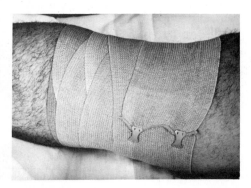

Figure 27.18

ACTION

Spica: This is the same as a figure 8 bandage, except that it usually covers a much larger area, such as the hip (Fig. 27-19).

RATIONALE

A spica bandage is particularly useful in bandaging the thumb, breast, shoulder, groin, and hip.

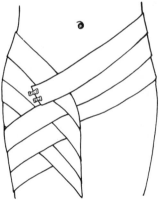

Figure 27.19

ACTION

Recurrent: The bandage is first positioned by two circular turns. The roll is then turned perpendicular to the circular turns and passed back to front and front to back, overlapping each time until the area is covered. It is secured by making two circular turns over the initial circular turns (Fig. 27-20).

RATIONALE

A recurrent bandage is used for anchoring a dressing on the head, a stump, or a finger.

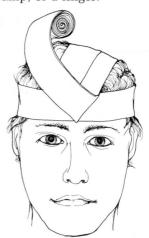

Communicative Aspects

OBSERVATIONS

1. Observe frequently for signs of restricted circulation. Check for blanching, erythema (redness), cyanosis, tingling sensation, edema, and coldness of the tissues (Fig. 27-21).

2. Unusual drainage or odor may indicate a pressure area or infection.

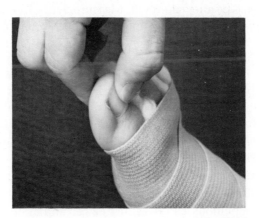

Figure 27.21

CHARTING

DATE/TIME	OBSERVATIONS	SIGNATURE
5/19 1500	Ace bandage applied to left leg from toe to groin. Rt. foot very edematous. States he had phlebitis in his left leg several years ago. Hospitalization was not necessary at that time. B/P 176/88, P 84, R 18, T 99.8	F. White RN
1515	Toes blanch on left leg. States that discomfort has decreased.	F. White RN

Discharge Planning Aspects

CLIENT AND FAMILY EDUCATION

1. Instruct the client and family on the technique for applying bandages if the client is to be discharged with bandages.

2. Inform the client and family about where to purchase bandages and how to wash them, if washable. Ace bandages are to be washed in mild detergent,

rinsed thoroughly, and allowed to drip dry. If a healing wound is located under the bandage, explain the technique and importance of first applying a sterile dressing to the wound before bandaging.

3. Instruct the client to elevate body parts if there are signs of impaired circulation, such as swelling, and there are no contraindications to such an action. Swelling may be a sign that the bandage is being applied too tightly. Advise the client to notify the physician if loosening the bandage and elevating the body part do not alleviate the situation.

4. Instruct the client to report changes in appearance of the affected part to the physician.

5. Inform the client that the bandage will be snug; however, if the bandaged part becomes numb, loses sensation, or becomes painful, the nurse should be notified at once.

REFERRALS

The client and family should be told what type of bandages they will need and where to purchase them.

Evaluation

Quality Assurance

Documentation should reflect the condition that warranted bandaging, progression of the client's condition in relation to bandaging the part, and the client's reaction to the technique. The type of bandage, as well as the amount of equipment and materials used in the bandage, should be noted periodically in the chart. Appearance of the bandaged part should be noted, with particular emphasis on comparison with previous reports or observations. The nurse should document possible complications that accompany bandaging and measures taken to make sure that these did not occur. If complications did occur, document signs taken to reverse or alleviate them. Measurement of vital signs and assessment of the client's overall condition should be reflected periodically.

Infection Control

1. Unclean bandages may cause infection if applied over a wound. Keep all materials used in bandaging clean. Reusable bandages should be washed thoroughly in warm, sudsy water and rinsed, dried, and sterilized before reapplication. When the client goes home, sterilization may become impossible. In this case, emphasize the importance of applying sterile dressings to the wound and keeping the bandage as clean as possible. If the bandage gets excessively soiled, it should be replaced.

2. Observe aseptic technique when applying a bandage. If a healing wound is present, apply a sterile dressing before the bandage.

3. Observe meticulous handwashing before and after applying a bandage. Discard soiled or disposable dressings in a paper bag, which is taped shut and labeled "Contaminated." If infection is present, double bag the discarded dressing according to isolation technique (See Technique No. 66, Isolation Precautions).

Technique Checklist

	YES	NO
Client understood what would happen before procedure was initiated	_____	_____
Sterile dressing was applied before bandaging	_____	_____
Bandaged part was placed in normal anatomical position	_____	_____
Padding applied to decrease friction between exposed skin areas	_____	_____
Bandage applied with pressure evenly distributed along length	_____	_____

Bandaged extremity checked frequently for impaired
   circulation   _____ _____

   How often? _____

Bandage accomplished desired purpose:

   Immobility _____

   Securing a dressing _____

   Securing a splint _____

   Providing support _____

   Pressure on an area _____

   Securing traction _____

   Enhancing cardiovascular status _____

Client and family given adequate instruction on bandaging
   prior to discharge   _____ _____

28   Baths, Cleansing

Overview

Definition

The medium and method of cleansing the body; types are as follows:

Complete bed bath: The entire body of the client is washed at the bedside by the nurse.

Abbreviated bed bath: Only the parts of the client's body that might cause illness, odor, or discomfort if neglected are washed. This includes face, axillae, genitalia, anal region, back, and hands.

Partial bath: Complete or partial bathing of the client's body at the sink or tub or in the shower.

Rationale

Cleanse the skin to remove accumulated perspiration, sercretions, microorganisms, and debris to prevent infection and preserve the integrity of the skin.

Provide comfort and relaxation to a tired, restless client.

Stimulate circulation, both systemically and locally.

Promote muscle tone by active or passive exercise.

Remove products eliminated by the skin.

Prevent lung congestion by stimulating drainage through changes of position.

Improve the client's self-esteem and self-image through improved appearance and feelings.

Terminology

Syncope: Faintness

Assessment

Pertinent Anatomy and Physiology

See Appendix I: *skin*.

Pathophysiological Concepts

1. The skin acts as an exchange surface for body heat and as a vapor barrier to prevent water from leaving the body. Body surface losses of sodium and water increase when there is excessive sweating or when large areas of skin have been damaged.

2. Moisture in contact with the skin for a prolonged period of time can cause irritation and predispose to the growth of bacteria.

Assessment of the Client

1. Assess the physical condition of the client to determine the type of bath that is needed. Assess the client's stamina and decide how much assistance is needed. Assess range of motion in determining the level of self-care possible during the bathing process.

2. During the bath, assess the condition of the skin. Determine the presence of rashes, bruises, scratches, and/or cuts and breaks in the integrity of the skin. Assess dryness of the skin and any special needs to determine the frequency of bathing and desirable cleansing agents to be used.

3. Use the opportunity for conversation afforded by the bathing procedure to assess the client's general frame of mind. Seek insights into the client's feelings about the illness.

Plan

Nursing Objectives

Promote hygiene and comfort for the client.

Observe the client's skin condition.

Assess the client's range of motion.

Encourage the client to be as independent as possible or allowed.

Assess the client's physical and mental status.

Establish between client and nurse a communication pattern that promotes health teaching and expression of client concerns.

Client Preparation

1. Before the bathing procedure is initiated, explain the procedure to the client. Allow the client to have a choice about the type of bath, if possible.

2. All necessary equipment should be gathered prior to beginning the procedure to avoid chilling the client during any delays.

3. For the bed bath, remove the top bed linen and replace it with a bath blanket to provide warmth and absorb moisture (Fig. 28-1). It is also less cumbersome. Close the windows and make sure that the client is not in a draft. Provide privacy for the procedure. Have the client void before beginning to ensure maximum comfort during the procedure.

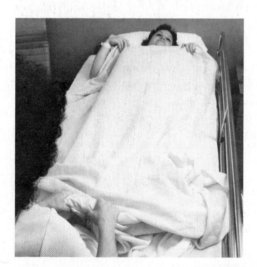

Figure 28.1

4. For the tub and shower bath, gather all articles prior to going to the bathroom. Be sure the client is physically able to perform the bath or remain in attendance to prevent falls.

Equipment

Bath towel

Washcloth

Soap

Lotion

Powder, if desired

Bath basin for bed bath

Toilet articles

Make-up for female clients

Implementation and Interventions

Procedural Aspects

ACTION

RATIONALE

Bed Bath

1. Fill the basin with water that is 110° to 115° F. Change the water as often as necessary to maintain the desired temperature.

Warm water tends to relax muscles and increase circulation by dilatation of blood vessels. Excessive heat may cause burns or diversion of blood from the vital centers of the brain, resulting in syncope.

2. Use soap to enhance cleansing unless the client is allergic, objects, or has excessively dry skin. Rinse the skin thoroughly so that all soap is removed.

Soap decreases surface tension and causes more efficient cleansing. Soap may irritate delicate tissues, such as the eye. When left in contact with the skin for a long period, soap is drying and can cause itching.

3. Fold the washcloth around the hand by laying the open hand palm side up on the cloth and folding each side over and the top down. Tuck the top under the palm side to secure it (Figs. 28-2 to 28-6).

The dangling ends of the cloth are annoying. Folding the cloth keeps it warmer longer.

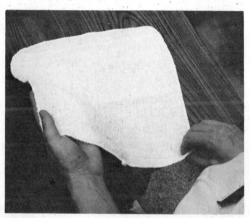

Figure 28.2

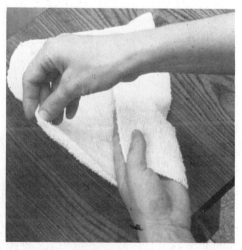

Figure 28.3

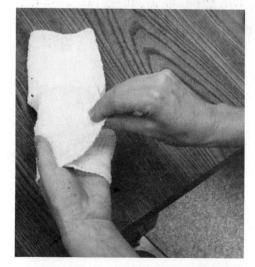

Figure 28.4

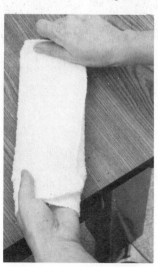

Figure 28.5

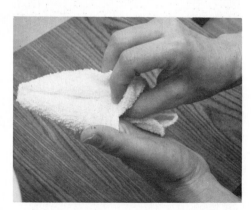

Figure 28.6

ACTION

4. Use firm, gentle strokes to cleanse the client's skin (Fig. 28-7). Cleanse the contaminated areas last. The suggested sequence for the bath is:

    Face
    Arms, hands, axillae
    Chest and abdomen
    Legs and feet
    Back
    Perineum
    Anal region

Place the towel under the limb to be cleansed (Figs. 28-8, 28-9).

RATIONALE

Firm, gentle strokes stimulate muscles and aid circulation. Following the suggested sequence will reduce the spread of microorganisms. Placing a towel under the limb protects the bed linen and facilitates drying.

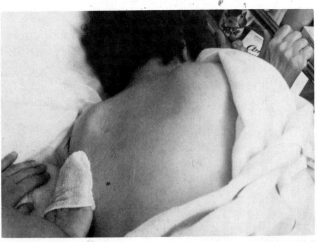

Figure 28.7

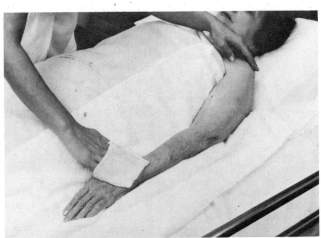

Figure 28.8

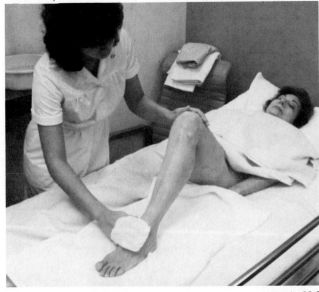

Figure 28.9

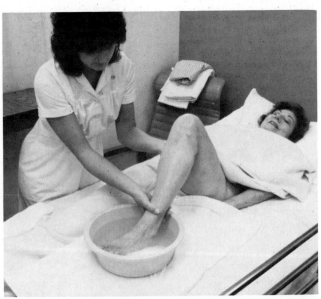

Figure 28.10

5. Immerse accessible body parts, such as the hands and feet, in the basin of bath water (Fig. 28-10).

Immersion aids in dissolving contaminants, removing debris, softens nails, and is refreshing to the client.

ACTION	**RATIONALE**
6. Move all body parts through their full range of motion during the bath, unless contraindicated (see Technique No. 80, Range-of-Motion Exercises).	Active and passive exercises prevent contractures and improve circulation.
7. Dry the skin thoroughly. Be careful not to scratch the client with long fingernails or rings. Apply lotion to the skin if the client wishes. Apply make-up to the female client if she desires and is able to tolerate it.	Thorough drying helps prevent decubitus ulcers and discourages bacterial growth. The integrity of the skin must not be compromised by accidental abrasions which can allow normal flora on the skin to penetrate into the body, where it is pathogenic. Lotion will also prevent drying and cracking of the skin and contribute to maintaining skin integrity.
8. The bath may be accompanied by shaving the male client, cleaning the nails, changing dressings, offering mouth care, shampooing the client's hair, and performing catheter care. Refer to the appropriate technique.	Bathing should promote a sense of well-being and should include all measures that the client can tolerate and desires.
9. Leave the client in a comfortable position and be sure the call light is within easy reach. Place the bed in low position.	Always ensure the safety of the client.

Abbreviated Bath

| The same principles apply as for the bed bath. However, only the parts of the client's body that might cause illness, odor, or discomfort if neglected are washed. Wash in this sequence:
    Face
    Hands
    Axillae
    Back
    Genitalia
    Anal region | When the client is too ill to tolerate a full bed bath, it is still important to complete minimum hygiene measures. |

Partial Bath

| The same principles apply as for the bed bath. Additional safety measures include the following: | |
| 1. Assist the client to and from the bathing area. Remain in attendance if the client is weak or unstable. If the client is left alone, be certain that the client knows where the call light is and how to use it. | Safety must always be of paramount importance. It is important to bathe the client; however, if there is any question about the safety of leaving the client in the bathing area, prudence would dictate bathing in bed rather than risking falls or other complications. |

ACTION	RATIONALE
2. Provide a chair in which the debilitated client can sit during the bath. Instruct the client in the use of the handrail and call light. Remain within close call of the client (Fig. 28-11).	Conserve the client's strength and make sure that safety needs are met.

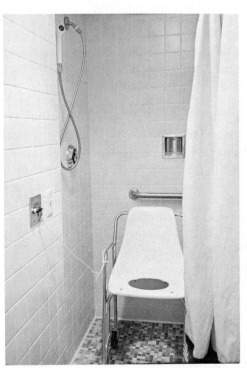

Figure 28.11

Special Modifications

Casts

1. When the client is in a plaster cast, avoid getting the plaster wet. Place a waterproof material over the cast when bathing the client. If a small part of the cast gets damp, it may be dried with an electric hair dryer. Observe or assist the client so that burns do not result (see Technique No. 37, Cast Care).	Plaster is a porous material, which breaks down when exposed to large amounts of water over a long period.

IVs

2. Bathe the client with an IV in the same way as any other client. However, the area around the infusion site will be covered with a sterile dressing. Bathe up to the dressing, being careful not to pull the tubing accidentally. The dressing on the infusion site should be changed using sterile technique every day (see Technique No. 65, Intravenous [IV]	The client with an IV risks infection from the break in skin integrity from the infusion. Skin care is very important to decrease the chance of infection. Since the presence of an infusion may also inhibit ambulation, the client may benefit from the activity of the bath and passive or active exercise program. Take care not to dislodge the infusion.

ACTION	RATIONALE
Infusion Administration). The IV bag or bottle should be passed through the sleeve of the hospital gown when the gown is changed in lieu of disconnecting tubing, which may lead to infection.	
3. When bathing the obese client, cornstarch may be used under the breasts and between overlapping abdominal folds to promote dryness and prevent skin breakdown. A cotton swab may be used to cleanse the umbilicus (Fig. 28-12).	Skin surfaces that are allowed to rub against each other are subject to skin breakdown and infection.

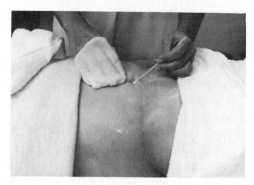

Figure 28.12

Communicative Aspects

OBSERVATIONS

1. Observe the client's activity, responses, mood, and general appearance.
2. Note skin changes, such as rash, discoloration, or other unusual chracteristics.
3. Check the progress of wound healing.
4. Observe areas around bony prominences and between skin folds, where the hazard of skin breakdown may develop from constant pressure or friction.
5. Observe the general hygiene habits of the client to determine areas needing health teaching.

CHARTING

DATE/TIME	OBSERVATIONS	SIGNATURE
7/30 0920	Reddened area observed over coccyx during complete bed bath. Area massaged gently. Skin is dry and has poor turgor. Lotion applied. States concern about surgery tomorrow. Explanation about surgery given. ————————	F. White RN

Discharge Planning Aspects

CLIENT AND FAMILY EDUCATION

1. Instruct the client and family about proper hygiene if deficiencies, such as the presence of fecal material on the buttocks or build-up of perspiration and debris between the folds of the skin, are discovered during the bath.
2. During the bath, converse with the client about physical condition and health potential. Use this time to answer questions and to offer health teaching.
3. If the client has a physical disability or will require help with bathing at home, teach the family proper technique, stressing safety precautions. Show the family how to do range-of-motion exercises and how to prevent skin breakdown.

Evaluation

Quality Assurance

Documentation should address the safety precautions taken. The client's condition and tolerance of the procedure should also be noted. Baseline vital signs should be reflected and used for comparison if complications arise. The documentation should reflect that the nurse was aware of the complications from prolonged bed rest and assessed the client to ensure prevention of these problems.

Infection Control

1. Cleansing the skin and drying it thoroughly help prevent the chance of infection by eliminating conditions favorable to bacterial growth. Cleansing should always proceed from the clean area to the contaminated area to prevent the chance of introducing pathogenic organisms into the clean area.

2. The skin is the natural protective barrier of the body. As long as it is intact, the risk of infection is minimized. The skin surfaces of hospitalized clients frequently become colonized with transient pathogenic organisms. Thorough bathing will help minimize the risk of these organisms entering the body through breaks in the skin or invasive devices such as urinary or intravenous catheters. The nurse should be careful not to scratch or otherwise traumatize the skin during bathing. Remove rings and shorten long fingernails before providing skin care.

3. Dead tissue associated with decubitus ulcer (a gangrenous process characterized by localized decaying and sloughing of skin) is an excellent medium for the growth and proliferation of infectious agents. The decubitus ulcer must be cleansed and cared for frequently (see Technique No. 78, Pressure Sore, Prevention and Treatment). Keeping the skin clean is an important measure in the prevention of decubitus ulcer.

Technique Checklist

	YES	NO
Explanation of procedure given prior to starting	———	———
Complete bed bath given	———	———
Chilling avoided	———	———
Condition of skin noted and charted	———	———
Range-of-motion exercises	———	———
Partial bath	———	———
Attendance while in bathing area	———	———
Complications avoided	———	———

29   Baths, Therapeutic

Overview

Definition

The medium and method of treating the body therapeutically by immersing the body or body parts in water of varying temperatures or in water with emollients added. Types of therapeutic baths are as follows:

Sitz bath: The immersion of the body from midthigh to iliac crest in water of a temperature from 100° to 115°F.

Emollient bath: The immersion of the body in a regular bathtub of water at 95° to 100°F containing one of the following:

Three cups of oatmeal

or

One pound of cornstarch

or

Eight ounces of sodium bicarbonate

or

Medication as ordered by the physician

Rationale

SITZ BATH

Promote phagocytosis through increased peripheral vasodilatation.

Stimulate formation of new tissue through increased blood supply.

Relieve pain by relieving pressure on nerve endings caused by deep congestion of blood.

Promote relaxation of local muscles.

Promote suppuration.

EMOLLIENT BATH

Soften and remove dermatologic crusts.

Relieve pruritus by protecting irritated skin from air currents or by coating skin with a palliative substance.

Apply medication to a large area of skin.

Protect skin lesions.

Terminology

Emollient A soothing and softening agent, applied locally

Palliative: Serving to relieve or alleviate without curing

Phagocytosis: Ingestion and digestion of bacteria and particles by a phagocyte

Pruritus: Severe itching

Suppuration: The process of pus formation

Assessment

Pertinent Anatomy and Physiology

See Appendix I: *skin.*

Pathophysiological Concepts

Pain is a personal, subjective, and unpleasant experience evoking unpleasant sensory, emotional, and motor responses. *Pain threshold* is the point at which stimuli begins to cause pain. *Pain tolerance,* on the other hand, is a measurement of the maximum intensity that one is willing to endure before willing something to be done about the pain. When it is not possible to eliminate the cause of pain, attempts must be made to moderate the reaction to pain. Drug therapy may be enhanced by palliative measures.

Plan

Nursing Objectives

Promote healing.

Relieve pain or pruritus.

Promote relaxation.

Promote pyschological comfort by soothing irritation.

Provide for cleanliness.

Client Preparation

1. Explain the reason for the bath and the actual procedure to be followed. Allow the client to ask questions to become more at ease about the procedure. Be sure the client knows the reason for the treatment.

2. Assemble all necessary equipment before taking the client to the bathing area.

3. Soiled dressings are contaminated. Remove these in the client's room prior to going to the bathing area and dispose of them according to proper technique. If an inner dressing adheres to the wound, it may be soaked off in the tub.

Equipment

Bath tub, sitz tub, or portable sitz tub

Water of indicated temperature

Bath thermometer

Medication, as ordered

Rubber or plastic ring for sitz bath, if indicated

Washcloths and towels

Implementation and Interventions

Procedural Aspects

ACTION	RATIONALE
Sitz Bath	
1. Run the water in a regular bathtub filled approximately one-sixth full. There are specially designed sitz tubs that allow the client to sit comfortably with hips and buttocks immersed in water. A portable sitz basin may be available for use in commode or chairs, or even in the bed. (Fig. 29-1).	The water should be warm enough to promote peripheral vasodilatation and comfort, but must not burn the client.

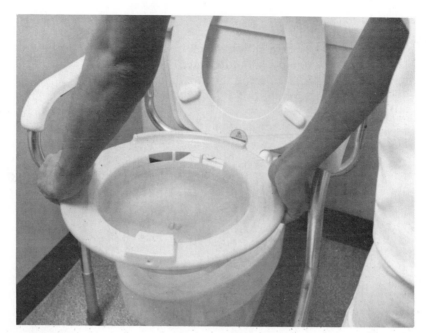

Figure 29.1

ACTION

If nothing else is available, a large basin may be used. The water should be 100°F to 115°F and should be measured with a bath thermometer.

2. Have the client sit on a rubber or plastic ring to relieve pain or the pressure and discomfort of rectal or perineal sutures.

3. Provide adequate assistance to and from the bathing area for the client. Ensure safety from falls and from anxiety by providing supervision based on the clinical condition and needs of the client.

4. The client's feet and legs should not, if possible, be immersed in the warm water. Seating the client in a specially designed sitz chair is preferable to seating in a bathtub.

5. A constant water temperature can be maintained by adding warm water as needed throughout the procedure.

6. The sitz bath should last approximately 10 to 20 minutes, or as ordered by the physician.

RATIONALE

Direct pressure on the operative area will cause increased pain.

Various aspects of the hospital regimen may predispose the client to weakness and fatigue. These include pain, surgical procedures, tension, anxiety, and medical treatments.

Local vasodilatation of the lower extremities will draw blood away from the perineal area.

Fluctuations in water temperature can cause cardiovascular stress.

Maximal benefit is obtained in the first 10 to 20 minutes. Prolonging the procedure tires the client and increases the risk of cardiovascular stress.

ACTION	*RATIONALE*
7. Place a bath blanket around the client's shoulders and over the knees during the sitz bath to prevent chilling (Fig. 29-2).	Chilling causes vasoconstriction, which counteracts the desired effect.

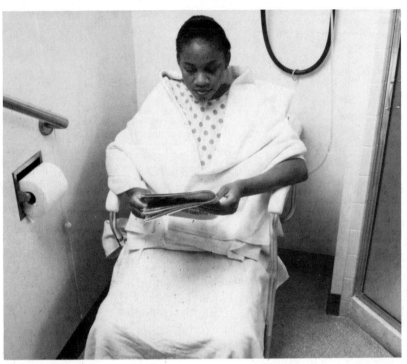

Figure 29.2

8. Check the client's pulse frequently during the sitz bath. If an irregularity occurs, return the client to bed at once.	Irregular or accelerated pulse may indicate cardiovascular stress.

Emollient Bath

1. Water temperature should be between 95°F and 100°F and should be determined with a bath thermometer.	Slightly warm water will prevent vasodilatation, which may increase pruritus.
2. Demonstrate acceptance of the client's skin condition by avoiding staring or showing signs of revulsion, by looking at the client rather than the lesion or affected area, and by allowing the client to verbalize feelings about disfigurement.	Unpleasant skin conditions create fear of disfigurement and rejection by others.
3. Apply the emollient solution in the bath to those areas of the client's skin that are not submerged. Use light, gentle strokes of the washcloth. Pat the skin dry without rubbing.	Rubbing causes irritation and increased warmth, which increases pruritus.

ACTION	RATIONALE
4. Allow the client to soak in the emollient bath for 20 to 30 minutes so that the skin is coated but chilling is prevented.	Clients with skin problems may be prone to chilling.

Communicative Aspects

OBSERVATIONS

1. Note the appearance of the treated area.

2. Record the amount and character of drainage.

3. Observe the client's reaction to the procedure, including level of tolerance and results obtained (e.g., relief of pain or pruritus).

CHARTING

DATE/TIME	OBSERVATIONS	SIGNATURE
9/21 1130	Sitz bath to perineal region at 115°F for 20 min. No change in pulse noted. Incision appears clean with no drainage. States pain is relieved since bath. B/P 138/70, P 82, R 16.	G. Ivers RN
4/2 2130	Red macular rash on trunk, inner aspects of arms and thighs, behind knees, and soles of feet. Cornstarch bath at 98°F for 30 min. Entire body surface except head and neck submerged in bath. Rash does not appear to have increased in area or intensity. States that itching is greatly relieved since bath. Dried with minimal rubbing. B/P 144/62, P 68, R 18	F. White RN

Discharge Planning Aspects

CLIENT AND FAMILY EDUCATION

Sitz Bath

1. Instruct the client to keep fingers away from wounds.

2. Instruct the client to take a sitz bath after every bowel movement and as needed for relief of pain after rectal surgery unless contraindicated by condition or physician's orders.

3. Emphasize the importance of correct water temperature.

4. Tell the client to expect that the initial sensation in the wound area during sitz bath will be unpleasant because of the tenderness already present. However, this should soon subside, and the sitz bath will provide an excellent means of relief from pain and discomfort.

Emollient Bath

1. Discourage the client from scratching affected areas.

2. Instruct the client to avoid temperature extremes and wearing tight clothing.

3. Reinforce the physician's instructions concerning diet and allergies, if appropriate.

4. Tell the client that an unpleasant sensation may be expected upon entrance into the water. This is due to the already irritated condition of the skin. However, reinforce the idea that the tub bath should relieve itching and discomfort and promote relaxation.

5. Explain the procedure for emollient baths to the client and family if they are to be continued at home. Emphasize the need to prevent chilling and to avoid rubbing affected areas.

Evaluation

Quality Assurance

Document the condition for which the bath is prescribed. The condition of the skin, lesion, or wound should be documented before the procedure is begun and after each bath to determine the effectiveness of the therapeutic baths. The client's reaction to the bath should be noted, as well as precautions taken to ensure the client's safety and comfort.

Infection Control

1. The sitz tub or basin should be scrubbed and disinfected each time it is used. Since the presence of skin lesions or wounds allows entry of infectious microorganisms, the soaking receptacle must be free of contaminants before the client is allowed to enter.
2. The presence of skin conditions with crusts and exudate allows a vehicle for entry of microorganisms. In addition, many skin conditions are considered contagious. For this reason, the tub must be disinfected before and after the client's bath.
3. Wash hands thoroughly before and after assisting with a sitz or emollient bath to help eliminate the chance of cross-contamination.
4. For the client with a disease process requiring isolation precautions, use a disposable or individual sitz bath basin rather than a bathing facility shared with other clients.

Technique Checklist

	YES	NO
Assessment of client's condition	_____	_____
Client understood method of and reason for the bath	_____	_____
Water temperature within proper range as measured by bath thermometer	_____	_____

Time client remained in the bath:

_____ minutes

Type of emollient added to bath:

Oatmeal _____

Cornstarch _____

Sodium bicarbonate _____

Other _____

	YES	NO
Desired result of bath accomplished	_____	_____
Complications:	_____	_____

_____

_____

30   Bedmaking

Overview

Definition

The process of applying or changing bed linens; the types are as follows:

Unoccupied (open) bed: The bedmaking process used when the occupant is not in the bed

Occupied bed: The bedmaking process used when the client must remain in bed

Surgical bed: The bedmaking process used to prepare the bed to receive a client after return from the recovery room

Rationale

Provide a suitable environment in which the client will be able to carry on normal body activities 24 hours a day when unable to be out of bed.

Provide a suitable environment for comfort and rest for the client who is able to be out of bed for periods of time.

Terminology

Draw sheet: A narrow sheet placed across the bed over the bottom sheet. It covers the area between the client's chest and knees and is stretched tightly and tucked under each side of the bed. The draw sheet protects the mattress and lower sheet and helps keep the client dry and comfortable.

Mitered corner: A means of anchoring sheets on a mattress. See Implementation and Interventions section for procedure.

Assessment

Pertinent Anatomy and Physiology

See Appendix I: *skeletal system, skin, vertebral column.*

Pathophysiological Concepts

1. The two layers of the skin are firmly cemented together. However, excessive rubbing of the skin may cause the two layers to become forcibly separated, allowing interstitial fluid to accumulate in the area. This is called a *blister,* In addition, continued friction may compromise the integrity of the skin, allowing entrance of microorganisms and infection.

2. Interference with the normal blood supply to the skin will cause death of cells and result in areas of ulceration. Decubitus ulcers may occur when pressure is extended over a long period against one area of the skin. Those areas of the body particularly susceptible to ulceration are areas over the bony prominences, including the spine and rib cage.

Assessment of the Client

1. Assess the physical condition of the client to determine the amount of mobility possible. Determine whether or not the client may be out of bed for bedmaking. Check physician's orders to learn if there are medical reasons for the client remaining in bed. The primary consideration is the tolerance level and safety of the client and not the convenience of the nurse.

2. Assess the level of fatigue and discomfort of the client prior to making an occupied bed. Turning required during bedmaking is strenuous and tiring to the client. Use judgment in determining when the client can best tolerate this procedure. Timing may enhance the client's tolerance and comfort (i.e., 30 minutes after a pain medication or after a dressing change or breathing treatment may be the optimal time to make the occupied bed).

Plan

Nursing Objectives

Provide a clean environment.

Promote physical comfort.

Promote psychological comfort by providing a neat environment in which the client can receive visitors.

Prevent cross-contamination.

Prevent undue strain for the client and nurse.

Client Preparation

1. The client should be bathed before the occupied bed is made. This provides a clean environment; however, consideration of the client's condition and fatigue must be considered. It may be necessary to wait for the client to rest before making the bed.

2. Explain what actions will be expected from the client to facilitate the bedmaking process. Have all equipment at hand prior to beginning to reduce unnecessary delays.

Equipment

Contour sheet or flat sheet

Top sheet

Pillowcase(s), as needed

Draw sheet, if needed

Spread and blanket

Implementation and Interventions

Procedural Aspects

ACTION	RATIONALE
Unoccupied Bed	
1. Use appropriate handwashing technique before and after making the bed. Avoid contact between the linens and the nurse's clothing.	Bed linens harbor microorganisms, which can be transferred by direct contact with the hands or clothing.
2. Strip the linens from the bed carefully, form them into a compact bundle, and place them in a hamper or pillowcase (Figs. 30-1, 30-2). Do not place the linens on the floor.	Fanning soiled linens can spread microorganisms through the air. Contact with the floor is unsightly and can also contribute to the spread of infectious agents.

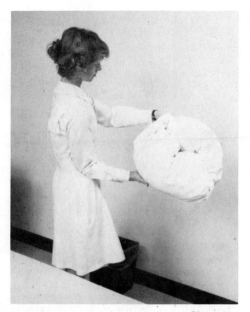

Figure 30.1

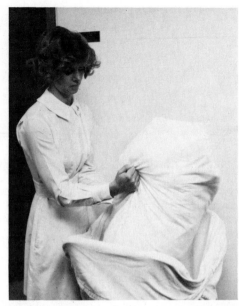

Figure 30.2

ACTION

3. Raise the bed to its highest position. Complete one side of the bed before moving to the other. Place the bottom sheet with its center fold in the center of the mattress.

   If it is a contour sheet, place the top and bottom corners on the nearest side over the corners of the mattress.

   If it is a flat sheet, align the end even with the foot of the mattress and secure the top with a mitered corner: place the end of the sheet evenly under the mattress (Fig. 30-3). The side edge of the sheet is then raised onto the bed (Fig. 30-4), and the remaining portion is tucked under the mattress edge (Fig. 30-5). The entire side section is then folded under the side of the mattress (Figs. 30-6 to 30-8). Both head and foot may be secured with mitered corners, if this is desired and the sheet is long enough.

   Place the center fold of the draw sheet in the center of the bed, and tuck the entire near edge securely under the mattress.

RATIONALE

Conserve time and energy as much as possible by avoiding unnecessary walking around the bed and working in a stooped position.

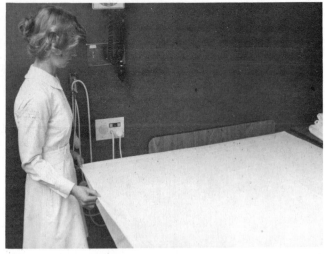

Figure 30.3

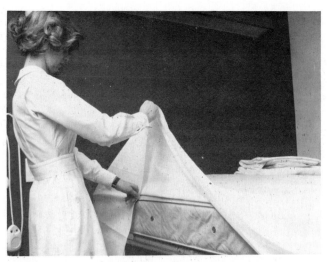

Figure 30.4

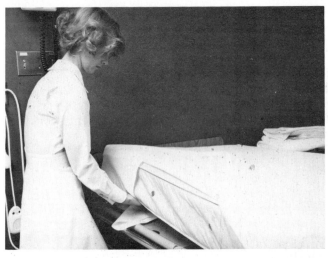

Figure 30.5

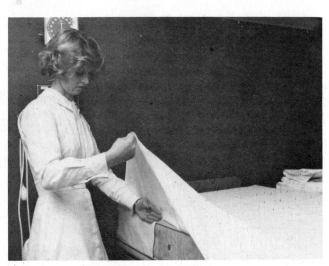

Figure 30.6

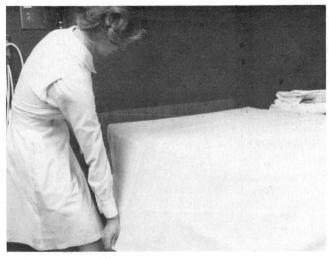

Figure 30.7

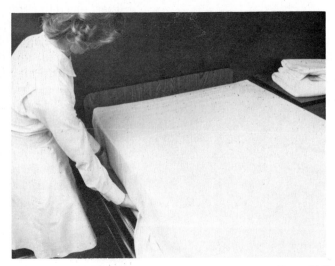

Figure 30.8

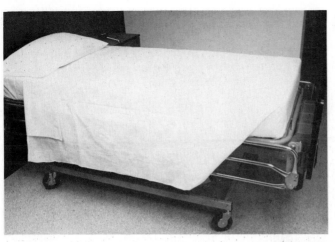

Figure 30.9

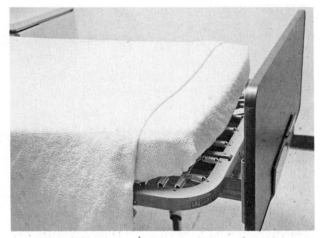

Figure 30.10

ACTION	RATIONALE
Place the center fold of the top sheet in the center of the bed and align the top edge even with the top of the mattress. Tuck the top sheet in at the nearest bottom corner of the mattress and secure with a mitered corner. To miter the foot section of the top sheet, the raised side edge is lowered to the side of the bed rather than tucked under, making a neat and serviceable corner (Fig. 30-9).	
Apply the spread in the same way as the top sheet. Move to the other side of the bed and repeat the entire process in the same sequence.	
4. Tighten the bottom sheet and the draw sheet and tuck them securely so that no wrinkles remain. Tighten the bedding, using the weight of the body applied through the large muscles of the legs and gluteals. Keep the back straight during this process.	A taut, wrinkle-free foundation lessens discomfort and pressure on the client. Using one's weight to counteract resistance from the sheets decreases the nurse's effort. Keeping the vertebral column straight prevents strain on the smaller, weaker back muscles.
5. Loosen the top linens. Finish the bed by forming a cuff, with the top sheet over the spread and a toe pleat at the foot of the bed (Fig. 30-10).	The top linens should not be tight, since this can exert pressure on the lower extremities of the client, resulting in discomfort and tissue breakdown.
6. The top linen may be fanfolded to the foot of the bed.	Lowering the top linens facilitates the client's return to bed.

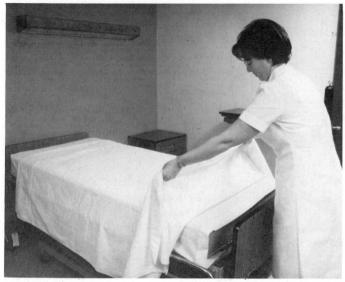

Figure 30.11

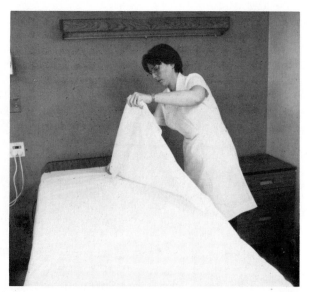

Figure 30.12

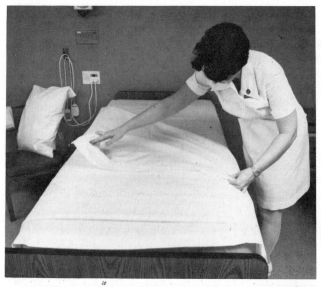

Figure 30.13

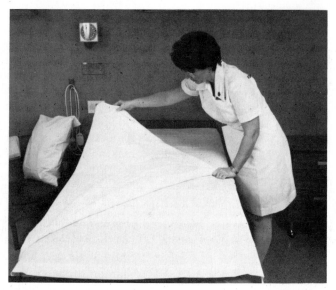

Figure 30.14

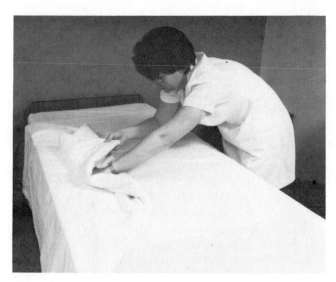

Figure 30.15

ACTION	RATIONALE

Surgical Bed

Prepare the same as an unoccupied bed, except the top linen. Do not tuck the top linen in at the foot of the bed. Fanfold it to the side of the bed away from the door through which the client will be returned from surgery (Figs. 30-11 to 30-15).

Fanfolding the linen facilitates transfer of the client from the stretcher to the bed without undue exposure or strain.

Occupied Bed

1. Raise the siderail on the side of the bed opposite the nurse. Roll the client to the far side of the bed. Encourage self help, if possible, by asking the client to hold onto the raised side rail. If the client is totally dependent, the draw sheet may be used to roll the client's body from one side to the other by lifting the opposite edge and letting the client roll by gravitational pull. Placing the client's near arm and leg across the midline of the body toward the opposite side will facilitate rolling. Be sure the siderail is up so that falls are prevented.

Rolling requires less strain on both the nurse and the client than does pushing or pulling.

2. The client should make as few position changes as possible. Loosen the soiled linens on the vacated side of the bed and tuck them under the client (Fig. 30-16). Place the clean linen on the bed, secure it in place on the near side, and fanfold it as far under the client as possible (Fig. 30-17). In one movement, roll the client over the soiled and clean linens toward the clean side of the bed. Have the side rail up for the client to use for assistance and to prevent falls. Move to the other side of the bed. Remove the soiled linens (Figs. 30-18, 30-19) and finish making the bed (Fig. 30-20). The top linen is secured as for an open bed.

Limiting the amount of position change lessens strain and fatigue for both the client and nurse. Keeping the siderail up on the side of the bed toward which the client is leaning will aid in support and enhance safety.

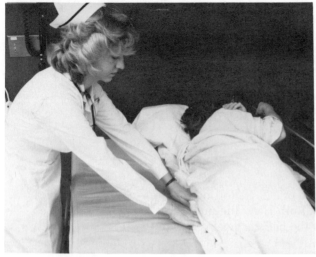

Figure 30.16

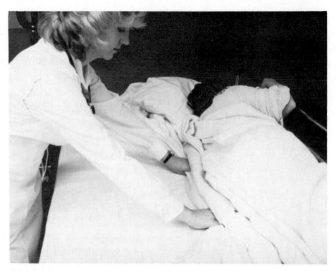

Figure 30.17

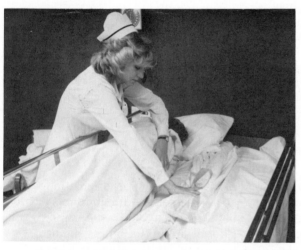

Figure 30.18

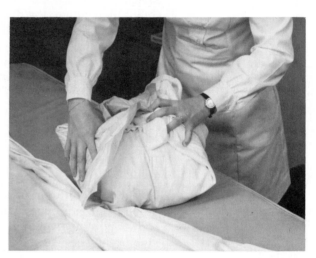

Figure 30.19

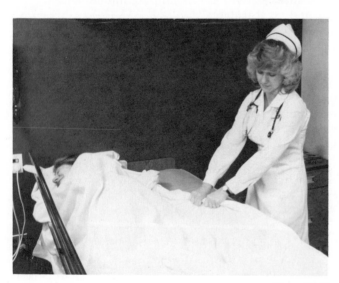

Figure 30.20

ACTION	RATIONALE
3. Protect the client's modesty and provide warmth by adequate draping during the procedure.	The client's ego may already be damaged due to the dependent nature of the condition. Attention to enhancing self-image by respecting modesty requires small effort and may prove vital to the client's emotional outlook.

Special Modifications

1. If the client is very weak or debilitated, obtain the assistance of another nurse in turning the client during the bedmaking process. The second nurse may also help hold the client in position while the opposite side of the bed is being made.	First and foremost, make sure that the client is not overly fatigued, strained, or jeopardized by the bedmaking procedure. Having assistance reduces the amount of participation required of the client.
2. Bed appliances should be applied before the client is placed in the bed, when possible. If the appliances must be applied with the client on the bed, secure the assistance of several other persons. Examples of bed appliances are foot board, air mattress, sheepskin, and eggcrate mattresses.	Adequate assistance in applying bed appliances will protect the client from falls or becoming overly fatigued. It will also protect the nursing personnel from strains.

Communicative Aspects

OBSERVATIONS

1. Observe the condition of the client's skin, with particular attention to the formation of pressure areas on the bony prominences of the heels and elbows.
2. Observe any limitations or problems with movement.
3. Observe the client's sensorium as evidenced by responses and by ability to follow instructions.

CHARTING

Chart anything unusual about the client noticed or occurring during the bedmaking procedure. It is usually not necessary to chart that the bed was made.

Discharge and Planning Aspects

CLIENT AND FAMILY EDUCATION

1. If the client will be confined to bed for a long period of time at home, show the family how to apply the draw sheet and the bottom sheet so that maximum comfort is provided.
2. Demonstrate to the family and client how to use proper body mechanics during bedmaking, to conserve energy and to minimize back strain.

REFERRALS

If a hopsital bed will be required by the client at home, refer the family to a hospital supply house where such beds may be rented or purchased.

Evaluation

Quality Assurance

If the client is very dependent, document safety precautions taken during bed-making to prevent falls.

Infection Control

1. Airborn microorganisms may be spread by shaking the linens during bed-making. Placing the linens inside a hamper or bag after they are removed minimizes the chance of contaminating the air.

2. Careful handwashing before and after making the client's bed is essential.

3. Removal of the linen from the room and the nursing unit should be done in a coordinated manner to make sure that others are not exposed to cross-infection through carelessness or poor technique. The linen should be transported to the general soiled linen room by chute or by covered cart. The cart should not be taken from room to room, since this may allow the spread of microorganisms. Linen may be wrapped in one of the sheets, taken to a central receiving area, and left in a covered container. Those handling soiled linen should wear gloves and protective covering over their clothing. Soiled linen should not be allowed to accumulate.

4. Some infectious processes requiring isolation may necessitate wearing a protective gown and gloves during the bedmaking procedure. Refer to Technique No. 66, Isolation Precautions.

Technique Checklist

	YES	NO
Procedure explained to client	————	————
Unoccupied bed		
Client able to be up without excessive fatigue	————	————
Occupied bed		
Client able to participate in turning during procedure	————	————
Assistance with turning required	————	————
Pressure areas noted	————	————
Location _____		
Family shown how to make an occupied bed	————	————

31

Bedpan and Urinal, Placing and Removing

Overview

Definition

Assisting the client with the processes of elimination through use of bedpan or urinal

Rationale

Maintain normal elimination patterns.

Promote healthful habits or regular bowel and urinary elimination.

Provide for accurate observation and measurement of the client's urine and stool.

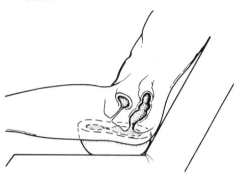

Figure 31.1

Terminology

Bedpan: A metal or plastic receptacle for receiving fecal and urinary discharges from the client confined to the bed (Fig. 31-1)

Bedside commode: A portable chair-type device with a container located beneath to receive the stool during elimination at the bedside

Fracture pan: A smaller bedpan with a sloping edge, which can be slipped under the client who cannot raise the hips sufficiently to sit on a regular bedpan

Urinal: A receptacle used to receive voided urine

Assessment

Pertinent Anatomy and Physiology

1. See Appendix I: *anus, bladder, genitalia (female), genitourinary system (male), kidneys, rectum, ureters, urethra, urination.*

2. The frequency of bowel elimination is variable. What is normal is the usual pattern for the individual person. Some persons defecate several times a day and some only three times each week. Defecation takes place when the sigmoid colon fills with feces, causing sensory stimulation of the internal anal sphincter. When this sphincter relaxes, feces are allowed to move into the rectum. Voluntary control relaxes the external anal sphincter to allow evacuation of the feces. The pressure exerted on the rectum by assuming the sitting position with the knees bent when defecating helps evacuate the bowel contents. If the need to defecate is ignored, the rectum eventually increases in size and loses some of its sensitivity to the stimulation to defecate; constipation is the result.

Pathophysiological Concepts

1. *Constipation* refers to difficulty in evacuating the stool. It is usually accompanied by straining and feelings of fullness in the lower abdomen. Causes may be indiscriminate use of laxatives, decreased fluid intake, ignoring the need to defecate, lack of exercise, some medications, and unbalanced diet. Prolonged retention of fecal material can result in fecal impaction. The feces become a hardened mass, which must be removed manually. Liquid stool often is passed around the mass. Prolonged blockage of the bowel results in bowel obstruction.

2. *Diarrhea* results when the bowel contents move along the digestive tract so quickly that liquids are not absorbed. When the stool reaches the rectum, it is still very liquid. Diarrhea often is accompanied by abdominal cramping and a sense of urgency. Causes of diarrhea may be certain medications, nervousness, indiscriminate use of laxatives, poor nutrition, and some diseases such as Crohn's disease and ulcerative colitis.

3. The *p*H of the urine is variable. When excess acid is present in the body, the kidneys excrete more hydrogen ions in the urine. For each hydrogen ion excreted, a bicarbonate ion is reabsorbed. Thus, acid is excreted and base is conserved in order to maintain the optimal hydrogen ion concentration in the extracellular fluid. Acidification of the urine depends on the active secretion of hydrogen ions in the kidneys. The kidneys are unable to produce a urine more acid than a *p*H of 4.4. The presence of urinary buffers prevents a sharp drop in the urinary *p*H but increases the amount of acid that can be excreted. The most important buffers in the urine are phosphate and ammonia. An increase in the amount of alkali in the body results in an elevated plasma bicarbonate concentration. When the amount of bicarbonate surpasses the amount of hydrogen ions available, the excess bicarbonate results in alkaline urine.

Assessment of the Client

1. Assess the ability of the client to get on and off the bedpan. Assess degree of mobility in determining whether to use a standard bedpan, a fracture pan or a bedside commode. Assess the ability of the client to hold the urinal in place and determine how much assistance is needed. Assess the client's awareness of the need to use the urinal or bedpan. Assess the steadiness of the client when sitting unassisted and the ability of the client to successfully pivot before placing the client on the bedside commode.

2. Assess the urine and feces of the client to determine presence of pathologic states. Assess the amount of feces in relation to the nutrition and activity level of the client. Assess the amount of urinary output in relation to the intake. Discrepancies should be noted and assessed as to possible pathology.

3. Assess the condition of the client's skin around the buttocks and the perineal area. Sitting on the bedpan for extended periods can lead to pressure and skin breakdown. Check the condition of the skin and determine pressure areas early so that padding can prevent breaks in the skin.

4. Assess the client in relation to cultural background. In some cultures, persons outside the family are not allowed to assist with elimination needs. In those circumstances, assess the ability of the family to meet elimination needs and the amount of teaching required to ensure safety.

Plan

Nursing Objectives

Establish a routine of elimination by offering the bedpan or urinal at regularly scheduled times or at the client's request.

Allay the embarrassment and guilt that may occur when the client must be dependent on others for fulfillment of this private, basic need.

Client Preparation

1. If the client will need assistance with placement of the equipment, explain initially exactly where the bedpan or urinal will be placed, how this will be accomplished, and what is expected of the client.

2. If the client will get up to the bedside commode, be certain that the receptacle for catching the stool is securely in place. Move the bedside commode to a convenient place near the side of the bed. Before the client arises, obtain any equipment needed for sitting up on the bedside commode, such as pillows, slippers, or robe.

Equipment

Clean, labeled bedpan

Bedside commode

Toilet tissue

Washcloth, towel, soap, and water

Clean, labeled urinal (the female urinal has a flared, cuplike top to fit the female anatomy; the male urinal simply has an opening in the top)

Cover

Aerosol air freshener, if the client has no allergies to such preparations

Linen protector

Implementation and Interventions

Procedural Aspects

ACTION	RATIONALE
1. If possible, have a person of the same sex assist the client with elimination needs. Provide privacy.	Normal functions of elimination may be inhibited by feelings of dependence and embarrassment.
2. Elimination will be enhanced if the head of the bed is elevated to as near a natural position as possible, if this is not contraindicated by the client's condition. Warm the bedpan by running warm water over it (Fig. 31-2). *Note:* The metal bedpan retains heat; be careful that it is not hot enough to burn the client. Dry the bedpan and powder the edges to facilitate insertion and removal by reducing friction.	Proper elimination may be hampered because the client cannot assume a normal physiologic position for elimination. The bedpan or urinal may be unfamiliar and uncomfortable.

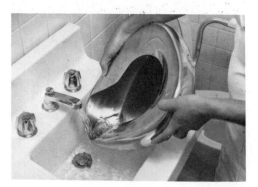

Figure 31.2

ACTION

3. Some clients can assist in placement of the bedpan and urinal. Ask the client to raise the hips from the bed and assist in the proper positioning of the bedpan as much as possible. (Fig. 31-3). Place padding under the lumbosacral area to promote comfort. (Figs. 31-4, 31-5). Hand the client the urinal and assist in raising the bedcovers while maintaining the client's privacy and modesty.

RATIONALE

A position of comfort with adequate support may facilitate elimination.

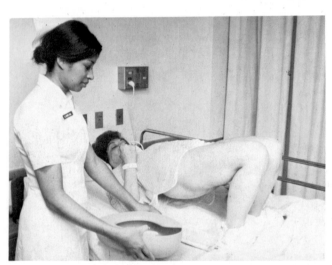

Figure 31.3

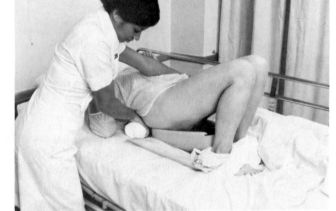

Figure 31.4

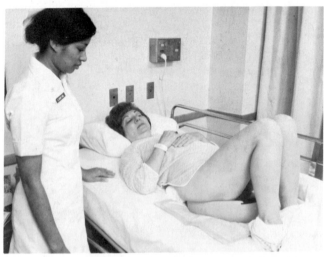

Figure 31.5

ACTION

4. If the client is weak and needs some assistance, place the linen protector, bedpan, and rolled towel within easy reach. Assist the client in the removal or rearrangement of clothing, gowns, or pajamas. Explain to the client about flexing both knees while keeping both feet flat on the bed. Assist the client to elevate the buttocks by placing one hand under the client's sacral area. Using the trunk muscles and elbow for leverage, assist the client to lift up while placing the linen protector, bedpan, and rolled towel with the free hand. Assist the client in lowering onto the bedpan gently (Figs. 31-6 to 31-8).

RATIONALE

Some clients cannot turn to the side easily because of casts, equipment, or debility. Lifting the hips may be more effective in conserving energy and promoting comfort.

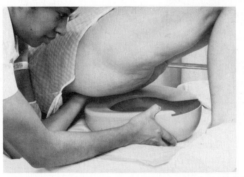

Figure 31.6

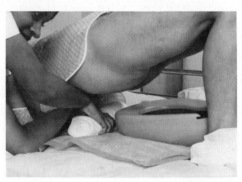

Figure 31.7

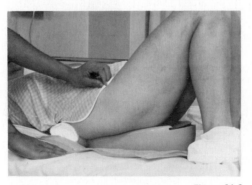

Figure 31.8

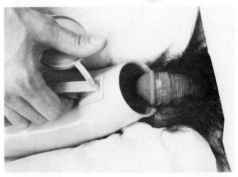

Figure 31.9

5. For the client who cannot assist in placement of the urinal, do this for the client in a matter-of-fact way. Place the urinal in position with minimal exposure. (Fig. 31-9). Tell the client when the urinal is in place and assist by holding the urinal if necessary. Keep the client draped and avoid exposure.

Protect the client's modesty, privacy, and self-respect by projecting a professional attitude, and a sense of caring by providing adequate screening and draping.

ACTION

RATIONALE

6. For the client who cannot assist in placement of the bedpan: If no lifting movement is possible, roll the client toward the opposite side of the bed. Place the bedpan against the client's buttocks in the proper position and hold it in place as the client rolls back over onto the bedpan. (Figs. 31-10 to 31-12). Again, pad the back for comfort.

A rolling motion creates less strain and exertion for both the client and the nurse than does a lifting or pushing motion.

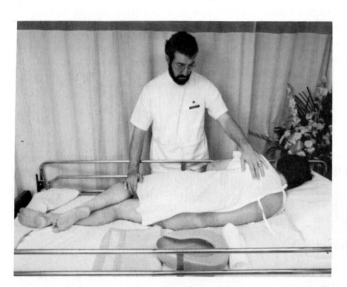

Figure 31.10

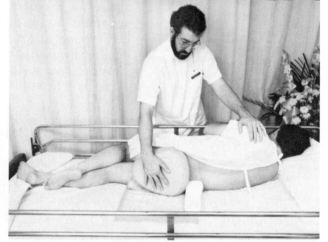

Figure 31.11

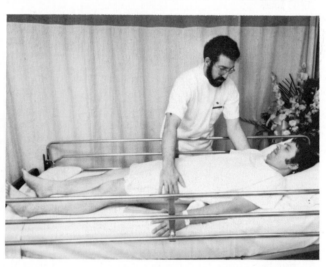

Figure 31.12

ACTION

RATIONALE

7. Place the call button within easy reach of the client and answer it promptly. If the client is weak or confused, remain nearby in case help is needed.

8. Allow the client to do self-cleaning after using the bedpan. If the client is unable to do self-cleaning, offer water and a washcloth for hand-washing (Fig. 31-13). Assist the client if necessary. Cleanse the rectal and perineal area with minimal exposure. For the female, always cleanse the perineum from *front to back*. If the skin is not cleansed thoroughly with toilet tissue, use warm water and soap and dry thoroughly.

Prompt attention to the signal call bolsters the client's confidence in the staff and prevents unnecessary time spent on the bedpan, with the possibility of creating a pressure area. Self-care enhances self-esteem. Teaching proper bowel habits is an important function of the staff while the client is hospitalized. Everyone should engage in handwashing after each bowel movement. The perineum is always cleansed from front to back to prevent contamination of the vaginal area or the urethral area with fecal material. Proper cleansing is needed to reduce the number of micro-organisms present and to promote the comfort and well-being of the client. Perineal irritation and/or infection can occur from improper cleaning.

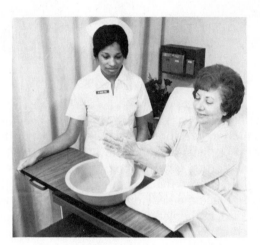

Figure 31.13

9. Note the contents of the bedpan or urinal. Cover it and take it to the bathroom to empty. If a specimen is needed, collect it and send it to the laboratory. Clean the bedpan or urinal and store all equipment properly.

Proper cleansing and storage promote a clean and healthful environment.

ACTION

RATIONALE

Special Modifications

1. For the client in a lower-limb cast or traction who cannot raise the hips, a flattened bedpan (fracture pan) may be used (Fig. 31-14). Powder the pan and slip it under the client, who may raise one hip as much as possible (Fig. 31-15). Position a pad under the client in case of spillage. Cleanse the client well and be sure the linen is dry.

The flattened pan will slide more easily under the client who cannot bend at the waist or at the knees. Proper cleansing after the procedure is essential to prevent irritation and infection.

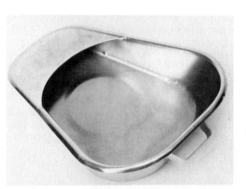

Figure 31.14

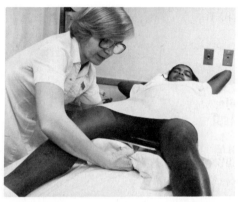

Figure 31.15

2. For the client who has only minimal locomotion capabilities or who is weak, a bedside commode may allow a normal elimination posture while conserving strength (Fig. 31-16). Place the bedside commode next to the bed and assist the client to be seated on it, using the pivot technique (see Technique No. 76, Position, Change of). Be sure that the client is not too weak to sit on the commode. Leave the call button within easy reach. Remain with the client if there is any question of the client's safety on the bedside commode. After the client finishes, allow the opportunity for handwashing, assist in cleansing the client's buttocks, and assist the client back to bed. Empty the stool immediately and rinse the receptacle. Store the commode chair nearby, out of sight, if possible.

The bedside commode offers the capability of allowing the client to sit in the normal position for elimination. It can be moved to the best place to facilitate client transfer. The stool should be emptied immediately to provide a pleasant environment for the client.

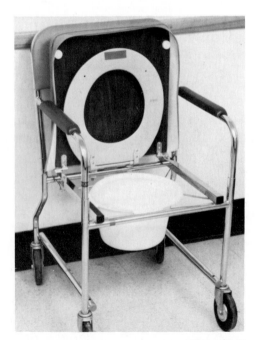

Figure 31.16

Communicative Aspects

OBSERVATIONS

1. If intake and output must be recorded, measure the urine accurately and chart the amount. Also, observe the color, odor, and consistency of the urine.
2. If the client has passed feces, note the color, consistency, odor, and amount. Report anything unusual, such as the presence of blood or worms.
3. Observe the skin around the buttocks and perineal area for signs of pressure from using the bedpan.
4. Observe the method used by the client to get on and off the bedpan. Determine if there is a better way. Seek input from the client. Observe the client on the bedside commode for signs of fatigue.

CHARTING

DATE/TIME	OBSERVATIONS	SIGNATURE
3/1 1000	Large, softly formed brown stool in bedpan. States he feels much better now and that added roughage to his diet seems to have helped with passing the stool.	G. Ivers RN

Discharge Planning Aspects

CLIENT AND FAMILY EDUCATION

1. Prolonged bed rest may adversely alter normal patterns of elimination. Explain that these changes are usually temporary and related to lack of activity, changes in diet, and medications. Normal regularity usually resumes when the client's health improves and normal activities are resumed. Factors that promote normal regularity are adequate fluid intake, roughage in the diet, and laxative juices such as prune or apricot juice.
2. Instruct the client and family to inform the physician when serious problems with elimination arise so that medication or treatment to correct the problem can be prescribed to prevent severe complications.
3. Some clients are not aware of what constitutes regularity and feel that if they do not have a daily bowel movement, something is wrong. Teach the client and family that the normal pattern of elimination varies greatly among individuals. For one person, two or three stools daily may be normal, whereas for another, a stool every other day is normal.
4. Instruct the client about how variations from the normal pattern of living, such as hospitalization, vacations, and emotional stress can temporarily affect elimination.
5. Teach the family the techniques of using the bedpan, bedside commode, and urinal if the client will not be able to resume normal activities when discharged.
6. Emphasize to all female clients and to parents of female children the great importance of cleansing the female perineum from front to back.

Evaluation

Quality Assurance

Each hospital should have a system of handling eliminatory processes that ensures prevention of contamination of other persons: for example, methods of assignment of bedpans and urinals should be specified, sewage should be processed so that infectious organisms do not enter the public sewage; bathroom facilities should be available to all clients; and terminal cleansing of reusable bedpans and urinals should be done in a consistent and efficient manner. Any problems with using the bedpan and urinal should be noted in the chart. It is not necessary to note each time that a bedpan or urinal is used; however, the chart should reflect attention to adequate intake and output and to adequate bowel elimination.

Infection Control

1. All equipment used consecutively by different clients should be disinfected after each client's use. When the bedpan is emptied, it should be cleaned with hot water and washed free of all fecal material, which could be a breeding ground for pathogenic bacteria.

4. After defecation, the debilitated client's anal and perineal area should be cleansed with warm water and soap to remove all fecal material. The person in a weakened state is particularly susceptible to infection.

3. Handwashing before and after assisting the client is necessary for the nurse. Assist the client to do handwashing after the bowel movement, even if the client did not do self-cleaning, in an effort to form or reinforce good hygiene habits. The client should also be offered the opportunity to do handwashing after using the urinal.

4. After use, the bedpan should be cleaned with hot water. Any remaining fecal material should be scrubbed free with a brush specifically designated for this purpose. The bedpan should be stored in the client's bathroom and properly labeled with the client's name and room number. The bedpan should not be stored in close proximity to any area where eating or oral care is done, such as above the sink.

Technique Checklist

	YES	NO
Client understood the procedure before bedpan, beside commode, or urinal was offered	_____	_____
Adequate output noted	_____	_____
Bedpan used by client	_____	_____
Placed by client	_____	_____
Placed by nurse	_____	_____
Pressure areas on hips and/or buttocks	_____	_____
Irritation and infection of rectal area prevented	_____	_____
Family understood how to care for client's elimination needs at home	_____	_____

32

Binders, Application of

Overview

Definition

A broad bandage encircling the abdomen or chest; types are as follows:
Straight abdominal binder
Scultetus (many-tailed) binder
T-binder

Rationale

Secure dressings.
Provide abdominal support.
Prevent tension on sutures and wounds.
Prevent irritation when client is allergic to adhesive.

Terminology

Sanguineous: Bloody

Vulva: The external female genitalia

Assessment

Pertinent Anatomy and Physiology

1. See Appendix I: *genitalia (female), genitourinary system (male), skin.*
2. The major organs located in the abdominal area include the liver, stomach, spleen, gallbladder, pancreas, large and small intestines, and kidneys (Fig. 32-1).

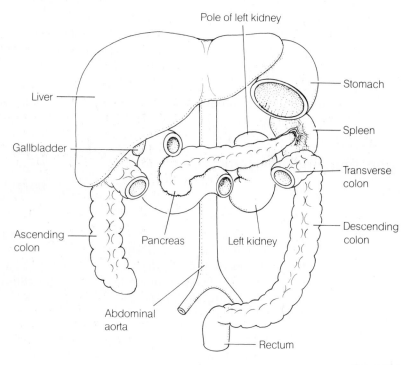

Figure 32.1

Pathophysiological Concepts	1. The function of the male scrotum is to regulate the temperature of the testes. The optimal temperature for sperm production is about 2° to 3° below body temperature. If the temperature is too low, the scrotal muscles contract, causing the testes to be brought up tight against the body. When the testicular temperature rises, these muscles relax, allowing the scrotal sac to fall away from the body. Tight-fitting clothing may hold the testes against the body and contribute to infertility.
	2. The Bartholin's glands in the female genitalia may become infected, causing bilateral or unilateral swelling and pain. Purulent discharge may indicate gonococcal infection. Infection may progress to formation of an abscess, which requires surgical intervention.
Assessment of the Client	1. Assess the extent of the wound or incision in relation to the activity level of the client to determine which type of binder will best achieve the desired purpose.
	2. Assess the skin under the binder at frequent intervals to ensure its integrity. Determine whether the binder is too tight or wrinkled. Also, check for the proper anatomic alignment of body parts.
	3. Assess the allergy status of the client. If the client is allergic to adhesive tape, a binder may offer a satisfactory alternative. However, since many allergies may be present in the same person, a complete allergy history is appropriate.

Plan

Nursing Objectives	Reduce tension on sutures and wounds.
	Keep the dressing(s) in place.
	Offer an alternative to tape for an allergic client.
	Alleviate incisional discomfort.
Client Preparation	1. If the purpose of the binder is to secure a dressing, the underlying dressing should be changed using sterile technique unless contraindicated by physician orders.
	2. Explain the expected effects of the binder application so that the client will understand and possibly be more cooperative.
	3. Gather all equipment before beginning. It might be helpful to show the client what the binder looks like and how it will be applied.
Equipment	Binder of appropriate type
	Safety pins or clamps, if needed

Implementation and Interventions

Procedural Aspects

ACTION	RATIONALE
Straight Abdominal Binder	
1. Place the binder under the client, with the lower border well under the hips. Fasten binder edges firmly to avoid friction. Begin fastening the binder at the bottom (Figs. 32-2, 32-3).	Maximal support is provided when pressure is equally distributed. Friction can cause irritation. Support from below reduces tension on the wound and adjacent parts.

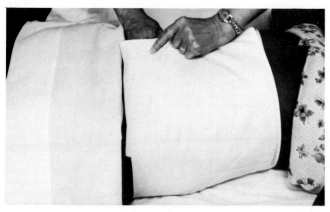

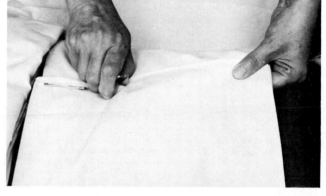

Figure 32.2

Figure 32.3

ACTION

2. Make darts where necessary so that the binder will fit snugly but allow adequate room for breathing. If the binder extends above the waistline, loosen it slightly to avoid interfering with respirations. Many binders fasten with a self-adhesing material, which allows the binder to be fit to the contours of the client's body.

Scultetus (many-tailed) Binder

1. Place the binder well under the hips, with no wrinkles. Bring the lower strap straight across the body and tuck at the opposite side. Bring the remaining straps across the center one by one, alternating sides and slanting to achieve a fishtail effect. The final two straps come straight across the body, as do the first two. Secure the top strap with two safety pins placed horizontally. Take care to apply the same amount of pressure to each strap (Figs. 32-4, 32-5).

RATIONALE

A tight binder may reduce chest expansion during respirations. However, the binder must be tight enough to provide support.

Maximal support is achieved when pressure is equally distributed. Uneven pressure can interfere with circulation and cause discomfort.

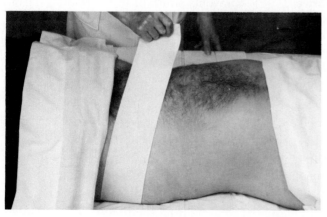

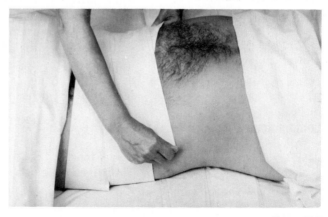

Figure 32.4

Figure 32.5

ACTION

RATIONALE

2. Examine the client carefully for the compression of tubes and drains.

Tubes and drains depend on patency to function properly. Compression inhibits the drainage capabilities.

T-binder (Fig. 32-6)

1. The T-binder is used to secure dressings in the perineal area. A single T-binder is used for women, and a double T-binder is used for men. If surgery has been extensive and the dressing is large, a double T-binder may be used for the female client.

The scrotal sac and penis are very sensitive. The double T-binder allows the dressing to remain secure without exerting pressure on the male genitalia.

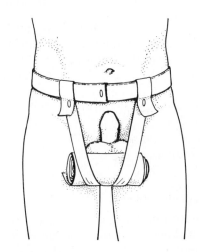

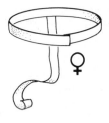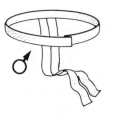

Figure 32.6

2. Secure the T-binder around the waist, bring the strap(s) forward between the legs and secure to the waistband. Because of the sensitivity of the genitals, care must be taken to make sure that the binder is comfortable and secure and is fulfilling the purpose.

Anchoring the binder from the waist prevents strain or pressure on the genitalia.

Communicative Aspects

OBSERVATIONS

1. Check for drainage under the binder, noting both amount and characteristics. The appearance of sanguineous drainage calls for close observation and appropriate measures to prevent extensive blood loss.

2. Observe for any strong or foul odors emanating from the binder. These may indicate infection.

3. Observe the client during periods of activity to make sure that the binder is secure and snug. Determine proper positioning of the binder.

4. Observe the client's skin under the binder for pressure or chaffed areas.

5. Observe for patency of tubes and drains.

CHARTING

DATE/TIME	OBSERVATIONS	SIGNATURE
4/29 1330	T-binder applied to retain scrotal dressing after bilateral orchidectomy. Incision cleansed, slight redness and no drainage. Binder secured with no statements of discomfort at this time. ————————	F. White RN

Discharge Planning Aspects

CLIENT AND FAMILY EDUCATION

1. Instruct the client to notify the nurse if the binder is loose or uncomfortable in any way. Stress the importance of reapplying the binder to avoid pressure areas or irritation. Stress the fact that after a period of time, the binder may begin to cause irritation. This should be reported to the nurse. After initial application, the binder may feel constricting and uncomfortable, but this should subside. If initial discomfort does not subside in 10 to 15 minutes, it should be reported to the person in charge.

2. Inform the client and family of the reason for the binder. Tell the client the desired effect of the binder and elicit cooperation in assessing the success of the procedure.

REFERRALS

If binders will be needed after discharge from the hospital, tell the client and family where these may be purchased and how to care for them. The American Cancer Society may provide assistance in obtaining binders for the client diagnosed as having cancer.

Evaluation

Quality Assurance

Document the reason for the binder and the client's understanding and acceptance of the procedure. The documentation should also reflect the nurses' knowledge of possible complications resulting from incorrect positioning of the binder, poor alignment of anatomy beneath the binder, and improper application technique, as well as the measures taken to prevent these complications. The results of the binder application should be reflected as compared with the desired results. If the desired results were not obtained, evidence of notification of the physician and further measures should be reflected. The reaction of the client, both physically and psychologically, should be noted.

Infection Control

1. Thorough handwashing should be carried out prior to and after application of the binder.

2. The binder should be cleaned whenever it becomes soiled. If the client is experiencing a large amount of drainage, it may be necessary to have two binders so that one can be cleaned while the other is being worn. Most binders are cleaned by washing in a mild detergent, rinsing thoroughly, and drying. If the drainage is infected, the binder should be bagged and sterilized to kill infectious organisms, in addition to being cleaned.

3. Dressings under the binder should be changed frequently, or as ordered by the physician, to decrease the risk of the wound becoming infected. All dressings should be sterile.

Technique Checklist

	YES	NO
Procedure explained to client	————	————
Sterile dressing applied prior to binder application	————	————
Normal anatomic alignment ensured before applying the binder	————	————
Tubes and drains patent after binder applied	————	————
Drainage noted on binder	————	————
Drainage reported to physician	————	————
Desired effect of binder accomplished	————	————
Family and/or client taught how to apply binder:		
Demonstrated ability to apply binder	————	————
Understand where to obtain binders	————	————
Understand how to care for binders	————	————

33

Bladder Irrigations

Overview

Definition

The process of introducing a stream of solution into the bladder by means of a catheter and draining it by natural or artificial means

Rationale

Relieve inflammation of the bladder wall.

Prevent or treat infection.

Minimize formation of blood clots.

Maintain patency of urinary drainage system.

Terminology

Catheter: A tube for evacuating or instilling fluids

Closed system: A urinary drainage system in which the catheter is not separated from the tubing

Intermittent irrigation: The process of introducing and emptying solution from the bladder through a closed system at designated intervals

Manual irrigation: A single process of introducing and emptying solution from the bladder

Open system: A urinary drainage system in which the catheter is separated from the tubing

Three-way catheter: A double lumen tube consisting of an inflation tube, an irrigation tube; and a drainage tube (Fig. 33-1)

Tidal (through-and-through) irrigation: An automatic continuous process of introducing and emptying solution from the bladder through a closed system

Two-way catheter: A single lumen tube consisting of an inflation tube and a second tube through which irrigating solution is introduced and urine is allowed to drain (Fig. 33-2)

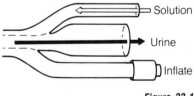

Figure 33.1

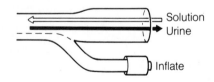

Figure 33.2

Assessment

Pertinent Anatomy and Physiology

See Appendix I: *bladder, urethra.*

Pathophysiological Concepts

1. In the male the urethra is completely surrounded by the prostate gland. When this gland begins to enlarge, as it frequently does in elderly men, it compresses the prostatic urethra and interferes with the flow of urine. Resection of the enlarged prostate usually is followed by irrigation to ensure that clots do not lodge in the drainage system during the healing process.

2. Urinary tract infections are a frequently seen form of infection. These infections range from bacteria in the urine, to cystitis (infection of the bladder) and pyelonephritis (infection of the kidney). Cystitis is especially common in women owing to the short urethra and the proximity of the vagina and rectum, which provides easy access to the urinary system for microorganisms.

Assessment of the Client

1. Assess the client's urine before the irrigation to determine the presence of blood, clots, or unusual appearance. This baseline data offers a comparison against which to judge the effectiveness of the irrigation.

2. Assess the client's understanding of the procedure and willingness to cooperate.

3. Assess the effectiveness of the irrigation periodically to determine whether modifications should be made.

Plan

Nursing Objectives

Provide emotional comfort to the client.

Maintain a sterile bladder drainage system.

Preserve patency of bladder drainage system.

Observe characteristics of urinary drainage.

Instruct the client and family in the indicated method of irrigation.

Client Preparation

1. Before manual or intermittent irrigation, the client should be told that a feeling of fullness and desire to void may occur when the fluid is instilled. Deep breaths may help aid in relaxing and overcoming this feeling. During continuous tidal irrigation, the client should be told to expect a feeling of slight fullness.

2. Occasionally a clot may stop up a three-way catheter causing distention and spasms of the bladder if not relieved. Tell the client to notify the nurse at once if excessive fullness or pain during tidal irrigation is experienced.

3. Place a linen protector beneath the client's hips to prevent the bed linen from becoming wet from leakage or spills during manual irrigation.

Equipment

MANUAL IRRIGATION

Closed system

    Sterile container for solution

    Cotton balls and disinfectant

    Sterile drape

    Syringe (30 ml–50 ml) with an 18-gauge needle

Open System

    50-ml irrigating syringe (Asepto or bulb)

    Sterile drape

    Sterile drainage tube protector

    Sterile solution, as ordered

    Sterile container for solution

    Cotton balls and disinfectant

    Sterile drainage receptacle

INTERMITTENT IRRIGATION

Intermittent bladder irrigation setup

Heavy IV standard

Sterile solution, as ordered (2000-ml bags)

Catheterization tray with three-way catheter (if not already in place)

TIDAL (THROUGH-AND-THROUGH) IRRIGATION:

Tidal irrigation setup

Heavy IV standard

Sterile solution, as ordered (2000-ml bags)

Drainage containers

Large basin

Implementation and Intervention

Procedural Aspects

ACTION

RATIONALE

Manual Irrigation

Open system technique:

1. Use strict aseptic technique during manual irrigation. When disconnecting the drainage tubing to irrigate the catheter, avoid contaminating the ends of either the catheter tubing or the drainage system. Disinfect the catheter ends and separate the catheter from the tubing. Place a sterile tubing protector over the end of the tubing to prevent contamination. Hold the catheter tubing at least 2.5 cm (1 in) from the end during irrigation.

The bladder tissue is very susceptible to injury and infection. The urinary tract offers a favorable environment for the multiplication of microorganisms because it is dark, warm, and moist.

2. Irrigate the bladder with a sterile solution, usually normal saline or an electrolyte solution. Pour the solution into a sterile container and draw the desired amount into a sterile syringe (Fig. 33-3).

By the process of osmosis, irrigating fluids may be reabsorbed into the bloodstream, causing dilution of the blood. It is desirable for the irrigating solution to be as near the same molecular density of the blood as possible.

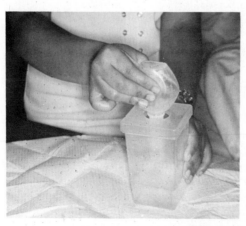

Figure 33.3

ACTION

3. Gradually instill a total of 100 ml of solution in 30 ml amounts unless otherwise ordered. Take extreme care not to contaminate the tip of the syringe, the end of the catheter, or the solution (Figs. 33-4 to 33-6).

RATIONALE

Increase in the pressure on any portion of a confined liquid is transmitted undiminished to all parts of that liquid. As the volume of urine rises to about 250 ml, the pressure in the bladder becomes 130 mm, which is sufficient to initiate nerve impulses to produce pain or the desire to void.

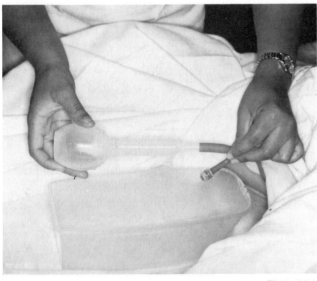

Figure 33.4

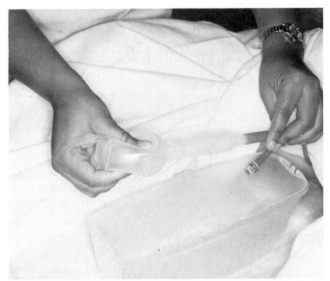

Figure 33.5

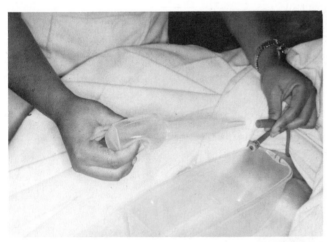

Figure 33.6

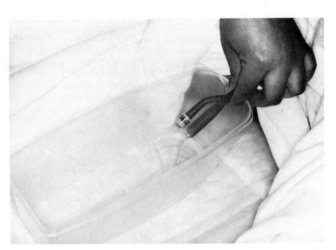

Figure 33.7

4. Allow the fluid in the bladder to return by gravity by holding the catheter over a basin below bladder level (Fig. 33-7). If no return is obtained, use the syringe to initiate or complete gentle withdrawal of the irrigation fluid. Reattach the tubing to the catheter, taking care not to touch or otherwise contaminate the urinary drainage system.

Siphonage is produced when the free surface of the liquid in one vessel is lower than the surface of the liquid in the other, causing a difference in pressure.

ACTION	**RATIONALE**
5. Remove the equipment and leave the client in a clean and comfortable environment.	Procedures involving the eliminatory process may be embarrassing to the client. Attention to the physical environment after irrigation may distract the client and help to ease anxiety.
Closed system technique:	
1. Record the amount of urine in the bag.	The amount of urine at the beginning of the procedure will be used as a baseline measurement against which to measure urine excreted after irrigation.
2. Clamp the drainage tubing. Open the irrigation setup taking care to maintain sterility. Place the drape under the end of the catheter.	Clamping the tubing will force the irrigation fluid into the bladder as intended instead of allowing it to run down the drainage tubing into the drain bag.
3. Don the sterile gloves. Using sterile technique, aspirate the desired amount of sterile irrigating solution into the syringe. Attach the needle. Disinfect a small section of the catheter about 2 in to 3 in below the attachment to the drainage tubing and away from the insertion port for inflating the balloon. This is the area through which the solution will be injected. (Fig. 33-8) Insert the needle into the catheter and gradually inject the solution. To irrigate the catheter only, 50 ml of solution is adequate. To irrigate the bladder, 150 ml to 250 ml are needed.	Disinfecting the entry port of the catheter helps to eliminate the possibility of transmitting microorganisms.

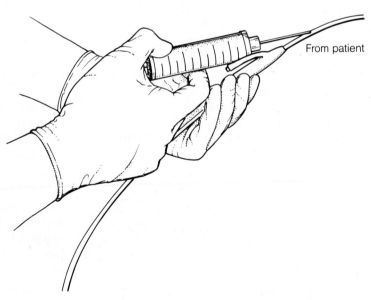

From patient

Figure 33.8

ACTION

4. Remove the needle from the catheter. For catheter irrigation, immediately lower the catheter. If the intention is bladder irrigation, wait a few minutes and lower the drainage tubing. The drainage tube must be unclamped before the solution can drain.

RATIONALE

Lowering the catheter allows the irrigation fluid to flow by gravity out of catheter. Unclamping the tubing accomplishes the same thing for bladder irrigation.

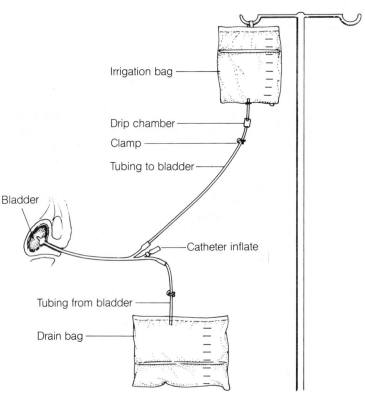

Irrigation bag

Drip chamber

Clamp

Tubing to bladder

Bladder

Catheter inflate

Tubing from bladder

Drain bag

Figure 33.9

Intermittent Irrigation (Fig. 33-9)

1. To initiate intermittent irrigation, remove the covering from the large bag of sterile solution (usually 2000 ml) and attach the drip chamber of the irrigation tubing to the outlet opening. (Fig. 33-10).

2. Hang the bag of sterile solution on an IV standard and adjust it to place the drip chamber 2½ ft to 3 ft above the level of the bed.

3. Before the tubing from the irrigation fluid is attached to the client's catheter, flush the tubing with solution. (Fig. 33-11). Then

Maintaining a closed system decreases the chance of contaminating the urinary system. The intermittent irrigation system is used when frequent irrigation is needed so that the closed system will not have to be opened frequently for manual irrigation.

The pressure of water in a container for irrigation has been established as approximately 1/2 lb for every foot of elevation. Low pressure is utilized for bladder treatments because of the bladder's musculature and ability to expand.

Instillation of air into the bladder may cause painful distension and cramping.

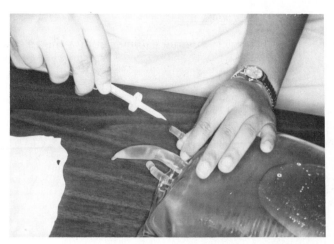

Figure 33.10

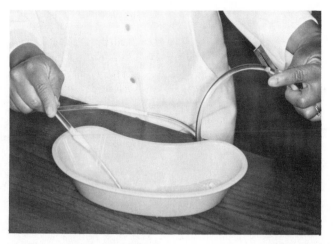

Figure 33.11

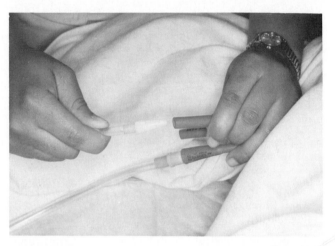

Figure 33.12

ACTION	**RATIONALE**
close the clamp below the drip chamber and attach the tubing to the inlet of a three-way catheter (Fig. 33-12). Connect the drainage system to the catheter outlet. Secure the tubing to the bed linen so that it is not accidentally pulled or kinked, causing disruption of the patency of the system and pain and discomfort for the client.	
4. To irrigate the bladder, open the tubing from the irrigation solution to the bladder and allow 100 ml of solution to flow into the bladder by gravity. Close the clamp and allow the solution to remain in the bladder 15 to 20 minutes or as ordered by the physician. After the specified time, open the drainage clamp and allow the irrigation fluid to drain into the receptacle provided for this purpose. Leave the clamp on the drain tube open.	Irrigation solution flows by gravity into and out of the bladder to protect the delicate lining and prevent discomfort for the client.

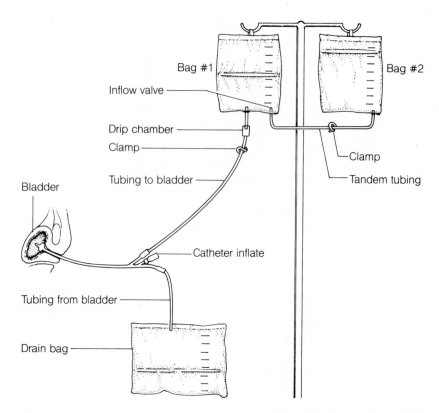

Bag #1

Inflow valve

Drip chamber

Clamp

Bag #2

Clamp

Tandem tubing

Tubing to bladder

Bladder

Catheter inflate

Tubing from bladder

Drain bag

Figure 33.13

ACTION	RATIONALE
Tidal (through-and-through) Irrigation (Fig. 33-13)	
1. To initiate irrigation, remove the covers from two large bags of sterile irrigation fluid (usually 2000 ml). Insert a drip chamber of the irrigation tubing into each of the bags. Close the clamps on each of the tubes and hang the bags from a tandem IV standard or appropriate apparatus to keep the bags in the desired position.	Continuous tidal irrigation is used when constant bathing of the inner aspects of the bladder is necessary.
2. If air is noted in the irrigation tubing, flush the tubing by disconnecting it from the catheter, releasing the appropriate clamp and allowing the fluid to run through the tubing until all air is removed. Clamp the tubing and reconnect it to the catheter. Be sure that any exposed ends of the system are closed with a sterile cover during flushing.	Air in the bladder can cause distention. Opening the closed system provides an avenue for the entrance of infectious microorganisms and should be done only if absolutely necessary.
3. To start or restart the irrigation of the bladder, release the clamp on one of the bags of irrigation solution enough to allow the desired rate of flow to be maintained. Be	If the solution is allowed to run into the bladder without a means of emptying, it will soon fill and distend, causing discomfort and pain. Having the drainage bag below the level of

ACTION	***RATIONALE***
certain that the tubing draining the fluid from the bladder is open so that the bladder will not be distended. The irrigation fluid drains into a large bag that is attached to the bed in a position lower than that of the bladder.	the bladder allows the fluid and urine to drain by gravity.
4. Secure the drainage tubing to the bed so that accidental pulling or jerking is avoided, patency is maintained, and the client is able to move about as freely as possible in the bed.	Tubing should not be secured so tightly that the client cannot turn and change positions easily.
5. Empty the drainage bag each time a new bottle is hung. Record each on the intake and output (I&O). Empty the bag by releasing the clamp at the bottom of the bag and allowing the fluid to run into a graduated container so that accurate amount may be ascertained.	By measuring accurately the amount of solution entering the bladder in relation to the amount drained, the amount of urine being excreted can be determined.

Communicative Aspects

OBSERVATIONS

1. Observe the color, appearance, and amount of urinary drainage.
2. Check tubings frequently to ensure patency of drainage system (e.g., no kinks, twists, loops below bed level).
3. All tubes leading from the bladder should be below bladder level.
4. Observe the client for any discomfort. Assess the cause(s) of the discomfort. Before giving any pain medication, be certain that the catheter is draining adequately. Overfilling the bladder is very painful and easily relieved by allowing the bladder to drain. In this case, pain medication may not be needed.

CHARTING

Record intake and output measurements on an I&O form. Follow the protocols of the hospital for determining I&O during bladder irrigation. For accurate calculation of urinary output during tidal irrigation, empty the drainage system each time the new bag of fluid is hung. Enter the 2000 ml on the intake portion and the amount in the drainage bag on the output portion. This allows the nurse to obtain an accurate measurement of the amount of urine being excreted.

DATE/TIME	OBSERVATIONS	SIGNATURE
4/9 1230	Foley catheter irrigated with 30 ml sterile normal saline at room temperature. System remained closed. 30 ml solution returned by gravity, yellow, no sediment. Expressed no pain or discomfort. ——————————	G. Ivers RN
6/12 0730	Bladder irrigated with 100 ml of KMnO4 1:1000 at room temperature. Solution remained in bladder for 15 min, then returned by gravity. Irrigation return contained many small particles. Expressed slight sensation of fullness during the procedure. ——————————	G. Ivers RN
9/15 1400	Continuous through-and-through irrigation started with 2 bags (4000 ml) room temp. solution hanging 3 feet above bladder level. Dripping slowly, return is pale pink. Stated some feelings of fullness, but no pain or discomfort. B/P 138/64, P 64, R 16, T 97.8°F. Siderails up, cautioned to remain in bed. Call light in reach. ——————————	G. Ivers RN

Discharge Planning Aspects

CLIENT AND FAMILY EDUCATION

1. Instruct the client that tubing should be free of kinks, twists, bends, and pressure from body parts so that the urine can drain by gravitational pull.

2. Tell the client never to disconnect the tubing because touching could contaminate the drainage system.

3. Offer instructions concerning the importance of adequate fluid intake if the client's condition allows.

4. If bladder irrigation is to be done at home, the client or family will need specific instructions and demonstrations.

5. Preoperatively, the client should have been prepared for an indwelling catheter with the expectation that a feeling of urgency and desire to void are normal during the first postoperative hours. Explain that straining and trying to void around the catheter will only increase tissue irritation and cause fatigue.

6. The client should know to expect a feeling of slight fullness during irrigation. Should pain or spasm occur, however, the nurse should be notified at once because a clot may be blocking the catheter or the tubing may be twisted or kinked. A greatly distended bladder is very dangerous for clients who have recently undergone urologic surgery.

REFERRALS

If bladder irrigation is to be done at home, a public health or visiting nurse referral may be needed.

Evaluation

Quality Assurance

1. Adherence to aseptic technique during manual irrigation is vital to the client's safety and progress. Institutional policy should reflect a method of maintaining the sterility of the open and closed urinary drainage system. Documentation should be available to indicate that all nurses have access to the proper policy. Audits of the procedure will help determine compliance with the policy. Documentation in the chart should reflect the amount of fluid instilled and frequency of irrigation. The client's reaction to the irrigation procedure also should be reflected. If the client will require irrigation after discharge, teaching efforts should be documented with the nurse's evaluation of the level of understanding and proficiency of the person who is being taught to do the irrigation.

2. For intermittent and continuous tidal irrigation, document the amount of irrigation fluid used and the amount and character of return. Note the client's reaction to the irrigation. Documentation should reflect the nature of the teaching efforts directed to client and family as well as an evaluation of their level of understanding. Note any side-effects, as well as an evaluation of those side-effects that are common to this procedure but did not occur. Nursing interventions to prevent or manage complications should be noted.

Infection Control

1. The threat of infection is very great in urinary tract techniques. Instilling a foreign matter into the bladder, in this case the irrigation fluid, has inherent dangers of introducing infectious organisms at the same time. Meticulous handwashing is essential before and after irrigating the bladder. If the sterility of the irrigation equipment cannot be guaranteed, use new equipment.

2. In intermittent and continuous tidal irrigation, maintaining a closed system is essential to protect the client from infection. When hanging new bags of solution and emptying the drainage bag, care must be taken to ensure the integrity of the sterile system. Careful handwashing is essential before handling the irrigation system.

Technique Checklist

	YES	NO
Manual irrigation	_____	_____
Frequency _____		
Results _____		
Client and family understand reasons for irrigation	_____	_____
Sterility of catheter system maintained	_____	_____
Accurate I&O reflecting irrigation	_____	_____
Technique taught to family member who will irrigate catheter at home	_____	_____
Intermittent irrigation		
Client and family understand the reasons for procedure	_____	_____
Sterility of system maintained	_____	_____
Frequency of irrigation _____		
Appearance of return noted each time irrigation done	_____	_____
Tidal (through-and-through) irrigation		
Client and family knew in advance what the irrigation would entail and why it was necessary	_____	_____
I&O kept current and accurately	_____	_____
Sterility of system maintained	_____	_____
Frequent notation of appearance of irrigation return	_____	_____
Complications _____		
_____		

34   Body Mechanics

Overview

Definition

The efficient use of the body, applying the principles of physical science for optimal use of energy and movement

Rationale

Avoid unnecessary muscle strain and possible injury.

Assist in locomotion of the client in and out of bed with minimal strain for nurse and client.

Perform everyday activities safely and properly by using correct principles of body mechanics.

Terminology

Alignment: The proper relationship of body segments to one another

Atony: Decrease or absence of normal muscle tonus

Atrophy: Decrease in size and loss of normal function of a muscle resulting from or related to disuse

Balance: Stability or steadiness

Base of support: The area on which an object rests

Center of gravity: The point at which the mass of an object is centered

Contracture: a permanent contraction state of a joint resulting from the tightening and lengthening of opposing muscles, which cause the joint to fix in an unusual position permanently

Fulcrum: The fixed portion of a lever, which allows movement

Gravity: The force that pulls objects toward the earth

Lever: A rigid bar that moves on a fixed axis called a fulcrum

Posture: Body alignment

Tonus: The normal status of a healthy muscle consisting of a partial steady state of contraction while awake

Torsion: Twisting

Assessment

Pertinent Anatomy and Physiology

See Appendix I: *skeletal muscles, skeletal system, vertebral column.*

Pathophysiological Concepts

1. The bones of primary importance in body mechanics are the vertebral column and the large bones in the legs, arms, and pelvis. Abnormal stress on the bone results in structural problems. In good alignment no undue strain is placed on the joints, muscles, or bones and connective tissue. Common problems of the musculoskeletal system often relate to misalignment and abnormal curvatures of the vertebral column. Poor posture places pressure on the vertebral column, frequently straining the muscles of the back and leading to backache.

2. The human body functions best in the vertical position. The lungs function optimally when the diaphragm is allowed to contract down into the abdominal cavity. A body in balance or equilibrium is stable, secure, and unlikely to tip or fall. The body maintains balance by nerve impulses received in the semicircular ducts of the inner ear. Diseases of the inner ear upset balance and equilibrium.

Assessment of the Client

Assess the client for understanding and use of proper body mechanics and identify deficits so that proper body mechanics can be taught during hospitalization.

Plan

Nursing Objectives

Teach the client, family, and co-workers the proper use of the body as a machine of activity, using proper principles to prevent injury.

Recognize and change incorrect habits of body mechanics, substituting proper activities in their place.

Reinforce correct behavior.

Client Preparation

In this text, client preparation for proper body alignment and body mechanics is reviewed for each individual technique as appropriate.

Implementation and Interventions

Principles of Body Mechanics

1. The *center of gravity* is the point at which the whole weight of the body may be considered to be concentrated. In humans, the center of gravity is considered to be in the center of the pelvis at the level of the second sacral vertebra. The feet form the supporting base of the body. The greater the supporting area and the lower the center of gravity, the more stable the body will be. Therefore, a more stable base of support can be achieved by spreading the feet.

2. Good posture is the key to body mechanics and involves more than just standing erect. It keeps the center of gravity as nearly as possible in the same vertical line when standing, sitting, or squatting (Fig. 34-1).

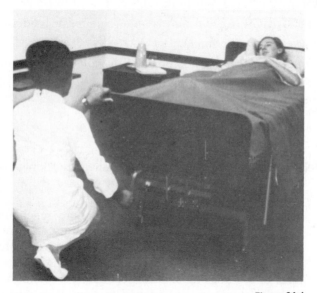

Figure 34.1

3. When a force acting on the body tends to rotate the body in one direction or another, the principle involved is called *torque*. The direction of torque is either clockwise or counterclockwise. For the body to be in equilibrium and not rotate, a force of equal resistance in the opposite direction must be applied. The major factor in determining torque deals with the distance between the center of gravity and the object causing resistance. This explains why those positions that require less energy and cause less strain are better than others for work activities. For example, when one is lifting an object from the floor, stooping requires greater strain because the distance from the center of gravity to the object is greater than that resulting from bending at the knees and picking up the object.

4. Laws that govern balance in the standing position also apply when the body is in motion. To prevent strain, proper contraction of the muscles to counteract gravitational resistance is necessary. For example, carrying a heavy object at arm's length produces far greater strain than carrying it close to the body, which allows correct body alignment. Lifting a client by bending forward at the waist produces unnatural body alignment and possibly will result in back strain. Lifting by flexing the hips and knees, placing one foot forward (broadens the base of support), and keeping shoulders in the same plane as the pelvis reduces the amount of energy necessary to accomplish the task with much less strain on the body muscles (Fig. 34-2).

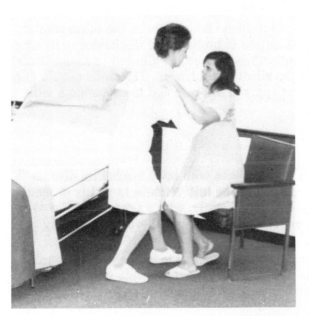

Figure 34.2

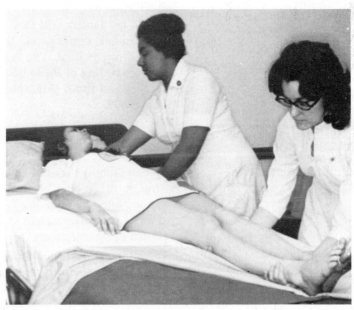

Figure 34.3

5. Many simple laws of physics can lighten the nurse's workload. It is easier to slide an object than to life it (Fig. 34-3). Sliding the object on an even surface requires less energy than moving it on an incline. Friction increases the amount of energy required to accomplish a task. Friction can be reduced by application of an intermediate object (*e.g.*, a draw sheet on a bed). When lifting, face the work situation and avoid rotary movements of the spine. Utilizing smooth, continuous movements requires less energy than continually stopping and starting movements.

6. Teach the client how the use of proper body mechanics can promote comfort and prevent strains and problems associated with prolonged bedrest. For example, encourage the client to use the siderails and bend both knees, pushing the heels into the mattress when pulling up in bed. Lifting items from the bedside table should be done with a bent elbow for added involvement of the muscles of the upper chest, shoulder, and upper arm, rather than with the arm straight using only the muscles of the upper arm. When raising oneself to a sitting position in bed, allow the arms to pull (as on the siderails) or to push (as from the mattress) rather than letting all of the strain be borne by the lower back muscles.

Communicative Aspects

OBSERVATIONS

1. Note the client's posture as well as any unusual curvatures of the spine or other abnormalities.

2. Observe all clients, especially those with orthopedic problems, for proper knowledge and application of correct body mechanics.

Discharge Planning Aspects

CLIENT AND FAMILY EDUCATION

1. All clients should be taught proper posture and body mechanics. The best method is the nurse's good example during execution of daily tasks.

2. When the family will care for a bedridden client at home, the nurse should explain and demonstrate the principles of proper body mechanics in turning and lifting a client. The family member(s) should be allowed to demonstrate understanding of these before the client is discharged. The client should also understand those principles that apply to self-care and to cooperation with caregivers.

Evaluation

Quality Assurance

1. Documentation should reflect any problems with body mechanics demonstrated by the client, as well as any nursing interventions to rectify or modify them. Note any teaching provided to the family, with a synopsis of the nurse's impression of their level of understanding and evaluation of any return demonstrations.

2. In-service education should reflect ongoing efforts to ensure that all employees practice use of proper body mechanics. A hospital-wide program might help to reduce time lost because of injury and might increase productivity.

Technique Checklist

	YES	NO
Principles of proper body mechanics explained to client and family	_____	_____
Understanding of principles of body mechanics demonstrated by client and family	_____	_____

35 Braces, Application and Removal

Overview

Definition

A leather, fabric, plastic, or metal appliance used to support a specific body part

Rationale

Provide support for the body weight.
Prevent deformities.
Correct deformities.
Prevent extraneous or abnormal movements.

Terminology

Alignment: The proper relationship of body segments to one another
Balance: Stability or steadiness
Center of Gravity: The point at which the mass of an object is centered
Posture: Body alignment

Assessment

Pertinent Anatomy and Physiology

See Appendix I: *skeletal system, vertebral column.*

Pathophysiological Concepts

1. The bones usually involved with braces are the vertebral column and the long bones in the legs. Abnormal stress on these bones results in structural problems. In good alignment no undue strain is placed on the joints, muscles, or bones and connective tissue. Common problems of the musculoskeletal system often relate to misalignment and abnormal curvatures of the vertebral column. Poor posture places pressure on the vertebral column, frequently straining the muscles of the back and leading to backache.

2. Bracing the back and long bones may enable the client to ambulate earlier. The benefits of early ambulation include decreasing the chances of cardiovascular problems, such as orthostatic hypotension, edema, and thrombus formation; preventing respiratory problems, such as shallow breathing, fluid accumulation in the lungs, and respiratory infections; preventing gastrointestinal (GI) problems, such as constipation and impaction; and preventing urinary problems, such as stasis of urine, kidney stone formation, urinary retention and incontinence, and urinary infections.

3. The human vertebral column is a versatile arrangement of bony segments that are linked in a series by ligaments. Not only does it provide the strength and rigidity necessary for support of the head, trunk, and upper extremities, but it is also flexible. In addition to its supporting function, this hollow cylinder of bones effectively surrounds and protects the soft spinal cord as well as the origins of the 31 pairs of spinal nerves. Fractures of the vertebrae (broken neck or broken back) may result in paralysis or death. Another less serious but extremely painful injury to the neck is the herniated disk (also called slipped or ruptured disk).

Assessment of the Client

1. Assess the client for proper fit of the brace. If the brace is worn incorrectly, the purpose of the brace may not be accomplished.

2. Assess the presence of bony prominences under the brace. Observe the skin areas on the upper and lower edges of the brace for irritation, redness, swelling, tenderness, or callouses.

3. Assess the working condition of the brace itself. Inspect the device for missing screws, hooks, or parts. If parts are supposed to be movable, check to see whether they move freely or need lubrication.

Plan

Nursing Objectives

Restrict motion of a joint.

Support muscles weakened by trauma or disease.

Prevent contracture.

Ensure the safety and comfort of the client.

Maintain proper body alignment during recuperation.

Client Preparation

1. Provide a screened area for application of the brace to protect the client's privacy.

2. To prevent soiling and promote comfort, many braces are put on over clothing. If appropriate and allowed, assist the client in donning a soft cotton shirt to be worn under the back brace or a stocking under the leg brace.

3. If the brace requires lubrication of the hinges with grease or oil, apply these substances before the brace is applied to the client.

Equipment

Brace

Implementation and Interventions

Procedural Aspects

ACTION	RATIONALE
Back Brace	
1. Roll the client to one side. Ensure that the neck and back are in proper alignment.	In proper alignment, no undue strain is placed on the joints, muscles, or the bones.
2. Place the brace against the client's back with the upper and lower edges of the brace in place. Be sure that the brace fits the curvature of the back with the spine in the center. Push the straps or supportive material under the brace and client as far as possible. (Fig. 35-1, 35-2)	The brace has been measured and tailored to fit the client exactly. It must be in proper position to provide necessary support and to prevent complications.
3. Roll the client back into the supine position while maintaining proper alignment of neck and back. Pull the straps from under the client. Check to be certain that the spinal column is still in the center of the brace and proper alignment has been achieved. Fasten the straps so that the brace fits securely. If there are straps on each side of the brace, they should be pulled and fastened simultaneously.	A snug, secure fit will ensure that the brace does not rub and chafe the client because of friction between the brace edges and the skin. Simultaneous closure of straps will help to ensure that equal pressure is applied to each side.

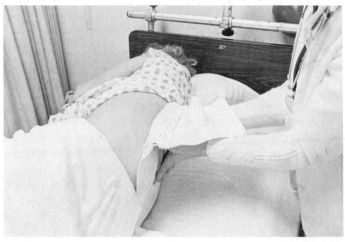

Figure 35.1

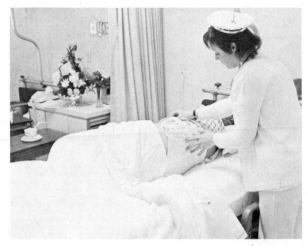

Figure 35.2

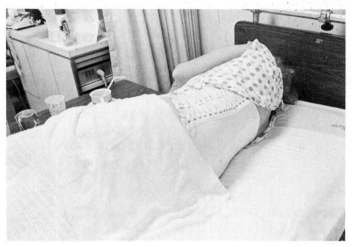

Figure 35.3

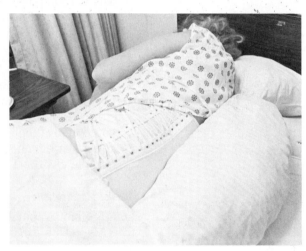

Figure 35.4

ACTION	*RATIONALE*
4. Check for pressure areas created by the brace or straps. Pay particular attention to the bony prominences, such as the iliac spines, scapulae, and the sternum. Leave the client in a comfortable position with adequate support to maintain alignment (Fig. 35-3, 35-4).	Prolonged contact with a noxious or irritating article will cause skin breakdown and pain.
5. To remove the back brace, assist the client to the supine position in bed. Unfasten the front straps and tuck the nearer ones under the client. Turn the client toward one nurse while the other removes the brace. Be certain that proper alignment of neck and body are maintained throughout. Assist the client into a comfortable position. Store the brace in its proper place.	Attention must be given to maintaining proper body alignment during removal of the brace.

ACTION	*RATIONALE*
Leg Brace	
1. Assist the client into the sitting position on the edge of the bed. After the client has dressed, apply the brace.	Clothing under the brace may promote comfort and prevent soiling the brace with perspiration.
2. If the brace has a shoe attached to it, place the client's foot into the shoe. Be certain that the foot fits completely and correctly into the shoe in its natural anatomical position. Fasten the shoe securely but not too tightly.	Extreme tightness may interfere with normal circulation. The client may have impaired sensation in the foot. Be sure that the toes are not curled up under the foot or caught in the material of the shoe in an abnormal position.
3. Secure the remaining portions of the brace around the calf, knee, or thigh. The brace should be snug but not tight. Check the brace for pressure especially over the bony prominences of the ankle, knee, and hip.	Snugness is necessary for proper fit; however, tightness may cause irritation, pain, and impaired circulation. Pressure may cause tissue breakdown.
4. To remove the leg brace, unfasten the cuff and shoe with the client sitting securely on the side of the bed. Remove the brace and shoe and assist the client into a comfortable position.	Removal of the weight of the brace will cause a shift in the client's center of gravity, which may result in a fall if the client is not sitting down securely when it is removed.

Special Modifications

Long leg braces may be applied while the client is supine in bed. Apply the braces using the same principles as when applying the back brace.	The intent is to apply the braces securely and safely with a minimum of discomfort to the client. Also emphasize maintenance of proper

Communicative Aspects

OBSERVATIONS

1. Observe the client's adaptablility to the brace including successful ambulation with the brace, proper body alignment and posture while in the brace, and psychological reactions to wearing the brace.

2. Observe the condition of the client's skin under the brace. Note particularly the presence of any reddened or irritated areas, which signify improper fit or application of the brace.

3. Observe the proper positioning of the brace when the client is in bed. Check again after arising to be certain that the brace has not shifted or twisted during change of position.

CHARTING

DATE/TIME	OBSERVATIONS	SIGNATURE
9/4 1100	Back brace applied and seems to fit securely with no pressure points. Able to ambulate in brace for 10 min without fatigue. No problems turning in bed during application. Technique demonstrated to wife————————	C. Green RN

Discharge Planning Aspects

CLIENT AND FAMILY EDUCATION

1. Ensure that the client and family know how to apply the brace correctly and how to care for it. Tell them what side-effects to watch for such as reddened area, tissue breakdown, and bruises.
2. The client should be told to reevaluate the fit of the brace continuously if it is to be worn for an extended period. Weight loss or gain may alter the fit of the brace. In addition, wearing of the brace material itself may alter the fit.

REFERRALS

The client and family should be referred to a reliable orthopedic appliance technician or physical therapist to ensure proper fit of the brace.

Evaluation

Quality Assurance

Document the reaction of the client to the brace, the mobility of the brace, and an assessment of the proper fit evidenced by presence of pressure indications. Documentation should further indicate that the nurse knew what the potential side-effects were and the measures taken to avoid them. Note in the documentation efforts and the reaction of the client and family to these.

Infection Controls

1. Wash hands thoroughly before and after applying or assisting with application of the brace.
2. The immobilized client is susceptible to infections resulting from stasis of body fluids such as urine and fluid in the lungs. Encouraging mobility to the extent tolerable to the client may help prevent such complications.
3. Pressure areas and resulting skin breakdown offer excellent breeding grounds for bacteria and infectious agents. Note pressure areas early to prevent tissue destruction.

Technique Checklist

	YES	NO
Brace fits snugly in all areas	____	____
Bony prominences under brace checked after each wearing	____	____
Reddened areas noted	____	____
Pressure areas massaged	____	____
Bruises noted	____	____
Tissue breakdown noted	____	____
Client understands and accepts the need for the brace	____	____
Client or family demonstrated ability to apply brace properly	____	____
Client or family know how to care for and maintain the brace	____	____
Client or family understand signs of complications	____	____
Referral to orthopedic appliance technician or physical therapist	____	____

Cardiopulmonary Resuscitation (CPR)

Overview

Definition

The act of manually restoring the action of the heart and lungs

Rationale

Restore normal heart and lung function after an unexpected failure of these organs.

Maintain adequate circulation until definitive treatment can be instituted.

Terminology

Anoxia: Deficiency of oxygen

Arrhythmia: Abnormality of the heart beat

Assessment

Pertinent Anatomy and Physiology

1. See Appendix I: *heart.*
2. Failure of the heart to pump blood normally is particularly damaging to the brain. The blood carries oxygen, which is necessary to the vital centers of the body. When the supply of oxygen to the brain is interrupted, death of the tissue begins within 4 minutes.
3. The thorax is a cone-shaped bony cage that is narrow at the top and broad at the bottom. Twelve pairs of ribs form the outer perimeter of the cage, which encloses the heart and lungs. The sternum lies in the midline in the front of the thorax. It is a flat, narrow bone about 6 in (15 cm) long. The lower portion is called the xiphoid process (Fig. 36-1). The ribs are slender, curved and fairly flexible. Some of the ribs join the sternum by means of the costal cartilage, which allows flexibility of the rib cage during breathing.

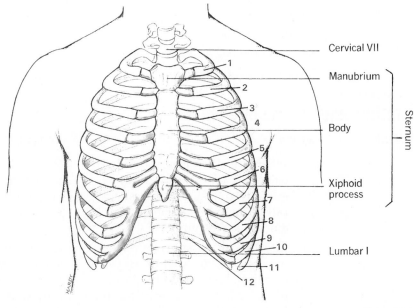

Figure 36.1

Pathophysiological Concepts

1. *Cardiac arrest* is the term for the situation in which the heart stops beating and the organs of the body are deprived of blood. Breathing ceases and unconsciousness follows. After 4 to 6 minutes, the lack of oxygen supply to the brain causes permanent and extensive damage. The signs of cardiac arrest are apnea and an absence of a carotid or femoral pulse.

2. The ribs are attached to the sternum by cartilaginous material that allows flexibility of the thorax, a state unlike that of most bones of the body. It is therefore possible to compress the sternum to such a degree that pressure is placed on the heart in sufficient quantity to pump the blood and to maintain a blood pressure around 100 mm Hg systolic. During resuscitation, the sternum must be compressed. If the xiphoid process is pressed forcefully, it may injure the liver.

3. Lactic acidosis occurs quickly during cardiac arrest. Lactic acidosis is the end product of anaerobic metabolism of glucose and is seen most often in cases of acute cellular hypoxia. The serum pH may decrease dramatically. Sodium bicarbonate may be given to correct the acidosis.

Assessment of the Client

1. Assess the client according to the ABC rule: **A**irway must be cleared of obstruction so that the client can breathe; **B**reathing must be assisted to prevent oxygen deprivation to the brain and other vital organs; **C**irculation must be maintained by external cardiac massage.

2. Assess the presence of wounds or injuries that may cause a modification in the usual method of administering cardiopulmonary resuscitation.

Plan

Nursing Objectives

Prevent anoxia to the brain.

Maintain adequate ventilation and circulation.

Client Preparation

1. Cardiac arrest is usually sudden and unexpected. When arrest occurs, cardiopulmonary resuscitation (CPR) must be initiated promptly. The best preparation is knowledge of the correct procedure.

2. When a client is suspected of being in cardiac arrest, attempt to arouse the person. If there is no response, turn the client carefully to the supine position. CPR is ineffective if the client's head is above the level of the heart.

Equipment

Airway

Cardiac arrest board

Self-inflating bag and mask device

Intravenous infusion equipment

Implementation and Interventions

Procedural Aspects

ACTION	RATIONALE
1. When the client is suspected of being in a state of cardiac arrest, establish unresponsiveness and call for help immediately. Check quickly for respirations.	Cardiac arrest is usually sudden and unexpected. Time is of the essence because brain damage can occur in 4–6 min.
2. Clear the air passages by removing any foreign material. Hyperextend the neck with the head tilted back. Pull the jaw upward. Using mouth-to-mouth or bag	An obstructed air passage prevents adequate ventilation of the lungs and hampers adequate gaseous exchange. Provision of a constant source of oxygen in the lungs is essential to oxygen-

ACTION

inflation, quickly inflate the client's lungs four times (Fig 36-2). When using mouth-to-mouth resuscitation, take a deep breath and make a tight seal over the client's mouth while pinching the client's nostrils. Breathe into the client's mouth four times, taking a complete breath between each time to ensure that fresh oxygen is being forced into the client's lungs. Give these breaths in rapid succession. An inflated bag attached to a mouthpiece may be used if immediately available. The mouthpiece may cover the client's mouth and nose (in which case, it must be pressed firmly against the client's face to prevent air leaks) or may be attached to an adapter to fit onto an endotracheal or tracheostomy tube. Each time the bag is squeezed, air is forced into the client's lungs. Tilt the client's head and hold the bag in place with one hand while the other hand squeezes the bag. If two persons are available for respiratory assistance, one person should compress the bag while the other uses both hands to ensure an open airway and an airtight seal over the client's nose and mouth.

RATIONALE

ation of the blood and maintaining the brain and other vital organs. The inital four breaths are building breaths; they are given in rapid succession so the client's lungs do not deflate fully after each breath.

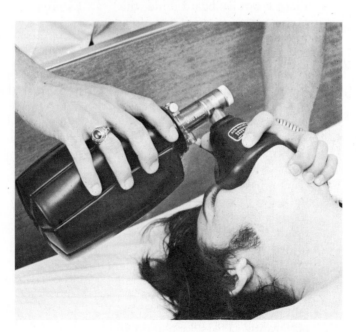

Figure 36.2

ACTION

RATIONALE

3. Establish lack of pulse. Palpate the carotid pulse (Fig. 36-3).

The carotid is the most accessible pulse point in adults.

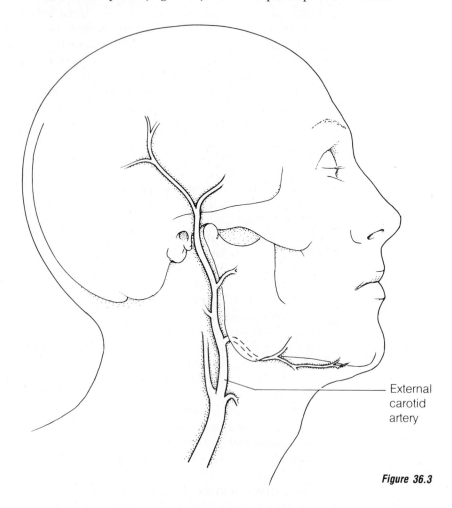

External carotid artery

Figure 36.3

4. Place a cardiac board under the client's chest if one is not already in place or if the client is not lying on a hard surface.

5. Place the heel of one hand on the lower third of the sternum, over the heart. Place the other hand over the first (Fig. 36-4). Compress the sternum 1½ in to 2 in. (2.5 cm–5 cm) directly downward in the adult. Administer sufficient pressure to compress the heart but do not compress too hard as internal injury may result. Weight should be transmitted vertically during compressions with the elbows straight and the shoulders over the hands. The mnemonic device to maintain rhythm when one rescuer is performing CPR is "one-and-two-and-three-and-four-and...."

External cardiac compression is effective only when the client is on a hard surface that allows for counterpressure.

Too much pressure on the sternum may cause the xiphoid process to injure the liver. Pressure on the ribs on either side of the sternum may cause a rib fracture, which might result in a punctured lung and pneumothorax.

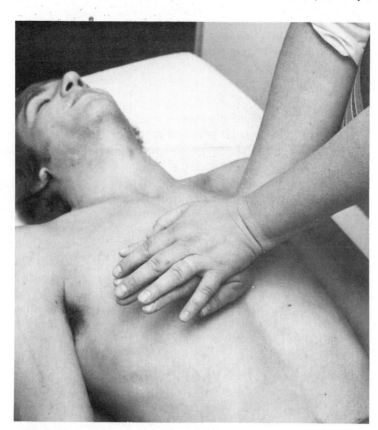

Figure 36.4

ACTION

6. Maintain assisted ventilation and circulation at a rate of 12 respirations/min and 80 cardiac compressions/min. When one person is giving CPR, 2 inflations of the lungs should be interspaced with 15 consecutive cardiac compressions. When help arrives, the ratio should be 1 inflation to every 5 compressions. The mneumonic for chest compressions with *two* rescuers is "1—1000, 2—1000...."

7. When switching places, the compressor at the client's chest calls for the change. The compressor replaces the mnemonic with, "Change—1000, 2—1000, 3—1000, 4—1000, 5—1000." On the fifth count, the rescuer at the head gives one breath and moves to the victim's chest, locating the position to compress the heart. The rescuer at the chest moves to the victim's head and checks the pulse and breathing for 5 seconds. If no pulse is felt, CPR continues at the two-rescuer rate.

RATIONALE

The normal heart rate is 72 beats/min; the normal respiratory rate is 14 to 20/min. Adequate ventilation and circulation can be maintained with the 2:15 or the 1:5 ratio.

When switching to the two-person technique or switching places during the process of CPR, the goal is to keep the rhythm regular and to maintain the client's circulation and respirations.

ACTION	RATIONALE
8. An intravenous infusion should be started as soon as possible. Sodium bicarbonate usually is administered to prevent or reverse acidosis.	The arrested heart may respond more quickly with the intravenous administration of cardiogenic drugs.
9. If closed-chest massage produces no response, the physician may wish to defibrillate the heart mechanically. Lubricate the paddles of the defibrillator with electrode paste (Fig. 36-5). Place the paddles on the client's torso, one on the upper left side of the chest slightly toward the midline and the other somewhat below the left axilla. Instruct all members of the resuscitation team to stand clear when the current is released.	Most defibrillators work on the principle of passing an electrical current through the heart muscle in an effort to reestablish normal rhythm. The electrode paste prevents burning the skin. The exact location of the paddles will vary with the size of the client. The desired effect is to pass the current through the heart muscle. This current is transmissible to other persons who might be in contact with the client at the time the current is released.

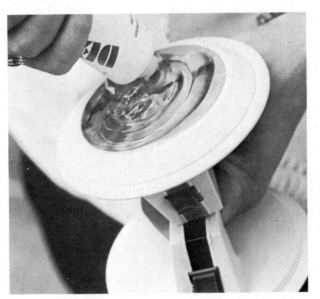

Figure 36.5

10. Place a plastic oral airway into the client's mouth. Endotracheal intubation may be done by using a laryngoscope to visualize the trachea. An endotracheal tube is slipped past the epiglottis into the trachea (Fig. 36-6). This procedure should be performed only by specially trained personnel. Assist with anchoring the tube when it is in place with ties or tape to ensure that it does not slip out. Assisted breathing may be done through the endotracheal tube using an inflation bag device.	The endotracheal tube ensures a direct opening into the trachea so that air may be forced into the lungs to ensure inflation.

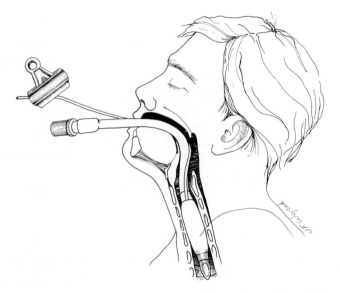

Figure 36.6

ACTION

11. Have a suction device ready in case of vomiting. Remove the vomitus from the oral area. If suctioning equipment is unavailable, use the index and middle fingers to sweep the emesis from the client's mouth. Turn the client's head to the side to prevent aspiration.

12. Periodically reassess the client to determine the effectiveness of CPR. Successful cardiac activity can be determined by the return of the carotid pulse, by pupil movement (constriction), and possibly by spontaneous return of respirations. Reassessment should be done after the initial four cycles of CPR, on the arrival of a second person, and periodically during the resuscitation efforts.

RATIONALE

During assisted **ventilation**, the stomach may become dilated by air forced down the esophagus. Gaseous distention of the stomach can cause the gastric contents to be vomited through the mouth. If this substance is not removed at once, the client may aspirate. Oral suctioning may alleviate the problem until a nasogastric tube can be inserted.

Once the heart starts beating, blood supply to the brain is reinstituted and vital functions return.

Communicative Aspects

OBSERVATIONS

1. Observe the signs and symptoms of cardiovascular problems that preceded the arrest.

2. Observe the reaction of the client to resuscitation efforts. Carefully note the time of arrest, the duration of resuscitation, and the time at which the client reacted or was pronounced dead. Circulation must be restored within 4 minutes to prevent irreversible brain damage or death.

3. Keep a record of the following: when resuscitation began, when the physician arrived, when resuscitation ended, drugs administered, techniques used, and the outcome of the procedure.

CHARTING

DATE/TIME	OBSERVATIONS	SIGNATURE
4/19 1015	No palpable pulse or noticeable respirations. Placed on cardiac board. Resuscitation given by RN and LVN at ratio of 5 compressions to 1 respiration. "Code 99" called.	F. White RN
1020	Weak femoral pulse felt. Pupils constricted. Skin cool, moist, and pale.	F. White RN
1025	Dr. K. here. Meds given as ordered.	F. White RN
1045	Femoral pulse 72. Good volume and regular rhythm.	F. White RN
1050	Spontaneous resp 12/min. Radial pulse 76/min. Color good. Reacts to verbal stimuli. B/P 92/60. Pupils react readily and equally.	F. White RN
1055	Physician explained emergency to family.	F. White RN
1115	Condition remains stable. Family in room. B/P 110/88, P 72, R 16.	F. White RN
1200	Vital signs stable. Sleeping at this time.	F. White RN

Discharge Planning Aspects

CLIENT AND FAMILY EDUCATION

1. Because time is a key factor during a cardiac arrest, all teaching of the client and family is done after resolution of the emergency. The family should be notified of the arrest as soon as possible.

2. Instruct the family to maintain a calm attitude when visiting the client after the cardiac arrest.

3. Reinforce physician instructions regarding resumption of previous activities after cardiac emergency.

4. Answer, as simply as possible, any questions the client and family may have regarding the cardiac arrest. Encourage the family members to take a CPR course in case this emergency should arise at home.

Evaluation

Quality Assurance

Document the precipitating factors before the cardiac arrest. The chart should reflect a progressive record of the arrest, its resolution, those persons involved, the techniques and medications used, and the outcome. Follow-up care of the client should reflect assessment for signs of cardiac emergency. Support and education of the family should be noted.

Each hospital should have a consistent method of certifying employees in the latest techniques of CPR at least yearly. The agency should also have a standard procedure for external cardiac massage and a protocol for obtaining skilled assistance in case of cardiopulmonary arrest. Nurses should know where the emergency equipment is kept and how to use it. If the agency has a special team to assist in CPR, the method for notifying and assisting them should be known to every employee. Biomedical technicians should have a consistent means of ensuring that all emergency equipment is in proper working order.

Infection Control

Equipment that will be used for consecutive clients should be cleaned between uses. This is particularly important for emergency equipment. There is no time to clean the equipment before use in an emergency situation. Often in the tension and anxiety of the emergency atmosphere, cleaning of equipment may be overlooked. It should be an assigned responsibility to see that all equipment is cleaned and ready for use as soon as possible after cardiovascular emergency.

Technique Checklist

	YES	NO
Time CPR started _____		
Time CPR ended _____		
Outcome		
Vital signs restored	_____	_____
Client pronounced dead	_____	_____
Time _____		
External cardiac massage	_____	_____
Assisted respiration		
Mouth-to-mouth _____		
Inflation device _____		
Endotracheal intubation	_____	_____
Tracheostomy	_____	_____
Record of times, techniques, and medications on chart	_____	_____
Cardiac defibrillation (no. of times) _____		
Family notified at _____		

37   Cast Care

Overview

Definition

Observations and nursing interventions that prevent or alleviate complications resulting from the application of a cast

Rationale

Maintain desired anatomical position.

Provide traction for reduction of a fracture.

Prevent or correct contractures.

Terminology

Blanching: A method of pressing the skin or nailbed to ascertain circulatory impairment. The nail should whiten momentarily, then quickly return to normal color. Continuous blanching is abnormal.

Fracture: A break in the continuity of a bone. Types include

Avulsion: Muscle damage with separation of small fragments of bone cortex at the site of attachment of a ligament or tendon (also called a "chip" fracture or sprain fracture)

Capillary: A fracture appearing on x-ray film as a fine, hairlike line; sometimes seen in fractures of the skull

Colles': A break in the lower end of the radius

Comminuted fracture: The bone is broken in more than two places or is splintered with multiple fragments

Complete: A fracture involving the entire cross section of the bone

Compound fracture: An open fracture in which there is a skin wound and the potential for infection

Compression: A fracture resulting when one bony surface is forced against an adjacent surface

Greenstick fracture: The bone is not broken all the way through but instead is bent and partially broken along the transverse plane of the bone (most common in childhood when the bones are more pliable and less brittle)

Impacted: A fracture is which a portion of the fractured bone is driven into another portion

Monteggia's: A fracture in the proximal half of the shaft of the ulna with dislocation of the head of the radius

Oblique: A fracture occurring at a 45° angle to the bone shaft

Pathologic: A fracture occurring in diseased bone with little or no trauma involved

Pott's: A fracture of the lower part of the fibula, with serious injury of the articulation of the lower tibia

Simple fracture: The bone is broken in only one place and the skin has no wound; the most common type of fracture (also called a closed fracture).

Spiral: A fracture that twists around the bone shaft

Fiberglass cast: A cast made of fiberglass material that performs the same function as the plaster cast but is lighter

Full-leg cast: A cast extending from midthigh to toes

Hanging cast: A cast extending from axilla to fingers, usually with a bend in the elbow

Plaster of paris: Quick-drying cast material, used in rolls

Short-leg cast: A cast extending from below the knee to the toes

Spica cast: A cast involving a great portion of the main trunk of the body, front and back, and possibly one or more extremities

Spreaders: An instrument used to spread or loosen a cast that is too tight

Stockinette: A soft, cloth material used under the cast, next to the skin, to protect delicate tissues

Assessment

Pertinent Anatomy and Physiology

See Appendix I: *bone repair, skeletal system.*

Pathophysiological Concepts

1. During fracture repair, osteogenic cells move into the area in a relatively short period and fill the gap between the bone parts. If this does not occur, fibroblasts will enter the area and fill the gap with fibrous tissue. Such tissue has no affinity for calcium, resulting in nonunion of the fracture ends.

2. There must be appropriate amounts of both organic and inorganic constituents to have functional bone tissue for support and protection. A dietary deficiency of calcium and phosphate interferes with normal calcification and results in a condition called *rickets.* This condition, found in infants and children, is usually the result of a deficiency of vitamin D. Elderly persons are subject to a generalized loss of cortical bone substance called *osteoporosis.* This condition is believed to result from excessive bone resorption, probably caused by an inadequate intake of dietary calcium. Frequent sideeffects are bone pain and pathologic fractures.

3. Emboli are foreign particles moving through the bloodstream. They are usually clots, which may block major vessels, causing ischemia and tissue death. Fat emboli are also possible, especially after fracture.

Assessment of the Client

1. Assess the location and appearance of the fracture or the cast. Assess the amount and location of any pain the client is experiencing. Assess the amount of physical limitation caused by the cast and its potential effect on the client.

2. Assess the client's history to determine how much experience there has been with broken limbs and casts. If this is the client's first experience with a broken bone, assess the amount of additional time and techniques needed to promote familiarization with the healing process.

Plan

Nursing Objectives

Ensure immobilization and desired anatomical position.

Prevent impairment of circulation.

Prevent pressure areas under the cast.

Prevent pressure on nerves.

Record observations of extremities in a cast.

Teach the client and family observations that should be made while in the hospital and after discharge.

Client Preparation

1. Handle the affected limb as little as possible on admission to the nursing unit. Remove clothing from the injured limb last or in any manner that will disturb the injury least.

2. Firmness and support keep the cast in correct conformity until drying is complete. Preparation of the bed should include bedboards, if indicated, to prevent sagging, and enough plastic-covered pillows to support the base in the desired anatomical position.

3. Tell the client that the affected limb will feel warm immediately after cast application because the plaster or fiberglass is dipped in warm water to make it moldable to the limb. Emphasize the need to lie still until the cast dries to prevent misshaping the new cast and possibly causing pressure areas. The client should expect some discomfort, but pain and continuous localized pressure should be reported. Tell the client to expect to compensate for the alteration in the center of gravity when getting up with a cast because of the added weight of the cast. Advise that pressure from the hanging cast is to be expected when standing erect as well as soreness because of reduced mobility of the affected part.

Equipment

Cast application materials, which may include a container filled with warm water, stockinette and plaster in all sizes, or fiberglass casting material, and any other supplies requested or used routinely by persons applying the cast

Implementation and Interventions

Procedural Aspects

ACTION

1. Keep the extremity in correct alignment until the cast is completely dry, usually about 24 hours. Keep bed covers off of the cast until it is dry. If the cast must be lifted, the palms of the hands should be used, rather than the fingertips (Figs. 37-1, 37-2). Exposing the cast to the circulating air (e.g., using a blow dryer, if allowed) will hasten drying. A casted extremity should be turned every 2 hours to ensure even drying. The cast is completely dry when it no longer feels damp or slightly soft to the touch.

RATIONALE

The goal of casting is to hold the extremity or bone immobile until healing is complete. The cast is applied to fit snugly but to allow adequate circulation necessary for proper healing. Pressure areas impair circulation and must be avoided.

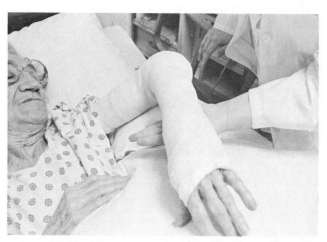

Figure 37.1

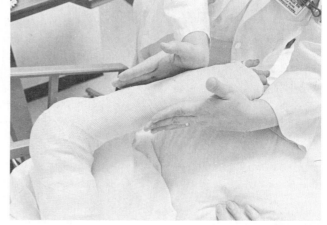

Figure 37.2

ACTION	RATIONALE
2. Place extra padding, such as moleskin, over the rough edges of the plaster cast. Be careful not to impair the circulation to the foot or hand.	The rough edges of the plaster cast may traumatize the skin, especially in children. The pressure of the rim of the cast may also cause bruises.
3. Place a protective covering, such as a plastic bag, over the cast during bathing if allowed. Make an effort to keep the cast as dry as possible.	Plaster is porous and will absorb water readily. The plaster cast must be dried if it becomes wet.
4. Elevate casted extremities with all contours supported to prevent cracking. Ice may be applied to the cast to prevent or reduce edema (Fig. 37-3).	Poor venous return is common to an injured part. Cold applications constrict blood vessels, anesthetize nerve endings and aid in blood coagulation.

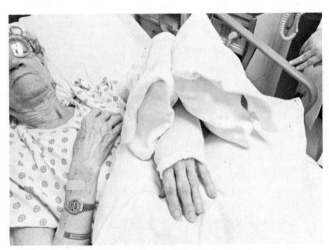

Figure 37.3

5. Check the toes or fingers frequently, especially during the first 24 hours, for early signs of circulatory impairment. These signs include numbness and tingling, unusual color (pale or cyanotic), skin cool to the touch, obvious edema, and continuous blanching of nailbeds. If seepage of blood should occur through the cast material, encircle its exact perimeter. Write the date and time so that further seepage can be evaluated (Fig. 37-4). Any drainage and its progression must be called to the attention of the physician and noted in the chart.	A cast is not flexible and shrinks slightly as it dries; it may inhibit circulation and result in swelling in the fracture area. Documentation will provide a baseline against which future developments may be weighed to determine the degree of seriousness of swelling and drainage.

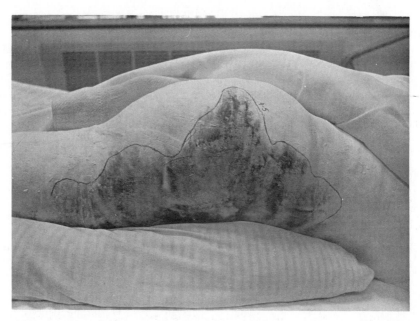

Figure 37.4

ACTION

6. Proper body alignment and positioning are extremely important to the client in a cast. To promote maximum comfort, change the client's position frequently. Avoid pinching of skin and formation of pressure areas on bony prominences. Maximum chest expansion also must be facilitated.

7. Foreign particles under the cast may precipitate skin irritations and infections. Discourage the client who wishes to relieve itching under the cast by scratching with some object. If the physician allows such a practice, devices used for scratching under the cast must be well padded and used with extreme care.

8. Exudates and secretions on the skin after cast removal should be removed carefully and gently so that trauma to the delicate skin is prevented. Wash the skin gently with mild soap and warm water.

9. For bathing a client with a cast, refer to the Technique No. 28, Baths, Cleansing.

RATIONALE

Abnormal stress on the bones results in structural problems. In proper alignment, no strain is placed on the joints, muscles, or bones and connective tissues.

Scratches under the cast can become infected because of the warm, dark, moist environment. A musty odor coming from under the cast may indicate pus formation.

After cast removal, the skin will be flaky, and the muscles will be sore and stiff.

ACTION	**RATIONALE**
10. The cast usually is supported by some means when the client is out of bed. Crutches or a sling are frequent aids to ambulation with a cast. A small wrist sling may be all that is allowed for the hanging cast (Fig. 37-5).	Unnecessary strain is undesirable during recovery from a fracture. The purpose of a hanging cast is to exert pressure from gravitational pull to keep the fracture of the humerus aligned.

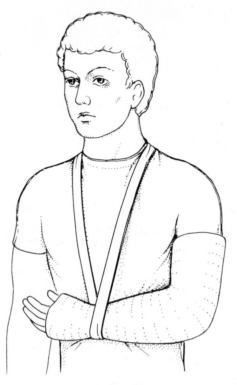

Figure 37.5

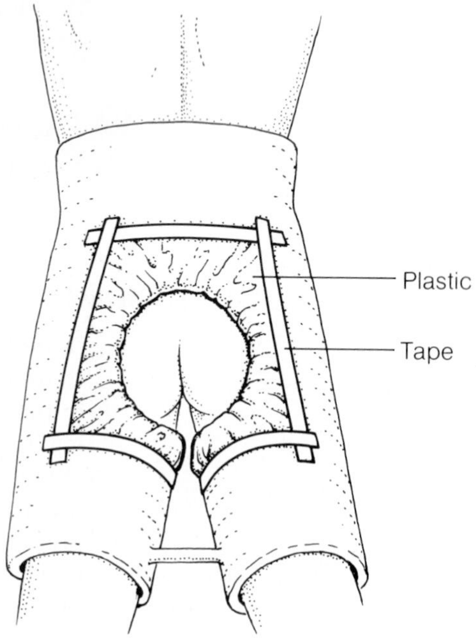

Plastic
Tape

Figure 37.6

Special Modifications

Spica Cast

1. Four persons are needed to turn a client in a drying spica cast to decrease the chance of cracking the cast. The cast is completely dry when it no longer feels damp or slightly soft to the touch.	Because of the amount of body mass involved, the client is unable to participate in the turning procedure. There must be adequate assistance to prevent the possibility of cracking the cast.
2. Elimination usually presents a problem to the client in a hip spica because it is difficult to use a bedpan. In an attempt to preserve the cleanliness and freshness of the cast, place sheets of plastic around the open perineal edges (Fig. 37-6). For females an emesis basin may be the best receptacle in which to urinate.	Plastic will help to protect the cast from dampness and soiling. However, the skin around the open area must be watched closely for signs of any reaction to the plastic.
3. Place bedboards under the mattress of the client in a spica cast.	Firm support is needed because of the extent of the casted area.

Communicative Aspects

OBSERVATIONS

1. Observe the client for signs and symptoms of aseptic inflammation that normally follow fracture of a bone:

   Elevated temperature within a few hours

   Increased white blood cell count

   Swelling at the fracture site

   Pain in the area of the fracture

   Bruising in the fracture area

2. Observe the client hourly for symptoms of nerve and circulatory impairment until all symptoms are negative. Check toes or fingers for:

   Color

   Blanching

   Sensation (increased numbness or tingling since cast application)

   Edema

   Temperature of distal extremities

   Mobility

   Pain

   Skin irritations at the edges of the cast

3. Bleeding may occur if there is a wound or incision. Observe for bleeding at frequent intervals, and chart and report any excessive or unexpected observations.

4. Bony prominences, such as the heels, ankles, wrists, elbows, and feet, may develop pressure areas if allowed to remain in contact with the bed for prolonged periods. Check frequently and relieve pressure areas by positioning or padding.

5. Observe the cast frequently for signs of a foul odor or a "hot spot" on the cast, signs that may indicate the beginning of infection.

CHARTING

DATE/TIME	OBSERVATIONS	SIGNATURE
8/14 1300	Short-leg cast applied to r. leg by Dr. B. Toes of right foot are swollen almost twice the size of the left foot. Color of toes is pink and they are partially movable. Expresses no tingling in the toes or foot and no pain at this time. Toenails blanch easily. Cautioned to keep cast on pillow. Call light in reach and siderails up. Instructed to call nurse if pain or loss of feeling occurs in casted foot. B/P 144/82, P 88, R 18, T 100.2° F———————	P. Dillon RN

Discharge Planning Aspects

CLIENT AND FAMILY EDUCATION

1. Teach the client and family the signs of nerve or circulatory impairment, such as numbness and tingling in the extremity, discoloration, failure of the nails to blanch, and swelling.

2. Teach the client and family the signals of possible pressure areas under the cast or on adjacent bony prominences, such as pain, a foul odor, or drainage from under or through the cast.

3. Emphasize the importance of exercising the unaffected extremities to prevent atrophy.

4. Explain the method and importance of isometric exercises. These exercises involve flexing and relaxing muscles of the extremity in the cast to build and maintain muscle tone. Isometrics involve no joint movement.

5. Demonstrate padding techniques and other pertinent information to the person who will be caring for the cast after discharge.

REFERRALS

Give the client and family the name(s) of available orthopedic appliance suppliers in the event that they may need to replace items such as slings, crutch pads, or traction equipment after discharge. If the client will need further assistance, referral to a home health nurse may be beneficial.

Evaluation

Quality Assurance

Document the client's initial reaction to the cast application. Appearance and condition of the affected area should be noted both before and after application. The documentation should reflect that the nurse knew the signs of circulatory impairment and took precautions to avoid, recognize, or alleviate them. Document the client's adaptation to the cast. Note progression of any side-effects and their management. Note psychological as well as physical responses. Document health teaching to both the client and the family. If demonstrations of care were offered and returned, assess the degree of understanding and anticipated compliance with medical restrictions after discharge. Note actions taken to avoid complications.

Infection Control

1. Handwashing is essential before and after handling the client in a cast. Transmission of hospital-acquired infections must be avoided.

2. If a wound or incision is present under the cast, it is dressed using sterile technique before the cast is applied. The cast must be observed closely for signs of infection as healing progresses.

3. Scratching under the cast may cause tissue breakdown and result in infection. Pressure on surrounding parts may also result in breakdown and eventual infection of otherwise healthy tissue.

Technique Checklist

	YES	NO
Cast application and restrictions explained to client and family	_____	_____
Extremity checked every _____ min for _____ hr		
Color _____		
Sensation _____		
Edema _____		
Temperature _____		
Mobility _____		
Pain _____		
Skin irritation _____		
Signs of bleeding on cast noted during hospitalization	_____	_____
Bleeding or drainage reported to physician	_____	_____
Date first noted _____		
Date reported to physician _____		
Cast dried without incident	_____	_____
Client mobile with cast	_____	_____
Discharge instructions on cast care at home	_____	_____

38 Catheter (indwelling), Care of

Overview

Definition

Cleansing of the indwelling catheter and meatus to prevent urethral irritation and inflammation

Rationale

Prevent infection or inflammation of the perineal area, meatus, and urethra.

Reduce the possibility of urinary tract infection.

Terminology

See Technique No. 39, Catheterization, Urethral.

Assessment

Pertinent Anatomy and Physiology

See Appendix I: *bladder, genitalia (female), genitourinary system (male), urethra.*

Pathophysiological Concepts

1. Urinary tract infections are a frequently seen form of infection. These infections range from bacteria in the urine, to cystitis (infection of the bladder) and pyelonephritis (infection of the kidney). Cystitis is especially common in women due to the short urethra and the proximity of the vagina and rectum, which provides easy access to the urinary system for microorganisms. Some conditions of the genitals are highly contagious (e.g., genital herpes).

2. Most inflammations of the penis involve the glans and prepuce. Balanoposthitis (inflammation of these areas because of staphylococcus, coliform bacillus, or, less often, gonococcus) is often seen in males whose foreskin is intact because of the secretions and debris which accumulate there. The surface of the glans becomes reddened, swollen, and itches. The viral condition called condyloma acuminatum is the most common form of benign penile growth. It can be transmitted to other parts of the body or to other persons. Leukoplakia is another common complication resulting in chronic irritation and inflammation of the penis. It is considered precancerous.

3. Inflammations are relatively common in the lower genitourinary tract of women because this area is readily accessible to infectious organisms, and the moisture and warmth of these tissues provide an excellent environment for growth of pathogens. Vulvitis is a nonspecific disorder subsequent to local and systemic disorders. Treatment includes cleanliness, avoiding harsh soaps and bubble baths, elimination of tight-fitting pantyhose and panty girdles, and possibly hydrocortisone creams. Candidiasis, yeast infection, thrush, and moniliasis are all names for the inflammation caused by the fungus *Candida albicans.* These organisms are present in healthy people; however, certain conditions and medications can upset the normal balance, resulting in an overgrowth of this fungus with resulting symptoms. Fungicidal creams, ointments, and tablets are effective in treating this condition.

Assessment of the Client

1. Assess the client's perineal area for signs of inflammation and swelling, particularly around the urinary meatus. Note any discharge around the catheter from the urinary meatus. Inquire about past and present complaints of irritation or discomfort.

2. Assess the client's previous experience with catheters. Determine if the client has received catheter care previously and knows what to expect.

Plan

Nursing Objectives

Provide mental and physical comfort to the client.

Reduce or eliminate the presence of microorganisms.

Instruct the client and family on the care of the catheter system if the catheter must remain indwelling after discharge from the hospital.

Observe characteristics of the perineal area to determine existing or potential pathology.

Client Preparation

1. Wash hands thoroughly before performing this technique.

2. Explain to the client the method and importance of frequent catheter care. Answer any questions before initiating the procedure.

3. Screen or drape the client adequately to protect privacy and preserve the client's dignity.

Equipment

Container of cotton balls with antibacterial cleansing agent

Gloves

Washbasin with water

Soap

Hand towel and washcloth

Implementation and Interventions

Procedural Aspects

ACTION	RATIONALE
1. Perineal care may be given with soap and warm water. To administer catheter care, cotton sponges saturated with an antibacterial cleansing solution are required. Catheter care usually is performed twice daily, or as often as needed to keep the area clean. Wear gloves when performing catheter care.	The skin and mucosa harbor pathogenic microorganisms. The urinary tract offers a favorable environment for such microorganisms which may fulminate into urinary problems.
2. To perform catheter care, hold the catheter taut, but avoid pulling or jerking.	Pressure on the urethral–vesical area may stimulate the neural system of the bladder and cause bladder spasms and pain.
3. For men, raise the penis and retract the foreskin approximately ½ in to 1 in. Cleanse the urinary meatus with one cotton ball. Cleanse the catheter from the point of insertion outward with another cotton ball (Fig. 38-1). Do not contaminate the area by any contact with anal secretions. Repeat the procedure with a fresh cotton ball each time until all secretions and crusts are removed. When finished, clean the foreskin with soap and water and rinse well. Do not leave cleansing solutions under the foreskin. Be sure to pull the foreskin back down into place when finished.	The mucous membranes of the genital area must be kept clean and free from possibly infective exudates and secretions. Cleansing should always progress from the clean toward the contaminated, never the opposite. Leaving strong, cleansing solutions under the foreskin for extended periods may cause irritation. If the foreskin is not replaced to its natural position, inflammation and stricture may occur.

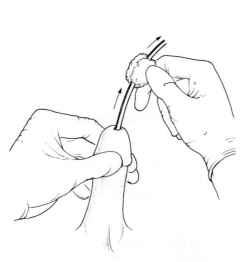

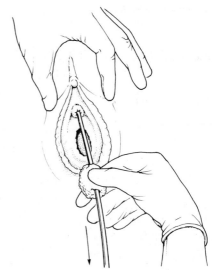

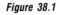

Figure 38.1   *Figure 38.2*

ACTION	RATIONALE
4. For women, separate the vulva by placing the thumb and first forefinger between the labia minora. The urethral meatus is cleansed with cotton balls from front to back using a fresh one for each stroke. The perineum is cleansed from the meatus downward and outward with fresh cotton balls. The catheter is also cleaned from the meatus outward until no exudate remains (Fig. 38-2).	The female perineum must be kept free of secretions, feces, and menstrual flow. Discharge that accumulates at the meatus soon becomes colonized with bacteria. It is essential to progress from the clean area toward the contaminated area when cleaning the catheter.
5. Leave the client in a comfortable environment. Pin the drainage tube to the sheets with no tension or twisting so that it will not be accidentally jerked. Tape the catheter to the female client's leg with some slack between the point of entry and the point of taping so that the catheter does not pull during leg movement. Tape the male client's catheter to the inner aspect of the leg or to the abdomen so that fistula does not develop below the penis.	Pulling the catheter causes pain and trauma to the delicate lining of the bladder and urinary tract. When two skin surfaces are allowed to rub against each other for an extended period, skin breakdown results. The penis should be taped so that it is not allowed to lie against the scrotal sac continuously.

Communicative Aspects

OBSERVATIONS

1. Observe the skin and urinary meatus for signs of redness, skin eruption, or swelling at the insertion site or surrounding area.

2. Inspect the proximal end of the catheter and meatus to be certain that the area is free from dried crusts and blood.

3. Observe the perineal area for signs of inflammation and accumulation of discharge.

CHARTING

DATE/TIME	OBSERVATIONS	SIGNATURE
4/3 0900	Foley catheter cleaned with antiseptic solution. Perineum cleansed, appears clear with no rash or redness. No swelling around catheter noted. Patent, draining yellow urine. ———————————————	P. Dillon RN

Discharge Planning Aspects

CLIENT AND FAMILY EDUCATION

1. If the client will have an indwelling catheter remaining after discharge, the family or client must know how to care for it properly. The method and frequency of catheter care should be discussed. The person who will care for the catheter at home should demonstrate proficiency in the technique for cleaning the catheter and should understand the basic principles behind the procedure.

REFERRALS

The client who will be dismissed from the hospital with a catheter in place should be referred to a visiting nurse for follow-up to ensure that the catheter is cared for properly and to determine potential problems as early as possible.

Evaluation

Quality Assurance

Documentation should reflect consistently the provision and results of catheter care regardless of the frequency. Note the appearance of the meatus and surrounding tissue. Note education efforts directed toward the client or family, as well as an evaluation of the acceptance and understanding of those taught.

Infection Control

1. The ultimate goal of this procedure is the prevention of infection. Because the urinary tract is particularly susceptible to infection, the cleansing of the catheter, meatus, and surrounding tissue is vitally important. Stress to the client, family, and co-workers the importance of cleansing from noncontaminated to contaminated areas to avoid spreading harmful microorganisms to susceptible areas.

2. Handwashing is extremely important in providing catheter care. Before the procedure it is essential so that microorganisms are not transmitted accidentally to the client through contact. Gloves should be worn to protect the nurse and the client. Because many conditions, such as genital herpes, are transmitted by direct contact, the routine use of gloves and meticulous handwashing before and after the procedure are essential.

3. Catheter care includes the care of the catheter tube as it enters the client's body, as well as the tissue surrounding the entry point. This is the area that is to be kept free of microorganisms that might cause pathology if allowed to proliferate and enter the body. The catheter system is not to be opened during this procedure. The chances of infection are great because of the presence of microorganisms. Irrigation and other techniques of the urinary system should be performed at another time under sterile conditions.

Technique Checklist

	YES	NO
Procedure explained to client	_____	_____
Frequency of catheter care _____		
Catheter care noted in chart each time performed	_____	_____
Maintained cleanliness of catheter and surrounding tissue	_____	_____

39 Catheterization, Urethral

Overview

Definition

Introduction of a tube into the urinary bladder; types are (Fig. 39-1):

Nonretention: Plain or straight catheter, for temporary intubation

Retention: Bulb-tipped catheter for prolonged intubation and continuous free drainage

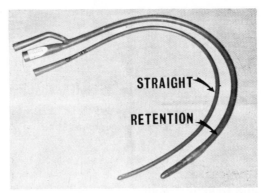

STRAIGHT

RETENTION

Figure 39.1

Rationale

Facilitate the evacuation of urine.

Obtain a sterile urine specimen.

Control urine flow.

Irrigate the bladder.

Instill medications.

Determine the amount of residual urine.

Prevent strain on the pelvis or abdominal wounds from a distended bladder.

Terminology

Catheter: A tube for evacuating or instilling fluids

Closed system: A urinary drainage system in which the catheter is not separated from the tubing

Condom catheter: A rubber or plastic sheathlike device applied externally to the penis and used as a means of catching urine. Figure 39-2 shows a disposable condom catheter.

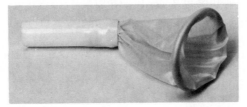

Figure 39.2

Manual irrigation: A single process of introducing and emptying solution from the bladder

Open system: A urinary drainage system in which the catheter is separated from the tubing

Three-way catheter: A triple lumen tube consisting of an inflation tube, an irrigation tube, and a drainage tube. Figure 39-3 shows a cross-section of a three-way catheter.

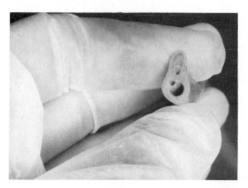

Figure 39.3

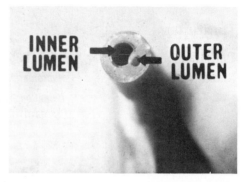

Figure 39.4

Two-way catheter: A double lumen tube consisting of an inflation tube and a second tube through which irrigation solution is introduced and urine is allowed to drain. Figure 39-4 shows a cross-section of a two-way catheter.

Assessment

Pertinent Anatomy and Physiology

See Appendix I: *bladder, kidneys, genitalia (female), genitourinary system (male), ureters, urethra.*

Pathophysiological Concepts

1. Urinary tract infections are a frequently seen form of infection. These infections range from bacteria in the urine, to cystitis (infection of the bladder) and pyelonephritis (infection of the kidney). The urethra of both men and women has a continuous mucous membrane lining with the bladder and the ureters. Thus, an infection of the urethra can extend readily through the urinary tract to the kidneys.

2. The male urethra is surrounded completely by the prostate gland. When this gland begins to enlarge, as it commonly does in elderly men, it compresses the prostatic urethra and interferes with the flow of urine. Another condition that may interfere with the ability to empty the bladder is stricture, or narrowing of the urethra as a result of adhesions. Most inflammations of the penis involve the glans and prepuce.

3. Inflammations are relatively common in the lower genitourinary tract of women because this area is readily accessible to infectious organisms, and the moisture and warmth of these tissues provide an excellent environment for growth of pathogens. Cystitis is especially common in women because of the short urethra and the proximity of the vagina and rectum, which provide easy access to the urinary system for microorganisms.

4. Urinary obstruction may result from congenital defects, stones, pregnancy, benign prostatic hypertrophy, infection, and certain neurologic disorders. Obstruction results in increased risk of infection and stone formation from urine pooling.

Assessment of the Client

1. Assess the client for urinary problems in the past. Determine if the client has ever been catheterized before and what feelings may exist about catherization.

2. Assess the presence of urinary retention, which is evidenced by distention below the umbilicus or at the level of the umbilicus if the distention is serious. Other symptoms of urinary distention are discomfort, voiding small amounts, or professed inability to void.

3. Assess the ability and willingness of the client to cooperate with the catheterization procedure.

4. Assess the client's bladder control and skin condition to determine if insertion of a catheter or application of a condom catheter is necessary to preserve the integrity of the skin and prevent breakdown.

Plan

Nursing Objectives

Allay fear and anxiety of the client regarding the physical condition and the procedure itself.

Control the presence of microorganisms on the skin to prevent the chance of infection.

Minimize trauma to the urinary tract.

Instruct the client and family about the reason for and care of the catheter system.

Client Preparation

1. Explain the procedure to the client and elicit as much cooperation as possible. Because this procedure can be embarrassing to the client, screen and drape adequately as necessary. Place a sign on the door to minimize the possibility of interruptions.

2. If the catheterization is to determine the amount of residual urine, ask the client to void before catheter insertion (Technique No. 20, Residual Urine, Measurement of).

3. If the purpose is to obtain a sterile specimen, be sure the client has not voided for 30 minutes before the procedure.

4. Gather all equipment before approaching the client.

Equipment

Catheterization tray, including sterile gloves, specimen container, lubricant, cleansing solution, and cotton balls

Appropriate catheter

Appropriate drainage system (for retention types)

Bath blanket

Sterile perineal pad (if needed)

Gooseneck lamp

Forceps (optional)

Implementation and Interventions

Procedural Aspects

ACTION	RATIONALE
1. Position the female client in the recumbent position with knees flexed and separated. Position the male in the supine position. Place the lamp in such a position that maximum visualization is afforded being careful not to burn or injure the client. Thorough handwashing *must* precede the catheterization procedure.	Relaxation of the abdominal and perineal muscles during insertion of the catheter greatly enhances the client's comfort during catheterization. Positioning should be done only to the extent the client's physical condition permits, however. The reduction of as many microorganisms as possible is accomplished by thorough handwashing.

ACTION

2. In the postpartum client or any client with vaginal or meatal discharge, remove the perineal pad and administer routine perineal care before beginning catheterization. Wash hands again after administering perineal care.

3. Catheterization is performed under sterile conditions. Establish a sterile field by opening the catheterization setup. Maintain the sterility of the inner aspect of the wrapper and don the sterile gloves (Fig. 39-5). (Refer to the open-glove method in Technique No. 58, Gown and Glove Procedure, Sterile). Pour the cleansing solution over the cotton balls.

RATIONALE

The human skin and mucosa harbor pathogenic microorganisms. The urinary tract offers a favorable location for multiplication of organisms, which can proliferate into urinary pathology.

As long as the inner aspect of the wrapper does not come in contact with anything nonsterile, it maintains its sterility. Likewise, touching a sterile surface with another sterile surface does not contaminate either surface.

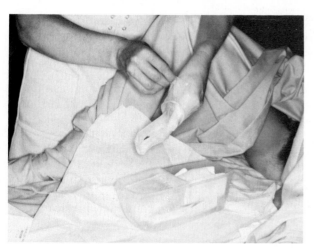

Figure 39.5

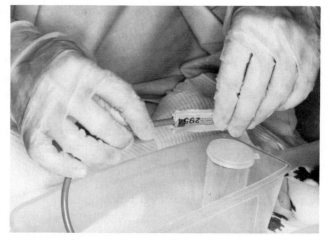

Figure 39.6

4. Apply a sterile, water-base lubricant, such as K-Y jelly, to the distal 3 in of the catheter (Fig. 39-6).

5. *Female:* Prepare a container to receive the urine and place the drapes under the buttocks and over the perineum. Folding the corners of the sterile lower drape around the gloves as the drape is pushed under the client will help maintain the sterility of the gloves (Fig. 39-7).

Male: Prepare the container to receive the urine and place the drapes over the pubis and under the penis.

Lubrication decreases friction between the catheter and urethral tract, minimizing mechanical injury to tissue.

Placement of sterile drapes provides a sterile area in which to perform catheterization.

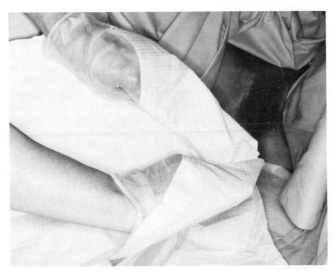

Figure 39.7

ACTION	**RATIONALE**
6. If a retention catheter is being inserted, prepare a syringe with the proper amount of sterile water for balloon inflation.	Having the syringe ready will eliminate delays during the procedure. Sterile water is used to inflate the balloon in case the balloon breaks.
7. *Female:* Separate the female vulva with the thumb and forefinger between the labia minora. This hand is now contaminated. With the forceps in the other hand, pick up a saturated cotton ball. Clean the urinary meatus and surrounding tissue with the cotton ball, using a single downward motion (Fig. 39-8). Repeat, using a new cotton ball each time. Identify the urinary meatus at this time (Fig. 39-9).	Cleansing will help remove contaminants that may lead to urinary infection. The urethra of a postpartum client is edematous, and the entire perineal area is tender; great care and gentleness should be used in cleansing and catheterizing. Always cleanse from an area of least contamination toward the contaminated area. Using forceps will prevent contamination of the sterile field.

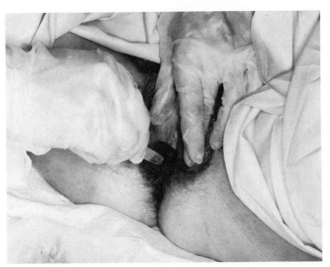

Figure 39.8

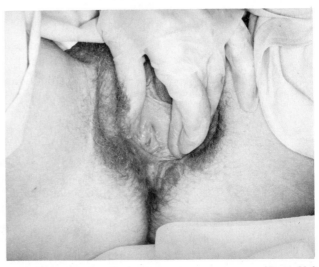

Figure 39.9

ACTION   **RATIONALE**

Male: In the male client, elevate the penis to a 60° to 90° angle with one hand, which is now contaminated. Retract the foreskin with the contaminated hand and cleanse the meatus with the cotton balls held by the sterile forceps. Start in the meatus area and move outward in circular motions (Fig. 39-10).

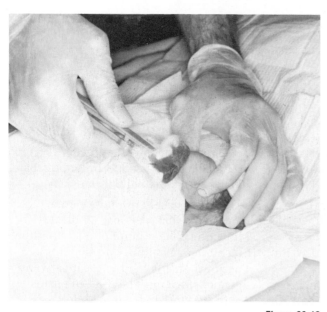

Figure 39.10

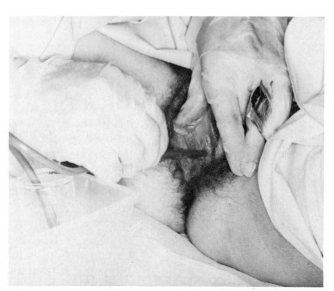

Figure 39.11

8. The contaminated hand may not be reintroduced into the sterile field. Using the sterile hand, remove the catheter from the tray. Leave the drainage end in the receptacle to prevent spilling when the bladder starts to drain after the catheter is introduced into the bladder.

   Female: Reidentify the urinary meatus. Holding the catheter in the sterile hand, slowly insert it into the bladder (Fig. 39-11). Encourage the client to breathe deeply as the catheter is inserted. Never force the catheter; if difficulty is encountered, notify the supervisor or physician. If the catheter is inserted accidentally into the vagina, discard it and use a new, sterile one.

Maintain sterility throughout the procedure. A degree of voluntary relaxation of the urinary sphincter can be produced by deep inspiration and slow exhalation. Obstructions of the urethra may require surgical intervention. Attempts to force the catheter into the blocked urethra will cause trauma and pain.

Deep breathing helps relax the sphincter and eases pain associated with insertion.

Vaginal flora may be pathogenic when introduced into the urinary system.

ACTION

RATIONALE

Male: Lift the penis perpendicular to the body and exert slight traction (Fig. 39-12). Insert the catheter slowly and steadily (Fig. 39-13). Twist the catheter to bypass slight resistance at the sphincters. Slight delay may be necessary for the sphincters to relax. Deep breathing may help relax the bladder muscle and sphincters. If great resistance is met, discontinue the procedure and report to the supervisor or physician.

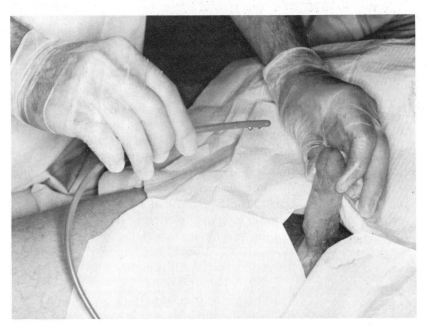

Figure 39.12

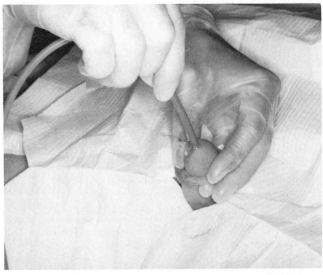

Figure 39.13

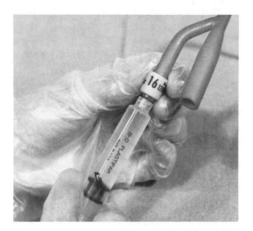

Figure 39.14

ACTION

9. Access to the urinary bladder is ensured when urine returns. If the catheter is to be retained in the bladder for a period of time, insert it another inch and inflate the balloon with the sterile water already drawn into the syringe (Fig. 39-14). Be certain that the proper amount of water is inserted to inflate the balloon. Over-inflation may cause the balloon to burst. Proper placement of the catheter is at the junction of the bladder and the urethra (Figs. 39-15, 39-16). Normal tension on the catheter will pull it to this junction, where it will be retained by the blocking action of the inflated balloon.

RATIONALE

Inflation of the balloon while the catheter is still in the urethra causes great discomfort. Ensure that the balloon portion of the catheter is in the bladder area before inflating.

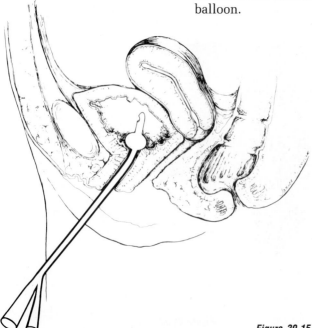

Figure 39.15

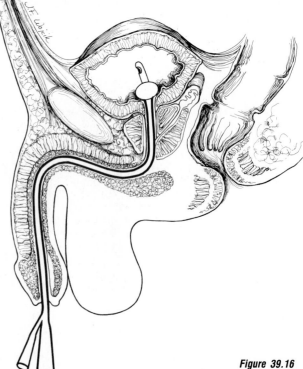

Figure 39.16

ACTION	**RATIONALE**
10. If a sterile specimen is needed, place the open end of the catheter in a sterile collection container. Allow the desired amount of urine to flow into the container. Take the specimen to the laboratory as soon as possible.	Sterile specimens may become contaminated if allowed to remain standing at room temperature for an extended period.
11. Remove the nonretention catheter by pinching the tubing and withdrawing gently.	Pinching will prevent urine from dripping on the client and linen during removal.
12. Connect the end of the retention catheter to a urinary drainage system. Do not pull the catheter while connecting to the tubing. Tape the catheter to the leg so that slack is left between the site of insertion and the site of taping. In the male, the catheter may be taped to the abdomen to prevent irritation on the underside of the penis.	Pressure on the inner bladder area caused by pulling the catheter will overstimulate the neural bladder, causing spasms and pain. Taping the catheter helps prevent unnecessary pulling.
13. Urinary drainage systems must protect the sterility of the urinary tract. The system may be open or closed. The closed system does not allow separation of the catheter from the drainage tube. The open system allows the catheter to be disconnected from the tubing, but this practice is discouraged. The distal end of the drainage tubing is connected to a drainage bag. The bag should be secured to the bed at a level below the bladder (Fig. 39-17).	Opening the urinary drainage system allows pathogenic microorganisms access to the urinary system. Urine drains from the bladder by gravity. Once the urine leaves the body, it is no longer sterile. If the bag is raised above the bladder level, gravity will cause the urine to flow into the bladder where it may cause infection. Obstruction of the tubing may cause urinary retention and stasis in the bladder.

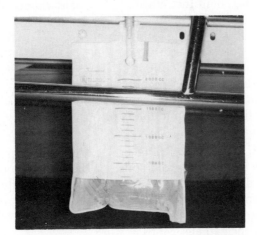

Figure 39.17

ACTION   **RATIONALE**

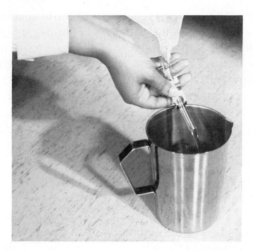

Figure 39.18

Make sure that the tubing is not kinked or twisted and is secured to the bed linen. When the drainage bag is emptied, it is opened from the bottom and allowed to drain into a graduated container for measurement (Fig. 39-18).

14. If the bladder is overly distended, drain the urine in increments of 1000 ml to 1500 ml. In the postpartum client, the bladder should be emptied completely before the straight catheter is removed.

Decompression of an overly distended bladder may cause shock or hemorrhage if accomplished too suddenly, from the rupture of vessels resulting from the rapid change in bladder pressure.

15. After completion of the catheterization, leave the client in a clean, comfortable environment. Situate the beside table to facilitate easy reach of needed articles. Reassure the client that movement will not dislodge the catheter. The initial burning sensation and discomfort will subside shortly. Record the amount of urine on the intake and output record and on the chart. Label and send the specimen to the laboratory, if necessary.

The retention balloon is sufficient to anchor the catheter securely in the bladder. Movement within the client's physical limitations is desirable to prevent the complications that accompany immobility for extended periods.

16. To remove the retention catheter, clamp the catheter to avoid spilling urine during removal. Deflate the balloon by withdrawing the sterile water through a syringe. Withdraw the catheter gently from the urethra. Place the catheter in a basin and discard as soon as possible. Cleanse the meatus with cotton balls if needed.

All fluid must be withdrawn from the inflated balloon to prevent trauma to the urethra during removal.

ACTION

RATIONALE

Special Modifications

1. Condom catheter application: For some men who are incontinent, the condom may be preferable to the retention catheter. Roll the condom smoothly over the penis with 1 in between the end of the penis and the collecting tube. The condom may be secured by application of an adhesive foam strip or a skin-bonding preparation and plastic tape (Fig. 39-19). The condom must be anchored securely but care must be taken not to restrict the blood supply to the penis. Attach the urinary drainage system to the collecting tube of the condom.

The condom does not enter the urethra, and therefore the risk of infection is minimized. The condom drainage system should be secured in such a way that the client is mobile but the tubing is not in danger of being pulled or disengaged from the penis.

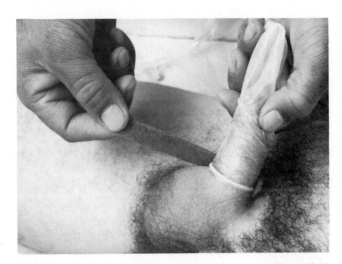

Figure 39.19

2. For catheterization of the pediatric client, location of the meatus is often difficult. An extra pair of gloves and adequate assistance may be necessary.

Adequate restraint of the child is essential. If the gloves touch the child's skin, they are contaminated and must be changed.

3. In pediatric catheterization, cleansing must proceed without delay. If voiding occurs during introduction of the catheter, continue to pass the catheter rapidly and gently.

The child may void before or on introduction of the catheter because of the stimulation of the urethral sphincter.

Communicative Aspects

OBSERVATIONS

1. Note color, appearance, and amount of urine removed.
2. Observe the client for unusual discomfort during insertion and removal of the catheter.
3. Observe for efficiency of the drainage system: tubing is free of kinks, twists and pressure from resting body parts; tubing is below bladder level to facilitate gravitational flow; tubing is above the urine receptacle level.
4. Note signs of inflammation or accumulation of discharges in perineal area.
5. Observe amounts of urine output in relation to fluid intake to evaluate adequacy of kidney function.

CHARTING

DATE/TIME	OBSERVATIONS	SIGNATURE
2/13 1200	No. 16 Foley catheter inserted and connected to gravity drainage system. 500 ml of yellow urine obtained. Explanation and reason given before and during procedure. Expressed concern about activity limits. Instructed concerning ambulation with catheter, keeping I&O record, and catheter care. Left in Fowler's position, reading. Sterile urine specimen to laboratory for culture.	G. Ivers RN

Discharge Planning Aspects

CLIENT AND FAMILY EDUCATION

1. Nonretention catheterization:
   a. Instruct the client or family to report any difficulty or change in voiding after catheterization.
   b. Instruct the client in the importance of increased fluid intake to assist in production of urine for at least 8 hours after catheterization.
2. Retention catheterization:
   a. Offer instructions concerning maintenance of the system while ambulatory and in bed.
   b. Emphasize the importance of adequate fluid intake.
   c. If the client will be dismissed with the catheter, instruct the person who will care for the client's catheter about the techniques for irrigation and replacement.
3. Tell the client to relax as much as possible during insertion of the catheter. Inform the client that there will be a burning sensation that may continue for several minutes but will subside gradually. If the catheter is to remain in place, offer reassurance that the discomfort will subside in a few hours.

REFERRAL

If the catheter must remain in place after the client is discharged from the hospital, the client should be referred to a visiting nurse for follow-up care. The client and family should be told where to purchase catheter supplies.

Evaluation

Quality Assurance

Documentation should include the measures taken to prevent infection. Any difficulty passing the catheter should be noted. The client's reaction to the procedure should be noted in addition to teaching and reassurance efforts by the nurse. Daily observation of the urine drainage and the catheterization site should be reflected in the record. Safety precautions taken to prevent complications should be noted. The intake and output (I&O) record should reflect the adequacy of the urinary drainage system. Account for any discrepancies. Descriptions of the urine and any deviations from the baseline standards should be noted.

Infection Control

1. Prevention of urinary tract infection is vital to the catheterization procedure. Meticulous handwashing is essential. Strict adherence to sterile technique during the procedure is also necessary. Cleansing the area around the meatus must be done from front to back in the female and from the meatus outward in the male to avoid contamination of the urinary meatus. When connecting the drainage bag to the catheter, the ends of both tubes should not be touched any closer than 2 in from the end.

2. Daily catheter care is essential. (See Technique No. 38, Catheter [Indwelling], Care of). If the system is closed, it will not be accessed from the outside. If the system is open, it may be accessed. Opening the system is discouraged, however, and should be preceded by cleaning the ends with a bactericidal agent.

3. The Center for Disease Control (CDC) does not recommend a specific time sequence for changing urinary catheters. Each client should be evaluated to determine when the catheter should be changed according to the amount of sediment in the urine and the amount of encrustation around the catheter. Hold the catheter several inches from the insertion point and roll it between the fingers and thumb. If the catheter feels gritty or encrusted, it should be changed. The overall goal is to prevent infection and provide for the safety and comfort of the client.

Technique Checklist

	YES	NO
Procedure explained to client	_____	_____
Sterile technique maintained throughout insertion	_____	_____
Catheter passed without difficulty	_____	_____
Sterile specimen obtained	_____	_____
Time obtained _____		
Time to lab _____		
Appearance of urine noted in chart	_____	_____
Catheter drainage system remained patent throughout duration of catheter retention	_____	_____
Complaints after catheter removed	_____	_____
Client voided after catheter removed	_____	_____
Care taught to family member or client	_____	_____
Referral to visiting nurse	_____	_____

40   Central Venous Pressure (CVP)

Overview

Definition

Measurement, in centimeters of water, of the pressure in the vena cava or right atrium, using a catheter threaded into the subclavian vein

Rationale

Determine the blood volume.

Evaluate the effectiveness of the pump mechanism of the heart.

Evaluate vascular tone.

Terminology

Hypervolemia: Increased volume of circulating blood

Hypovolemia: Decreased volume of circulating blood

Vena cava: The major vein returning blood to the right atrium of the heart

Assessment

Pertinent Anatomy and Physiology

1. See Appendix I: *blood vessels, heart.*

2. *Arterial pressure* is the pressure exerted to push the blood from the heart into the arterial system. It is greatest in the aorta, which is the main artery leaving the left ventricle of the heart. The diameter of the aorta is so large that it exerts very little peripheral resistance to the flow of the blood, which also predisposes to greater arterial pressure. As the blood gets farther from the heart, the pressure decreases until the blood enters the capillary system with very little pressure. By the time the blood enters the venules from the capillaries, it exerts very little pressure on the walls of the veins. Venous pressure varies with the location of the vein and the position of the body (i.e., standing, sitting, or lying). Venous pressure generally is considered to decrease as the blood travels through the peripheral veins toward the heart. *Central venous pressure* (CVP) is the pressure of the blood within the vena cava and the right atrium.

3. During normal breathing, the pressure in the thorax is negative. When the thorax enlarges during inspiration, the pressure increases. This expands the thin-walled intrathoracic veins, producing a suction effect that causes blood to flow into those vessels and then into the heart. During expiration, the venous inflow is reduced as the intrathoracic pressure is increased. This phenomenon aids in venous return to the heart. This phenomenon also is detected when the client breathes during CVP determination, causing fluctuations in the falling solution.

Pathophysiological Concepts

1. Right-sided heart failure is characterized by an accumulation of blood in the systemic venous system. This causes an increase in right atrial and peripheral venous pressures, with the development of edema in the peripheral tissues and congestion of the abdominal organs. Heart failure occurs when the heart fails to pump sufficient blood to meet the metabolic needs of the tissues.

2. In the upright position, gravity tends to interfere with the return of blood from the lower portions of the body. The muscles exert a squeezing action on the veins, which forces blood away from the area of activity toward the heart. The veins contain small valves which permit the blood to flow in only one direction. Thus, any activity causes blood to move toward the heart without backflow. There is some active contraction of the vein walls themselves which helps propel the blood back to the heart. When a person must stand in a steady position for extended periods, blood tends to accumulate in the extremities causing them to feel uncomfortably full and swollen. If the person remains in this immobile position for extremely long periods, venous return becomes inadequate and the heart does not receive sufficient quantities of blood to supply oxygen to the brain; fainting is the result. This can be prevented by doing isometric leg exercises, such as tightening and relaxing the calf muscles.

Assessment of the Client

1. Assess the level of consciousness and understanding of the client in determining how much explanation to offer. Assess the anxiety level of the family when explaining the procedure.

2. Assess the CVP reading in relation to the condition of the client, the vital signs, and intake and output. Assess the presence of edema. Determine breath sounds and heart sounds.

3. Assess the physical condition of the client. Determine past history of coronary symptoms. Assess for history of chronic lung disease, hypovolemia, or right-sided heart failure because these conditions will affect the CVP readings.

Plan

Nursing Objectives

Obtain an accurate CVP reading.

Allay the client's and family's fears and anxieties about the procedure.

Prevent infection.

Maintain fluid and electrolyte balance.

Prevent air embolism.

Protect the integrity of the intravenous infusion system.

Client Preparation

1. Allay anxiety and promote the cooperation of the client and family by explaining why the readings must be taken. Explain that the client will not feel anything during the reading, but that it is necessary for the client to lie flat in bed to prevent distortion of the reading by the force of gravity.

2. A central line connected to the right atrium or vena cava acts as an extension of the client's vascular system. The venous pressure set, with a three-way stopcock, is connected to the subclavian intravenous line. Set up the CVP set according to the instructions accompanying the equipment.

3. An inaccurate zero point results in inaccurate CVP readings. The zero point on the centimeter scale must be at the level of the client's right atrium. This is approximately midway between the anterior and posterior chest walls when the client is in the recumbent position (Fig. 40-1).

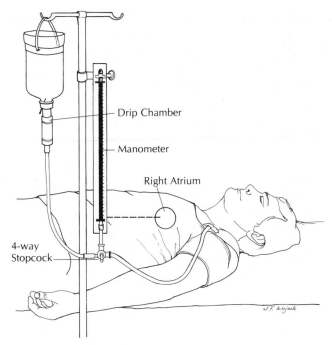

Figure 40.1

4. Circulatory dynamics are most stable while the client is supine because the arteries and veins are oriented horizontally at near-heart level. The client should be flat in bed, with no pillows. If the client's respiratory status is compromised by being flat in bed, however, lower the head of the bed as far as the client can tolerate and take the CVP reading. Note the angle of the bed in the chart so the reading can be taken with the client in the same position each time.

Equipment

Disposable venous pressure set, connected to IV infusion

Manometer with centimeter scale attached to IV standard

Implementation and Interventions

Procedural Aspects

ACTION

1. Fill the venous pressure tubing with fluid to remove *all* bubbles from the tubing. Turn the stopcock to the open position between the solution and the client but do not connect the tubing to the client's catheter until the tubing is flushed free of air (Fig. 40-2).

RATIONALE

Air in the line will interfere with the CVP reading and could cause an air embolism.

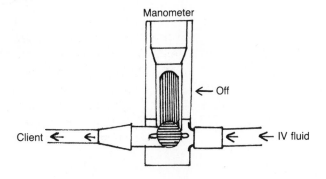

Figure 40.2

ACTION	**RATIONALE**
2. Keep all connections sterile while setting up the tubing. Apply a sterile dressing to the skin at the site of insertion of the venous catheter.	Introduction of pathogens into the vascular system may cause infection and emboli.
3. Have the client lie flat in bed with respirators detached during CVP reading, if possible.	External ventilators increase inspiratory pressure in the chest and may cause a higher CVP reading.
4. Fill the manometer with IV solution by turning the stopcock to open between the IV and the manometer (Fig. 40-3). Allow the fluid to run into the manometer to a level above the anticipated CVP level. It is not necessary to fill the manometer full of fluid.	By viewing the free fall of the fluid, the CVP can be determined more accurately.

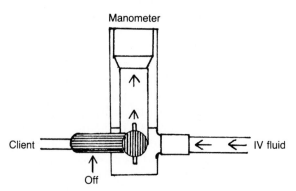

Figure 40.3

5. Turn the stopcock to the position communicating with the client's vascular system to measure the venous pressure (Fig. 40-4). View the fluid as it drops in the manometer. The fluid should fluctuate with each phase of respiration.	The fluid in the manometer will drop until its hydrostatic pressure is equal to the client's venous pressure. During expiration, the venous inflow into the thorax and heart is reduced as the intrathoracic pressure is increased.

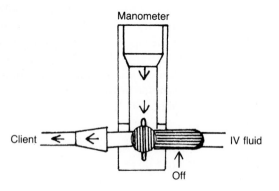

Figure 40.4

ACTION	RATIONALE
6. Read the scale on the manometer at eye level at the point where fluid descent ends. The level of the fluid will fluctuate with respirations. Read at the level of the meniscus when it is at its highest point after the free fall of the fluid has leveled. The usual pressure in the vena cava is 6 cm to 12 cm of H_2O and in the right atrium is 0 cm to 4 cm of H_2O.	Variations in the reading can occur if the scale is viewed from different angles. The point where the descent of the fluid stops signifies the pressure equal to that of the venous pressure in the vena cava or right atrium. The absolute value of a CVP is less informative than the upward or downward trend over a period of time. The CVP reflects the dynamic interrelationships among cardiac activity, vascular tone, and effective blood volume.
7. Reposition the stopcock so that the line is open between the client and the solution. Leave the fluid running at the rate prescribed by the physician.	A continuous flow of solution is necessary to keep the IV catheter patent.

Special Modifications

If the client cannot be lowered into the flat position to measure CVP, place the client in as low a position as can be tolerated. Mark the exact position on the care plan so that it can be duplicated each time the reading is taken.	As long as the CVP is measured under the same conditions each time, trends may be determined.

Communicative Aspects

OBSERVATIONS

1. If the fluid in the manometer drops rapidly, without the normal fluctuations during respirations, check for a leak in the tubing or attachment points.

2. If the fluid does not fall, drops sluggishly, or drops and stops intermittently, the catheter may be partially or completely occluded. Notify the physician. Do not irrigate the catheter. Be sure that there are no kinks in the tubing and that the stopcock is open in the proper direction.

3. Observe the actions of the client during CVP reading. A position change or equipment change may cause a variation of more than 2 cm to 3 cm of H_2O, resulting in an inaccurate reading.

4. Check the dressing on the subclavian catheter insertion site for bleeding or dampness, which may occur if the catheter becomes disconnected from the IV tubing.

5. Venous pressures usually are not taken with whole blood infusions because the blood may clot in the stopcock and cause mechanical difficulties.

6. Observe and record each CVP reading. Notify the physician of any drastic increases or decreases in the usual CVP rate. An elevated CVP may indicate hypervolemia, whereas a low CVP may indicate hypovolemia.

CHARTING

DATE/TIME	OBSERVATIONS	SIGNATURE
10/9 0900	CVP is 4 cm to 5 cm; respirator removed during CVP measurement. Bed flat; no respiratory problems. Client turned to left side. IV infusing at 33 gtt/min. HOB elevated slightly at client's request. Awake and alert. SCIV dressing dry.	G. Ivers RN

Discharge Planning Aspects

CLIENT AND FAMILY EDUCATION

1. Explain why the CVP readings must be taken. Tell the client and family how often the readings will occur and the preparations that will occur, such as having the client lie flat. If the client will be removed from the respirator during the reading, reassure to the client and family that this action will not compromise the client's health and safety.

2. Instruct the client and family about the need to maintain the sterility of the system. The client and family should not handle the tubing, dressing, or other equipment. Restraint of the client's hands may be necessary to ensure that the sterility of the system is not compromised.

Evaluation

Quality Assurance

Each hospital should develop a system for the accurate and timely reporting of CVP readings in a manner so that trends and fluctuations can be determined quickly and accurately. A graphic recording or sequential form may be used. The data may be placed into documentation either manually or by computer. Standard procedures for maintaining the sterility of the tubing and insertion site should be a part of the hospital procedure manual and should be familiar to every nurse who handles CVP systems.

Infection Control

1. Prevent the introduction of pathogenic organisms into the vascular system. Maintain the sterility of the system at all times.

2. The catheter dressing should be changed regularly, usually every 48 hours, using aseptic technique. If the dressing becomes wet, soiled, or loosened from the site, it is considered contaminated and must be changed. A sterile pad and cleansing solution are used to cleanse the site. An antimicrobial solution is applied to the site working from the venipuncture site outward. A sterile dressing should be applied according to hospital policy.

3. The tubing should be changed at regular intervals to prevent the colonization and proliferation of pathogenic organisms. Check hospital policy for frequency of tubing change.

4. Thorough handwashing should be performed before and after the measuring the CVP, changing the dressing, or changing the tubing.

Technique Checklist

	YES	NO
Procedure explained to client and family	_____	_____
CVP measured q _____ hours		
CVP measurement recorded on chart	_____	_____
Client able to lie flat for CVP measurement	_____	_____
If not, angle of head of bed during reading _____		
Client on respirator during measurement	_____	_____
Intake and output record reflects balance of fluid	_____	_____
SCIV site changed q _____ days		
Dressing changed q _____ days		

41

Chest Drainage (Closed)

Overview

Definition

The evacuation of air or fluid or both from the pleural cavity through a closed drainage system; types are:

Closed chest drainage without suction (by gravity)

Closed chest drainage with suction

Rationale

Reestablish subatmospheric pressure in the pleural cavity, thereby permitting reexpansion of the lung.

Terminology

Atelectasis: A state in which air can neither enter nor leave a lung segment, most often caused by trauma or surgery

Pleural cavity: Potential space between the two pleura covering the lungs

Subatmospheric pressure: Pressure below that of the atmosphere

Assessment

Pertinent Anatomy and Physiology

See Appendix I: *bronchial tree, lungs.*

Pathophysiological Concepts

1. The two membranes surrounding the lungs are the visceral pleura, which lines the chest cavity, and the parietal pleura, which covers the lungs. These two membranes are lubricated so that they glide against each other. The space between these two membranes has a negative pressure and contains neither air nor fluid. Collection of either of these substances in this cavity can interfere with breathing and may cause the lung to collapse. Problems in the pleural cavity include pneumothorax (air in the cavity), hemothorax (blood in the cavity), hemopneumothorax (both blood and air in the cavity), and atelectasis (the collapse of lung tissue).

2. Exchange of oxygen and carbon dioxide in the lungs depends on effective ventilation and adequate circulation of blood through both lungs. The amount of surface area available for diffusion greatly affects gaseous exchange. Ventilation brings oxygen into the lungs where it is released into the alveoli in exchange for the carbon dioxide which has been deposited by the capillaries. If ventilation is not uniform throughout both lungs, the rate of oxygen replenishment is reduced, leading to hypoxia. This situation occurs in pneumothorax. This type of perfusion problem is also common as a result of chronic heart failure, asthma, pneumonia, and chronic obstructive pulmonary disease (COPD).

Assessment of the Client

1. Assess the client's respiratory status. Auscultate both lungs to assess the presence or return of breath sounds. Assess the client's color (e.g., discoloration of the fingernails or around the lips) to detect signs of hypoxia. Observe for bilateral chest expansion.

2. Assess the patency of the system. Determine if all connections are secure and whether the tubes are draining.

Plan

Nursing Objectives

Maintain an airtight system, preventing complications and infections.

Relieve the client's anxiety and discomfort.

Teach the client the importance of turning, deep breathing, and coughing.

Prevent postural deformities and contractures.

Record observations accurately.

Promote adequate gaseous exchange.

Client Preparation

1. Explain to the client and family why the chest tube is being inserted and inform them about measures taken to prevent complications, such as avoiding kinked tubing, leaks in the system, and elevating the drainage bag above the level of the client's chest.

2. Place clamps in a convenient and conspicuous place for use after insertion should the airtight system develop a leak.

Equipment

Sterile chest drainage set (self-contained, disposable variety or 2,000 ml glass bottle(s) with rubber stoppers and tubing)

1 liter sterile water

Tape

Thoracic pump or wall suction

Chest bottle protector (if the glass bottles are used)

Clamps

Implementation and Interventions

Procedural Aspects

ACTION	RATIONALE
1. Wash hands thoroughly before touching the client or equipment.	Handwashing reduces microorganisms which might cause infection.

ACTION

RATIONALE

2. Produce a water-sealed drainage system by attaching the drainage tube(s) from the client to the tubing that is attached to the submerged portion of the drainage system. The tube is to be submerged at least at least 1 in under the water (Fig. 41-1). Tape all connections to prevent separation, which would allow air to be drawn into the lung causing further damage.

Water-sealed drainage facilitates escape of air and fluid from the pleural cavity. The water acts as a seal and keeps air from being drawn back into the chest by the negative pressure which is normally found in this area.

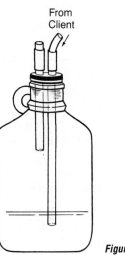

From Client

Figure 41.1

3. Be sure that the air escape tubing from the water seal compartment is patent. This tube is open to air or suction and is not submerged beneath the level of the water.

As drainage accumulates in the drainage bottle, the pressures eventually will equalize unless the air displaced by the accumulating fluid is allowed to leave the confined area. This promotes the negative pressure atmosphere, which continues to drain the fluid from the pleural cavity.

4. Mark the original fluid level with adhesive tape or sticker for measurement.

The amount of drainage may be indicative of the effectiveness of the system. Knowledge of the amount of fluid may assist in evaluation and treatment.

ACTION	**RATIONALE**
5. Arrange the tubing so that it does not interfere with the movements of the client. Ensure that no kinks, loops or pressure points are present to interfere with the proper drainage of the tubing. Tape the tubes in place to provide maximum security of the system. Fasten the tubing to the sheet with a plastic clamp to ensure proper positioning.	Kinking of the tubing may result in obstruction. Looping or pressure on the tubing may produce retrograde pressure forcing drainage back into the pleural cavity. Movement of the client is desirable and should not be inhibited by the presence of the tube.
6. Every hour, "milk" the tubing to prevent obstruction by compressing the tubing manually, progressing from the client toward the drainage system.	The tubing may become obstructed by clots and fibrin. Manual expulsion of these materials will aid in keeping the tubing patent.
7. Check the patency between the pleural cavity and the drainage system frequently by assessing the continuation of drainage and by viewing the oscillation of the water level. Oscillation will decrease as the lung reexpands and may cease before complete reexpansion because of clots and fibrin sealing off the tube.	Oscillation during respiration indicates a patent drainage system from the lung.
8. Never elevate the drainage bottle above the level of the client's chest.	Gravitational pull will allow fluid to flow back into the chest causing contamination and further compromising the pleural area if the bottle or bag is elevated above chest level.
9. Stabilize the bottles in a protective rack to prevent damage. Secure the plastic chest drainage set safely and securely in its stand. The bed is usually left in the high position. A hissing noise may indicate a leak. Caution the client and visitors to avoid handling the tubing or equipment.	If any part of the apparatus is damaged, the closed system is destroyed. If negative pressure is lost, atmospheric pressure in the pleural space will collapse the lung.
Keep clamps in a convenient and conspicuous place for clamping the chest tube as close to the client's chest as possible if the apparatus should become damaged. If the chest tube should become dislodged, apply immediate pressure over the area with a hand, sheet, or any material close by. Notify the physician at once. Sterile Vaseline gauze may be applied to prevent air leakage.	Clamping the chest tube near the point of insertion into the chest wall will decrease the possibility of air entering the pleural space.

ACTION	**RATIONALE**
10. Suction may be applied to the system by connecting the tubing leaving the drainage system to a thoracic suction pump or wall suction. The amount of suction will be ordered by the physician. A two- or three-bottle system may be used. Figure 41-2 shows a two-bottle system. Figure 41-3A illustrates a three-bottle system for a client with one chest tube; a three-bottle system for a client with two chest tubes is shown in Figure 41-3B. Disposable systems, such as Pleur-evac, are commonly used.	Suction may be prescribed to hasten reexpansion of the lung or to compensate for a persistent air leak in the closed system.

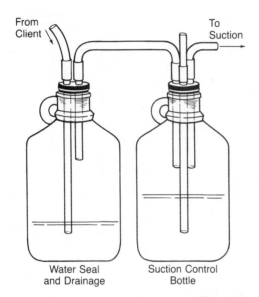

Figure 41.2

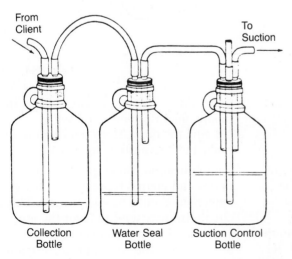

Figure 41.3A

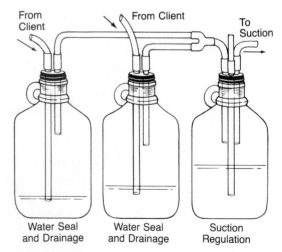

Figure 41.3B

ACTION

RATIONALE

Figure 41-4 illustrates a disposable, water-sealed drainage system. In this figure, arrows indicate the flow of air when the lung is reinflated. In the three-bottle chest drainage setup, the depth of submersion of the tube, which is open to the atmosphere, determines the amount of suction pressure. To increase suction pressure, the tube is submerged to a greater depth.

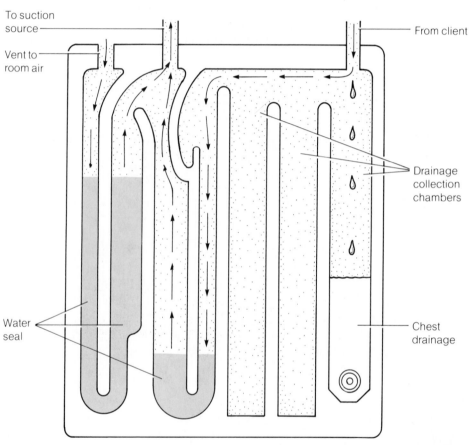

To suction source

Vent to room air

From client

Drainage collection chambers

Water seal

Chest drainage

Figure 41.4

11. Encourage the client to cough and deep breathe hourly.

Coughing and deep breathing assist in raising the intrapleural pressure, clearing the bronchi, expanding the lung, and preventing atelectasis.

12. Encourage proper body alignment. Put the limbs, especially on the affected side, through range of motion exercises several times daily. Allow the client to lie on the side where the tube is located. Be sure the tube remains patent and is not kinked or compressed by the client's body weight. Change position frequently.

Immobilization causes postural deformities and contractures. Proper body alignment should be encouraged. The client also may tend to favor the arm and shoulder on the affected side to prevent pain and discomfort. Aeration of the unaffected lung is maximized when the client lies on the affected side.

ACTION	*RATIONALE*
13. If the thoracic pump is disconnected or malfunctioning, the chest drainage system must be vented to the atmosphere while maintaining the water seal until suction can be reapplied safely.	The thoracic pump acts as a seal when it is not functioning.

Special Modifications

If the drainage bottle or bag becomes full, it must be changed under negative-pressure conditions. The tube should be clamped, according to the physician's instructions, near the chest wall and the drainage apparatus changed during the inhalation phase of the respiratory cycle. Use sterile technique.	If the drainage apparatus is full, the negative pressure is neutralized because no more fluid can be drained out of the lung.

Communicative Aspects

OBSERVATIONS

1. Observe the client for signs of respiratory distress, such as severe pain in the chest, shallow respirations, cyanosis, asymmetrical chest (mediastinal shift may occur when one lung collapses and the sternum is displaced to the side), and level of consciousness.

2. Observe the chest drainage system to ensure that air leaks are prevented. Constant bubbling in the water-sealed bottle may indicate air leaks in the system. Observe the drainage bottle to ensure that the tube from the client remains below the water level. Observe the suction bottle to see that the submerged tube remains at the same depth to ensure consistent suction pressure. Watch the disposable system to see that adequate water levels are maintained; refilling with sterile water may be needed.

3. For the first 2 hours after insertion of the chest tube, observe the fluid every 15 minutes. Observe the drainage every hour during the first 24 hours. After that time, observe the color, consistency, and amount of drainage every 8 hours. The amount can be estimated by marking a tape on the bottle each time it is measured. Determine the need for and success of procedures to "milk" the drainage from the tubing.

4. Include the amount of drainage on the intake and output (I&O) record.

CHARTING

DATE/TIME	OBSERVATIONS	SIGNATURE
5/22 0900	Chest tube in R. chest attached to sterile water-sealed drainage. 20-cm suction with electric pump applied. 200 ml bright red drainage obtained initially. Fluid fluctuating in tube. B/P 120/80, p 80, R 32; no cyanosis noted. Respiration shallow. Breath sounds diminished in R. side and L. side normal. Client encouraged to breathe deeply.	P. Dillon RN
0905	Continues to have shallow respirations. Turned to left side, P 88, R 26. IM med for discomfort given.	P. Dillon RN
0920	Respirations improving, deeper, R 18. Explanation given to client and wife regarding chest drainage (need to turn frequently and breathe deeply). Seems to understand why tube is in place and states understanding of the need to leave the apparatus alone. Drowsy at this time.	P. Dillon RN
1000	Tube remains patent. Total 250 ml red fluid returned thus far. Resting quietly at this time. B/P 118/68, P 72, R 18.	P. Dillon RN

Discharge Planning Aspects

CLIENT AND FAMILY EDUCATION

1. Explain the reasons for and principles of the drainage system to the client and family. Answer any questions regarding the equipment and expectations of client behavior.
2. Caution the client and family not to handle the equipment. Tell them what complications to watch for and report (e.g., loose connections or constant bubbling in the water-sealed bottle).
3. Encourage the client and family to report any problems or symptoms of respiratory difficulty at once. Sudden, sharp pain or abrupt changes in respiratory rate and depth may indicate complications and should be reported.

Evaluation

Quality Assurance

Documentation should include the amount, color, and presence of clots in the drainage. Document any abnormalities in the system and interventions. The current respiratory status, including rate, rhythm, and breath sounds should be noted and compared with previous measurements. The frequency of chest tube milking and the success of this procedure also should be noted. Note the reaction of the client to the procedure, as well as the amount of explanation and the apparent level of understanding and acceptance by the client and family.

Infection Control

1. Scrupulous handwashing should be done before and after handling the chest drainage equipment.
2. The chest drainage procedure should be carried out under sterile conditions. The opening into the chest wall provides a means of access for pathogenic organisms. Cover the wound with an antiseptic substance and sterile dressings.
3. The water in the chest drainage apparatus must be sterile to prevent the chance of contamination.

Technique Checklist

	YES	NO
Procedure explained to client and family	_____	_____
Closed chest drainage to		
Gravity flow _____		
Suction flow _____		
Amount of suction _____		
Coughing and deep breathing q _____ hr		
System remained air tight throughout time it was used	_____	_____
Drainage bottle kept below chest level	_____	_____
Reexpansion of lung accomplished	_____	_____
Complications		
Break in system _____		
Accidental dislodgement of chest tube _____		
Reported to physician	_____	_____
Total amount of drainage from chest _____		
Amount and appearance charted	_____	_____

42 Colostomy Care

Overview

Definition

The diversion of waste products through an artificial opening on the abdominal surface; specifically, care of an opening of the colon through the abdominal wall (Fig. 42-1)

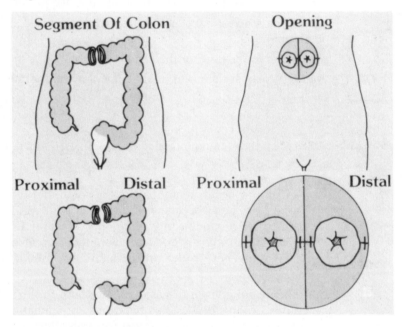

Figure 42.1

Temporary orifice: An opening formed in transverse segments of the colon to permit the escape of feces, known as a transverse loop or double-barreled colostomy (Fig. 42-2)

Figure 42.2

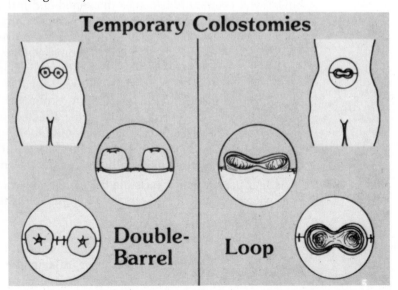

Permanent orifice: The rectum or lower sigmoid portion of the large intestine is removed, and an artificial orifice is created from the remaining or proximal end of the bowel.

Rationale

Establish regularity in the emptying of the colon of gas, mucus, and feces so the client can go about social and business activities without fear of fecal drainage.

Prevent excoriation by maintenance of clean, dry skin.

Cleanse the intestinal tract and prevent obstruction.

Prevent obstruction by regular evacuation of fecal material.

Terminology

Defecation: The voluntary act of eliminating feces from the body

Distal: Farthest from the center

Feces: Body waste discharged from the bowels

Ileostomy: Creation of a surgical passage through the abdominal wall into the ileum

Ileum: The lower third of the small intestine

Proximal: Nearest the point of attachment or midpoint

Assessment

Pertinent Anatomy and Physiology

See Appendix I: *anus, intestine (large), intestine (small), rectum, sigmoid colon.*

Pathophysiological Concepts

1. Cancer may occur in any part of the colon, but it is found most commonly in the rectum. Usually cancer of the colon and rectum are present for a long time before producing any symptoms. Bleeding is a highly significant symptom of colorectal cancer. Other symptoms are changes in bowel habits and a sense of urgency or incomplete emptying of the bowel. Pain is the last symptom.

2. Inflammatory bowel disease includes both Crohn's disease and ulcerative colitis. Crohn's disease is a recurrent, inflammatory disease of the gastrointestinal (GI) tract. It is progressive, relentless, and often disabling. Lesions usually are found in the terminal ileum or ileocecal area of the bowel. The colon is the second most common site involved. Crohn's disease is characterized by lesions that are surrounded by normal-appearing mucosal tissue. The bowel wall eventually becomes thickened and inflexible. Principal symptoms include intermittent diarrhea, colicky pain (usually in the lower right quadrant), weight loss, malaise, and low-grade fever. Treatment includes dietary modifications and alleviation of symptoms. Surgery usually is indicated for the treatment of complications. Ulcerative colitis usually begins in the rectum and spreads to the left colon, but may involve the entire colon. It is similar in symptomology and progression to Crohn's disease. Ulcerative colitis tends to involve the entire surface of the affected area, whereas Crohn's disease involves patches. Rectal bleeding and bloody diarrhea are common in ulcerative colitis. Surgical treatment as a last resort may involve removal of the rectum and entire colon with the creation of an ileostomy.

3. Intestinal perforation is possible because of obstruction of the bowel, chemical irritations, and acute infections. These are usually corrected or alleviated by colostomy.

Assessment of the Client

1. Assess the history of the client with emphasis on past bowel habits and problems. Note family history of cancer or inflammatory conditions of the bowel.

2. Assess the current physical status of the client. Assess the nutritional condition of the client, degree of discomfort, presenting symptoms, and depth of understanding on the part of the client and family regarding the condition.

3. Assess the appearance of feces, noting the presence of blood, the consistency (diarrhealike or formed), frequency, and the color. Assess the condition of the client's anal area, especially if diarrhea has been present.

Plan

Nursing Objectives

Know the client as an individual with individual needs.

Encourage early participation by the client and family in care of the colostomy.

Maintain an attitude of patience, concern, and support while the client learns to accept and care for the colostomy.

Observe the stoma for discoloration and stenosis.

Keep the skin clean and prevent excoriation.

Demonstrate colostomy irrigation and be available for return demonstrations to answer questions and to teach use and care of the irrigation appliance.

Assist the client in establishing a regular pattern of evacuation by seeing that irrigation is carried out at the same time each day.

Teach the client and family the importance of resuming normal diet and activities as soon as possible.

Client Preparation

1. Preparation for colostomy irrigation should begin well in advance of the actual procedure, if possible. The drastic alteration to physical appearance is a dreaded and frightening experience. With a little encouragement and opportunity, the client may be able to verbalize the hostility, fear, and frustration that are being experienced. A willingness to listen and answer questions is the nurse's best tool in helping the client cope with this difficult period.

2. A presurgical and postsurgical visit by a capable ostomy volunteer may be an excellent psychological lift for the client.

3. The client with a colostomy faces a tremendous threat to body image. Time will be required for adjustment to altered physical and emotional images. Do not try to hasten the client into acceptance. Each person progresses toward acceptance at an individual rate; some people never accept the alteration of the body image fully. Demonstrate a positive and patient attitude with emphasis on what the client can rather than cannot do. Involve the client in care of the colostomy as early as possible.

4. Describe the involutional changes that will occur in the stoma over time. Explain to the client that the stoma that will be seen immediately after surgery will not be indicative of the size or shape the stoma will assume later. It will become smaller, less obvious, and more nearly the color of the rest of the skin.

Equipment

Irrigation appliance (various commercial ones are available)

Irrigating solution:

Tapwater	Towels and washcloths
Saline solution	Clean colostomy bag or dressing
Soap solution	Paper bag
Bedpan or commode	Water-soluble lubricant
Stand to hold irrigating solution	Bath thermometer
Protective pad for bed	

Implementation and Interventions

Procedural Aspects

ACTION

RATIONALE

1. If the client is physically able, perform the irrigation in the bathroom with the client sitting in a chair (Fig. 42-3) or on the commode. If the client is unable to sit up, the side-lying position will suffice. The client should turn to the side on which the colostomy is located. Elevate the head of the bed slightly.

Normal body position for bowel evacuation provides psychological comfort and well-being.

2. The equipment should be completely assembled and conveniently arranged before the client enters the bathroom. Offer a full explanation of what will happen and why. Wash hands thoroughly before beginning.

Delays in progressing with the procedure only add to the client's anxiety. A complete explanation will reduce anxiety and enhance cooperation.

3. The temperature of the irrigation solution should be 105° F. Check it with a bath thermometer. Close the flow control clamp so the solution will not run out until ready. Fill the irrigation bag with the type and amount of solution prescribed by the physician. The first irrigation is usually only 250 ml. This may be increased daily up to 1500 ml. Place a stoma guard on the colon tube below the flow control clamp (Fig 42-4). Remove the bag or dressing present on the stoma and dispose of it in a plastic bag. Thoroughly clean the stoma and surrounding tissue.

If the temperature of the irrigation fluid is too cool, it may cause cramping; if it is too warm, it may injure the mucous lining of the colon. The initial irrigation will have little fecal material to remove since most was removed before surgery, and the client has been on an altered diet. As dietary consumption increases in bulk and amount, and as tissue repair of the colon continues, irrigation with larger amounts of water will be necessary to evacuate bowel contents. The stoma dressing should not be left in the client's trash basket. For microbiologic reasons it should be removed from the room in a paper bag and disposed of in the trash room.

4. The type of irrigation appliance may vary. The most common type consists of a gasket held over the stoma by a belt around the client's waist (Fig. 42-5). The gasket opens into a long plastic bag that is open at both ends. The upper opening is to allow the insertion of the irrigation tube into the stoma; the lower opening is placed in the commode or bedpan to allow evacuation of the feces (Fig. 42-6). Fas-

The stoma and surrounding tissue is particularly susceptible to breakdown due to contact with fecal material. The gasket should fit snugly enough to protect the surrounding-tissue from leakage but should not be painful to the client.

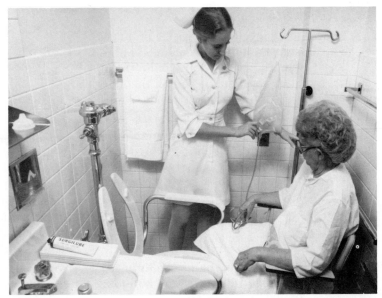

Figure 42.3

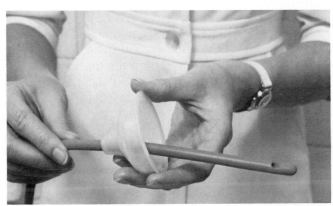

Figure 42.4

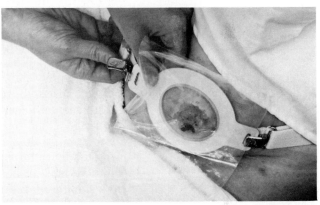

Figure 42.5

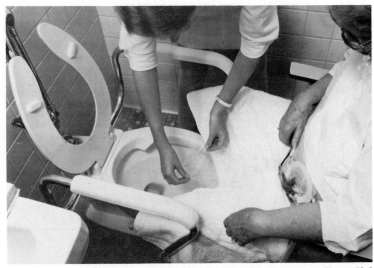

Figure 42.6

ACTION	*RATIONALE*
ten the belt to the gasket on one side and place the gasket over the stoma. Pass the belt around the client's waist and fasten on the other side of the gasket. The belt should fit snugly to prevent leakage.	
5. Fill the tubing with solution to expel the air. Lubricate the distal tip of the tube with a water-soluble lubricant, such as K-Y jelly (Fig. 42-7).	Air introduced into the colon adds to distension and discomfort. It also causes embarrassment when the air is passed to the outside because loud noises often accompany this expulsion. Lubrication of the tip reduces friction as the tube is inserted and decreases discomfort.
6. Introduce the colon tube through the guard into the stoma 2 in to 3 in, or as ordered by the physician (Fig. 42-8). Never use force. If resistance is met, pull the tube out slightly, release a small amount of solution, pause a minute, and again attempt insertion gently. If resistance cannot be overcome, notify the physician. When the tubing is inserted properly, slide the stoma guard against the skin (Fig. 42-9). Open the clamp and allow water to flow into the colon. Hang the irrigation bag on an IV standard, rack, or hook at the client's shoulder level. Be certain it is secure and stable.	Forcefully pushing the tube into the colon may result in perforation of the bowel, an extremely serious complication. If the solution is being blocked by fecal material, releasing a small amount of irrigation fluid should dilute it enough to allow instillation of the remainder of the solution. The stoma guard prevents the solution from being forcefully expelled from the stoma during instillation.
7. If the client expresses a cramping feeling, lower the irrigation container, clamp the tubing, and allow the client to rest before resuming irrigation at a slower rate.	The amount of pressure on the flowing water is determined by the height of the bag; the higher it is held, the greater the pressure.
8. After all of the fluid has been instilled, clamp the tubing and remove the tube. Clamp the top of the drainage bag so that bowel contents do not splash out on the client during evacuation, which may be somewhat forceful. Solution may remain in the colon approximately 5 to 15 minutes. The bowel contents can usually be evacuated in 30 minutes. After evacuation, assist the client in cleansing the stoma and surrounding tissue with soap and warm water and dry it completely (Figs. 42-10, 42-11).	The client will learn the physical signs and feelings that will indicate that evacuation is complete. Because of the moist environment, tissue is susceptible to breakdown. Keeping the skin surrounding the stoma clean and dry helps preserve its integrity.

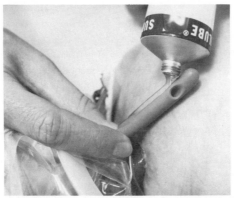
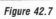

Figure 42.7

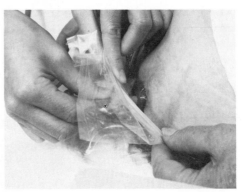

Figure 42.8

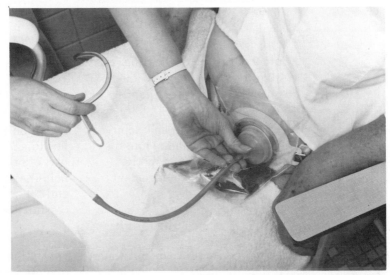

Figure 42.9

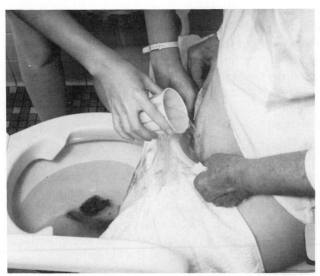

Figure 42.10

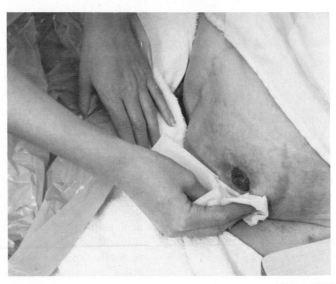

Figure 42.11

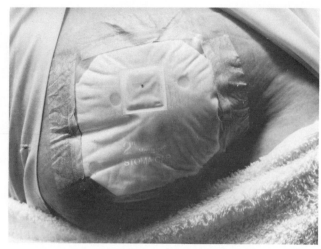

Figure 42.12

ACTION

RATIONALE

Apply a clean bag or dressing (Fig. 42-12). Both the client and the nurse should wash their hands carefully.

9. Leave the client clean and comfortable. Wash, dry, and store the irrigation equipment properly. Offer praise and encouragement freely.

Attention to the client's emotional health and well-being is an important part of optimal recovery. Praise will help the client to gain the confidence and self-assurance needed to deal successfully with the colostomy.

Dressing Change

1. Clean the skin with soap and water each time the dressing is changed. Dry the area thoroughly and gently. Apply medicated ointment, if allowed.

Prevention of excoriation and irritation are vital to successful colostomy adaptation. Skin breakdown can delay the fitting and wearing of a permanent device.

2. Gauze pads may be placed over the stoma, with a larger, more absorbent dressing over them. Secure the dressings with Montgomery strips to prevent skin irritation due to frequent removal of adhesive tape (See Technique No. 49, Dressings, Surgical). Ostomy bags may be applied as soon as ordered.

Stoma dressings are intended to absorb the liquid part of the stool and to prevent soiling clothes and bed linens. Integrity of surrounding tissue must be maintained.

3. Stoma bags are available for the client to wear and may be held in place by a belt or may be self-adhering to the skin. As soon as the colostomy is evacuating satisfactorily, apply a bag and give the client instructions about care of the colostomy appliance. Most colostomy bags have a round opening in the upper portion that fits over the stoma. Thus, the evacuated contents are allowed to fall

It is very important to keep the skin around the stoma clean and dry. The appliance should provide protection from social embarrassment for the client and also should not compromise the integrity of the skin.

ACTION   **RATIONALE**

into the bag. The bags should be
changed as needed. The irrigation
bag can be rinsed with warm soapy
water, then in clear water, and
dried in room air. The belt also
may be washed in warm soapy
water and should be rinsed
thoroughly and allowed to dry
completely before reapplication.
Hands should be washed
thoroughly before and after this
procedure.

Communicative Aspects

OBSERVATIONS

1. Observe the client and environment to determine self-perception and self-concept, particularly in relation to alterations in body image. Observe for expressions of self-doubt, self-assurance, autonomy, orientation toward family and friends, and adaptive ability.

2. Observe the fecal return for appearance, color, and consistency.

3. Observe the skin around the colostomy for signs of redness or excoriation.

4. Observe the colostomy for any change in appearance.

5. Observe for signs and symptoms of fluid and electrolyte imbalance.

CHARTING

DATE/TIME	OBSERVATIONS	SIGNATURE
5/15 0945	Colostomy irrigated with 500 ml of tap water. No difficulty inserting the tube. Returned dark brown, formed stool and liquid. Stoma pink; client looked at the stoma for the first time today and asked questions about the irrigation procedure. Appears ready for teaching. Dressings applied.	F. White RN

Discharge Planning Aspects

CLIENT AND FAMILY EDUCATION

1. The nurse should be familiar with the following information to assist the client in maximizing rehabilitation potential:

   How soon after surgery is the colostomy irrigated?

   How often and when should the irrigation take place?

   What constitutes adequate nutrition?

   What foods may adversely affect colostomy functioning?

   What effect does dehydration have on proper colostomy function?

   How often and what kind of bowel movements should be expected?

   What is the best and most economical irrigating device for this particular client?

   How and where will irrigation be performed at home?

   How is equipment kept clean and odor-free?

   How and where is new equipment obtained when needed?

   What other family member can be taught colostomy care to ensure proper care if the client cannot perform self-care?

   Why are periodic follow-up visits essential?

   What unusual signs should be called to the physician's attention immediately?

   What community resources are available?

2. Explain before the operation, if possible, what is involved in the surgery and how it will affect normal living circumstances. However, overpreparation may serve to frighten or upset the client and family. Direct teaching toward the client's response and acceptance, which are measured by questions and degree of interest. In teaching, stress the remaining function rather than that function that will be lost.

3. After surgery, encourage the client to look at the stoma and to participate in its care. If resistance or hesitation is met, however, do not push or insist. Let each client progress at an individual pace.

4. Explain to the family and client that the size of the stoma is exaggerated at first because of swelling. It will diminish in time.

5. The low-residue diet of the first few weeks will progress to a normal diet in most cases. Advise the client to chew all food thoroughly. Some foods may need to be avoided, such as onions, beans, cabbage, and nuts, all of which are known to be gas forming; spicy or irritating foods which may cause diarrhea; and certain drugs, such as antibiotics, which will upset the normal flora of the bowel. It may be helpful for the client to keep some kind of anti-diarrheal medicine on hand.

6. Reassure the client that once regulated, he or she may resume normal activities. Caution the client against overrestriction. The colostomy client should avoid severe dietary restriction. There is no reason to limit social and traveling ventures or to take excessive supplies or clothing when going out. Emphasize the return to normalcy.

7. Encourage the client to maintain medical follow-up as suggested by the physician.

Evaluation

Quality Assurance

Documentation of the irrigation should include the results of the procedure as well as the client's participation and acceptance. Each irrigation should include a description of the return, problems with insertion of the tube, and amount of client participation. The time of the irrigation should be noted as well as any problems at other times, such as unplanned evacuation and leakage. For the client to resume normal activities, the goal of regular irrigation is to pattern the bowel to evacuate at the same time each day. Documentation should include how successfully this goal was met. Colostomies may be temporary or permanent. Usually the client will spend at least some time at home with the colostomy even if it is temporary. Teaching of the colostomy client is vital. All teaching efforts directed toward the client and family members should be documented. The response and demonstrated ability to do colostomy care should also be noted. Alteration to body image involves serious psychological readjustment. Documentation should include reactions voiced by the client and family.

Infection Control

1. Rectal surgery is preceded by thorough cleansing of the bowel to create as clean an environment as possible. The dressings placed on the surgical area after surgery should be sterile just as for any other surgical wound. After evacuation of feces begins, the equipment should be kept clean. Thorough cleansing of the stoma and surrounding tissue promotes the integrity of the skin and reduces the chances of infection.

2. Thorough handwashing is essential for the nurse and the client before and after colostomy irrigation.

Technique Checklist

	YES	NO
Procedure explained to client before proceeding with irrigation	_____	_____
Initial irrigation		
In bed _____		
In bathroom _____		
Tube inserted in stoma without difficulty	_____	_____
Results obtained	_____	_____
Procedure taught to client and family	_____	_____
Client able to perform irrigation	_____	_____
Family member able to perform irrigation	_____	_____
Bowel evacuates on a regular schedule	_____	_____
Stoma and tissue healthy and intact	_____	_____
Client seems to accept colostomy	_____	_____
Return to normal activities anticipated by client and family	_____	_____

43 Contact Lenses, Insertion and Removal

Overview

Definition
Insertion or removal, by the nurse, of corneal or scleral lenses of a client who is injured or incapacitated

Rationale
Insert lenses into the eye without trauma.
Remove lenses from the eye without trauma.

Terminology
Corneal lens: The most widely used type of contact lens covering only the cornea

Hard lenses: A lens that fits directly over the cornea; one that is not pliable, but hard and curved, with a fixed shape

Presbyopia: Visual defect involving loss of accommodation owing to loss of elasticity of the crystalline lens; also called farsightedness

Scleral lens: A larger lens that covers both the sclera and cornea, about the size of a quarter

Soft lens: A contact lens that is pliable and can be cupped before insertion

Assessment

Pertinent Anatomy and Physiology
See Appendix I: *eye (external), eye (internal).*

Pathophysiological Concepts
1. A *cataract* is an opacity of the lens or its capsule. Light rays cannot pass through the lens or are distorted before they reach the retina. The lens must be removed and corrective lenses used to see clearly. The cataract is often visible on gross examination of the eye and on ophthalmoscopic examination.
2. Binocular vision is vision with two eyes. The images from the two eyes blend to give an impression of depth and solidity. If the images are to be brought to identical points on the two retinae, various processes must be coordinated perfectly. These include eye movement, equal constriction or dilatation of pupils, and equal accommodation of lenses. Failure of any of these processess may result in defective vision. If the refractive power of the eye is too weak or the eyeball too short, the images fall back of the retina; this condition is called hyperopia (farsightedness). If refractive power is too great or the eyeball is too long, the images fall in front of the retina; this condition is called myopia (nearsightedness). With age the lens loses its elasticity causing presbyopia.

Assessment of the Client
1. Assess the visual history of the client, if possible. Determine what type of lenses the client wears, and any problems with removal or insertion. Determine whether the lenses are hard or soft.
2. Assess the physical condition of the eyes. Trauma to the orbit or eyeball may make removal difficult. Observe carefully the condition of the lens in the case of head trauma. If the lenses are hard contacts, they may be out of position or broken.

Plan

Nursing Objectives	Prevent injury to the eyes.
	Avoid loss or damage to the lenses.
	Successfully insert or remove the lenses.

Client Preparation

1. If the client is conscious but incapacitated, explain that the lenses will be inserted or removed carefully by the nurse. Request guidance from the client (if practical).

2. Lenses should be stored only in containers especially designed for this purpose. Differentiate between the left lens and the right lens. In an emergency situation when no container is available, prepare two receptacles containing water in which to place the lenses. Mark the receptacles "LEFT" and "RIGHT" so that the contacts can be identified. Carefully identify these containers so that they are not thrown away inadvertently during cleaning procedures.

Equipment

Lenses

Cleanser for lenses

Suction cup for removing contact lenses

Case for storage of lenses

A specially designed container to hold the contact lenses, labeled with the client's name, and containing separate compartments that are labeled "RIGHT"and "LEFT" for each corresponding lens.

Implementation and Interventions

Procedural Aspects

ACTION	RATIONALE
1. Wash hands thoroughly before cleaning contact lenses. All soap must be rinsed completely from the hands. Consult the client or family about the preferred method of cleansing the lenses and the type of solution recommended.	Soap film from the hands is transferred to the lenses, causing visual distortion.
2. Cleanse the lenses well before insertion. Place a stopper in the sink drain before beginning. Open the lens container carefully; remove one of the lenses with the tip of the forefinger. Identify whether it is right or left. Wet the lens with slowly running tap water and squirt a small amount of the lens cleaner on both sides. Rub the cleaner into both sides gently with the thumb and forefinger. Rinse with tap water. Insert this lens before cleaning the other one in the same manner (Fig. 43-1, 43-2).	If the lens is dropped, it easily may flow down the drain unless precautions are taken. The container must be opened carefully to avoid losing the lenses, which are difficult to find if dropped. The cleanser must be washed off of the lens, as it is irritating to the eye. Some lenses are marked so the right one may be differentiated from the left. some are not. It is important not to get the two confused since each lens is made to correct the vision in the eye for which it is intended, and they are not interchangeable.

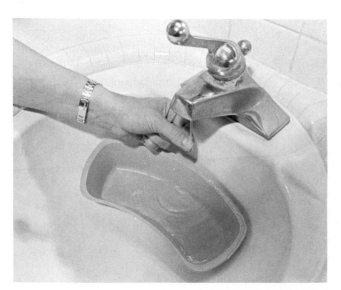

Figure 43.1

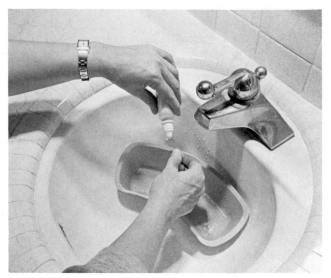

Figure 43.2

ACTION

3. To insert the lens, hold the soft lens at the edge between the thumb and the index finger. Apply a drop of wetting solution. Flex the lens slightly with finger pressure (Fig. 43-3). The hard lens is balanced on the index finger. A drop of wetting solution on the lens is spread to both sides with a gentle massaging motion between the index finger and thumb. Position the lens on the tip of the index finger (Fig. 43-4).

RATIONALE

Lenses must be moistened before insertion into the eye to facilitate placement and decrease discomfort once the lens is in place.

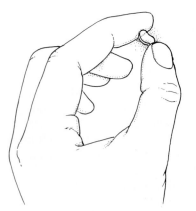

Figure 43.3

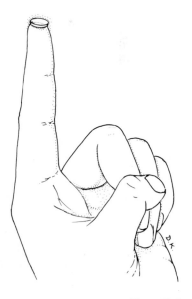

Figure 43.4

ACTION	*RATIONALE*
4. Position the client with head tilted backward. Separate the upper and lower eyelids of the appropriate eye with the thumb and index finger of the hand not holding the lens. Gently place the lens on the cornea directly over the pupil covering the iris, the colored portion of the eye (Fig. 43-5). Ask the client to blink a few times and to assess the situation of the lens. Visual assessment also will reveal appropriate lens position.	With the client looking upward at the ceiling, placing the lens directly in the desired location is easier. Insert gently and quickly before involuntary blinking occurs, which may interfere with placement. The hard lens looks like a clear disc on the eye and can best be seen at the edges of the lens.

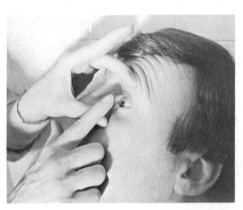

Figure 43.5

5. If the hard lens is not in the proper location, it may be moved by gently pushing on the eyelids to guide the lens into position.	Care must be taken not to injure the eye surface, but the lens floats on a thin watery layer and will move easily if pushed gently. It is made to fit directly over the iris and when in proper position, should stay without problem.

Removal

1. Manual removal is used for corneal lenses only. Place the tip of the forefinger of one hand horizontally on the lower lid below its margin. Place the top of the forefinger of the other hand on the upper lid above its margin and observe to determine if the lens is visible. Manipulate the two lids against each other in scissoring motion while the client closes, opens, and rolls the eye. The lens should slide out between the lids (Fig. 43-6).	Care must be taken that the lens does not pop out and get lost. Even the gentle pressure exerted by the nurse's fingers may be enough to cause the lens to flip out of the eye.

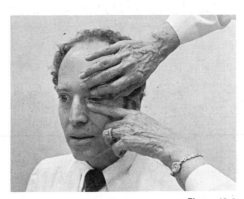

Figure 43.6

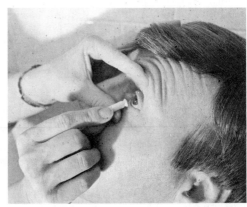

Figure 43.7

ACTION

2. Removal of the hard contact with a rubber suction cup is recommended when the client cannot participate in the removal. The surface of the suction cup must be free of dirt and grease. Pull the lower lid of the client's eye downward gently. Place the suction cup on the center of the lens. All edges of the cup should be in contact with the lens. Release the pressure on the suction cup and allow it to adhere to the lens. Do not pull the lens directly from the eye. Use a gentle rocking motion to release the suction between the lens and lower surface of the eye. Remove the lens from the eye by gently pulling outward and downward (Fig. 43-7).

RATIONALE

Dirt and grease will adhere to the lens and cause discomfort when lenses are reinserted later. The lower lid must be pulled gently so that the upper lid will not place pressure against the top of the contact lens, inhibiting its gentle removal. Only enough suction to adhere the cup to the lens is necessary. Greater suction may cause harm to the delicate outer layers of the eye. All edges of the suction cup must be in contact with the lens for it to adhere. The rocking motion to break the suction is very important to prevent eye injury. Removing the lens outward and downward prevents dropping it back into the eye accidentally.

Special Modifications

1. With some types of soft lenses, tap water is not used. Sterile distilled saline is the preferred cleansing solution. Often these lenses are cleaned in a special heating unit in which they soak overnight. Sterile normal saline is the solution used in most of these units.

Some persons are allergic to the cleansing solutions. Some types of lenses are harmed by the use of tap water.

2. If difficulty is encountered in breaking the suction from the bottom portion of the lens, raise the client's upper eyelid and break the suction at the upper edge. Remove the lens from under the lower lid by pulling gently outward and upward. If the client has excessively dry eyes, a drop of wetting solution before removal may help in releasing the suction.

Suction is spread evenly over the two surfaces, which are adhered. Breaking suction at any edge releases the pressure and facilitates removal.

Communicative Aspects

OBSERVATIONS

1. If the contact lens cannot be removed with ease, discontinue removal efforts and consult a physician. An ophthalmologist may need to be called.

2. Note the condition of the eyes before and after insertion and removal of contact lenses. Watch for redness and excessive tearing.

3. Unrelenting pain or excessive tearing may indicate a piece of dirt or an eyelash under the lens. Sometimes this debris can be observed. If this occurs, tearing may wash away the substance, or a drop of wetting solution may help. If the problem remains, the lens must be removed, cleansed, and reinserted.

CHARTING

DATE/TIME	OBSERVATIONS	SIGNATURE
9/18 0745	Corneal lenses removed and placed in special container. Given to wife to keep until after surgery.	G. Ivers RN

Discharge Planning Aspects

CLIENT AND FAMILY EDUCATION

1. The client usually will have had contact lenses before entering the hospital and should be familiar with the care and wearing procedures. People tend to become somewhat careless after they have become accustomed to caring for their lenses. Such undesirable habits as wetting the lenses with saliva and storing them in containers other than the contact case can result in eye infection and loss of eyesight. A review of various aspects of care may be needed with emphasis on proper storage when lenses are not in use. Emphasis should be on infection prevention.

2. If the client has not had contact lenses before, gentle guidance and encouragement may help to facilitate the transition to wearing them.

3. If the client has problems with the lenses, an appointment should be made with an optometrist or ophthalmologist.

Evaluation

Quality Assurance

Documentation should include removal procedure, storage of lenses, and the client's response. The nurse should document awareness of the possible complications of contact lens removal with a suction cup, and the measures taken to avoid them. Documentation should include evaluation of the client's habits in relation to wearing and caring for contact lenses.

Infection Control

1. The lenses should be soaked as recommended by the manufacturer when not being worn. A separated case is usually available from the manufacturer to facilitate the cleaning and storage process. Soap or disinfectant made especially for contact lenses should be used periodically to ensure that eye infections are not transmitted. Careful handwashing with soap should precede contact lens insertion and removal.

2. The mouth contains normal flora that may be pathogenic if introduced into the eye. Caution the client never to moisten lenses by placing them in the mouth.

3. Lens containers should *never* be borrowed from other persons because this may spread eye infection.

Technique Checklist

	YES	NO
Type of contacts		
Hard _____		
Soft _____		
Insertion		
Procedure explained to client	_____	_____
Careful handwashing prior to insertion	_____	_____
Lens cleaned before each insertion	_____	_____
Eye tissue healthy and without damage	_____	_____
Removal		
Suction cup	_____	_____
Complications _____		
Manual removal	_____	_____
Complications _____		
Lenses stored in proper container	_____	_____
Client educated or reeducated about proper care and handling of contacts	_____	_____

44 Crutchwalking

Overview

Definition

Aiding the disabled person in increasing stability and reducing body weight on one or both of the lower extremities

TYPES OF CRUTCHWALKING

Four-point gait: Weight-bearing is permitted on both legs; the pattern is as follows: right crutch, left foot; left crutch, right foot (Fig. 44-1). This is the normal reciprocal walking pattern with crutches.

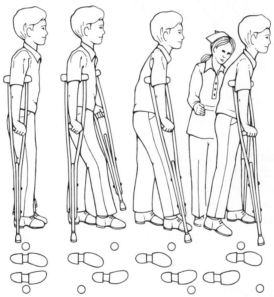

Figure 44.1

Two-point gait: Weight-bearing is permitted on both legs, and the pattern is a speed-up of the four-point gait: right crutch and left foot forward at the same time, left crutch and right foot forward at the same time (Fig. 44-2).

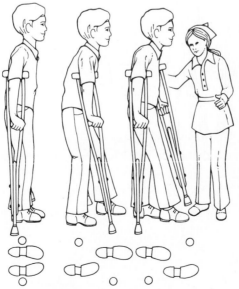

Figure 44.2

Three-point: Weight-bearing is permitted only on one leg; the other leg cannot bear weight but acts as a balance in the process of ambulation. This gait also is used when partial weight-bearing is allowed on the affected extremity. The pattern is as follows: both crutches and the impaired leg go forward; then the unimpaired leg follows through as weight is borne on the palms. The crutches and impaired leg are brought forward immediately, and the pattern is repeated (Fig. 44-3).

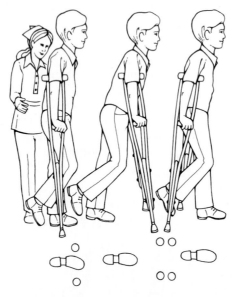

Figure 44.3

Swing-through gait (swing-to gait, tripod gait): The body is supported on the hands and crutches, and the body is then brought through the crutches in a swinging motion. Both crutches are advanced simultaneously while bearing body weight on both legs. The client leans forward, transferring body weight onto the extended crutches. The legs are swung up to the crutches or beyond (Fig. 44-4). This gait is used by paraplegics and those with braces on both legs.

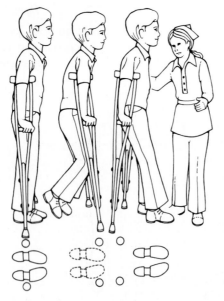

Figure 44.4

Rationale	Promote mobilization.
	Promote client independence through ambulation.
	Prevent injury to affected limb(s).
Terminology	*Alignment:* The proper relationship of body segments to one another
	Balance: Stability or steadiness
	Center of gravity: The point at which the mass of an object is centered
	Posture: Body alignment

Assessment

Pertinent Anatomy and Physiology

1. See Appendix I: *skeletal muscles, skeletal system*
2. The chief muscles involved in ambulation are those of the legs and thighs. The normal walking pace for adults is 70 to 100 steps per minute. Elderly people generally have a slower pace.
3. The major muscles involved in crutchwalking are the flexor muscles of the arm (to move the crutches forward), the extensor muscles of the forearm (to support the elbows while "swinging through" the crutches), the finger flexors (used to grasp the crutch grips), the shoulder muscles (which support the weight while the body is in midair), and the wrist muscles (which position the hands on the grips).

Pathophysiological Concepts

1. Muscle tone often is reduced when one is in poor health, particularly if prolonged bed rest is necessary. With inactivity, muscles decrease in size and strength. When clients are immobilized and unable to exercise, their muscles become weak and atrophied.
2. Changes in the joint result when the surrounding tissue is immobilized. When muscle movement decreases, the connective tissue in the joints, tendons, and ligaments becomes thickened and fibrotic. Chronic flexion or hyperextension of the joints can cause permanent contracture. Hyperextension results in pain and discomfort for the client and abnormal stress and strain on the surrounding ligaments and tendons of the joint.
3. Learning to use crutches properly may enable the client to ambulate earlier. Early ambulation decreases the chances of cardiovascular problems such as orthostatic hypotension, edema, and thrombus formation. Ambulating as soon as the client is able may prevent respiratory problems, such as shallow breathing, fluid accumulation in the lungs, and respiratory infections. Gastrointestinal (GI) problems, such as constipation and impaction, and urinary problems, such as stasis of urine, kidney stone formation, urinary retention and incontinence, and urinary infections, also may be prevented by early mobilization.

Assessment of the Client

1. Assess for dizziness or faintness as the client arises to the vertical position. This assessment may be made while the client is sitting on the side of the bed. Assess the client's sense of balance, and note any signs of weakness or fatigue.
2. Assess the client's postoperative progress in relation to wound healing and pain in the incision site. Assess the site for proper closure and adequate tension before undertaking crutchwalking.
3. Assess the client's posture for alignment during ambulation. The well-aligned posture is head erect, vertebral column straight, toes and patellae pointing forward, and elbows slightly flexed. Include in this assessment the normal gait of the client in relation to the prescribed crutchwalking gait.

4. Assess the client for weakness in the legs, back, and muscles, all of which are essential for crutchwalking. Assess the need for exercises to build up certain muscles to facilitate the crutchwalking experience. Assess the client's ability to take steps. Determine how much weight-bearing is allowed and can be tolerated. Assess balance in the client's upper body and ability to hold the body erect.

Plan

Nursing Objectives

Teach the client proper crutchwalking technique.

Alleviate fear and anxiety about crutchwalking.

Prevent development of faulty habits when walking on crutches.

Record daily progress.

Client Preparation

1. Active and passive exercises may prepare the client for crutchwalking. Isometric exercise, which may be performed while the client is lying in bed, involves tensing the muscles, holding them for a specified time (5–10 sec), and relaxing. This may be useful in building body tone and strengthening body parts. Other preconditioning exercises include quadriceps sitting, gluteal sitting, sit-ups, push-ups, raising arms, and pull-ups. Muscles which should be strengthened are the muscles of the shoulders, chest, arms, hands, and back.

2. Because of the dependent nature of the client's condition, ensure safety and prevent further injury from falls or incorrect use of crutches. Place a safety belt on the client until stability is gained. The client should wear nonskid shoes or slippers. Give adequate instruction before any attempts at crutchwalking. A nurse or therapist must accompany the client on early crutchwalking attempts.

Equipment

Adjustable crutches

Rubber crutch tips

Axillary arm pads

Nonskid shoes or slippers

Safety waist belt

Tape measure

Implementation and Interventions

Procedural Aspects

ACTION

1. To measure the client in the standing position, measure 1½ in to 2 in from the axillary fold to a position on the floor 4 in in front of the client and 6 in to the side of the toes. Allow a 2–finger-width insertion between the axillary fold and the armpiece. If the client must be measured lying down, measure from 2 in below the axilla to 4 in to 6 in out from the sole of the foot.

RATIONALE

Adjustable crutches are practical because the disease may cause structural changes or the client may improve and progress to a different crutch base and gait. Measurement should be taken with the client in the standing position so that as near to normal walking posture as possible can be ensured.

ACTION	**RATIONALE**
2. Start the first day adhering to proper techniques for balancing. Start with the tripod position formed by the client's body and the two crutches. Direct the client to stand with feet slightly apart and crutches placed forward and out from the body in such a fashion that a line drawn between them would form the base of a triangle, the apex of which would be the client's feet (Fig. 44-5).	Balance is emphasized from the first day to give the client a feeling of security and safety. Correct standing position is essential for maintaining balance.

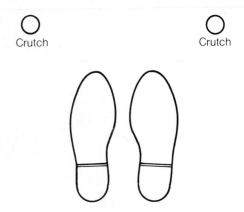

Figure 44.5

3. Teach the client to extend and stiffen the elbows and to place the body weight on the palms.	Pressure on the brachial plexus in the axilla may cause temporary or permanent paralysis of the arm.

General Guidelines for Determining Gait for Most Orthopedic Clients

When the client may bear partial weight on each limb, teach the four-point or two-point gait.	The type of disability usually determines the crutchwalking gait. Generally, this is ordered by the physician.
When the client may bear little or no weight on one extremity, teach the three-point gait.	
When there is complete paralysis of hips and legs, teach the swing-through gait.	

Special Modifications

1. To sit in a chair, the client with crutches stands with the back of the legs centered against the chair. Both crutches are held by the hand grips in one hand and the other is placed on the arm of the chair. The client leans forward, flexes the knees and hips, and lowers the body slowly into the chair (Fig. 44-6). To rise, the client places both feet in a wide stance with the crutches on the outside of the feet and to the front. The client rises by placing a hand on each crutch grip and pushing down during standing (Fig. 44-7).	The tips of the crutches must be spaced far enough apart for a wide base of support. The rubber tips must be firmly secured to the crutches to prevent slipping.

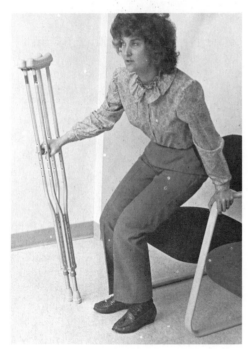

Figure 44.6

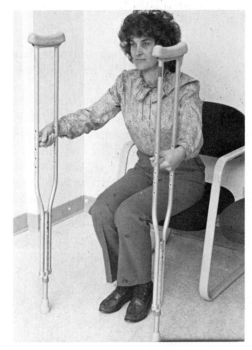

Figure 44.7

ACTION

2. To go up stairs, the client puts the unaffected leg on the next step to hold the weight of the body while the crutches and affected limb are brought up (Fig. 44-8). To go down, the crutches are placed on the next step to hold the weight while the unaffected and the affected limb are lowered to the step.

RATIONALE

It is essential to provide an adequate base of support during the transition from one step to another.

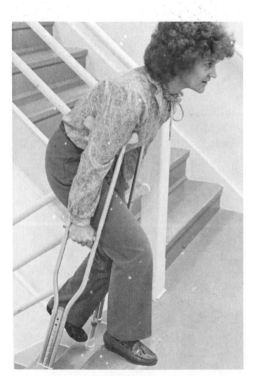

Figure 44.8

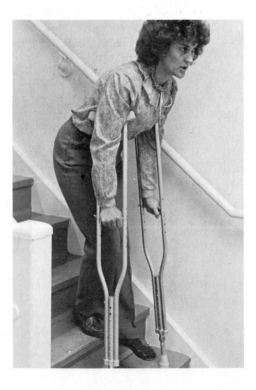

Figure 44.9

Communicative Aspects

OBSERVATIONS

1. Anxiety and fear experienced by the client may interfere with the ability to learn to walk on crutches. Observe for signs of depression and reluctance to try to walk on the crutches.
2. Observe for correct balance, posture, and gait to prevent complications and falls.
3. Physical tolerance should be considered in relation to the crutchwalking program. Note adequacy of muscle strength and need for increased conditioning.

CHARTING

DATE/TIME	OBSERVATIONS	SIGNATURE
2/14 0930	Crutch training begun. Ambulated with crutches for the first time. Used two-point gait. Posture poor; proper posture was demonstrated. Became very fatigued after going to nurses' desk and back. Expresses willingness to stand straight and seems eager to try again. Will resume crutch training after rest period.	J. Day RN

Discharge Planning Aspects

CLIENT AND FAMILY EDUCATION

1. Instruct the client in the proper method of using the prescribed crutch gait.
2. Instruct the client in the importance of correct posture in crutchwalking.
3. Instruct the client and family in safety measures (e.g., no wet spots, loose rugs, or other obstacles that are hazards to the person on crutches). The client should wear nonskid footwear when ambulating with crutches.
4. Tell the client and family where orthopedic supplies may be purchased after discharge so that items such as crutch tips and crutch pads may be replaced as needed.

Evaluation

Quality Assurance

Documentation should include the method of crutchwalking prescribed, the education of the client and family, and the response. The ability of the client to master the techniques should be noted as well as any difficulties experienced. The nurse should reflect awareness of possible safety hazards and efforts made to protect the client in the hospital and after discharge. Discharge teaching and status of crutchwalking ability should be noted before the client leaves the hospital.

Infection Control

Handwashing before and after assisting the client will help eliminate cross-contamination. Any device shared by clients, such as safety belt or crutches, should be cleaned between uses.

Technique Checklist

	YES	NO
Crutchwalking procedure explained to client and family	_____	_____
Client measured for crutches while standing	_____	_____
Safety belt used for first crutchwalking attempts	_____	_____
Nonskid footwear worn	_____	_____

Gait used by client

    Four-point _____

    Three-point _____

    Two-point _____

    Swing-through _____

	YES	NO
Client sent home with crutches	_____	_____
Family and client aware of safety hazards and care of crutches at home	_____	_____
Complications in hospital	_____	_____
Discharge instructions given to client and family	_____	_____

45

Death, Care of the Dying and the Dead

Overview

Definition

Care of the client in the final stages of life; care and consideration of the family of the dying client; and preparation of the body of the deceased for the mortician

Rationale

Offer care, comfort, and support to the dying client.

Provide solace and support for the family of the dying client.

Meet the emotional and spiritual needs of the living.

Show respect for the deceased.

Aid in preserving the normal appearance of the deceased.

Safeguard the belongings of the deceased.

Terminology

Autopsy: Examination of the body internally and externally in an attempt to determine cause of death

Shroud: A large piece of plastic or cotton material in which the body is wrapped after death

Assessment

Pertinent Anatomy and Physiology

1. Grief is an emotional response to loss. The stages of grief have been described by George Engle. *Shock and disbelief*—the first response is a refusal to believe, accept, or comprehend that the death has occurred. This period has been described as one of numbness, in which one attempts to insulate oneself against the stress of acknowledgment of the death. The second stage, *developing awareness*, occurs in the time, several minutes or hours, in which anguish and a sense of loss are felt. Crying, anger, and a sense of helplessness may accompany this stage. The third stage is the stage of *restitution*, during which the normal rituals are carried out, such as the funeral or wake, which initiate the recovery phase. *Resolution* occurs next, during which the grieving person attempts to come to grips with the loss, is at first consumed with thoughts of the lost loved one, and gradually becomes aware of self once again. Finally, the grieving person is able to think and talk about the deceased. This often leads to idealization, a condition in which only those positive memories of the dead person are remembered. The grieving process may take a year or more.

2. The stages of dying have been described by Elisabeth Kübler–Ross. The first stage is *denial*, in which the dying person refuses to believe that death is a possibility. This is a defense mechanism and is used to give the person time to adjust to the fact that death is inevitable. The second stage is often *anger* at having to give up life. The emotion may be directed at persons or objects. The third stage is *bargaining*, in which the dying person attempts to strike a bargain with God in return for more time to live. *Depression* generally follows, which may actually be a period of grieving for self. The final stage is

acceptance, when death is accepted as inevitable. Support is still needed and hope is still felt in every stage, even in acceptance.

Pathophysiological Concepts

The clinical signs of impending death are

1. Reflexes gradually disappear.
2. Respirations become accelerated and labored.
3. Skin feels cold and clammy.
4. Body temperature changes.
5. Blood pressure decreases.
6. Pulse rate increases and becomes weak.
7. Pupils become dilated and fixed.
8. Physical and mental capabilities deteriorate.
9. Corneal reflex is absent.

Assessment of the Client

1. Recognize the impending signs of death and prepare the family when death is approaching.
2. Assess the family for acceptance of the inevitability of the death. Assess the stage of grieving of each member and anticipate methods of assisting them toward resolution.

Plan

Nursing Objectives

Minimize the client's discomfort and anxiety.

Recognize the physical symptoms of death.

Provide for the spiritual needs of the client and family.

Offer support and comfort to the bereaved family and loved ones.

Meet legal requirements quickly and accurately.

Aid in keeping the body tissue in the best possible condition, so that problems in preparing the body for viewing are minimized.

Return personal belongings to the family.

Client Preparation

1. A visit from a clergy member of the client's faith or the hospital chaplain may be appreciated by the client. On the other hand, it may increase anxiety. Discuss this action with the family and the client before arranging such a visit.
2. If the family wishes to view the body, they should be prepared briefly for what they will see. Great tact and kindness is essential. Support for the family probably will be needed. Accompany the family and provide chairs if needed. Provide a time of privacy and quiet but remain available to offer comfort and answer questions.
3. If there is another person in the room with the deceased, the roommate should be moved to another room as quickly as possible. Consider the individual needs and anxiety level of the roommate when deciding how much information about the situation to provide. Generally, the roommate should be told the reason for the move and what is happening. Details are not necessary, but the feelings and sensitivities of the roommate should be considered.

Equipment

Postmortem care

Shroud	Identification tags
Bath equipment	Cotton balls or gauze pads
Dressing tray, if necessary	Saline
Clean linens, if necessary	

Implementation and Interventions

Procedural Aspects

ACTION

Care of the Family

1. Direct attention toward the family when death occurs. A clergy member may be called if requested by the family.

2. If the members of the family are extremely emotional or have physical manifestations such as fainting, the physician may be notified.

Care of the Deceased (Postmortem Care)

1. Raise the head and shoulders of the deceased with a pillow or elevate the head of the bed.

2. Maintain normal positioning of the body (Fig. 45-1). Arrange the body in straight alignment. Place the dentures in the mouth as soon as possible after death and close the mouth. Oral care should be given as thoroughly as possible. Close the eyes naturally by applying gentle pressure with the fingertips for a moment. If the eyes will not stay closed, place a moist pad or cotton ball on each. A folded towel may be placed under the chin to keep the mouth shut.

RATIONALE

The verbalization of feelings permits an outlet for emotion, which may help reduce initial mental anguish.

The impact of death on the family members will be exhibited in different forms of stress and shock.

Elevating the head will prevent blood from pooling in the face and causing discoloration.

Arrangement in normal positioning will prevent distortion of the face and body. The appearance of normal sleep is achieved with the eyes closed naturally. Oral care should eliminate mouth odors because the family may wish to be close to the client during viewing. Odors add to the distress.

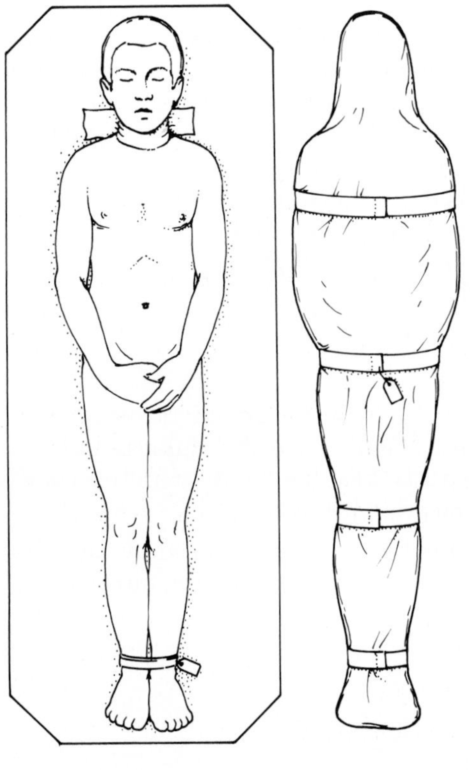

Figure 45.1

ACTION	RATIONALE
3. Prevent the loss of personal items. Gather the clothing and valuables of the deceased, label them, and give them to the next of kin. Note on the chart what was gathered, to whom it was given, and any jewelry remaining with the deceased. Be certain that the family has signed all of the necessary consent papers before leaving the hospital.	Loss of personal items can add to the anguish and sorrow of the family.
4. Apply the shroud while maintaining the dignity of the deceased. Cleanse the body if needed, change dressings, and pad areas of drainage, such as the buttocks and wounds. Remove any drains, tubes, and equipment. Make the body as presentable as possible if the family wishes to view the deceased before leaving the hospital. Do not apply the shroud until the family has gone. Wash and dry the deceased's face and comb hair. Leave the siderails down and elevate the bed to an accessible height so that the family can touch the body if they wish. Apply the shroud or a hospital gown. Attach an identification tag to the client (ankle or wrist) and to the shroud.	Cleansing the body and changing dressings will reduce the possibility of odors caused by microorganisms. The deceased should look as natural as possible for the family viewing period. It is essential that the body be accurately identified to prevent disastrous emotional trauma to the family, legal ramifications, and embarrassment to the hospital. Many times the family will wish to touch or kiss the deceased before parting.
5. Transport the body to the morgue. Cover the body completely with a sheet and blanket. Transport the deceased to the morgue quietly and inconspicuously. Service elevators and seldom-used corridors provide the desired route. Store the body in the appropriate area until it is picked up by the funeral home or the autopsy is performed.	The sight and knowledge of a death in the hospital can be upsetting to clients who are recuperating. Decorum and discretion in removing the body to the morgue will help to avoid upsetting other clients and visitors.

Communicative Aspects

OBSERVATIONS

1. The nurse should make every effort to convey a sense of caring and concern for the family. Avoid false cheerfulness and false reassurance; these will only lead to distrust. Treat the family with respect and compassion. Answer questions and be available to them.

2. After the client is pronounced dead by the physician, the mortician should be called. This may be done by the nurse, or by the family if they prefer.

3. If the deceased's head had been shaved for surgery, send the hair with the body to the funeral home.

4. Avoid discussing the death of a client with other clients or visitors.

5. Have a permission slip signed for removal of the body, autopsy consent, and whatever other consents are required by the institution or state of residence. In some states, the consent for the autopsy is the responsibility of the physician. Adhere to the proper witnessing procedure as well. Consult the policy manual to determine who is responsible for signing and witnessing consents.

6. If there is a delay in the arrival of the funeral home representative, or if the deceased is in the room with another client, remove the body to the location stipulated by hospital policy.

CHARTING

DATE/TIME	OBSERVATIONS	SIGNATURE
4/20 1100	Large amounts of projectile emesis. Vital signs no longer detectable. ———	J. Day RN
1110	Dr. B notified. Family at bedside. ———	J. Day RN
1125	Pronounced dead by Dr. B. Family remains at bedside. Daughter states that she is glad the suffering is finally over. Clergyman with family. ———	J. Day RN
1140	C. Funeral Home notified at daughter's request. Clothing, watch, and golden wedding band given to daughter, Mrs. G.H. Family left hospital to go to Mrs. H's home. ———	J. Day RN
1205	Postmortem care completed. Body to morgue. No jewelry. Identification tag on left wrist and on shroud. ———	J. Day RN

Quality Assurance

1. The time at which the vital signs stopped and anything unusual associated with the death should be noted in the chart.

2. The time at which the physician was notified, and who pronounced the client dead, as well as the time at which death was pronounced, should be noted.

3. The name of the funeral home notified and the person who requested the particular mortuary service should be noted.

4. Signatures and witnesses on the various permits and consents should be noted in the chart.

5. Disposition and inventory of the personal belongings and valuables of the deceased and whom these were given to should be reflected in the chart.

6. Disposition of the body, as well as the time and the name of the person or mortuary service removing the body should be noted.

7. Reactions of the family members should be reflected insofar as it required nursing interventions. These interventions and their results also should be noted. Attempts to prepare the family for the impending death and their level of acceptance should be noted.

Infection Control

The dead body offers an excellent medium for the growth of pathogenic organisms. Embalming prevents much of the damage that would otherwise occur before burial. It is essential that the nurse treat dressings and wounds as contaminated and dispose of the dressings properly, however. Scrupulous handwashing is essential after caring for the deceased. Wearing of gloves is in order when performing postmortem care in the presence of large amounts of drainage.

Technique Checklist

	YES	NO
Client expressed acceptance of death	_____	_____
Family at what stage of grieving process?		
_____		
Vital signs ceased at _____		
Physician notified at _____		
Pronounced dead at _____		
Postmortem care		
Body cleansed	_____	_____
Dressings changed	_____	_____
Alignment maintained	_____	_____
Eyes closed	_____	_____
Dentures in mouth	_____	_____
Clothing and valuables given to		
_____		
Body identified	_____	_____
Funeral home called	_____	_____
Name _____		
Clergy member called	_____	_____
Name _____		
Shroud placed on deceased	_____	_____
Body removed to morgue	_____	_____
Permits and consents signed	_____	_____

46

Dentures (Artificial), Care of

Overview

Definition

Cleaning of a person's artificial teeth

Rationale

Maintain cleanliness and comfort.
Prevent infection of the mouth.
Prevent bacteria from traveling to the digestive tract.

Terminology

Dentifrice: A preparation intended to clean and polish the teeth
Gingiva: The tissue surrounding the necks of the teeth; the gums
Stomatitis: Inflammation of the mouth
Vulcanite: Porous material used in making dentures

Assessment

Pertinent Anatomy and Physiology

See Appendix I: *mouth, teeth.*

Pathophysiological Concepts

1. *Dental caries* are the localized destruction of tooth tissue by bacterial action. There is demineralization of the enamel, which allows entry to the dentin and pulp. Streptococcal infection is a common cause of tooth decay.
2. Peridontal disease, or pyorrhea, is characterized by red, swollen gingiva and bleeding. Inflammation of the gums is called gingivitis.

Assessment of the Client

1. Assess the oral status in relation to how long the client has had artificial dentures, how they fit, and the condition of the gums.
2. Assess the condition of the dentures, any loose or chipped teeth, the extent of artificial dentures (whether full dentures or a partial plate), and any cracks, chips, or missing teeth on the artificial dentures.

Plan

Nursing Objectives

Teach proper care of artificial teeth to the client.
Prevent complications associated with inadequate cleaning of the mouth and teeth.
Handle the artificial dentures with care to prevent breakage.

Client Preparation

1. If the client is alert and able to perform self-care of dentures, provide the proper equipment at the bedside or in the bathroom for the client's use.
2. If the client is unable to perform self-care, cleaning the dentures will be an integral part of daily hygienic care.
3. If the client is unconscious, remove the artificial dentures from the mouth and place them in a labeled dental container covered with water or normal saline solution to keep the dentures moist.

4. To give mouth care, raise the head of the bed to Fowler's position unless medically contraindicated. If the client is unable to sit up for mouth care, it may be done with the client turned to the side facing the nurse.

5. Offer a thorough explanation of what will happen during the cleansing procedure. Ask the client how the dentures are usually removed, how the dentures are cleaned at home, and the easiest and most comfortable way to reinsert the dentures.

Equipment

Denture brush or toothbrush

Container for dentures

Dentrifice or denture cleaner of client's choice

Gauze pad (if needed) to clean client's mouth

Lemon and glycerine swab

Towel and curved basin

Implementation and Interventions

Procedural Aspects

ACTION

1. Always clean the dentures when giving mouth care to the client. Use only warm water to clean the artificial dentures.

2. Wash hands thoroughly before assisting with care of the dentures. If the client cannot remove artificial dentures, remove them in the following manner:

   Grasp the upper denture with the thumb and index finger on each hand (Fig. 46-1). Move the upper denture up and down gently to break the seal of the vacuum between the denture and the roof of the mouth. Once the seal is broken, slip the upper denture out of the mouth.

RATIONALE

The mucous membrane lining of the mouth must be kept clean. Hot water will damage the denture material.

Handwashing helps prevent cross-infection.

The upper denture is held in place by a vacuum seal. Release of a seal at any point breaks the vacuum and allows release by the entire surface.

The lower denture does not adhere to the gums by a vacuum.

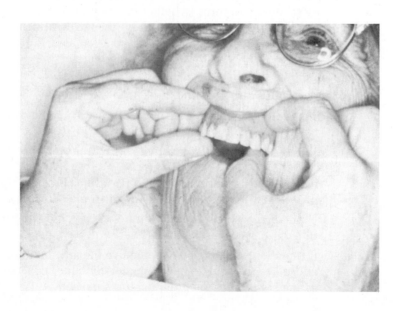

Figure 46.1

ACTION   **RATIONALE**

Remove the lower denture by
grasping the denture firmly with
the thumb and index finger of each
hand and lifting gently out of the
mouth (Fig. 46-2). During actual
removal, take care to rotate the
lower denture slightly to prevent
stretching the mouth.

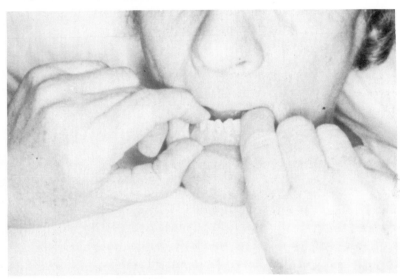

Figure 46.2

3. Place the artificial dentures in a
   basin. Remove the basin to the
   sink, where the dentures will be
   washed (Fig. 46-3).

Transporting the dentures by hand
offers an opportunity to drop and
break them. The basin offers protection.

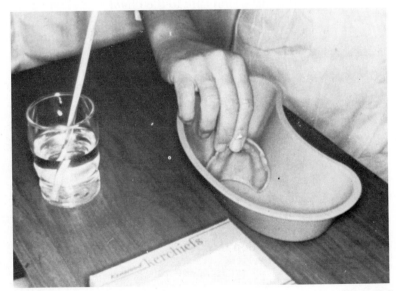

Figure 46.3

ACTION

RATIONALE

4. Use a brush and denture powder to clean the artificial dentures by applying a brushing motion. Brush the upper dentures in a downward motion, and the lower dentures in an upward motion. While the dentures are being cleaned, hold them over a soft towel or a basin of water with a washcloth in the bottom (Fig. 46-4). Rinse the dentures with running warm (not hot) water.

Brushing removes most of the accumulated debris, which is harmful and unpleasant when left in the mouth. If the dentures are cleaned over a soft surface, they are less likely to break if dropped.

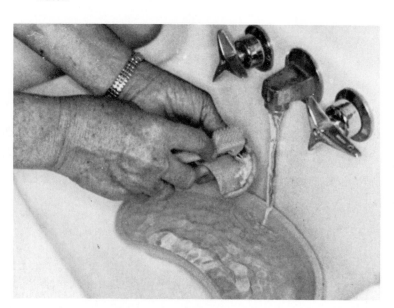

Figure 46.4

5. Administer oral care to the client (see Technique No. 69, Oral Hygiene). After the artificial dentures have been cleaned, replace them in the client's mouth, unless contraindicated, in the following manner:

Elevate the upper lip with one hand while the other inserts the denture (Fig. 46-5). Once the upper denture is in place, press it gently to ensure that the vacuum seal has been made (Fig. 46-6). Follow the same procedure for the lower denture, applying pressure in a downward motion (Fig. 46-7).

The vacuum seal is the mechanism by which the upper denture is held in place in the mouth.

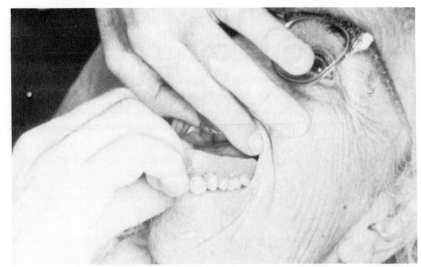

Figure 46.5

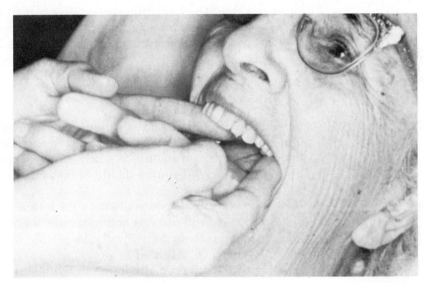

Figure 46.6

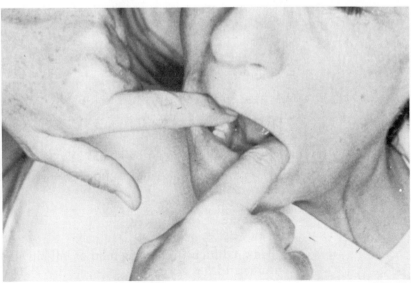

Figure 46.7

Communicative Aspects

OBSERVATIONS

1. Observe carefully the condition of the mouth when the artificial dentures are removed. Signs of redness or abrasion indicate poorly fitting dentures.

2. Note the condition of the dentures, with attention to cracks, chips, missing teeth, or excessive wear in any particular spot.

CHARTING

DATE/TIME	OBSERVATIONS	SIGNATURE
10/23 2115	Dentures removed from mouth and placed in covered container in bathroom to soak. Gums are pink with no signs of redness or pressure areas. Mouth has food debris throughout and foul odor. Oral care given. Dentures left out at client's request.	G. Ivers RN

Discharge Planning Aspects

CLIENT AND FAMILY EDUCATION

1. Teach the client and family the importance of proper mouth and denture care

2. Stress the importance of artificial dentures that fit properly. Teach the client that when the dentures are left out of the mouth for extended periods of time, the gum line will change, increasing the chances for improperly fitting dentures.

Evaluation

Quality Assurance

Documentation should reflect the condition of the client's mouth and the artificial dentures. Any problems with removal or insertion should be noted. The frequency of mouth care should be noted. Any teaching about the care of the mouth or the artificial dentures should be reflected in the chart.

Infection Control

1. Normally the teeth are covered with a thick film called dental plaque, which consists of masses of bacteria and nutrients. If not removed, these bacteria metabolize the carbohydrates available, producing acids that destroy the enamel of the teeth. Allowed to grow unchecked, these bacteria, as well as the other pathogens normally found in the mouth, may cause gum infection.

2. Careful handwashing is important before and after administering mouth care to any client.

3. Cleansing and stimulation of the circulation of the gums helps to prevent gingivitis, or inflammation of the gums.

Technique Checklist

	YES	NO
Type of artificial dentures		
Total _____		
Partial _____		
Procedure explained to client	_____	_____
Condition of dentures noted on chart	_____	_____
Insertion and removal of dentures progressed without complication	_____	_____
Oral hygiene given	_____	_____
Frequency _____		
Client had no difficulty chewing food or talking after denture care	_____	_____
Proper mouth care taught to family and client	_____	_____

47   Documentation Guidelines

Overview

Definition

The chart is a written record of the care administered by hospital personnel to a consumer of health care services. The record is to include

The health history and assessment of the client;

Observations and symptoms of the client;

Nursing care administered; and

Therapy and response.

Purpose

The client record is kept to provide

A means of communication;

A basis on which therapy is prescribed;

An aid to the physician in diagnosis;

Evidence of continuance;

Material for research and education; and

A legal document, admissible in courts as evidence.

General Guidelines

1. All entries on the chart must be accurate and factual. Exactness is essential in charting times, effects, and results of treatments and procedures. Full dates, including year, should be used. (The year is omitted from dates in charts in this textbook.)

2. Entries may be printed or in script but must be written legibly in ink.

3. Each entry must be followed by the writer's first initial, last name, and title, e.g., J. Doe, RN. All last names, including physicians, hospital staff, clients, and relatives should be spelled out in full. (Names are initialed in the charts of this textbook only to avoid associations with real people.)

4. Ditto marks and erasures are not acceptable. They may lead to legal questions should the chart be used in court proceedings. Errors are corrected by drawing a single line through the incorrect material and writing in the correct entry as close to the mistaken entry as possible. The erroneous material must not be obliterated, merely marked through. Many institutions do not advocate writing the word "error" because this connotes the idea that a mistake was made in care rather than in documentation. Refer to the hospital policy manual for direction. Suggested method for correcting a chart entry follows:

   ~~1000 Amb in hallway~~

   1000 Amb in room

5. Lines should not be left completely or partially blank in the client record. If a line is skipped or not filled completely, draw a single line through the remainder to prevent charting by someone else.

6. Descriptions are essential when charting about drainage, stools, vomitus, pain, and any other diagnostically valuable occurrence.

7. The time should be recorded on all entries.

8. Only abbreviations accepted by the institution are allowed on the client record.

9. Each page of the chart must be identified with the name of the client, hospital identification number, and any other data required by the institution.

10. Some hospitals have computer generated records that include such items as nurses' notes, care plans, and diagnostic test results. Although the use of the computer greatly enhances the speed and convenience of charting, it is nonetheless essential that all information entered on the chart be accurate. The professional nurse remains accountable for the entries made on the nurses' progress notes regardless of the manner of entry.

11. The reliance on diagnostic-related groups (DRGs) as a means of reimbursement for health care facilities has placed increased emphasis on the need for accurate documentation. Of particular importance are the dates of entries, the admitting diagnosis made by the physician, and justification of the length of stay and readiness to be dismissed. Emphasis is on continuity of care after discharge; referrals, health teaching, and discharge planning are also of particular importance.

12. The chart should reflect nursing assessment and nursing therapy prescribed by the professional registered nurse and reflected on the nursing care plan. Examples of nursing therapy are pain control, client education, and speed of progression of other therapies according to client tolerance.

Specific Guidelines

Physician's Orders

1. Each order should have the date and time it was written.

2. Some system of indicating which orders have been transcribed or carried out is necessary.

3. The licensed person who assumes responsibility for noting the orders must sign time, name, and title to verify notation of the orders.

Graphic Records, Treatment, and Procedure Sheets

1. Graphic records for temperature and pulse must reflect accurately the client's actual vital signs.

2. Discrepancies, such as elevated temperature or abnormally depressed pulse, should be reported to the nurse or physician responsible for the client's care.

3. All treatments and procedures must have the time at which they occurred. There also must be a place to chart client response, untoward side-effects, and outcomes.

Client Progress Notes (Nurses' Notes)

1. The client progress notes must reflect ongoing assessment, care, and response of the client. They should be client centered and comprehensive.

2. All entries should be meaningful and pertinent. Nonspecific phrases (e.g., "a good 8 hours") should be avoided.

3. Some specific situations follow (for others, see the particular technique):

   Dressings: Chart amount and appearance of drainage, appearance of wound, type of dressing applied, and the client's response.

   Hot and cold applications: Chart where and how long applied, appearance of skin before and after, safety precautions, and the client's response.

General care: Back care, decubitus care (size and appearance, drainage, type of care given), positioning, safety precautions, and response should be charted. A daily notation should be made of the client's sensorium regardless of the length of time the client remains in the institution.

Diagnostic tests: Time, type of test, side-effects, outcomes and response, interpretation of results, and the client's reactions should be charted.

Admission: Complete assessment of the client, method and time of arrival, instructions given, and client's response should be reflected in the documentation.

Discharge: Chart the discharge teaching and the client's response. Note the method and time of departure, equipment given to client before discharge, who accompanied the client out of the hospital, and the client's condition.

Discharge planning: From the time of admission, plans for discharge should be formulated so that continuity of care, efforts at education and nursing actions may be coordinated into realizing the client's potential. The chart is the logical, centralized location in which to document efforts to help the client reach the highest level of wellness and productivity possible.

The nurses' notes should reflect the nursing process as related to the following legal functions of nursing:

Application and execution of physician's legal orders

Observations of symptoms and reactions

Supervision of client

Supervision of those participating in care (except physicians)

Reporting and recording

Promotion of physical and emotional health by direction and teaching

48 Douche (Internal Vaginal Irrigation)

Overview

Definition

Irrigation or flushing of the vaginal canal

Rationale

Cleanse and disinfect the vagina and adjacent parts in preparation for surgery.
Relieve pain, soothe inflamed, congested tissue, and stimulate relaxed tissue.
Reduce offensive odors by deodorizing the vagina.
Apply medication to mucous surfaces.

Assessment

Pertinent Anatomy and Physiology

See Appendix I: *genitalia (female)*, *vagina*.

Pathophysiological Concepts

1. Vaginitis is an inflammation of the vagina characterized by discharge, burning, itching, redness, and swelling of the vaginal tissues. There is often pain on urination and with sexual intercourse. Vaginitis may be caused by chemical irritants, foreign bodies, or infectious agents.

2. Trichomonas is a genus of protozoa that normally inhabit the vagina in small numbers without causing any problems. If the normal environment of the vagina is altered, however, which happens with certain drugs or infections, the protozoa may proliferate with resulting symptoms including an irritating discharge with a foul odor, as well as itching and burning of the vaginal area. Other inflammations of the vagina include those caused by the fungus *Candida albicans*.

3. Vaginal carcinoma is relatively rare. Cervical carcinoma is a fairly common form of cancer of the female reproductive tract and also produces a foul discharge.

Assessment of the Client

1. Assess any odor or vaginal discharge, as well as other signs of inflammation such as redness, itching, and burning.

2. Assess the familiarity of the client with the douche procedure. Some women douche at home, whereas others may be embarrassed or uncomfortable about the douche. Determine how the client feels about the prospect and how much she will be able to assist.

Plan

Nursing Objectives

Reduce the client's anxiety during the treatment.
Provide for the client's comfort and privacy.
Observe the condition of the genitoperineal area.
Report the physical and emotional effects of the treatment.
Teach the client self-care.

Client Preparation

1. Explain the technique to the client. The douche is usually a relatively painless procedure that takes only about 10 minutes.

2. A distended bladder can cause discomfort during a vaginal treatment and predispose to trauma. Allow the client to void before the procedure.

Equipment

Vaginal irrigation tray (including douche container, tubing, douche nozzle, towels, gloves, cotton balls, and an antibacterial solution)

Water-soluble lubricant

Moisture proof drape

Irrigating solution (may be tap water, normal saline, sodium bicarbonate solution [1–2 tbsp sodium bicarbonate to 1000 ml water], vinegar [8 ml vinegar to 1000 ml water], or as ordered by the physician.)

Bath thermometer

Bedpan or commode

IV standard

Implementation and Interventions

Procedural Aspects

ACTION	RATIONALE
1. Fill the douche container with the ordered solution which should be 105° F.	Solution that is too hot may harm the mucous lining of the vagina.
2. With the client in the dorsal position on a bedpan, drape with a bath blanket in a triangular fashion as for a vaginal examination (Fig. 48-1). Be sure the body is aligned properly with all but one pillow removed. A linen protector may be placed under the client's hips to protect the bed linens.	Draping promotes privacy and reduces embarrassment. Normal body alignment facilitates relaxation.

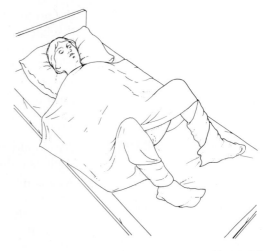

Figure 48.1

3. Give perineal care with soap and water before beginning.	Cleansing reduces the number of microorganisms normally found on the skin.
4. Place the douche tray on the foot of the bed and open onto a sterile towel. Set the container upright and clamp the tubing. Place a drape over the pubic area. Pour the antibacterial cleanser over the cot-	Although this is not strictly a sterile procedure because the vagina is not sterile, sterile equipment does reduce the number of pathogens in the area.

ACTION	RATIONALE

ton balls for cleaning the genitalia. Fill the douche container with 500 ml to 1000 ml of solution. Don sterile gloves.

5. Lubricate the douche tip with a water-soluble jelly. Separate the labia and cleanse the genitalia with a cotton ball in a downward motion from front to back using a new cotton ball for each of the motions. Repeat three or four times. Identify the vagina (See Appendix I, Fig. A16). Unclamp the tube and expel air from the tubing. Insert the douche nozzle into the vagina (Fig. 48-2).

Friction may cause trauma to delicate and inflamed tissue. Lubrication reduces friction. Always cleanse from the area of least contamination to that of most contamination. Insert the nozzle along the natural curve of the vagina.

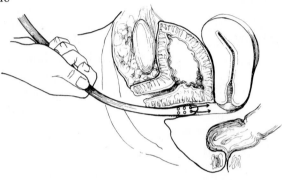

Figure 48.2

7. Hold or hang the irrigation container 12 in above the level of the vagina. Cleanse the folds of the vagina by gently moving the douche tip forward and backward along the vaginal tract.

Excess pressure may force infectious material into the uterus. Pressure is determined by the height of the bag.

8. Once all of the solution has been instilled, raise the head of the bed, unless contraindicated, to facilitate the return of the remainder of the solution. Remove the client from the bedpan and dry the genital area thoroughly. Rinse the equipment and store or dispose of properly.

Gravity will facilitate the return flow of the irrigating solution. Dry skin promotes comfort and healing, and reduces bacterial growth.

Special Modifications

Preferably, the douche is given with the client sitting on or standing over the commode. If the client is able to go to the bathroom, however, she will probably be able to administer her own douche. In this case the nurse assists as needed. The drainage may be collected in a container or bedpan placed inside the rim of the commode.

It is preferable to allow the client to engage in self-care as much as possible. This adds to feelings of self-confidence.

Communicative Aspects

OBSERVATIONS

1. Observe the appearance and condition of the vaginal area.

2. Observe the client during the procedure for excess fatigue, discomfort, or signs of emotional distress.

3. Observe the drainage for signs of blood, pus, tissue, or any other abnormalities.

CHARTING

DATE/TIME	OBSERVATIONS	SIGNATURE
4/28 1430	Vaginal douche given with client in dorsal recumbent position. Draped and perineal area cleansed with antiseptic solution. Solution returned in about 3–5 min, clear with no signs of bleeding. Perineal area remains reddened with no breaks in the skin. Perineal care given. ————————————	G. Ivers RN

Discharge Planning Aspects

CLIENT AND FAMILY EDUCATION

1. Caution the client about self-administration of douches, especially the scented commercial varieties, on a regular basis. They may upset the normal vaginal flora and may wash away protective secretions.

2. If douching is ordered for home use, instruct the client and family (if appropriate) about preparation of the solution, height of the container, and position to assume during douching. Explain how to care for the equipment.

Evaluation

Quality Assurance

Documentation should reflect the condition of the client's vaginal area, especially in relation to diagnosis or complaints prompting hospitalization. Results of the douche and the client's reaction to it should be noted. If the client will douche after discharge, evidence of instructions and the client's reactions to them should be noted.

Infection Control

1. Careful handwashing should precede and follow the douche procedure. Because the condition prompting douching is often related to some type of infection, great care must be taken not to spread this condition.

2. The procedure is not considered a sterile procedure; however, precautions should be taken not to infect the client or the nurse through carelessness.

3. Equipment must be cleaned thoroughly between uses. If the client is suspected of having an infection, the equipment should be bagged and returned for sterilization and decontamination. Disposable douches are available.

Technique Checklist

	YES	NO
Procedure explained to client	_____	_____
Douche performed without incident	_____	_____
Type of irrigating solution _____		
Desired results obtained	_____	_____
Observations noted in chart	_____	_____
Vaginal area	_____	_____
Discharge or drainage	_____	_____
Returned douche solution	_____	_____
Instructions for home douche given	_____	_____

49 Dressings, Surgical

Overview

Definition

The process by which a soiled dressing is removed, the wound cleansed, and a sterile dressing applied

Rationale

Absorb drainage.

Splint or immobilize wound and surrounding tissue.

Protect the wound from mechanical injury.

Promote hemostasis, as by a pressure dressing.

Prevent contamination by body excreta.

Provide physical and mental comfort.

Terminology

Sanguinous: Bloody

Assessment

Pertinent Anatomy and Physiology

1. See Appendix I: *skin*.
2. Tissue repair is accomplished by regeneration, which involves replacement of the destroyed tissue with similar or identical tissue, or by fibrous tissue formation, which results in the formation of a scar.
3. Wounds heal by primary or secondary union. Healing by primary union usually occurs when the tissue surfaces have been brought into close approximation by sutures, and regeneration occurs by sealing over the skin even when underlying tissues have not healed. Secondary union occurs when the wound is large and skin edges cannot be approximated successfully. A large amount of fibrous tissue usually results.

Pathophysiological Concepts

1. A wound is a break in the integrity of the body tissue. It may be internal (closed) or external (open). A wound is clean when it does not contain any pathogenic microorganisms (as opposed to a wound that is contaminated or infected). Wounds cannot be considered sterile owing to the normal flora inhabiting the skin, which are present in the wounds. The goal is to control the number and type of organisms to prevent contamination or infection.
2. The body's normal response to any type of injury is inflammation, a state that is characterized by swelling, redness, heat, pain, and impaired function of the involved part. Inflammation is a natural attempt of the body to destroy or dilute the invading agent, to repair damage, and to prevent spread of the condition.

Assessment of the Client

1. Assess the extent of wound healing, any potential or present problems, and the reaction of the client to the wound.
2. Assess the extent of the wound or incision in relation to the activity level of the client to determine which type of dressing will achieve the desired purpose best.
3. Assess the skin under the dressing frequently to ensure its integrity. Deter-

mine whether the dressing is too tight. Be alert for wrinkles in the dressing, and ensure the proper anatomical alignment of body parts.

4. Assess the allergy status of the client. If the client is allergic to adhesive tape, an alternative method of securing the dressing will have to be used, such as silk or paper tape, or a binder (See Technique No. 32, Binders, Application of). Many allergies may be present in the same person, however, so that a complete allergy history is appropriate. Check for allergies to iodine or shellfish if an iodine-based skin cleanser is used.

Plan

Nursing Objectives

Allay fear and anxiety regarding the wound.

Observe and evaluate the healing process.

Prevent or reduce infection.

Note and record wound size, appearance, and characteristics of drainage, as well as any complications (e.g., pain, fever, anorexia).

Client Preparation

1. Fear of the suture line breaking creates tension and anxiety and may predispose the client to immobility. The nurse should explain that sufficient tension has been applied to the wound by the sutures to prevent breaking when the client turns, coughs, or hyperventilates (See Technique No. 77, Preoperative, Perioperative, and Postoperative Care).

2. Explain to the client what will happen during the dressing change. Usually the client will not experience pain during the procedure, but knowing what will happen and how to cooperate will relieve anxiety. Tell the client not to move suddenly and to keep hands away from the incision area so the sterile field will not be contaminated.

Equipment

Dressing cart or dressing tray (containing supplies)

Sterile gloves

Tape

Dressings, as indicated

Suture set (sterile tray with hemostat, forceps, and scissors)

Antiseptic solution

Waxed or plastic bag for disposal of contaminated dressing

Implementation and Interventions

Procedural Aspects

ACTION

1. Prevent contamination of the wound by careful handwashing before and after the dressing change. Loosen tape and remove the outer dressing by touching the surface only (Fig. 49-1). Open the dressing tray or the suture tray. Place a sterile towel on the side of the incision opposite the side on which the nurse is standing. Remove the inner dressing with forceps (Fig. 49-2). These forceps are now contaminated. If the dressing adheres to the wound, it may be moistened with saline to facilitate removal.

RATIONALE

The wound dressing is considered contaminated and anything that comes in contact with it is considered contaminated as well. The sterile towel should be placed in such a position that the nurse does not have to lean over it during dressing change.

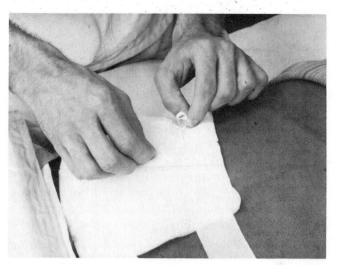

Figure 49.1

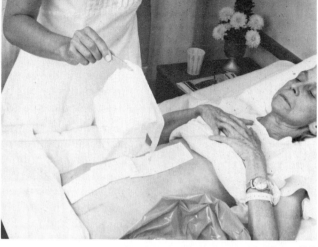

Figure 49.2

ACTION	**RATIONALE**
2. Place the removed dressing in a waxed bag for discarding. If the wound is infectious, use a plastic bag (Fig. 49-3).	Plastic prevents fluid from leaking through the sides of the bag and contaminating other surfaces.

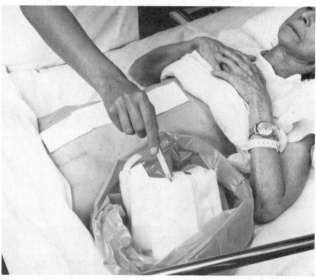

Figure 49.3

ACTION	**RATIONALE**
3. Don sterile gloves. Use an antiseptic to disinfect the area around the wound. If the physician permits, clean the wound with a sterile cotton swab, cotton ball or gauze pad and antiseptic solution. Work from the wound outward for an area of 2 in. Use a new sterile swab for each stroke (Fig. 49-4).	Avoid contaminating the wound. The use of a disinfectant on and around the wound decreases the number of microorganisms and lessens the danger of infection

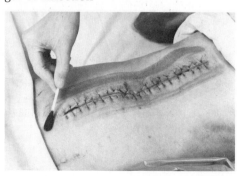

Figure 49.4

ACTION

RATIONALE

Sterile forceps may be used for this cleansing process. Remember that the forceps used originally to remove the dressing are contaminated and may *not* be used for cleansing the wound.

4. Cover the wound with a dry, sterile dressing; sterile forceps may be used to do so. A nonpenetrable or nonstick substance, such as a Telfa pad, may be used next to the skin to prevent the dressing from sticking to the wound (Fig. 49-5). The next layers of the dressing should contain enough thickness to absorb drainage (Figs. 49-6, 49-7). Large, bulky dressings should be avoided. Change the dressing more frequently if necessary, using moderately sized dressings. Extra padding may be needed over drains.

A dry, sterile dressing inhibits the spread of microorganisms by inhibiting capillary action. If the wound can be prevented from sticking to the dressing, there will be less trauma to the wound when the dressing is removed. Large, bulky dressings inhibit movement, are uncomfortable, and encourage the growth of microorganisms if not changed frequently.

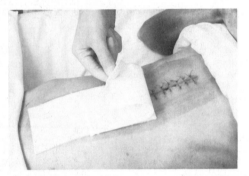

Figure 49.5

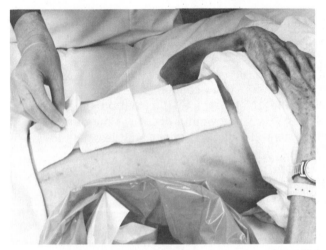

Figure 49.6

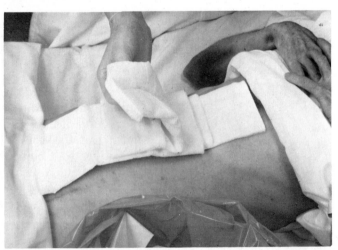

Figure 49.7

ACTION

5. Secure the dressing with some type of tape (Fig. 49-8). Silk and paper tape cause less skin reaction and are removed more easily than adhesive. If frequent dressing changes are necessary, Montgomery strips should be applied. Place the strips on both sides of the wound with the holes facing the wound. Lace gauze strings through the holes and tie them in the center to secure the dressing. To remove the dressing, untie the gauze, change the dressing, and replace. These strips are commercially available or may be made from 1-in or 2-in tape (Figs. 49-9, 49-10).

RATIONALE

Frequent dressing changes can result in skin breakdown because of recurrent pulling and reapplication of tape.

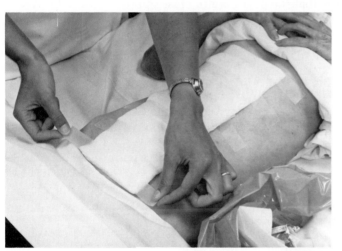

Figure 49.8

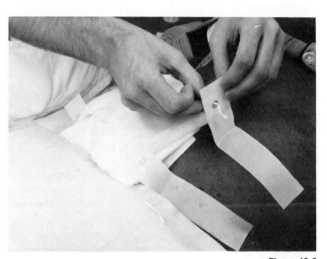

Figure 49.9

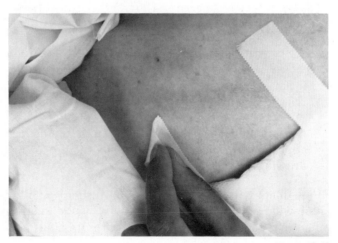

Figure 49.10

ACTION	RATIONALE
6. Leave the client in a clean and comfortable environment. Remove the waxed bag containing the soiled dressing to a covered container outside the client's room.	A clean environment enhances feelings of well-being and encouragement. Expedient removal of the soiled dressing prevents the growth of microorganisms in the trash receptacle.

Special Modifications

Some agencies recommend wearing sterile gloves during the dressing change; some recommend wearing clean, disposable gloves. Regardless, scrupulous handwashing is essential before and after dressing change. If the wound is infected, sterile gloves are necessary.	Wearing gloves has the advantage of protecting both the client and the nurse from possible cross-infection.

Communicative Aspects

OBSERVATIONS

1. Observe the wound to see that the edges are in close approximation. Observe for signs of infection, stage of healing, and proper functioning of involved body part.
2. Observe the character of the drainage, including appearance, amount, and odor.
3. Observe the client for cooperation and discomfort during dressing change.
4. Observe for signs of infection (e.g., redness, heat in the wound, and drainage). If any of these occur during the recuperation period, notify the physician.

CHARTING

DATE/TIME	OBSERVATIONS	SIGNATURE
3/5 0915	Dressing on abdomen changed. Incision cleaned with antiseptic solution. Moderate amount (soaked 1½ large dressing pads) serosanguineous drainage. Wound edges in close approximation with no signs of inflammation. Sterile dressing applied and secured with nonallergic tape. ————	J. Day RN

Discharge Planning Aspects

CLIENT AND FAMILY EDUCATION

1. Instruct the client and family to keep fingers away from the wound and from the part of the dressing next to the wound.
2. If the client is to go home with dressings, explain and demonstrate the procedure for changing the dressings to the person who will assume this responsibility at home. Emphasize sterile technique and the need to prevent infection. Instruct the client and family to report *any* change in drainage or wound appearance to the physician. Relate the proper method of discarding soiled dressings.

REFERRALS

If the client will need dressings after discharge, tell the family member responsible what type of dressings to get and where they may be purchased. If the client has cancer, some assistance with dressings may be obtained from the local chapter of the American Cancer Society.

Evaluation

Quality Assurance

1. Documentation should reflect the course of wound healing, with baseline descriptions of the wound and daily comments on the healing process. The amount and character of drainage should be noted as well as all measures taken to prevent infection. The nurse should reflect in the notes on the chart an awareness of the possible complications of wound healing and measures taken to recognize or prevent them.

2. Teaching of family and client in preparation for discharge should be reflected in the chart, with an evaluation of their readiness to learn and comprehension of information shared.

Infection Control

1. Infection is a constant threat to surgical wounds. The primary responsibility of the nurse changing the dressing is to prevent the spread of infection. Adherence to sterile technique is important in infection control.

2. Meticulous handwashing before and after the dressing change cannot be overemphasized. When teaching the family, do not assume that they know how to wash their hands. Teach how to cleanse hands thoroughly and when to do so, and stress the benefits to both the client and the family.

3. Note at the beginning of a dressing change whether an infectious process is suspected or present. If so, take proper isolation precautions in changing and disposing of the soiled dressings (See Technique No. 66, Isolation Precautions).

Technique Checklist

	YES	NO
Procedure explained to client	_____	_____
Sterile technique maintained	_____	_____
Normal healing progression without complications	_____	_____
Dressing discarded properly	_____	_____
Notation in the chart each time the dressing is changed	_____	_____
Client and family taught how to change dressing correctly at home	_____	_____
Client told where to obtain dressings after discharge	_____	_____

50

Elastic Stockings, Donning and Removing

Overview

Definition

The act of applying or removing snug-fitting hosiery to the feet and legs to counteract circulatory problems

Rationale

Promote venous return to the heart and prevent venous stasis.

Decrease or prevent swelling of the lower extremities.

Prevent distension of the superficial veins as occurs in varicose veins.

Assessment

Pertinent Anatomy and Physiology

See Appendix I: *blood, blood vessels, heart.*

Pathophysiological Concepts

1. Veins are low-pressure, thin-walled vessels that rely on the ancillary action of skeletal muscle pumps and changes in abdominal and intrathoracic pressure to return blood to the heart. Unlike the arterial system, veins are equipped with valves that prevent backflow of the blood. The structure of the venous system enables it to serve as a storage area for blood; however, it also makes the system susceptible to problems related to stasis and venous insufficiency.

2. By the time the blood returns to the heart, the pressure exerted by the blood on the vein walls is very small. Venous pressure varies with the location of the vein and the position of the body. The pressure within the vena cava and the right atrium, known as the central venous pressure (CVP), usually reflects the lowest ebb of venous pressure in the body. An increase in the venous blood pressure is indicative of heart failure. The heart fails to pump the blood effectively, and a buildup occurs in the right atrium and vena cava. The blood then backs up in the veins. This results in an abnormally high filtration pressure in the capillary beds, and fluid begins to accumulate in the interstitial spaces (*edema*).

3. Varicose veins result from prolonged dilatation and stretching of the vascular wall because of increased venous pressure. Blood in the legs collects in the superficial veins and is transported to the deeper venous system for transportation back to the heart. Activities such as walking and isometric exercises facilitate return of the blood to the heart. Prolonged standing promotes venous stasis. Because there are no valves in the inferior vena cava or in the common iliac veins, any change in pressure or decrease in activity increases the chance of pooling of venous blood in the extremities. Gravity further complicates this problem. The venous valves in the area become incompetent, allowing pooling of blood, which is responsible for the unsightly appearance of superficial varicose veins.

Assessment of the Client

1. Assess the client's feet and legs. Note any swelling or discoloration. Assess the temperature of the feet and legs by touching. Assess the presence of pedal and femoral pulses. Determine the presence of pain, numbness, tingling, or any other problems with the feet and legs. Note the presence of cuts, bruises, or any broken skin area on the feet or legs.

2. Assess the presence of varicose veins. Determine the extent of the discoloration. Determine the onset of the problem. Assess the type of work the client does and whether it requires long periods of standing.

3. Assess the client's physical condition. Determine if the client is severely or moderately overweight, which might contribute to inactivity. Assess the presence of other conditions that might predispose to circulatory problems, such as smoking, high salt intake, and lack of exercise.

Plan

Nursing Objectives

Properly apply the elastic stockings in such a manner that they are wrinkle-free and pressure is distributed evenly.

Reduce peripheral edema.

Promote the comfort of the client.

Teach the client and family the proper technique for application of elastic stockings.

Client Preparation

1. Explain the technique for application of the elastic stockings. Explain the purpose and elicit the client's cooperation.

2. Elevate the bed to a comfortable working level. Ensure the client's privacy by closing the door or pulling curtains. The client should be in the supine position with the legs even with or slightly above the plane of the body. Bathe, dry, and powder the client's legs and feet before applying the stockings.

3. Obtain the proper size stockings. For below the knee stockings, measure from the heel to the popliteal space directly behind the kneecap. Measure the circumference of the midcalf. For full-length stockings, measure the midthigh and midcalf circumference; measure length from the heel to the gluteal fold. Charts are available with the stockings to determine which size to select based on the client's measurements.

Equipment

Elastic stockings

Implementation and Interventions

Procedural Aspects

ACTION	RATIONALE
1. Identify the correct stocking for each leg. Holding the foot and heel portion of the first stocking, invert the remainder of the stocking over the hand and arm so that most of the stocking is inside out with the exception of the foot portion (Fig. 50-1).	Stockings fit the contour of the appropriate leg. The right stocking must be placed on the right leg and the left stocking on the left leg.
2. Have the client lie flat in bed. Lift the client's foot from the bed and support it at the heel.	If the foot and lower leg are in a dependent position, the blood will pool in the veins by gravity.
3. Slip the stocking foot over the toes, foot, and heel. Pull the leg portion	The foot portion must be applied securely and snugly to form a

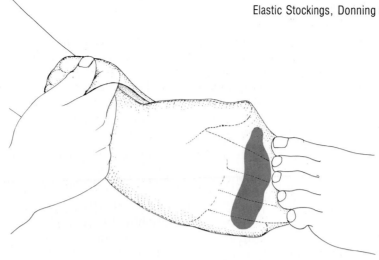

Figure 50.1

ACTION

of the stocking up the leg in a smooth, even motion to its full length.

4. Inspect the stockings to see that they are on evenly and straight. Observe the lines of the material to see that the stockings are not twisted.

5. To remove, grasp the top of the stocking with both hands and pull it smoothly down to the foot. Support the foot with one hand and pull the hose over the heel and off of the foot with the other hand.

6. Lower the bed to the lowest position after application or removal of the stockings.

RATIONALE

wrinkle-free anchor for application of the rest of the stocking. Because the stockings fit firmly against the skin, wrinkles can cause pressure and must be avoided.

Twisting can cause uneven pressure and impede the return of the blood to the heart.

The leg should not be left unsupported as this is uncomfortable and could cause structural damage or strain to the thigh and calf muscles.

Keeping the bed in low position may prevent falls or injury.

Communicative Aspects

OBSERVATIONS

1. Observe the position of the stockings. Check to see that they do not slip down, causing wrinkles. Observe to see that the stockings have been applied straight and evenly.

2. Observe the extremities above the level of the stockings to determine if edema is present. If the toes are not enclosed in the stockings, observe them for adequate circulation. Swelling, discoloration, and immobility may indicate that the elastic stockings are too tight.

3. Observe the feet and legs under the stockings to see that pressure areas do not form. The stockings should be removed two or three times a day for 30 minutes.

CHARTING

DATE/TIME	OBSERVATIONS	SIGNATURE
3/9 0930	Elastic stockings to both legs before sitting in chair. Principles of stocking application and why they must be worn explained to client and wife. Expressed understanding and willingness to keep hose on when up after discharge. Laundry instructions given. Edema of feet and ankles is much less than yesterday. Able to wiggle toes without problem. B/P 188/92, P 82, R 18. Remains hypertensive but breathing is much easier. ————	P. Dillon RN

Discharge Planning Aspects

CLIENT AND FAMILY EDUCATION

1. Explain to the client and family why the stockings are to be worn. Explain the basic physiology of venous return to the heart and the part that gravity plays in this phenomenon. Explain why it is better for the client to put on the stockings before arising.

2. Tell the client to report any problems with the feet and legs to the physician after discharge. The client and family also should be alerted to report cardiovascular symptoms, such as pain in the chest, difficulty breathing, discoloration in the feet and toes, and fainting.

3. Tell the client and family how to care for the stockings after discharge. Instruct them that the stockings may be washed in warm water with a mild detergent. They should be rinsed thoroughly, and excess water should be removed by rolling the stockings in a towel. Wringing the stockings may damage the material or stretch or distort the shape. The stockings may then be hung up or laid on a flat surface to dry.

Evaluation

Quality Assurance

Consult the agency policy regarding the need to chart the application and reapplication of elastic stockings. Some agencies may have a checklist or the presence of stockings may be noted once a day or once a shift. Any problems or abnormalities associated with the stockings should be noted. The chart should reflect the initial application of the stockings and the client's reaction. Evidence of ongoing assessment for complications resulting from wearing the stockings should appear in the chart. Teaching of the client and family should be documented.

Infection Control

1. Thorough handwashing should precede and follow application of elastic stockings.

2. Any breaks in the skin which will be covered by the stockings should be noted and continuously monitored to see that infection does not occur. A sterile dressing over the area may help to prevent proliferation of harmful microorganisms.

3. The stockings should be washed every other day or as needed to prevent colonization with harmful bacteria. Warm water and a mild detergent are recommended for washing the stockings. If an infectious process is present, however, it may be necessary to have two pairs of stockings so that one can be sent for disinfection while the other is being worn.

Technique Checklist

	YES	NO
Need for and procedure for application of elastic stockings explained to client and family	_____	_____
Stockings fit properly	_____	_____
Client taught application technique	_____	_____
Complications of stockings noted		
Swelling above or below openings of stockings _____		
Pressure areas under stockings _____		
Complications reported to physician	_____	_____
Client discharged with stockings	_____	_____

51

Enema (Lower Bowel Irrigation) and Rectal Tube

Overview

Definition

The process of introducing a stream of solution into the rectum or lower colon and draining it off by natural or artificial means; the rectal tube facilitates expelling gas

Rationale

Cleanse or remove accumulated solids or gases from the lower bowel.

Stimulate peristalsis in the bowel.

Soothe and treat irritated mucosa.

Cleanse the bowel in preparation for x-ray examination.

Terminology

Harris flush (up-and-down flush): Lower bowel irrigation that promotes the expulsion of flatus from the intestines. This is especially helpful with postoperative clients whose intestinal tracts have been at rest and now must be stimulated into reestablishing normal peristalsis.

Feces: Body wastes, including food residue, bacteria, epithelium, and mucus discharged from the bowels by way of the anus

Flatus: Gas in the digestive tract

Hemorrhoid: A dilated blood vessel internally or externally located in the colon, rectal, or anal region

Impaction: Retention of hard, dried stool in the rectum and colon

Nonretention enema: Solution given with the intention of being expelled within a few minutes with feces, gas, and any other substances in the bowel

Peristalsis: The wavelike movement of the intestinal tract that is responsible for the onward movement of intestinal contents

Polyp: A growth with a pedicle, usually found in a vascular area such as the nose, uterus, or rectum

Retention enema: Solution introduced into the lower bowel but not expelled

Assessment

Pertinent Anatomy and Physiology

1. Appendix I: *anus, intestine (large), rectum.*
2. Peristalsis is controlled by the autonomic nervous system (ANS).
3. The adult colon has a capacity of about 750 ml to 1000 ml of solution.

Pathophysiological Concepts

1. A common symptom of abnormalities of the bowel is diarrhea. Large-volume diarrhea results from an increase in the water content of the stool, and small-volume diarrhea from an increase in the peristaltic action of the bowel. Small-volume diarrhea usually is characterized by cramping as well as frequent, explosive stools. This form of diarrhea often is associated with intrinsic disease of the colon, such as ulcerative colitis.

2. A bowel problem may manifest itself in the form of an impaction. Fecal impaction stimulates secretion of mucous in the portion of the bowel proximal to the blockage. This results in watery, diarrhealike stools as the body attempts to evacuate the mass. Impaction may indicate a problem with the peristaltic ability of the bowel or may result from dietary or mobility changes. The resulting inability of the bowel to evacuate leads to increased reabsorption of water from the stool and compounds the impaction problem. If not relieved, the impacted stool becomes a bowel obstruction and may have to be removed surgically.

Assessment of the Client

1. Assess the client in relation to the reason for hospitalization. Assess past bowel habits and when the last bowel movement occurred.

2. Assess the client's familiarity with the enema procedure. Determine the amount of teaching needed to meet each client's individual needs.

3. Assess the appearance of fecal material before the enema for indications of impaction, blood in the stools, and other pathology of the bowel.

Plan

Nursing Objectives

Carry out the treatment as quickly and efficiently as possible to prevent trauma, undue discomfort, and embarrassment.

Educate the client and family in principles of establishing and maintaining normal, regular bowel habits.

Observe and record carefully the client's reactions and the results of treatment.

Ensure a safe atmosphere and optimal cooperation by proper positioning and use of siderails, organizing and checking equipment beforehand, and adequate instruction of the client.

Client Preparation

1. Position the client on the left side, flat in bed, if not contraindicated. Explain the procedure to the client. If the client is unable to retain the solution, the enema may be given with the client on the bedpan. Have the client flex both knees, placing the top one higher than the bottom one.

2. If the client will retain and expel the enema on a bedpan, a pad placed under the hips and buttocks before beginning the procedure may prevent soiling the bed linens.

Equipment

Disposable enema bag

Bath thermometer

Linen: hip pad, towel, bath blanket

Bedpan, bedside commode, and tissue (if client cannot go to the bathroom for expulsion)

Solutions as ordered:

  Amount: 750 ml to 1000 ml

  Temperature: (adult enema) 105° F to 110° F

  Types

    Liquid soap: 1 packet to 1000 ml water

    Saline: 2 drams salt to 1000 ml water

    Olive oil: 2 oz to 5 oz olive oil, warmed to 100° F. Retain 3 minutes.

    Glycerine and water: 3 oz glycerine in 4 oz of water

    Commercial solutions: give as directed on package

Rectal tube

Water-soluble lubricant

Bath thermometer

Implementation and Interventions

Procedural Aspects

ACTION	*RATIONALE*
1. Be certain that the correct type of enema is being administered according to the physician's orders and the desired outcome.	Each agent or type of enema produces a specific action on the client.
2. Agents used to stimulate peristalsis must be mixed thoroughly and correctly before administration.	Peristaltic stimulants act as mucosal irritants. Incorrect or incomplete mixing may cause harmful local irritation.
3. Check the temperature of the solution with a bath thermometer. Proper temperature is 105° F to 110° F.	Heat is effective in stimulating nerve plexuses in intestinal mucosa. The temperature of the environment, the length of the tubing, and the rate of fluid flow will influence the temperature of the solution. Solutions entering the rectum at or very slightly above body temperature will not injure normal tissue.
4. Lubricate the final 2 in to 3 in of the enema tube with a water-soluble lubricant, such as K-Y jelly (Fig. 51-1).	Friction is reduced when a surface is lubricated.

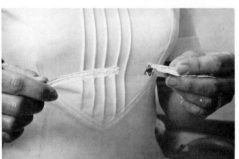

Figure 51.1

5. Expel air from the tubing before insertion into the rectum by allowing solution to run to the tip of the tubing (Fig. 51-2).	Air introduced into the colon before the solution may overly distend the walls causing additional discomfort and peristalsis.

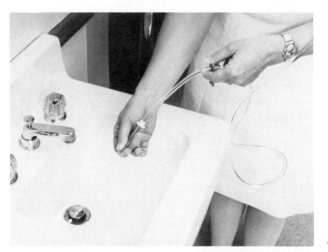

Figure 51.2

ACTION

RATIONALE

6. The anal canal is approximately 1 in to 1½ in long in the adult. Separate the buttocks gently with one hand and instruct the client to take a deep breath and slowly exhale. Insert the enema tube 4 in to 5 in (Fig. 51-3). If any resistance is met, *do not* force tubing. Allow a little solution to flow and then continue insertion of tubing. If continued resistance is encountered, discontinue efforts and notify the physician.

Slow insertion of the lubricated tube minimizes spasm of the intestinal wall. If fecal material is blocking the tubing, a small amount of solution should dilute and diffuse it enough to allow insertion to continue.

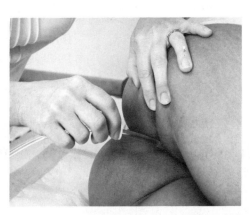

Figure 51.3

7. Hold the enema solution above the client so that it will instill by gravitational flow. The maximum elevation for an adult is 18 in to 24 in. Release the clamp and elevate the bag slowly to initiate flow. Rotate the tubing gently to avoid contact with the colon wall.

Gravity causes the solution to flow from the reservoir into the rectum. The higher the fluid is elevated, the faster the rate of flow and the greater the pressure in the rectum.

8. If the client complains of cramping or premature desire to evacuate the enema solution during instillation, clamp the tube or lower the bag until the feeling subsides, then resume instillation. In a retention enema, it is particularly important not to stimulate peristalsis because the enema should not be expelled.

Distension and irritation of the intestinal wall produce strong peristaltic action, which is sufficient to empty the bowel.

9. Clamp the tubing after most of the solution has entered to prevent instillation of air.

Air in the colon causes additional discomfort.

ACTION

RATIONALE

10. *Harris flush:* Lower the enema bag below bed level before all of the solution has entered the colon and allow it to siphon back into the bag from the colon. Continue raising and lowering the bag alternately until gas bubbles cease or the client feels more comfortable, and abdominal distension appears relieved (Figs. 51-4, 51-5).

Allowing the solution to flow in and out of the colon provides a means of relieving distention due to gas accumulation. Gravity provides the force to push the water into and out of the colon; this is achieved by positioning the bag higher or lower than the rectum.

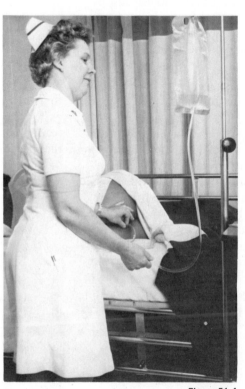

Figure 51.4

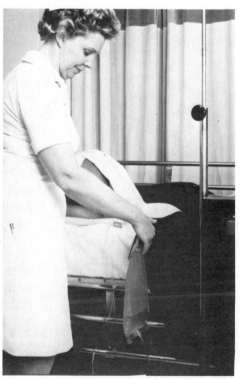

Figure 51.5

11. Solutions should remain in the colon the desired or prescribed length of time.

The effect of the enema will be enhanced if the solution is retained the prescribed length of time.

Nonretention enema: Assist the client to retain the enema for 5 to 10 minutes by offering encouragement and positioning the client to facilitate comfort and minimize pressure on the rectum. Have the bedpan ready or be prepared to assist the client to the bathroom when expulsion is inevitable.

Retention enema: Encourage the client not to expel the enema for the time span ordered by the physician or until the solution is absorbed.

ACTION

RATIONALE

12. If the client is in bed, be sure that the signal light and tissue are within easy reach. If the client is allowed to go to the bathroom, place the call light nearby and provide instructions on how to use it. Be sure that the client and linens are left clean after the enema. Allow a rest period since the enema procedure can be very tiring. Label reusable enema equipment with the client's name and store in an appropriate place. Leave the bedside area neat and clean.

Even after the enema has been expelled, some subsequent expulsion is possible. The client should expect and be prepared for this.

13. *Rectal tube:* A tube is inserted into the rectum and left in place for the purpose of expelling gas and relieving distension. Lubricate the tip of the rectal tube and insert in to the rectum as with the enema tubing (Fig. 51-6). No fluid is instilled, however. The tube may be taped in place for approximately 20 minutes. Place the end of the tube under water to detect the presence of gas release by bubbling of the water. A plastic bag or container may be secured over the end of the tube in case liquid feces are returned (Fig. 51-7).

The rectal tube allows gas to escape the rectum without relaxation of the external sphincture, which is sometimes difficult during illness or recuperation.

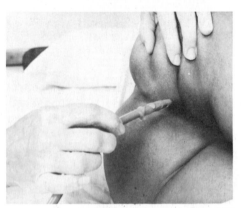

Figure 51.6

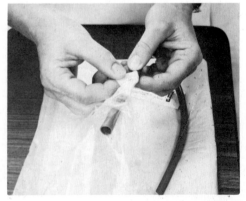

Figure 51.7

Special Modifications

If there has been no evacuation of the nonretention enema after 1 hour, place the client on the right side near the edge of the bed with the bedpan on the chair next to the bed. Remove the tubing from the enema bag and place it in the bedpan. Reinsert the rectal end into the client as before.

An enema may not be expelled if there is reduced neuromuscular response. Leaving the solution in the colon may result in absorption into the bloodstream, with resulting cardiovascular problems, however. Manual assistance with expulsion may be necessary.

ACTION	RATIONALE
Allow the solution to run out of the rectum by gravitational flow, measuring to make certain that all of the fluid is returned. If the solution does not return, attach a funnel to the end of the tubing and fill tubing with warm water (105° F). Reinsert the tube, allow a little fluid to run in, then quickly invert the funnel into the bedpan. Measure as previously mentioned.	

Communicative Aspects

OBSERVATIONS

1. When the enema is expelled, observe the color and consistency of the feces (hard, soft, loose). Observe the amount of fluid returned, general amount of flatus expelled (large or small). Note any unusual findings such as blood, mucus, pus, or worms in the stool.

2. Observe the reaction of the client to the enema procedure. Watch for signs of fatigue and exhaustion. Observe for signs that the client cannot tolerate more enema solution and signs that expulsion is inevitable. Note the client's general reaction to the procedure after completion.

3. If the enema was the retention type, note if the desired results were obtained.

4. If the client was unable to expel the nonretention enema, note the results of attempts to remove the fluid from the colon and the client's reaction.

5. *Rectal tube:* Note the amount of flatus and the relief experienced by the client. Observe the abdomen before and after to assess the success of the procedure.

CHARTING

DATE/TIME	OBSERVATIONS	SIGNATURE
6/30 1430	Saline enema given. Held solution for 6 min before expelling in bedside commode. Large amount of formed brown stool returned. States that he feels much better. Abdominal distension decreased. Resting quietly at this time ——	G. Ivers RN

Discharge Planning Aspects

CLIENT AND FAMILY EDUCATION

1. If the client will need enemas after discharge, teach the client or family the correct technique. Explain basic anatomy, how often to give enemas, and why.

2. Administration of an enema provides an excellent opportunity for health teaching. Teach the client and family what constitutes normal elimination patterns and that enemas should only be used for unusual problems. Reliance on enemas or over-the-counter laxatives for elimination is unnatural and dangerous. Explain the importance of adequate diet and fluids, exercise, and responding to the natural urge in the promotion of normal elimination. Emphasize the fact that "normal" does not necessarily mean *daily* bowel movements. Every person has a different pattern of normalcy.

Evaluation

Quality Assurance

Documentation should include the type of enema, and the desired and actual results. Any complications or unusual occurrences or outcomes should be noted, with steps taken by the nurse to resolve them. The client's reaction to the procedure, measures taken to preserve strength, and health teaching also should be reflected.

Infection Control

1. Any procedure dealing with the eliminatory processes has potential for cross-contamination. Careful handwashing before and after the procedure is essential.
2. When reusable equipment is stored, it must be labeled clearly to prevent the possibility of someone using it by mistake.

Technique Checklist

	YES	NO
Procedure explained to client	_____	_____
Type of enema given _____		
Amount of solution given _____		
Medication added _____		
Client held the enema for _____ minutes		
Desired results obtained	_____	_____
Complications		
_____		
Complications reported to physician	_____	_____
Client and family taught to administer enemas after discharge	_____	_____

52   Evening Care

Overview

Definition

Personal care for the client before sleep

Rationale

Promote the client's comfort, personal hygiene, and sleep.

Provide a clean, safe environment for the client during the night.

Assessment

Pertinent Anatomy and Physiology

Sleep is a state in which the cerebral cortex of the brain is totally active, but consciousness is lost. There are two different forms of sleep. One is non-dreaming, or slow-wave, sleep, which is characterized by diminished brain activity. The deepest sleep occurs about 1½ hours after going to sleep. The second form of sleep is rapid eye movement (REM) sleep, or paradoxical sleep. This occurs after about 2 hours of sleep and usually involves the dreaming period. Various physiological changes occur during sleep: muscle tone is diminished; heart rate and blood pressure are decreased; metabolic rate is diminished by about 10%; body temperature falls slightly; and respiration is slower and shallower.

Pathophysiological Concepts

Severe sleep deprivation results in varying degrees of mental deterioration and hallucinations; however, these symptoms vanish after the person has been permitted to sleep in 4-hour blocks of time. This is the amount of time required for a REM cycle to be completed.

Assessment of the Client

1. Assess the client's physical condition in relation to readiness for sleep. Is the client comfortable, in pain, anxious, or frightened?
2. Assess the client's usual pattern of preparing for rest. Determine when the client usually bathes or showers. Determine when the client usually retires, customary habits before sleeping, snacks or nourishments, diversionary methods for sleeplessness, and any other information pertinent to sleep habits.
3. Assess the client's potential for safety risks. Assess the state of confusion, sedation, ambulation difficulties, nocturia, history of falls at night, night vision problems, and any other problems that might place the client at risk in a strange environment at night.

Plan

Nursing Objectives

Make sure that the client is clean, safe, and comfortable.

Observe the client and evaluate the care given during the day; make adjustments and plans for care that will be required during the night.

Equipment

Washcloth and towel

Basin of warm water

Personal items (cosmetics, toothbrush, toothpaste)

Bedpan or urinal

Lotion or powder for backrub

Other items, according to need (fresh dressings, binders, linens, or gowns)

Implementation and Interventions

Procedural Aspects

ACTION	RATIONALE
1. Try to anticipate all of the client's needs during evening care. Offer the bedpan or urinal. Assist with handwashing, brushing teeth, and other toiletries as needed. Administer backrub (see Technique No. 26, Backrub). Change dressings (see Technique No. 49, Dressings, Surgical) and reapply binders or bandages (see Technique No. 27, Bandaging, and Technique No. 32, Binders, Application of). Tighten and smooth bed linens, changing if necessary to provide a clean and fresh environment in which the client will sleep. Fluff and turn the pillow and administer sleeping medication, if ordered. Turn off the radio and television if the client wishes. Dim the room light, making sure the call light is within easy reach and that the client knows how to use it.	A feeling of comfort and confidence will ease the client's mind and may facilitate sleep. Many people have difficulty sleeping in a strange place. Try to provide the client with a restful night so that energy can be channeled to the recuperation process.
2. Pay particular attention to safety precautions, especially at night. Lower the bed to its lowest position with the siderails raised. A night light should be on in every room. Ask the client to call for assistance when getting up rather than taking a chance on falling.	During the night the client's sensorium may be dulled by medication or fatigue. Many elderly become confused when awakening at night in a strange environment, and as a result may fall. Extra attention to safety precautions may prevent accidents and injuries.

Communicative Aspects

OBSERVATIONS

1. Note the client's readiness to settle down for the night, effectiveness of evening care, and anything significant in regard to physical or psychological condition or treatments. Record any significant observations in the chart.

2. Observe the client's condition in relation to procedures performed to facilitate sleep, such as dressing changes, application of binders, and backrub.

CHARTING

DATE/TIME	OBSERVATIONS	SIGNATURE
5/22 2130	Evening care given. Seems very restless. Backrub and other comfort measures seem to help somewhat. States that he is discouraged and wants to go home. Glass of warm milk given; states that this usually helps calm him down at home so he can rest. Reassurance about condition offered. ———	J. Day RN

Discharge Planning Aspects

CLIENT AND FAMILY EDUCATION

1. If the client will be dependent on others at home for care, inform the family about what constitutes adequate evening care to promote sleep and relaxation.

2. Specific teaching for the client depends on what is being done. Evening care provides an opportunity for reinforcement of teaching done previously, for answering questions, and for allowing the client to voice worries or complaints, which may then be addressed by the nursing staff.

3. If the client has a high safety-risk index, talk with the family about safety measures to take after discharge: siderails on the bed at home; night lighting; slippers with rubber soles; removal of small, slippery throw rugs; moving the bed closer to the bathroom; and a call or alarm for night use. These safety precautions, taken at home, decrease the chance of falls or injury.

Evaluation

Quality Assurance

Documentation should reflect the measures taken each night to prepare the client for sleep. In addition, those measures proven most effective should be noted as evidence of a coordinated, planned approach to care. Problems occurring during the night should be reflected, as well as the resolution of each problem. Evaluation of the safety risks and implementation of a plan to decrease these risks should be documented.

Infection Control

Handwashing should be done before approaching the client for evening care. Articles used in evening care should be labeled clearly for the client and used only for that person. The client should be taught proper hygiene (e.g., washing hands after voiding or defecation, and brushing the teeth each night). Hands should be washed again after evening care.

Technique Checklist

	YES	NO
Procedure explained to client	_____	_____
Bedpan or urinal offered	_____	_____
Hands and face washed	_____	_____
Teeth brushed	_____	_____
Backrub	_____	_____
Dressing changed	_____	_____
Linens clean, fresh, wrinkle-free	_____	_____
Sleeping medication	_____	_____
Call light in reach of client	_____	_____
Family instructed on evening care	_____	_____

53   Eye (Artificial), Removal and Insertion

Overview

Definition

Removal and reinsertion of the artificial prosthesis used to fill the orbit after enucleation of the eye

Rationale

Clean the socket, the surrounding tissue, and the prosthesis to prevent infection and discomfort.

Assess the integrity of the socket and surrounding tissues.

Examine the condition of the prosthesis.

Terminology

Prosthesis: Replacement of a missing part by an artificial substitute

Assessment

Pertinent Anatomy and Physiology

1. The orbit is the cavity that surrounds and protects the eye. The walls of the orbit are formed by the union of seven cranial and facial bones.
2. The eyelids are the protective movable sheaths of tissue located in front of the eyeball. The upper and lower lids meet at the outer canthi. The conjunctiva is a thin, transparent membrane that lines each eyelid and is involved with the secretion of mucus.
3. The lacrimal gland secretes tears, which are carried to the conjunctival sac through a network of short ducts. Tears bathe the surface of the eyeball and keep it moist at all times.

Pathophysiological Concepts

1. A variety of conditions affect the eyelids. A chalazion is a small tumor of the eyelid formed by the distension of one of the secretory glands. Infection of the conjunctiva is called conjunctivitis, or pinkeye.
2. Tears normally flow into the lacrimal sac and then into the nasolacrimal duct, which passes downward through a bony canal to open into the lower portion of the nasal cavity. Inflammation and swelling of the nasal mucosa, which occurs in the common cold, causes obstruction of the nasolacrimal ducts, and interferes with the normal drainage of tears.

Assessment of the Client

1. Assess the client for ability to assist with the insertion and removal of the eye prosthesis. Determine the usual method of cleansing the eye and the socket at home and follow the usual routine as much as is possible. If the routine is not considered to be in the best interests of the client's health, teach proper technique and methods of keeping the eye socket clean and healthy.
2. Assess the condition of the client's other eye. Determine what prompted the loss of the eye and, if the pathology could affect the remaining eye, assess the extent of damage.
3. Assess the condition of the eye socket and the eye prosthesis.

Plan

Nursing Objectives

Carry out normal eye care for the client regardless of the condition that prompted hospitalization.

Use measures to prevent infection and avoid further injury to the remaining eye.

Reinforce or teach proper techniques for the maintenance of the artificial eye and the body tissue into which it is inserted.

Client Preparation

1. Explain to the client what will happen. If the client is able, solicit assistance and carry out the procedure as closely to the normal routine as possible.

2. Many hospitals require removal of an artificial eye when the client goes for surgery. If the client is scheduled for surgery, explain in advance that the eye will have to be removed.

3. Respect the client's privacy. Many people do not wish the fact that they wear an eye prosthesis to be known. Provide a private area for the cleaning of the eye.

Equipment

Container

Warm saline (105°F to 110°F)

Soft gauze or cotton balls

Prosthesis container

Suction cup to remove the eye

Implementation and Interventions

Procedural Aspects

ACTION

1. Identify the eye to be removed. Unless the client has an alternative method, pull the lower eyelid down over the cheekbone with the thumb and exert slight pressure on the lower portion of the eyelid. (Fig. 53-1). An alternative is to use a small suction cup applied directly to the prosthesis. A slight rocking motion will release the suction. Once the suction is released, the prosthesis should pop out.

RATIONALE

The goal is to break the suction holding the artificial eye in place. Once released, the eye will pop out, so care must be taken not to scratch or drop the eye.

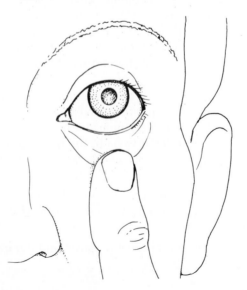

Figure 53.1

ACTION

RATIONALE

2. To clean the prosthesis, wash gently in warm normal saline and dry with gauze pads. If it will not be reinserted immediately, place the prosthesis in a container with a secure lid and label with the client's name and room number. Place the container in a secure place.

Remove all of the crusts and secretions from the eye, being careful not to scratch or break it. Adequate labeling reduces the chance of losing the eye.

3. To clean the socket, spread the lids apart and wash out the inside with cotton balls or gauze pads moistened with warm saline. Wipe from inner to outer canthus. Remove all crusts and secretions. Dry the surrounding tissue with dry pads in the same manner.

The reason for the enucleation of the eye will determine the extent of the removal of surrounding tissue. The lacrimal ducts may still be intact. Wiping from the inner to outer canthus reduces the chance of pushing debris into the ducts and moves debris away from the unaffected eye.

4. To insert the eye, separate the upper and lower lids gently with the thumb and forefinger. Holding the prosthesis in the other hand between the thumb and forefinger, place the eye gently into the socket in the natural alignment (Fig. 53-2).

Hold the eye firmly to avoid dropping it. The eye should fit easily into the socket.

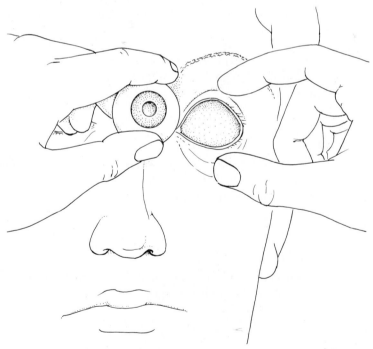

Figure 53.2

Communicative Aspects

OBSERVATIONS

1. Observe the condition of the socket and the prosthesis.
2. Observe the client's reaction. If the client is able to perform the removal, cleaning, and reinsertion or to help with the procedure, observe for proper technique and potential problems.

CHARTING

DATE/TIME	OBSERVATIONS	SIGNATURE
8/23 0815	L. eye prosthesis removed, socket cleaned, and eye reinserted. Some ex-udate found in socket but tissue appears intact. States that he has not felt like cleaning the eye since he became ill a week ago. Eye and socket cleaned and dried and eye reinserted. ————————————	D. Hill RN

Discharge Planning Aspects

CLIENT AND FAMILY EDUCATION

1. Instruct the client on the proper technique for cleaning the eye and desirable frequency only if errors in current methods are found.

REFERRALS

If the condition of the prosthesis is poor, a new one might be needed. Artificial eyes are quite expensive and should be obtained only from a reputable prosthetic expert.

Evaluation

Quality Assurance

Documentation should include a description of the condition of the socket and the prosthesis. An evaluation of the client's current methods of cleaning the eye and any education efforts should be noted. Any problems should be reflected in the chart as well as the attempts to resolve those problems.

Infection Control

Careful handwashing before and after the procedure is necessary. Although this is not a sterile procedure, it usually is done with sterile equipment in the hospital setting. The goal is to prevent the spread of infection to the other eye and to preserve the integrity of the tissues surrounding the artificial eye.

Technique Checklist

	YES	NO
Client able to do eye care	———	———
Client able to advise nurse about usual method of removing and cleaning artificial eye	———	———
Eye removed without problem	———	———
Socket tissue intact	———	———
Condition of prosthesis satisfactory	———	———
If not, referral made ———	———	———
Client knows how to care for the eye prosthesis and the tissue before discharge	———	———

54 Eye, Irrigation of

Overview

Definition

Washing out of the conjunctival sac with a stream of liquid

Rationale

Remove a foreign body.

Flush out an irritating chemical.

Treat an inflammation of the conjunctiva; remove inflammatory secretions.

Obtain antiseptic effects.

Produce specific temperature effects.

Prepare the eye for surgery.

Terminology

Accommodation: Adjustment of the eye for seeing at different distances; the adjustment of the eye whereby it is able to focus the image of the object on the retina. The contraction and relaxation of the ciliary muscles, which are reflex in nature, are necessary for accommodation.

Asepsis: A condition free from germs, free from infection, sterile

Bactericidal: An agent capable of killing bacteria

Canthus: The angle at either end of the slit between the eyelids; the external and internal canthus

Conjunctiva: Mucous membrane that lines the eyelids and is reflected onto the eyeball

Conjunctival reflex (blinking): An involuntary response; closure of the eyelids when conjunctiva is touched or threatened

Contamination: The introduction of disease, germs or infectious material into or onto normally sterile or clean objects

Dissemination: Scattered throughout an organ or the body (as applied to disease organisms)

Eyeball: The body of the eye; a spherical organ situated in a bony cavity called the orbit

Microorganisms: Minute living bodies imperceptible to the naked eye (usually refers to bacteria or protozoa)

Pathogen: A microorganism or substance capable of producing disease

pH: The hydrogen ion (H +) concentration; a symbol used to express the degree of acidity or alkalinity. (For example, the normal pH of the blood is 7.35 to 7.45.) The pH of a neutral solution is 7.0 at 25°C.

Plexus: A network of nerves or vessels

Assessment

Pertinent Anatomy and Physiology

1. See Appendix I: *eye (external), eye (internal).*

2. The eyelids are the protective movable sheaths of tissue located in front of the eyeball. The upper and lower lids meet at the outer canthi. The conjunctiva is a thin, transparent membrane that lines each eyelid and is involved with the secretion of mucus.

3. The lacrimal gland secretes tears, which are carried to the conjunctival sac through a network of short ducts. Tears bathe the surface of the eyeball and keep it moist at all times. Tears also protect the cornea, which will become hardened, like the epidermis of the skin, if exposed to air. Tears also wash away debris that enters the eye. A bactericidal enzyme in the tears, lysozyme, offers protection against certain microorganisms.

Pathophysiological Concepts

1. A variety of conditions affect the eyelids. A chalazion is a small tumor of the eyelid formed by the distension of one of the secretory glands. Infection of the conjunctiva is called conjunctivitis, or pinkeye.

2. Tears normally flow into the lacrimal sac and then into the nasolacrimal duct, which passes downward through a bony canal to open into the lower portion of the nasal cavity. Inflammation and swelling of the nasal mucosa, which occurs in the common cold, causes obstruction of the nasolacrimal ducts, and interferes with the normal drainage of tears.

Assessment of the Client

1. Assess the appearance of the eyes in comparison to each other, amount and character of any discharge, excessive tearing, redness, swelling of the eyelids, and size and reaction of the pupil.

2. Assess the client's history of visual and optical problems. Assess the client for complaints of itching, burning, visual disturbances, sensitivity to light, and any pain including location, duration, and intensity.

Plan

Nursing Objectives

Allay fear and anxiety.

Use measures to prevent infection and avoid further injury to the eye.

Provide an environment restful to the eyes.

Carry out the procedures as ordered by the physician expeditiously.

Teach the client and family proper care of the eyes and eye health.

Client Preparation

1. For maximum safety of the client, all equipment used and the solution introduced into conjunctival sac should be sterile. Use aseptic technique throughout the procedure. Take precautions to prevent dissemination of the infection to the other eye, as well as to other persons. Thorough handwashing is essential before and after the procedure. If the presence of infection is suspected, the nurse may wish to irrigate slowly and stand back during irrigation. The unaffected eye may be covered during the procedure.

2. Gravity will aid the flow of solution away from the affected eye. Position the client sitting comfortably or lying supine, with head tilted toward the side of the affected eye so that the solution will flow from the inner canthus toward the outer canthus.

3. Place a linen protector over the client's shoulders to prevent wetting the clothing and linen. If able to sit up and assist, the client may hold the basin at the edge of the eye to catch the irrigation solution. In the lying position, place the curved basin against the client's cheek on the affected side to receive solution.

Equipment

Prescribed irrigating solution

Eye irrigator

An eyedropper (if small amounts of solution are used)

A soft rubber bulb syringe, flask, or irrigating can (for larger amounts)

Commercially prepared plastic irrigating bottles containing sterile ophthalmic solution

Implementation and Interventions

Procedural Aspects

ACTION	*RATIONALE*
1. Check the physician's order for the specified solution, its amount, and the temperature. For cleansing purposes, physiologic saline usually is used.	Antiseptic solutions are usually selected for their effect on the causative agent.
2. Arrange the light in a position to afford optimal illumination of the working area without its shining directly into the client's eye. An eye pad may be ordered for wear between irrigations.	Photosensitivity, or an unusual sensitivity to light, is common in many eye conditions.
3. Gently separate the eyelids with the thumb and fingers of one hand to expose the conjunctival sac (Fig. 54-1). Slight pressure may be exerted on the bony prominences of the cheek and brow, never on the eyeball.	If the cornea or conjunctiva is touched, reflex blinking will occur. The eyelids must be held apart manually to prevent spontaneous closing of the eye during irrigation.

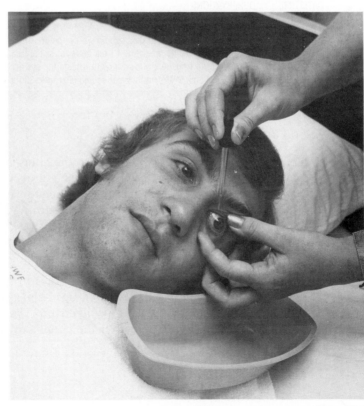

Figure 54.1

ACTION	*RATIONALE*
4. Irrigate the eye, using low pressure but with sufficient force to remove secretions from the conjunctiva gently. The solution should flow steadily. Repeat until the eye is free of debris.	Pressure should be sufficient to remove unwanted secretions but not so great that it stimulates the blinking reflex.
5. Do not touch the eyelid, lashes, or the eyeball itself with the irrigating instrument.	Any type of corneal stimulation gives rise to discomfort, pain, and the desire to blink.
6. Ask the client to close the eye being irrigated periodically throughout the procedure.	Movement of the eye beneath closed lids helps disengage and move secretions from the upper to the lower conjunctival sac.
7. Dry the surrounding area with a sterile cotton ball.	Drying will minimize the urge of the client to rub or wipe the eye after irrigation.

Communicative Aspects

OBSERVATIONS

1. Observe the client for squinting, excessive blinking, frowning, or rubbing the eyes.
2. Note the appearance of the eye(s). Look for the presence of redness, swelling, lacrimation (tearing), discharge (amount and appearance), and pupil size (unequal, pinpoint, or dilated). Observe the appearance of the irrigation fluid after irrigation to determine if the debris or secretions were removed.
3. Record any verbal statements (headache, burning, smarting, pain, photophobia, and visual disturbances such as blurring).

CHARTING

DATE/TIME	OBSERVATIONS	SIGNATURE
12/9 0930	Right eye irrigated with 30 ml sterile saline, 98°F. Returned cloudy. Large amount of yellow purulent discharge from eye before irrigation. Stated, ''My eye hurts most of the time, but it feels better after the treatment.'' Wife present during irrigation; shown how to irrigate the eye according to physician's directions. Will demonstrate technique at the 1330 irrigation. ————	J. Day RN

Discharge Planning Aspects

CLIENT AND FAMILY EDUCATION

1. Reinforce the physician's directions to the client and family. Reiterate the importance of following these directions and using the medicine for the length of time recommended by the physician even if the symptoms seem to be relieved. Stress the importance of returning for follow-up visits as directed.
2. Teach the client and family how to irrigate the eye and the importance of using correct technique to prevent injury to the eye and spread of infection.
3. Relate to the client's family and visitors ways in which they can aid in the client's recovery. Suggest that they engage in pleasant conversation near the client, including the client in the conversion. They should identify themselves when they enter the room if the client's eyes are bandaged.

Evaluation

Quality Assurance

1. Documentation should include eye treatments, why they were given, and what were the results. Condition of the eye should be noted on admission and at least daily until discharge. Any optic symptoms should be noted.
2. Teaching efforts directed toward the client and the family should be noted, as well as an evaluation of their effectiveness. If home care of the eyes is needed, the documentation should reflect who was taught to do the treatments and an assessment of their ability and willingness to do so.

Infection Control

Infection is often the reason for the eye irrigation in the first place. The goal of therapy is to prevent the spread of the infection to the client's other eye or to anyone else. Careful handwashing, wearing of gloves, and adherence to careful aseptic technique are all essential. Eye patches and dressings should be disposed of properly. If the eye is infected, the secretions in the irrigating fluid should be disposed of according to isolation procedure.

Technique Checklist

	YES	NO
Procedure explained to client	_____	_____
Eye irrigation accomplished with minimal discomfort	_____	_____
Debris or secretions removed from eye	_____	_____
Condition of eye improved at discharge	_____	_____
Irrigations to continue after discharge	_____	_____
Family member taught to do irrigation	_____	_____
Family and client understand follow-up care instructions	_____	_____

55

Fecal Impaction, Removal of

Overview

Definition

Manual removal of abnormal accumulation of fecal material that forms a hardened mass in the lower portion of the bowel

Rationale

Ensure the return of normal peristalsis.

Restore normal fluid and electrolyte balance.

Prevent rectal trauma and bleeding.

Relieve pain and discomfort of the client.

Terminology

Feces: Body wastes, including food residue, bacteria, epithelium, and mucus discharged from the bowels by way of the anus

Hemorrhoid: A dilated blood vessel internally or externally located in the colon, rectal, or anal region

Peristalsis: The wavelike movement of the intestinal tract that is responsible for the onward movement of intestinal contents

Polyp: A growth with a pedicle frequently found in a vascular area, such as the rectum

Stool: Evacuation of the bowels; waste matter discharged from the bowels

Assessment

Pertinent Anatomy and Physiology

See Appendix I: *anus, intestine (large), rectum.*

Pathophysiological Concepts

1. A common symptom of abnormalities of the bowel is diarrhea. Large-volume diarrhea results from an increase in the water content of the stool, and small-volume diarrhea from an increase in the peristaltic action of the bowel. Small-volume diarrhea usually is characterized by cramping, and frequent, explosive stools.

2. Another common bowel problem is impaction (Fig. 55-1). Fecal impaction stimulates secretion of mucus in the portion of the bowel proximal to the blockage. This results in watery, diarrhealike stools when the body attempts to evacuate the mass.

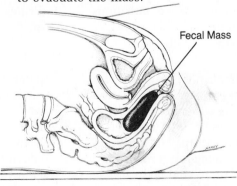

Fecal Mass

Figure 55.1

Assessment of the Client

1. Assess the onset of the present problem. Determine the date of the client's last bowel movement, presence of watery stool, hardness of abdomen, rectal pain, desire to defecate without results, and generalized malaise.

2. Assess the presence and severity of fecal impaction by digital examination of the rectum, unless contraindicated by client diagnosis or symptoms such as rectal bleeding.

3. Assess past bowel habits. Determine the client's normal elimination pattern. Note if there has been a change in bowel habits in the past few months or years. Assess usual dietary and exercise patterns.

4. Assess whether the client understands what an impaction is. Ask if the client has ever had an impaction before, and determine whether it was removed manually.

Plan

Nursing Objectives

Relieve the discomfort of impaction with minimal discomfort to the client.

Allow the client adequate time to rest and recover from the procedure.

Reassess the client's bowel habits and dietary regimen to prevent future impaction.

Teach the client and family measures that will prevent recurrence of impaction.

Client Preparation

1. A clear explanation of what impaction is and why it must be removed should precede initiation of treatment. Tell the client that manual removal will cause discomfort, but once the impaction is removed, the rectal fullness and pain will subside.

2. A mild sedative may be given 30 minutes before the removal of the impaction to lessen the severity of discomfort. Pad the bed well and protect the client's personal clothing from soiling.

Equipment

Linen protector

Bedpan

Clean gloves

Lubricating jelly

Enema equipment (see Technique No. 51, Enema and Rectal Tube)

Tissue or washcloth

Implementation and Interventions

Procedural Aspects

ACTION	RATIONALE
1. Fecal impaction is easier to prevent than to treat. Preventive measures include adequate fluid intake, proper exercise, nutritious diet, judicious use of laxatives, suppositories, and cleansing enemas.	Unless the client has been taking medicine to decrease peristalsis, the presence of a fecal impaction usually indicates less than optimal nursing care.
2. Elderly clients are especially prone to constipation and the formation of impactions; therefore, preventive measures should be undertaken early. Identify those clients at risk for impaction formation. Clients on prolonged bedrest may be predisposed to impaction for-	Regularity of bowel movements refers to amount as well as frequency of bowel movements. Often liquid stool will be discharged around the impaction and may be misleading. These stools are usually foul-smelling and uncontrolled. This is usually a sure indication of fecal impaction.

ACTION

mation. Barium sulfate used in various radiologic examinations may enter the bowel and harden. Mentally confused clients may disregard the natural impulse to defecate, hence impaction occurs. Monitor these clients to ensure regular bowel movements.

3. Fecal impaction is usually a dry, hard mass in the lower rectum. Softening and lubrication may be accomplished by suppositories or oil retention enemas. This usually is followed by cleansing enemas until the impaction is removed.

4. If enemas fail to remove the impaction, remove it by digitally breaking up the mass into smaller pieces and manually removing them from the bowel. Position the client in Sims' position. Place the bedpan nearby so that the fecal material may be placed in it. Place a pad under the client to preserve the linens on the bed. Don clean gloves. Lubricate the forefingers and gently insert them into the anal canal (Fig. 55-2). This will be uncomfortable for the client; offer encouragement and explanation during the procedure. Use the index finger to break the mass into smaller pieces. Remove it manually, one piece at a time, into the bedpan (Figs. 55-3, 55-4). If the

RATIONALE

The hard mass of fecal impaction results from a decrease in motility and advancement of the feces in the large bowel. During the delay caused by slow movement, unusually large amounts of water are reabsorbed into the intestine, resulting in a dried, hard mass.

Dilatation of the anal sphincture and discomfort from the procedure are exhausting to the client. If the impaction is very large and difficult to remove, arrange for several sessions to remove the entire impaction.

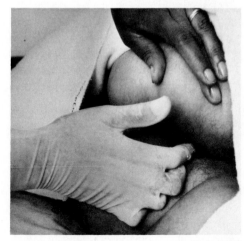

Figure 55.2

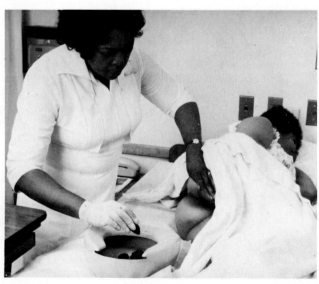

Figure 55.3

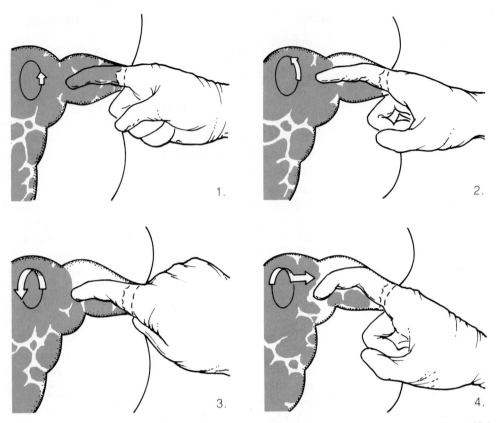

Figure 55.4

ACTION	RATIONALE
mass is very hard and large, it may be necessary to remove only a part of the total mass at one time.	
5. After the impaction is removed, clean the rectal area and allow the client to rest (Fig. 55-5).	The procedure is stressful as well as painful. Recuperation will vary with the individual client.

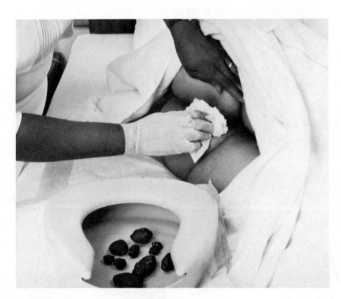

Figure 55.5

Communicative Aspects

OBSERVATIONS

1. Observe the client during digital removal of the impaction to assess tolerance of the procedure. It may be necessary to discontinue the removal for several hours to allow the client to rest.

2. Observe the rectal area after removal of the impaction to make sure that the manual manipulation did not irritate the mucosa or an internal hemorrhoid, resulting in rectal bleeding.

3. Observe the client for regular bowel movments to ensure that the impaction will not recur.

CHARTING

DATE/TIME	OBSERVATIONS	SIGNATURE
11/19 0700	Oil retention enema with 4 oz oil instilled. Instructed to retain the oil as long as possible. States she feels fullness in the rectal area but will hold the enema solution. ————————	P. Dillon RN
0810	Enema expelled with small amount of liquid stool. Hard mass felt on digital rectal examination. Large fecal impaction removed manually. Slight bleeding from small external hemorrhoid. Expressed a great deal of discomfort during removal of impaction; seems relieved now with less abdominal distension.—	P. Dillon RN

Discharge Planning Aspects

CLIENT AND FAMILY EDUCATION

1. Teach the client to observe stools for amount, consistency, and frequency if impaction is to be suspected in the future. A deviation resulting in less frequent stools or in uncontrolled, loose stools may indicate impaction.

2. Constipation with impaction occurs most frequently in immobilized or inactive clients who have inadequate water intake, seldom change position, and do not use their abdominal muscles for bearing down during bowel movement. Knowledge of these causes may enable the client to participate actively in impaction prevention by altering behavior and modifying diet to include sufficient fluids, bulk, and appropriate foods such as fresh fruits and vegetables to promote motility and propulsion.

3. Instruct the client and family on the dangers of becoming laxative dependent. Because of their availability and predictability, laxatives are often abused, especially by older adults. The importance of a balanced diet and adequate exercise should be stressed. Use of high-fiber foods, such as bran, may be substituted for continual laxatives use.

Evaluation

Quality Assurance

Documentation should include symptoms evidenced by the client or observed by the nurse. Success of preliminary efforts to remove impaction should be reflected. Amount of time necessary to remove the impaction, appearance of feces, and the client's tolerance of precedure should be noted. Any complications should be noted, as well as the ways in which these were resolved.

Infection Control

Fecal impaction removal is not a sterile procedure. Clean gloves should be worn by the nurse. Careful handwashing before and after the procedure is necessary.

Technique Checklist

	YES	NO
Procedure explained to client	_____	_____
Enemas and laxatives given	_____	_____
Results _____		
Sedation given to client before procedure	_____	_____
Impaction removed	_____	_____
Client tolerated procedure without problems	_____	_____
Instructions given to client and family about prevention of impaction in the future	_____	_____

56   Foot Care

Overview

Definition

Preventive measures taken to avoid deformities or infection of the feet

Rationale

Prevent deformities of the feet.

Prevent infection.

Maintain comfort and cleanliness.

Promote satisfactory peripheral circulation.

Promote improved metabolic functioning.

Terminology

Claudication: Limping or lameness

Intermittent claudication: A severe pain in the calf muscles occurring during walking but subsiding with rest; results from inadequate blood supply

Inversion: Movement that turns the sole of the foot inward

Ischemia: Deficiency of blood in a body part because of functional constriction or actual obstruction of a blood vessel

Footdrop: A deformity in which the foot is extended abnormally at the ankle in the direction of the sole of the foot

Assessment

Pertinent Anatomy and Physiology

See Appendix I: *foot.*

Pathophysiological Concepts

1. The tibialis anterior muscle flexes and inverts the foot dorsally. Injury to the nerve supply results in a condition known as *footdrop* (inability to pull the foot upward toward the shin). Persons with footdrop have a characteristic high step and flop of the affected foot because the foot fails to clear the ground when they step forward.

2. Because the feet are farther away from the heart than any other body part, they are the most compromised by vascular conditions that interfere with normal circulation. In diabetes, for instance, ulceration of the feet and toes is a constant threat. In advanced peripheral vascular disease, the color of the extremities is usually abnormal, and healing of lesions and wounds is very difficult.

3. Muscular involvement is limited by the capacity of the circulatory system to provide glucose and oxygen and to eliminate lactic acid and carbon dioxide. Claudication is often the result of poor circulation.

Assessment of the Client

1. Assess the condition of the client's feet and lower extremities. Palpate the dorsal and pedal pulses as an indication of the status of circulation to the feet. Be alert for wounds, lesions, blisters, callouses, ingrown toenails, and unnatural foot position. Assessment of the foot includes

   Examination of the skin and signs of nail disruption

   Palpation for any joint or phalangeal sensitivity

   Examination for stress areas in joints and phalanges

   Examination of the shoes for signs of abnormal wear

   Assessment of the mobility of ankles and toes

   Assessment of cleanliness of the feet

2. Assess the client's health history in relation to the presence of diseases that might predispose to foot problems, such as diabetes and peripheral vascular disease. In the diabetic client, a physician's order is needed to cut the toenails.

Plan

Nursing Objectives

Keep the client as comfortable as possible.

Prevent complications associated with prolonged bed rest.

Teach proper foot care to the client and family.

Client Preparation

1. Explain to the client what will happen during foot care. Solicit information about the usual methods of foot care used by the client.

2. Determine the range of mobility of the client. If able, the client may sit on the side of the bed or move to the bathroom for foot care.

Equipment

Footboard

Basin and toenail clippers

Lanolin or petrolatum-based cream

Implementation and Interventions

Procedural Aspects

ACTION	RATIONALE
1. To avoid the deformity known as footdrop, place a footboard at the end of the bed. Position the client with feet flat against the footboard in the natural position (Fig. 56-1). Add padding to the bony prominences of the foot and ankle to prevent the formation of pressure sores over these areas. The client should perform active and passive exercises involving the feet, toes, and ankles, at least twice daily.	Prolonged bedrest places a severe strain on all body parts, especially the feet. The footboard facilitates keeping the feet in the natural position and also keeps the bed linens from pushing the tops of the feet downward.

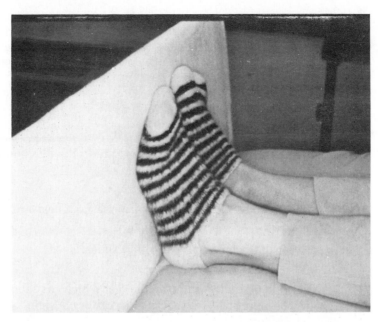

Figure 56.1

ACTION	RATIONALE
2. Keep the feet clean. Immerse the client's feet in water, even when a bed bath is given (see Technique No. 28, Baths, Cleansing). Rub an emollient gently on the feet each day to prevent drying and cracking.	Unclean feet can harbor micro-organisms that can invade broken areas and cause disease and illness. Warm water stimulates circulation.
3. Toenails can be a source of foot problems. Soak the foot first in a basin of warm water to soften the nails. Trim each nail carefully, straight across, and not too short. A physician's order is needed to trim the nails of a diabetic client or those with severe peripheral vascular disease. Check the institutional policy on trimming nails.	Careful trimming will help to prevent trauma and ingrown nails.
4. Advise the client to use a powder if the feet tend to perspire. Tight shoes are not only uncomfortable but predispose to ingrown toenails, corns, and poor circulation.	Properly fitting shoes are essential for good foot care.

Communicative Aspects

OBSERVATIONS

1. Watch for any cracking, breaks in the skin, and ingrown toenails. Attend to any of these conditions at once.

2. Be sure that the client's feet are flat against the footboard at all times.

3. Avoid large concentrations of linens at the foot of the bed because the weight rests heavily on the client's feet.

4. Be sure the heels and the ankle prominences are propped so that they do not lie directly against the mattress, predisposing to pressure sores.

CHARTING

DATE/TIME	OBSERVATIONS	SIGNATURE
3/8 2130	Toenails trimmed straight across after soaking in warm water for 5 min. No breaks in skin around toes or on other parts of the feet. Socks applied. Feet propped against footboard. ——————————————————	P. Dillon RN

Discharge Planning Aspects

CLIENT AND FAMILY EDUCATION

1. Explain the need for daily foot care to the client and family. Emphasize the need for the following:

   Bathe and massage feet daily.

   Inspect the feet for cuts, abrasions, scratches, and blisters.

   Lubricate feet daily with lanolin.

   Wear flat, ventilated well-fitted shoes.

   Wear socks free of lumps.

   Avoid externally warming the feet which may increase the metabolic demand beyond the level that the circulatory system can support, resulting in ischemic injury.

   Perform knee, ankle and foot exercises daily.

2. Demonstrate the proper method of cutting toenails, and encourage the client or family to follow this method at home. Extreme care must be taken to explain the special problems of a diabetic client. Because of poor healing, especially of the lower extremities, any kind of a cut or trauma on the feet is a potential crisis. Be certain the family and client understand diabetic implications for cutting toenails.

REFERRALS

For the client with compromised circulation, such as diabetic clients and those with peripheral vascular disease, a referral to a podiatrist may prevent trauma to the feet from unskilled trimming of the toenails.

Evaluation

Quality Assurance

Documentation should reflect the condition of the client's feet on admission and subsequent notations regarding the improvement or worsening of any foot condition. Procedures carried out on the feet should be reflected, as well as outcomes, and the reaction of the client. Teaching should be noted.

Infection Control

1. Clients with poor circulation have difficulty recovering from wounds and diseases of the feet. They also are predisposed to infection of the feet owing to compromised healing. Skin care of the feet is very important to prevent infection.

2. Careful handwashing should occur between the care of clients. When working with infection-prone clients, careful handwashing is especially important.

Technique Checklist

	YES	NO
Procedure explained to client	———	———
Feet soaked before foot procedures performed	———	———
Toenails cut straight across and proper length	———	———
Condition of feet noted in chart	———	———
Footboard applied to bed	———	———
Client able to keep feet flat against footboard	———	———
Proper foot care demonstrated to client and the family	———	———

57

Gastric Intubation (Decompression, Irrigation, Lavage, and Gavage)

Overview

Definition

The introdcution of a tube into the stomach for therapeutic or diagnostic purposes. Tube types are

Levin: A rubber or plastic, disposable, single-lumen tube

Salem-sump: A plastic, disposable, double-lumen tube with airway

Dobhoff: A thin, pliable, single-lumen tube of much smaller diameter (No. 8 French) than the Levin tube, with a small amount of mercury or tungsten in the end for weight

Rationale

Prevent or relieve abdominal distension.

Aid in diagnostic procedures.

Wash out the gastric system.

Instill nourishing fluid into the gastric system.

Aspirate or decompress the gastric system.

Terminology

Anorexia: Loss of appetite

Dysphagia: Difficulty swallowing

Endoscopy: Direct visual examination of certain natural openings or cavities by means of hollow, lighted instruments

Eructation: Raising of gas from the stomach (belching)

Gastric decompression (aspiration): The removal of gastric contents, foods, fluids, or gas by means of a syringe or electric suction machine

Gastric gavage: A method of artificial feeding by means of gastric intubation

Gastric lavage: The administration and siphoning back of a solution through a catheter passed into the stomach

Intermittent: Ceasing at intervals

Nares: The openings in the nose, the nostrils

Assessment

Pertinent Anatomy and Physiology

See Appendix I: *esophagus, intestine (large), intestine (small), stomach.*

Pathophysiological Concepts

1. Signs and symptoms of gastrointestinal (GI) tract disorders are often anorexia, nausea, vomiting, abdominal distension, constipation, diarrhea, decreased bowel sounds, and GI bleeding. Bleeding may be either in the vomitus or feces.

2. Pathology of the esophagus may manifest itself in dysphagia. If it is due to narrowing of the esophagus because of tumor encroachment or lesions, it may be detected by endoscopic visualization. An *esophageal diverticulum* is an outpouching of the esophageal wall caused by a weakness in the muscle layer.

3. *Esophageal varices* are dilatations of the esophageal veins and capillaries. They arise with persistent obstruction of blood flow through the portal vein, resulting in diversion of blood flow to the other venous channels, such as the gastric and esophageal veins. Esophageal veins are relatively small and inelastic and are therefore subject to rupture. The final outcome is often massive and fatal hemorrhage.

4. Total deprivation of food, or starvation, ultimately results in death. When food intake is restricted, the nutritional needs of the body are supplied by the body stores. The primary need is energy for vital functions. Muscle protein is catabolized and fat is mobilized from the adipose tissue. The initial weight loss during starvation is due to water loss. As starvation continues, weight loss slows and is mainly due to consumption of body fat. The caloric requirements of the body are reduced because the basal metabolic rate decreases and tissue served by metabolic energy is lost through protein breakdown.

Assessment of the Client

GASTRIC INTUBATION

1. Assess the knowledge and anxiety level of the client when deciding how much preparation is needed. Some persons want to know everything about anticipated treatments; for some, this will only increase the anxiety and dread. Assess past experience with gastric intubation and determine how much and when to prepare the client.

2. Assess the physical characteristics of the client. Determine if the client has ever had nasal surgery, a nasal injury, nasal polyps, or other nasal conditions that might interfere with the passage of the tube.

3. Assess the condition of the client in relation to the need for and expected results of the gastric technique. Take baseline vital signs. If the tube is being inserted to relieve gastric distension, measuring the circumference of the abdomen may give an indication of how much relief has been accomplished. If the tube is for the instillation of nourishment, assess the nutritional status of the client.

Plan

Nursing Objectives

Allay the fears and anxieties of the client.

Maintain medical asepsis.

Teach the client and family the purpose of the treatment.

Observe the signs and symptoms that might indicate displacement of the tube.

Observe and record accurately the effects and results of the procedure.

Maintain optimal client comfort and security throughout the procedure.

Observe for early signs and symptoms of complications, and take appropriate action.

Client Preparation

1. Before insertion begins, it may be helpful to show the client the tube as well as pictures or diagrams to enhance understanding of the reasons for the tube. Determine the client's readiness for this type of information. Regardless of the method used, offer the client an explanation before beginning insertion.

2. Place the tube in ice for 15 minutes before insertion or place in the refrigerator for several hours before use. Cold causes the tube to be more rigid and more easily directed during insertion.

3. When administering a nutritional formula by way of the tube, warm it to room temperature before administration to decrease excessive peristalsis and prevent regurgitation.

Equipment

Gastric intubation

Gastric tube, as ordered (adults, No. 12 to No. 16 F, depending on the size of the client)

Basin with ice, if a rubber tube is used

Disposable irrigation set

Water-soluble lubricant

Clamp

Adhesive tape (½ in)

Safety pin

Rubber band

Glass of water with straw (if permitted)

Stethoscope

Emesis basin

Wipes

Bath towel

Restraints for pediatric clients

In addition to the above, the following equipment is needed for each particular technique:

Gastric decompression

Suction apparatus capable of intermittent suction

Gastric irrigation

Solution (as ordered by physician)

Disposable irrigation set (with basin, 50-ml syringe)

Gastric lavage

Solution or antidote (as ordered by the physician or indicated by Poison Control)

Gastric gavage

Asepto or feeding syringe or formula bag

Formula pump

Formula, as ordered

Graduated cup

Water

Implementation and Interventions

Procedural Aspects

ACTION

RATIONALE

Gastric Intubation

1. Adhere to aseptic technique throughout the procedure. Use every precaution to prevent injury and infection.

   The gastric tract is lined with a delicate mucosa that can be traumatized during insertion and result in infection. Use gentleness and cleanliness to combat this possibility.

2. Pass the tube through the nasopharynx with the client in the sitting position. High Fowler's position is best, unless there are medical contraindications. Place a basin nearby in case the tube insertion stimulates vomiting. (A towel may also be placed over the client's chest). Lubricate the tip of the tube with a water-soluble jelly or water to facilitate insertion.

   Swallowing is easier and the gag reflex is decreased when the tube is passed through the nasopharynx rather than the mouth. Lubrication reduces friction between the tube and the nares and facilitates initial insertion.

3. Hyperextend the head and neck to allow the tube to fall readily into the nasopharynx. Place a pillow behind the back and shoulders to facilitate hyperextension.

   The tube should fall readily into the nasopharynx if the floor of the nasal passage is depressed.

4. Determine the approximate depth of tube to be inserted by measuring from the tip of the nose to the lower edge of the ear lobe; from the ear measure down to the lower tip of the sternum. (Fig. 57-1)

   The goal is to place the tube into the stomach but not into the esophagus or small intestine.

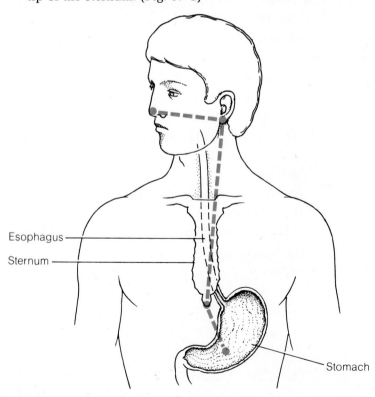

Esophagus

Sternum

Stomach

Figure 57.1

ACTION

5. Grasp the lubricated tip of the tube in one hand. With the other hand, elevate the tip of the nose to expose the nostril better. (Fig. 57-2) During insertion use the hand on the nose to anchor the tube while the other hand is being used to insert (Figs. 57-3, 57-4). Accomplish the actual passage of the tube in firm, steady progression. Ask the client to swallow as the tube is passed gently but steadily. Tell the client what is happening and how best to help with the insertion by turning of the head or swallowing. When the tube reaches the throat, offer a cup of water or ice chips to the client to aid in swallowing, if allowed. Pass the tube to the predetermined depth (Fig. 57-5).

RATIONALE

Once manipulation of the nasal passage has been accomplished, the only remaining obstacle is the gag reflex in the throat. Swallowing opens the passage and allows the tube to pass freely.

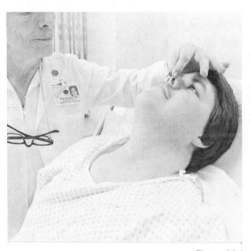

Figure 57.2

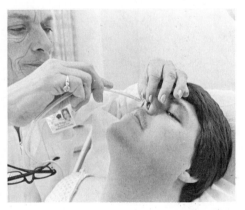

Figure 57.3

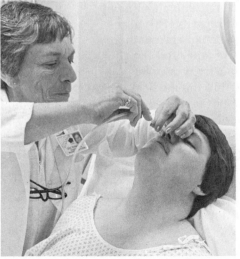

Figure 57.4

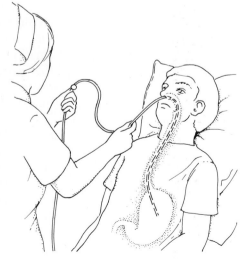

Figure 57.5

ACTION	**RATIONALE**
6. Never force the tube if an obstruction is encountered. Remove the tube and reinsert it in the other nostril if it cannot be passed through the first. If persistent obstruction or expression of severe pain occurs, cease the intubation attempt and notify the physician.	The mucous membrane of the GI tract is easily damaged and thus is a probable site for infection if injured.
7. Presence of the tube in the stomach can be verified by obtaining a small amount of gastric juice on aspiration with a syringe or by auscultation with a stethoscope over the epigastric area as air is inserted through the tube (Fig. 57-6). Attach the tube to the appropriate suction device or clamp as ordered by the physician.	Assurance of proper positioning of the tube in the stomach is essential. The stomach is never empty; it always contains a small amount of gastric juice.

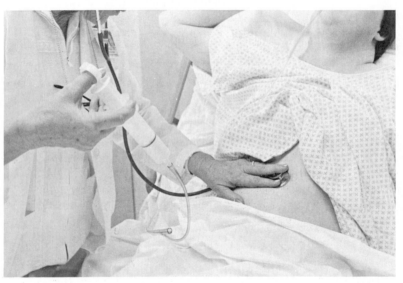

Figure 57.6

| 8. Leave the client with a feeling of comfort and security. Fasten the tube to the client's nose with a small piece of tape. Tell the client that normal activity may be resumed within the medical limitations of the physical condition only if the tube is not jerked or pulled. Frequent oral hygiene and lubrication of the lips will facilitate comfort. Return all equipment to the proper place; leave the irrigation syringe and basin at the bedside for future use. | Normal activities, such as turning or talking, will not dislodge the tube. Owing to the presence of the tube in the nose, there is a tendency for the client to breathe through the mouth, with a resulting dryness and parching of the mouth and lips. |

ACTION	**RATIONALE**

Gastric Decompression (Aspiration)

1. Gastric suction may be produced by mechanical suction. Ensure that the suction apparatus is functioning properly before attaching it to the client.

Suction will empty the contents of the stomach and relieve distension. While healing occurs in the abdominal area or when vomiting is undesirable, the stomach may be kept empty by means of suction.

2. Suction of ½ to 4 lbs/sq in may be used for gastric suction without causing injury to gastric mucosa. Usually the suction is left on the low position. The suction is intermittent; that is, it does not produce suction all of the time because this might injure the lining of the stomach.

The secretions in the stomach are usually very thin liquid if the client has not been eating solid food. It is relatively easy to withdraw these secretions from the stomach by low suction at frequent intervals.

3. Empty the suction bottle every 8 hours or as often as necessary. Evaluate the fluid intake in relation to the amount removed by the suction machine.

If the fluid removed is not replaced, electrolyte imbalance may result.

Gastric Irrigation

1. To ensure that the gastric tube remains open, remove particles and dilute secretions by instilling a liquid such as normal saline. Disconnect the tube from the suction equipment. Fill the irrigation syringe with the amount and type of solution ordered (usually 30 ml normal saline) and inject the solution slowly into the tubing. Disengage the syringe and allow the solution to drain back into a basin that is placed slightly below the level of the client's gastric area.

Gastric secretions tend to thicken as fluid is withheld by mouth. This makes it difficult for gastric content to drain easily through the nasogastric tube. Diluting the secretions with saline facilitates removal from the stomach and does not upset the chemical balance of the gastric area. The tube acts as a siphon to remove the irrigation fluid.

2. If the solution does not flow back into the syringe, gentle pressure may be applied by aspirating the syringe. This method should be used only to initiate the flow of solution. If it is necessary to remove all of the irrigation fluid by aspiration, take care to apply only gentle pressure to prevent harm to the lining of the stomach. When the instilled solution is returned, fasten the tubing again to the suction. Any amount over or under the amount instilled should be recorded as intake or output.

The nasogastric tube may lodge against the side of the stomach. Vigorous aspiration may result in trauma to the gastric lining, with resulting pain or hemorrhage. The pressure on the syringe must be gentle.

ACTION	RATIONALE
3. Some nasogastric tubes are irrigated by the insertion of air into the auxiliary tubing, the opening of which is near the opening of the drainage tube but separate from it. These tubes are fastened to continuous suction which is not usually released for irrigation (Fig. 57-7).	Insertion of a small amount of air is usually sufficient to propel the tube away from the side of the stomach to facilitate drainage. Liquid should never be injected into the auxiliary tube opening as leakage will result.

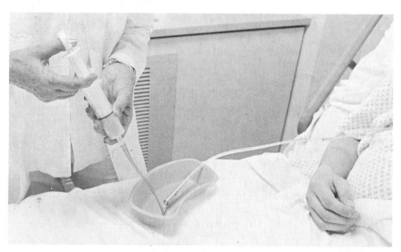

Figure 57.7

Gastric Gavage

1. A healthy nutritional state is maintained by the regular intake of a proper, balanced diet that supplies all of the needed nutrients in adequate amounts. Some clients require special formulas in special amounts, which they are unable to ingest by normal means. The gastric tube offers a means to nourish these clients. Place the client in as near normal position for eating as is possible considering the medical limitations. Raise the head of the bed if not contraindicated.	Even though the means of nourishment is not normal, preserving other outward signs of normal eating patterns helps to bolster the client's orientation and sense of self-esteem.

ACTION

RATIONALE

2. Nourishment may be administered by means of a smaller, more flexible feeding tube. The smaller tube is very pliable and has a small amount of mercury or tungsten in the tip to facilitate insertion and proper placement. Because the tube is so pliant, it usually is inserted with a stylet. After the tube is in place, an x-ray may be taken to ensure proper placement in the stomach. When placement is ensured, the stylet is removed and the tube taped in place. The stylet must be removed carefully so that the tube is not pulled out inadvertently at the same time. Peristaltic stimulation from the initial feedings will cause the tube to flow into the small intestine. Radiologic confirmation of intestinal placement is necessary. Feedings may be given intermittently or continuously with one bag following another. Continuous feeding usually is accomplished by pushing the formula into the stomach at a preset rate by means of a formula pump set at a certain rate. If the feeding will not flow into the tube, it must be checked for patency since these tubes may curl and knot up in the stomach. Irrigate the tube periodically with water or normal saline. For continuous feedings, irrigate every 6 hours; for intermittent feedings, irrigate every 3 to 4 hours.

The smaller, more flexible feeding tube is less traumatic to the gastrointestinal tract. The metal acts as a weight to keep the tube in place. If the feedings are continuous, consideration must be given to the fact that the stomach usually is not asked to digest continuously. The usual pattern in the healthy person is to eat at intervals, with the digestion process very active after a meal and tapering off to allow a rest period before the next meal. Continuous feeding means continuous digestion. Because of the small lumen of this tube, it will become clogged if not irrigated frequently.

3. Before instillation of any fluid into the tube, ascertain the proper position of the tube. Check for stomach location by aspiration of gastric content.

If the tube has become dislodged, it may have slipped into the lung. It is vital that no fluid be instilled into the lung area.

ACTION

RATIONALE

4. For bolus feeding, a 50-ml feeding syringe is filled with formula. Pour the formula slowly into the syringe, keeping it about half full as it enters the feeding tube. The higher the syringe is held, the faster the formula will flow into the stomach by gravitational pull. Slow instillation of formula is desirable (Fig. 57-8). Passage of formula through the tube is shown in Figs. 57-9 and 57-10.

Excess air entering the stomach will increase distension and discomfort. Keeping the tube partially full prevents air from entering between the portions of formula. Distension, nausea, and excessive peristalsis may be prevented by slow instillation of the formula.

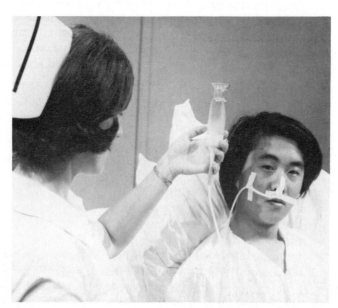

Figure 57.8

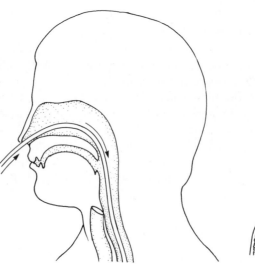

Figure 57.9

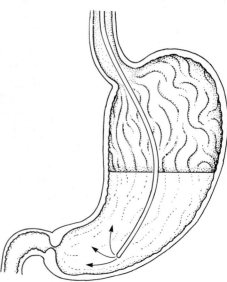

Figure 57.10

ACTION	*RATIONALE*
5. To maintain patency, flush the tube with 30 ml of water after the feeding, unless contraindicated. Remove the syringe and clamp the tube to prevent air entering or fluid leaking. Leave the client in a comfortable position. Clean and store the equipment for the next feeding.	Accumulation of the formula allowed to stand in the tube may cause a blockage of the feeding tube. Flushing leaves water in the tube to help maintain patency.

Gastric Lavage

ACTION	*RATIONALE*
1. Lavage of the stomach should be sufficient to reach all of the gastric surface. Inject lavage solution (approximately 500 ml for the adult) or the prescribe antidote through the nasogastric tube in quantities sufficient to cleanse or neutralize the stomach contents. Then aspirate or allow the lavage fluid to flow naturally (Fig. 57-11). To lavage effectively, a tube with a large lumen is required because of the size of the particles and thickness of gastric secretions. Continue lavaging the stomach until the return is consistently clear.	A large amount of solution is necessary to flatten out the rugae of the stomach so that the fluid may reach all parts of the mucous membrane. Addition of the lavage solution dilutes harmful substances, liquifies large or thick portions of matter, and facilitates removal of stomach contents.

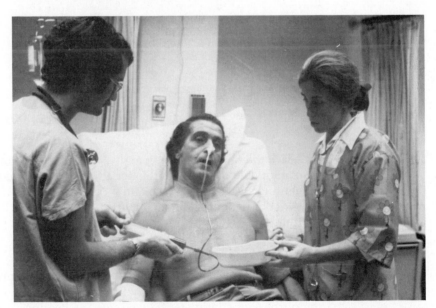

Figure 57.11

ACTION	**RATIONALE**
2. Unpleasant aftertaste may be eliminated with fluid intake or a sweet-tasting substance, if allowed. Administer oral care after gastric lavage.	Oral care will freshen the mouth and leave the client more comfortable.

Removal of the Nasogastric Tube

1. Explain to the client that the tube will be removed. Loosen the tape holding the tube in place. Don a clean glove on the hand that will pull out the tube. This is for purposes of cleanliness since the tube will be covered with secretions. Clamp or pinch the tube and withdraw it in one continuous motion (Fig. 57-12).	Clamping the tube cuts off air pressure and prevents any fluid from remaining in the tubing and entering the trachea.

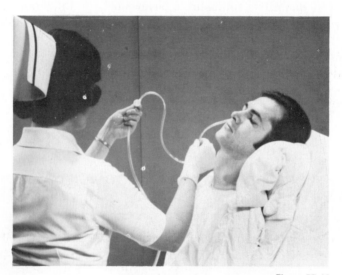

Figure 57.12

2. Leave the client in a clean and comfortable environment. Offer a cloth for washing the face and assist in removing the tape marks, if needed.	A clean environment and washing the face will contribute to a sense of well-being.

Special Modifications

A feeding tube may be inserted surgically into the jejunum directly for the purpose of administering feedings. Feedings may be continuous or intermittent. The tube is sutured in place.	Jejunostomy feedings allow the stomach to be bypassed to facilitate healing.

Communicative Aspects

OBSERVATIONS

Gastric Intubation

1. Examine drainage from the tube for color, consistency, and presence of abnormal components such as blood, or "coffee ground" material.

2. Observe the client for cyanosis, dyspnea, or coughing, any of which is an indication that the tube has entered the trachea or lung and must be removed immediately.

Gastric Decompression

1. Observe the client for nausea, vomiting, and distension, which indicate the suction is functioning improperly or inefficiently.

2. Observe for signs and symptoms of fluid and electrolyte imbalance. All signs and symptoms should be evaluated, investigated, reported, or treated with appropriate nursing measures.

3. To maintain appropriate suctioning, ascertain that the equipment is in proper working condition, check patency of the tube, and irrigate the tube properly if allowed.

4. Observe drainage for amount, character, and any abnormalities, which must be reported promptly.

5. Accurately measure and record amounts of all irrigation solution and fluid returned from the suction.

Gastric Gavage

1. Check the tube placement before beginning to be certain it is in the stomach. Aspirate a small amount of stomach contents or instill a small amount of air while auscultating the gastric area, where the air entering the stomach should be heard.

2. Observe for signs and symptoms of distension or regurgitation.

3. Observe the client's reaction to the procedure.

Gastric Lavage

1. Examine drainage from the tube for color, type, appearance, amount and the presence of the substance for which the lavage was ordered. Note any abnormalities in the stomach contents which might indicate trauma or injury, such as blood.

2. Observe the effect of the treatment on the client.

CHARTING

Gastric Intubation

DATE/TIME	OBSERVATIONS	SIGNATURE
12/3 1330	No. 16 Levin tube inserted with 120 ml clear fluid obtained. Procedure explained before insertion. No problems with insertion. States that he can feel the tube in his throat. Rinsed mouth with water. Tube secured to nose with tape and attached to wall suction, low, intermittent. ———————	P. Dillon RN

Gastric Lavage

DATE/TIME	OBSERVATIONS	SIGNATURE
5/17 1410	No. 18 Levin tube inserted without difficulty. Stomach lavaged with 1000 ml normal saline. 1500 ml greenish brown fluid returned. Tube removed. Appears calm and relaxed. States that he feels much better, less nausea. Given mouthwash. ———————	P. Dillon RN

Discharge Planning Aspects

CLIENT AND FAMILY EDUCATION

Gastric Intubation and Decompression

1. Explain the reason for and the expected results of the gastric intubation to the client and family.

2. Explain to the client that frequent position change will help to prevent irritation to the lining of the stomach. Talking and moving about in bed will have no effect on the tube. If allowed, the client may sit up and ambulate to the extent allowed by physical condition. Emphasize the importance of not pulling or jerking the tube.

Gastric Gavage

1. Explain to the client and family how the feeding will be done and why. Emphasize that the caloric needs of the client are being met even though no food is being taken orally.

2. If the client is to go home with a feeding tube, teach the family member responsible for feedings how to perform gastric gavage safely and properly. Stress the methods of assuring that the tube is in the stomach before proceeding with the feeding. Be sure the family knows how much and when to feed, recognizes complications, and knows how and when to change the tube.

3. *Referrals:* If gavage feeding is to be performed on a long-term basis and will be done by the family after discharge, follow-up visits by a visiting nurse may help allay the family's apprehension. The transition process from hospital to home may be enhanced by ensuring that the visiting nurse will assist with evaluating the client's nutritional status, changing the tube, and answering any questions that the family might have.

Gastric Lavage

1. If lavage is to remove poison from the stomach, explain the procedure to the family and client if time allows.

2. If lavage is for diagnostic study, explain the procedure and purpose before beginning. Relate the study to the symptoms presented by the client.

3. If lavage is for surgical preparation, be sure the client understands why it is necessary. Anxiety is common before surgery, and gastric intubation will increase that anxiety unless the client fully understands why it is necessary and how it is in the best interests of a quick return to health.

4. *Referrals:* If the lavage procedure was for the purpose of removal of a harmful substance, advise the family of the nearest poison control center and how to use those services, if appropriate. Without being judgmental, emphasize how knowledge of the poison control center can save lives.

Evaluation

Quality Assurance

1. The purpose of the procedure should be reflected clearly, and the outcomes should be related to the reason for the procedure. Intake and output (I&O) records should accurately reflect the amounts of irrigation or feeding instilled, or the amounts removed from the stomach. Clear descriptions of the return from the tube should be in evidence.

2. Explanations and education efforts for the family and client should be described in the record. Questions about the procedure should be reflected, as well as responses.

3. The reaction of the client to the procedure should be reflected. Any complications should be noted as well as efforts to relieve or resolve them. Any signs and symptoms exhibited by the client should be noted. All information passed on to the physician in relation to the procedure should be reflected in the chart.

Infection Control

1. The GI tract is not a sterile passageway. The natural enzymes and acids in the stomach and esophagus are usually sufficient to kill any problem micro-organisms. The lining of the GI tract is delicate, however, and insertion of the tube may traumatize the lining and allow an entrance for pathogens into the system. For this reason, it is essential to insert the tube gently and to avoid using force if resistence is met during insertion.

2. Careful handwashing is essential before and after insertion and irrigation of the nasogastric tube, and before and after administration of tube feedings.

3. The nasogastric tube should be changed periodically to prevent growth of pathogenic organisms on and around the tube itself. Refer to hospital policy about changing feeding tubes or the specific request of the physician involved.

Technique Checklist

	YES	NO
Gastric intubation		
Procedure explained to client	_____	_____
Tubing measured before insertion	_____	_____
Tube placement assessed by		
Aspiration of stomach contents	_____	_____
Auscultation of air inserted into the stomach through the tube	_____	_____
X-ray taken	_____	_____
Gastric decompression		
Tubing attached to suction	_____	_____
Gastric content measured every _____ hours		
Description of gastric content made each shift	_____	_____
Symptoms which prompted insertion of tube relieved and noted on chart	_____	_____
Tube removed without complication	_____	_____
Gastric gavage		
Procedure explained to client	_____	_____
Placement of tube checked before every feeding	_____	_____
Amount of each feeding recorded	_____	_____
Client reaction to each feeding recorded	_____	_____
Demonstration and education of client's family for caring for tube at home	_____	_____
Family educated about method of tube feeding, amount and possible complications when performing gastric gavage at home	_____	_____
Gastric lavage		
Procedure explained to client or family	_____	_____
Poison or harmful substance successfully removed from stomach	_____	_____
Trauma or injury to GI mucosa from poison or harmful substance	_____	_____
Stomach successfully cleansed in preparation for	_____	_____
Diagnostic study _____		
Surgery _____		

58

Gown and Glove Procedure, Sterile

Overview

Definition

Maintenance of a sterile environment by donning gown and gloves in such a manner as to cover nonsterile areas without contaminating the outside of the gown or gloves

Rationale

Maintain sterile environment.
Protect the client from contamination.
Minimize risk of infection.

Assessment

Pertinent Anatomy and Physiology

1. See Appendix I: *skin.*
2. Hair is considered an appendage to the skin. With certain exceptions, such as the palms, and soles of the feet, hair is present over most of the body surface.
3. The human body normally lives in harmony with a variety of bacteria in the mouth and pharynx, in the intestines, and on the skin.

Pathophysiological Concepts

When the integrity of the skin is broken, which happens in the case of a surgical incision, bacteria have a direct route to the internal tissues of the body. To prevent the spread of infection, a sterile field is produced and maintained during surgery.

Plan

Nursing Objectives

Don gown and gloves in such a manner as to ensure sterility.
Maintain sterility throughout the procedure.

Equipment

Sterile gown
Sterile gloves
Powder (optional)
Equipment pertinent to the procedure

Implementation and Interventions

Procedural Aspects

ACTION	RATIONALE
1. Thorough handwashing must precede donning gown or gloves. Preoperatively, a surgical scrub is done according to individual hospital policy.	Any sterile procedure depends upon the absence or reduction of microorganisms.

ACTION

2. *Sterile gown procedure:* Dry the hands with a sterile towel held away from the body and discard it after use (Fig. 58-1). Gowns are packaged inside out, therefore grasp the inside of the gown at the neck and let it tumble open while holding it away from the body (Fig. 58-2). Slip hands into armholes, touching *only* the inside of the gown (Fig. 58-3). Someone else will reach inside the sleeves and pull them on until the end of the sleeve continues to extend just past the end of the fingertips, still covering all of the skin of the hand. The second person ties the gown at the neck and waist from behind, being careful not to touch the front of the sterile gown. The closed glove procedure may now be done. If someone in sterile attire is available to assist with gloving by holding the gloves outstretched, the nurse may pull the gown sleeves over the hands and plunge each hand into the sterile gloves without touching the outer surface or the person holding the gloves.

RATIONALE

The front of the gown is considered sterile. Sterile objects become contaminated when touched by unsterile objects.

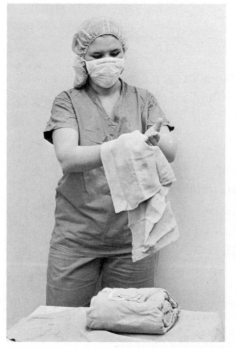

Figure 58.1

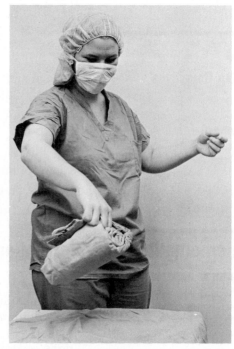

Figure 58.2

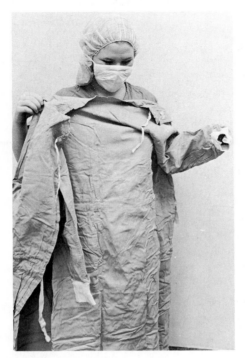

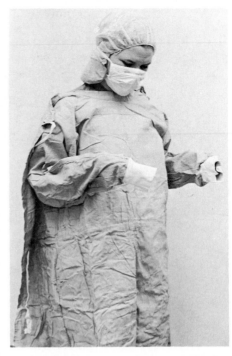

Figure 58.3

Figure 58.4

ACTION

3. *Closed-glove procedure:* Open the package of gloves with sterile forceps and leave them open on a sterile towel. Don the sterile gown and with hands extended only as far as the cuff seam, but not through the end of the cuff (Fig. 58-4), grasp one glove through the gown sleeve and place it thumb-side down on the palm side of the other arm. Position so the opening is toward the cuff end of the sleeve (Fig. 58-5). Grasp the edge of the glove cuff next to the wrist with the fingers of the hand to be gloved. Grasp the upper edge of the glove cuff with the still-covered free hand and pull over the fingers and hand being gloved (Fig. 58-6). Pull the sleeve on to place the cuff in the proper position at the wrist, automatically drawing the glove onto the hand. Apply the second glove in the same manner, using the gloved hand to assist (Fig. 58-7).

RATIONALE

To maintain sterility, the sterile surfaces must come in contact with only those objects and surfaces which are also sterile.

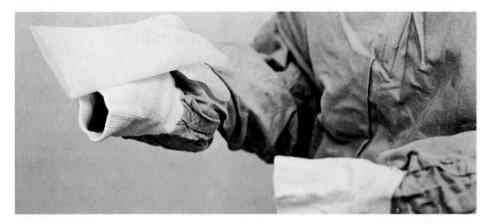

Figure 58.5

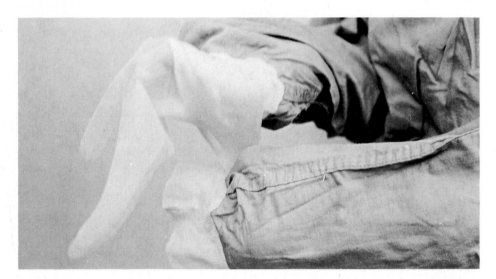

Figure 58.6

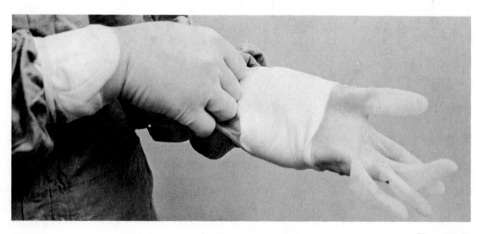

Figure 58.7

ACTION

4. *Open glove procedure:* Open the gloves (which must be cuffed). With one hand, grasp the cuff of the opposite glove and slip the fingers of the opposite hand inside the glove (Fig. 58-8). Pull the glove on by holding onto the cuff. Be careful not to contaminate the outside of the glove; leave the glove cuffed. Slip the gloved fingers under the cuff of the other glove and insert the ungloved fingers inside (Figs. 58-9, 58-10). Pull the second glove on, leaving the cuff turned (Fig. 58-11). The areas inside the folded cuffs is considered sterile (Fig. 58-12).

RATIONALE

The open glove method is used when a sterile gown is not worn, and sterility is being maintained chiefly for the hands, such as in a catheterization or dressing change procedure. Sterility is maintained as long as the bare hands touch *only* the inside of the gloves, which will be against the surface of the skin anyway when the glove is on the hand. The area under the cuff is sterile, so that the gloved hand is not contaminated when it reaches under the cuff to pull on the second glove.

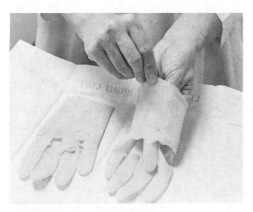

Figure 58.8

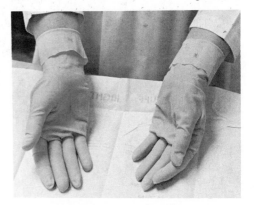

Figure 58.9

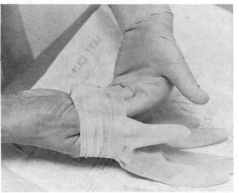

Figure 58.10

Figure 58.12

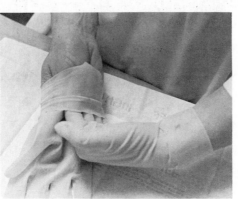
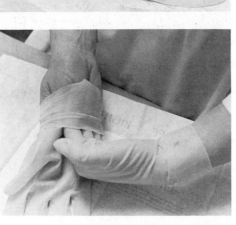

Figure 58.11

ACTION	*RATIONALE*
5. On completion of the procedure, be careful to keep the gloved hands in the sterile field.	The area from the waist up and to the front is sterile, as are the arms in the closed-glove method. In the open method, the gloved hands are sterile.

Communicative Aspects

OBSERVATIONS

1. Observe for breaks in sterile technique during gown and glove application.
2. Observe for tears or rips in the gloves and gowns. Observe also for any wetness soaking through or into the gown because this is considered a break in the sterile field.

Discharge Planning Aspects

CLIENT AND FAMILY EDUCATION

If the client will undergo procedures at home that require sterile glove procedure (e.g., catheterization), teach the family member who will perform this procedure how to don gloves and keep the field sterile. Explain what the sterile field is and why it is important in the particular procedure.

Evaluation

Quality Assurance

Maintenance of sterile technique is essential. Quality control methods must be developed for each institution. Breaks in sterile procedure must be considered very serious. Regularly scheduled in-service programs on proper technique and maintenance of sterile conditions should be a part of every hospital's teaching program.

Infection Control

The reason for this procedure is the prevention of infection by inadvertent transmission of microorganisms. Handwashing before donning sterile gloves reduces the number of pathogens in the field. Strict adherence to procedure is necessary to prevent accidental contamination of the sterile field. Most hospital-acquired infections are preventable.

Technique Checklist

	YES	NO
Sterile technique maintained	_____	_____
Gown on without contamination	_____	_____
Gloves applied by		
Open glove method _____		
Closed-glove method _____		

59 Hair, Daily Care and Shampoo

Overview

Definition

The daily care or cleansing of the client's hair and scalp

Rationale

Promote mental and physical comfort.

Maintain cleanliness of hair and scalp.

Prevent tangling and matting of hair from prolonged bed rest.

Increase circulation of the scalp.

Terminology

Baldness: Lack of hair on the head

Dandruff: A scaly material from or on the scalp, also called *seborrheic dermatitis*

Hair follicle: A pouchlike depression in the skin in which a hair develops from the matrix at its base and grows to emerge from its opening on the body surface

Hair shaft: The visible portion of the hair

Seborrheic dermatitis: A chronic disease that causes crusting or scaling spots on the scalp

Assessment

Pertinent Anatomy and Physiology

1. See Appendix I: *skin*.
2. Hair is formed by well-nourished germinal cells in the deepest part of the follicle. As these cells divide, the daughter cells are pushed upward, getting farther and farther away from their source of nourishment. Eventually all the cells die and become keratinized.
3. A hair usually consists of a central core, a medulla, surrounded by a cortex. Hair color depends on the quality and quantity of pigment (melanin) in the cortex. White hair has no pigment, but when mixed with pigmented hair, the result is gray hair.
4. The root of the hair is that part embedded in the follicle (usually slanting from the perpendicular), whereas the shaft projects above the surface of the skin. Two or more sebaceous glands are associated with each follicle. Each hair follicle goes through a growth cycle that includes three phases: anagen hair, catagen hair (the intermediate phase), and telogen hair (the involutional stage). The anagen stage on the scalp lasts about 3 years, whereas the telogen stage lasts only about 3 months. Once the hair follicle regenerates into the anagen stage, a new hair is produced. The process stops when the person becomes permanently bald. Protein shampoos affect only dead keratin and the hair follicle and therefore cannot prevent hair loss.
5. Hair loss is constant throughout life. The individual hair is replaced by the continued division of epidermal cells in the germinal area. Cutting or shaving hair has no effect on its growth; the maximal rate of growth is about 10 millimeters per month.

Pathophysiological Concepts	1. Seborrheic dermatitis commonly involves the scalp, eyebrows, ears, and anterior chest. The cause is unknown, but genetic factors are believed to be involved.
	2. Sebaceous glands secrete an oily substance called *sebum*. These glands are very numerous on the scalp. During adolescence, the glandular activity accelerates, and oily hair may occur.
	3. Certain therapeutic modalities affect the hair. Some antibiotics change the texture of the hair and may cause hair loss. Chemotherapy often causes loss of some or all of the hair. Hair generally returns after the chemotherapy has ended, however. Hypothyroidism may cause patchy hair loss or thinning of the hair.
	4. Nutrients are carried by the bloodstream to the scalp where they are picked up by the roots of the hair. Protein is important to healthy hair. Protein deficiency can cause dullness and may result in periods of slow growth.
	5. The aging process also affects the hair. Scalp hair may become thinner and grow more slowly. Baldness in both men and women may occur, although it is more prevalent in men and may occur at younger ages. Lack of nutrients because of diminished circulation may result in dullness and loss of color.
Assessment of the Client	1. Assess problems with the scalp such as dandruff, itching, hair fallout. Assess for scalp lesions, tumors, rashes, and other conditions that might alter the method of caring for the hair.
	2. Identify nits (eggs of lice) if present, differentiating them from dandruff. (See Technique No. 71, Pediculosis, Nursing Care)
	3. Assess the presence of any nutritional or hormonal problems that might attribute to scalp or hair loss. Observe the condition of the hair and scalp to assess condition.
	4. Assess how often the client shampoos at home and what type of shampoo is used.

Plan

Nursing Objectives	Maintain a healthy atmosphere through cleanliness.
	Promote a feeling of well-being through the cosmetic effects of hair care.
	Maintain adequate circulation to the scalp and hair follicles.
	Eliminate infestation and prevent the spread of pediculosis to others.
Client Preparation	1. Many people do not understand how hair can be shampooed while a person is flat in bed. Offer adequate explanation before initiating this technique to help the client understand and be more cooperative.
	2. To avoid chilling the client, protect against drafts. Replace the top covers with a bath blanket and tuck a towel around the client's neck and shoulders.

Equipment

Daily care
  Comb and brush
  Towel
Shampoo
  Shampoo basin
  Dryer
  Three bath towels and a small pad to protect the bed
  Two wash cloths
  Plastic sheet or apron
  Shampoo
  Wash basin (two or three)
  Pitcher
  Cup

Implementation and Interventions

Procedural Aspects

ACTION	RATIONALE
Daily Care	
1. Hair should be brushed daily. Encourage the client to comb or brush the hair thoroughly during morning care activities and throughout the day as needed. Assemble all necessary equipment on the bedside table within the client's reach.	Daily brushing aids in cleanliness, distribution of oil, and stimulation of circulation in the scalp. Self-esteem is enhanced if the client can provide self-care. The brushing action also encourages range-of-motion movement of hands and arms.
2. Provide hair care for the client who cannot comb, brush, or arrange hair. If assistance is needed, provide it in a way that recognizes the client's autonomy.	The client should feel as though some decisions about care have been retained, such as when the hair care occurs or how to style the hair.
3. Place a towel over the pillow and bath blanket over the client to prevent soiling the bed linens and to ensure that the client does not become chilled.	Protect the client from additional health problems related to the hospital stay.
4. Turn the client's head away from the nurse.	Hair can be brushed and combed more easily from the back.
5. Divide the hair into smaller sections and brush or comb each section starting near the scalp using an upward motion. Any comb used should have dull teeth.	Hair can be brushed and combed more easily from the back. The upward brushing motion will not split the shaft of the hair and is not aggravating to the scalp. Dull teeth on the comb will prevent scratching the scalp.

ACTION

RATIONALE

6. When brushing or combing long or tangled hair, keep the hair between fingers and brush or comb outward from the fingers (Fig. 59-1). If the hair is severely tangled or matted with blood or debris, cream rinse may be applied before combing. Hydrogen peroxide may be used to remove blood from hair and facilitate combing.

Anchoring the hair creates a counter-force to prevent undue pulling of the scalp. Application of substances to dissolve blood or remove tangles promotes the comfort of the client.

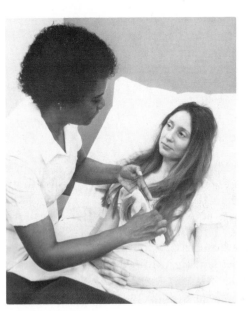

Figure 59.1

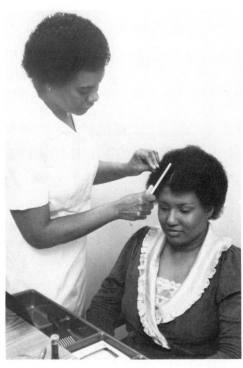

Figure 59.2

7. When providing hair care for persons with coarse or curly hair, use a wide-toothed comb. Comb small sections to remove tangles (Fig. 59-2). Apply small amounts of oil to dry or flaking areas of the scalp.

Coarse and curly hair become tangled more easily owing to the texture of the hair. Combing small sections provides comfort and ensures that the entire scalp will be reached.

8. When one side of the hair is finished, repeat the action on the other side. Arrange the hair in an attractive manner and remove the towel.

Enhance the client's self-esteem by attention to a pleasing personal appearance.

Shampooing the Hair

1. Place the client in a comfortable position. A pillow can be placed under the client's shoulders.

A properly positioned pillow will elevate and hyperextend the neck, allowing easier access to the scalp area while maintaining the client's comfort.

ACTION	*RATIONALE*
2. Place a plastic sheet between two towels. Slide this padding under the client's head. Place another pad on the edge of the shampoo basin.	Plastic will protect the bed linen but is hot and uncomfortable next to the client's skin; therefore, the plastic is padded to protect the client's skin and to prevent it from sliding once under the client. Padding on the shampoo basin promotes the comfort of the client.
3. Some shampoo basins have an open spout on one side. Place the shampoo basin under the client's head with the spout off the edge of the bed. Directly under the spout, at a lower level, place a wash basin to catch the water used to shampoo and rinse the client's hair (Fig. 59-3). Place a rolled bath towel under the client's neck.	The water flows by gravitational pull downward into the basin. The rolled bath towel is for the client's comfort and to absorb moisture.
4. Brush the hair and thoroughly wet it with warm (105° F) water (Fig. 59-4).	Brushing removes tangles. Water temperature above 105° F can injure the scalp.

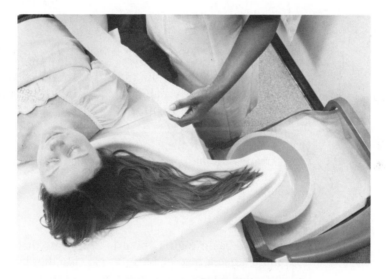

Figure 59.3

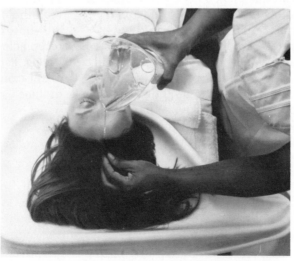

Figure 59.4

ACTION	*RATIONALE*
5. Apply shampoo and lather the hair well (Fig. 59-5). After a short rinse, shampoo the hair again. Rinse thoroughly after the second shampoo (Fig. 59-6). Work quickly so the client will not tire.	Shampoo left on the hair may cause itching and discomfort. The position of hyperextension of the neck is not normal alignment and cannot be tolerated for extended periods.

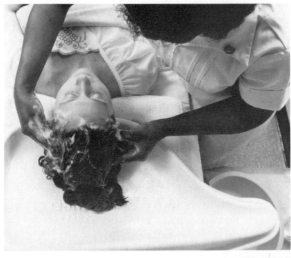

Figure 59.5

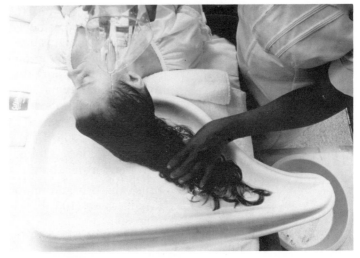

Figure 59.6

6. Test for cleanly rinsed hair by pulling a strand between the index finger and the thumb. Anchor the strand next to the scalp with the other hand before pulling.	Clean hair produces a squeaking sound. Anchoring will prevent hurting the client when the hair is pulled.
7. Dry the client's hair, neck, and ears. Arrange the hair in an attractive manner. Remove the towels and make the client comfortable.	Attention to personal appearance is an important aspect in preserving self-image.

Special Modifications

1. If a shampoo basin with a spout is unavailable, use a regular basin. Pad the client's head sufficiently to allow the water for wetting and rinsing the hair to run into the basin. Be sure that enough pillows are used to promote the client's comfort. Tuck a piece of plastic under the basin and allow it to fall over the side of the bed and into a wash basin to catch the water. Pad the side of the basin under the client's head slightly to tilt it toward the receptacle being used to catch the water. Wash and rinse the client's hair as described previously.	Using the principles of gravity, assemble the drainage system for the water so that each section is slightly lower than the previous one. The water then will flow down the plastic into the receptacle without wetting the bed linens. Padding is the key both to client comfort and to a satsifactory drainage system.

ACTION	**RATIONALE**
2. For clients with curly or coarse hair, apply a cream rinse before combing after a shampoo. Comb small sections with a wide-toothed comb.	Coarse and curly hair can be very delicate and cannot withstand pulling and straining to remove tangles. The cream rinse helps to remove the tangles and facilitates combing.
3. If the client has an oily scalp, more frequent shampoos will be necessary to promote comfort and cleanliness. The client with a dry scalp cannot tolerate harsh shampoos and frequent shampooing.	The sebaceous glands of some persons secrete more oil than others and soap (shampoo) emulsifies the oil so that it can be removed. Frequent washing increases dryness unless special shampoos, such as those rich in lanolin, are used.

Communicative Aspects

OBSERVATIONS

1. Observe the client's reaction to and tolerance of the process.
2. Lesions and tumors of the scalp should be noted.
3. Note the quantity of hair, distribution, pattern of loss, if any, and texture.

CHARTING

DATE/TIME	OBSERVATIONS	SIGNATURE
5/1 1030	Shampoo given in bed. Small reddened scalp abrasion noted in left temporal area. Dr. D. notified. Tolerated the procedure well; states she feels very refreshed.	G. Ivers RN

Discharge Planning Aspects

CLIENT AND FAMILY EDUCATION

1. Offer an explanation of the physiology of the hair to the client and family. Emphasize the importance of nutrition in hair growth and maintenance. Explain that the visible portion of the hair, the shaft, is supplied with nutrients (food) through the roots anchored in the scalp. The supply of nutrients is very important to the health of the hair. Poor diet deprives the hair, as well as the rest of the body, of needed nutrients.

2. Teach the client's family the objective of brushing and combing the hair: stimulating the circulation of the scalp, cleansing the hair shaft of dirt particles and dead cells, and bringing nutrients to the roots.

Evaluation

Quality Assurance

Document abraded or broken areas of the scalp. Any evidence of nits or pediculi should be recorded and reported so that immediate treatment can be accomplished. Note the client's tolerance of the procedure.

Infection Control

1. Great care must be taken during shampooing that the scalp is not injured from long fingernails or rings. Once the integrity of the skin on the scalp has been compromised, infection is possible.

2. Utensils for hair care, such as combs and brushes, should be used exclusively for one client. Items of hair care should not be shared because this is an excellent means of spreading infection and scalp conditions, such as pediculosis. Utensils that are designed for multiclient use, such as the shampoo basin, must be cleaned and disinfected thoroughly after each use.

3. Scrupulous handwashing is essential after caring for the client's hair.

Technique Checklist

	YES	NO
Procedure explained to client	_____	_____
Client and family understand the importance of nutrition to healthy hair	_____	_____
Client and family understand the technique for hair care at home	_____	_____
Daily care		
Hair brushed/combed daily	_____	_____
By client _____		
By family _____		
By nurse _____		
Client seemed pleased with styling and appearance	_____	_____
Shampoo		
Client positioned properly in bed with padding under head	_____	_____
Water temperature 105° F	_____	_____
Hair shampooed and rinsed twice	_____	_____
Head, hair, ears, and neck dried thoroughly	_____	_____
Hair styled	_____	_____

60 Handwashing

Overview

Definition
Mechanical removal of micropathogenic and macropathogenic organisms from the skin

Rationale
Provide a defense against the direct or indirect spread of microorganisms from one person to another.

Prevent self-contamination or alteration of resident flora.

Terminology
Asepsis: Absence of pathogenic microorganisms

Clean: Free from all discernible soil or dirt, sanitary

Contamination: In medical asepsis, contact with an object containing living organisms from someone other than the person handling the object

Detergent: Cleansing agent

Infection: Growth of pathogenic microorganisms, giving rise to signs and symptoms of disease

Medical asepsis: Efforts to prevent the transfer of pathogenic organisms from one person to another

Microorganisms: A microscopic living body that may or may not be capable of producing disease

Pathogenic microorganisms: Microbes capable of producing disease

Sterile: Free from living germs and microorganisms

Surgical asepsis: An attempt to render every object that comes in direct or indirect contact with a target area absolutely free from all microorganisms, sterile

Assessment

Pertinent Anatomy and Physiology

1. See Appendix I: *skin.*
2. Normal skin on the fingers and palms contains ridges and grooves. The ridges develop during the third and fourth months of fetal life. The unchanging pattern formed by these ridges is peculiar to each person; thus fingerprints are excellent means of identification. Normal flora on the fingers and hands may become pathogenic when introduced to a susceptible host.
3. The root of the nail is the part that is hidden in the nail groove. The part that shows is called the body. The white, crescent-shaped area in the body near the root of the nail is called the lanula. It may be slightly or completely overlapped by the cuticle, or eponychium. The rest of the nail appears pink due to the presence of underlying capillaries.

Pathophysiological Concepts	Every person has resident flora, microorganisms, that normally inhabit the body. These flora exist in a state of equilibrium with the body and normally do not cause disease. In altered physiologic states or introduced into different systems, however, these flora may cause disease. For example, *Escherichia coli* normally inhabits the bowel and rectum. However, *E. coli* in the blood is a serious abnormality that may lead to septic shock.
Assessment of the Client	1. Assess the need to wash hands. Hands should be washed before and after a procedure that involves direct or indirect contact with a client, after contact with any wastes or contaminated materials, before handling any food or food receptacle, or at any other time hands become soiled.
	2. Inspect the knuckles and under the nails where bacteria and germs may be harbored in the folds of the skin.
	3. Assess the condition of the hands. Eczema and dermatitis may follow frequent handwashing if a proper lotion is not used periodically to restore natural oils.

Plan

Nursing Objectives	Decontaminate or prevent contamination by the hands.
	Remove a maximum number of possible pathogenic organisms present on the skin.
	Prevent or reduce the incidence of cross-infection.
	Teach personnel, the client, and the client's family good personal hygiene.
	Maintain proper texture and integrity of the skin on the hands.
Client Preparation	1. Explain to the client when and how to accomplish thorough handwashing properly.
	2. Encourage frequent and effective handwashing as part of the client's hygiene before eating and after any activity in which the hands must come in contact with external genitalia, the anal region, body discharges, and known dirty areas (e.g., as the floor).
Equipment	Soap
	Running water
	Paper towels
	Lotion
	Orange stick or nail file
	Receptacle for soiled towels

Implementation and Interventions

Procedural Aspects

ACTION	RATIONALE
1. Remove all jewelry.	Bacteria may become lodged within any jewelry.
2. Stand in front of the sink with knees slightly bent. The soap and water controls should be within easy reach.	Adherence to proper body mechanics eases the strain on the back and leg muscles.
3. Water should be lukewarm	Warm water removes less protective oil from the skin than either hot or cold water, which tend to dry the skin.

ACTION   **RATIONALE**

4. Wet hands with water before   Application of soap to a wet skin sur-
using soap. Hold hands lower   face, followed by friction, produces an
than elbows (Fig. 60-1).   optimal amount of suds. Water drain-
                                      ing from the wrists to the finger tips
                                      carries bacteria from the skin into the
                                      sink.

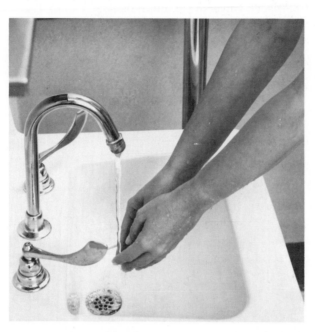

Figure 60.1

5. Use detergents that do not change   Normal skin acidity is a factor in con-
the pH of the skin (Fig. 60-2).   trolling bacterial growth and in pre-
                                       venting irritation.

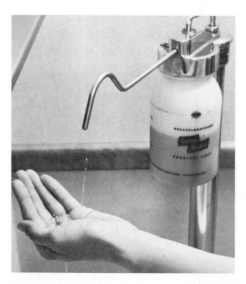

Figure 60.2

6. Interlace the fingers and thumbs   The interdigital areas are cleansed.
of both hands and move them   Micoorganism count is lower on the
back and forth.   smooth surfaces and higher in the
                                       folds and under the fingernails.

ACTION

RATIONALE

7. Wash the hands well for 30 seconds, using a rotary motion. Ten friction motions should be applied to each of the following: the palmar and dorsal aspects of the hands and fingers and the interlaced fingers (Fig. 60-3, 60-4, 60-5).

Friction aids in mechanical removal of bacteria and has been found to be more important in the removal of microorganisms than the type of detergent used.

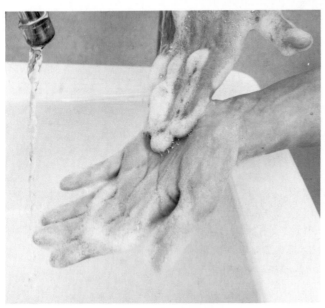

Figure 60.3

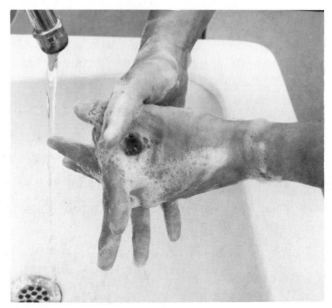

Figure 60.4

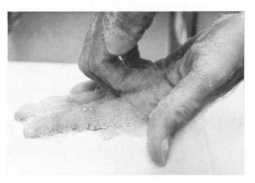

Figure 60.5

8. Rinse hands and wrists under running water allowing the water to flow from the elbows to the finger tips (Fig. 60-6).

Surface bacteria will run into the sink rather than up the forearm. Water aids in the removal of organisms.

9. Clean the fingernails with an orange stick or nail file (Fig. 60-7).

Clean, well-trimmed nails are essential to minimizing the opportunity for bacteria to accumulate and grow under the nails.

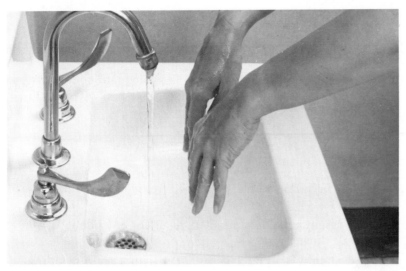

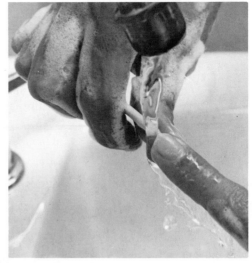

Figure 60.6

Figure 60.7

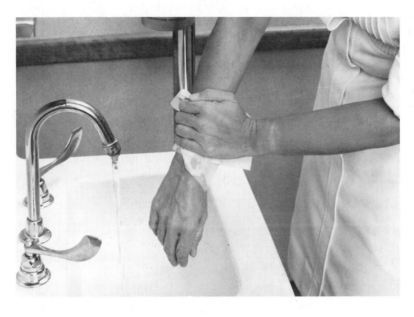

Figure 60.8

ACTION

10. Dry hands from the fingers toward the forearm with a clean paper towel (Fig. 60-8). Because the faucet handles are considered contaminated, turn them off with a paper towel.

11. Apply lotion, unless the handwashing was done in preparation for opening sterile packages or gloving (see Technique No. 58, Gowning and Gloving).

12. Return equipment to the proper area and dry all surfaces.

RATIONALE

Dry from the clean area toward the dirty. Prevent recontamination by contact with unclean surfaces.

Frequent handwashing destroys the natural oils and causes drying and cracking of the skin. If skin surface is kept intact, bacterial invasion and possible secondary infection may be prevented. If sterile packages are to be opened, the lotion should be applied after the procedure is finished.

Bacteria thrive on moisture.

Communicative Aspects

OBSERVATIONS

1. Note the condition of the client's or the nurse's hands. Note dryness or wrinkling that might indicate the need for moisturizing with lotions.
2. Note the technique of handwashing. If technique is inadequate, reminders, in the form of client education efforts or staff teaching programs, will help to reinforce proper technique.

Discharge Planning Aspects

CLIENT, FAMILY, AND HOSPITAL PERSONNEL EDUCATION

1. Handwashing is a must for all personnel on arrival to the unit and before leaving.
2. Handwashing is most essential before and after caring for any client as well as at indicated intervals during care.
3. Health care personnel should wear no jewelry, other than a plain wedding band with no jewels, and a watch since bacteria can become lodged in the crevices. The watch should have a stretch band that will allow it to be pushed up on the arm during handwashing and other procedures.
4. Teach the family and other personnel about manicuring and cleaning the fingernails. These tasks should be done before working hours as a part of daily hygiene. Manicuring also prevents hangnails and skin abrasions.
5. Stress the importance of keeping skin irritations to a minimum. When frequent handwashing is indicated, a change of assignment of health care personnel may be indicated if the irritation becomes severe. Skin irritation may also predispose to secondary infection. Plastic gloves may help to protect open skin areas from becoming infected.

Evaluation

Quality Assurance

A procedure regarding how and when to wash hands should be an important part of every hospital procedure book. A yearly in-service program is the minimal interval for education programs to remind personnel about the importance of proper handwashing technique.

Infection Control

1. A disease-producing bacteria generally found on the skin that plagues hospital and health agencies is staphylococcus (staph). When this bacteria gets into the body through a break in the skin, it causes local infection and can affect the entire body if it enters the bloodstream. Handwashing is an excellent way to minimize the risk of staph infection.
2. Pseudomonas aeruginosa is a pathogenic microorganism found in the diarrhea of infants, drainage from wounds, otitis media, and other conditions. Personnel must clean their hands well between these clients.
3. *Escherichia coli* is an organism commonly found in the alimentary tract and in the stool. Hands must be scrupulously washed after handling the bedpan, or after toileting or perineal care.

Technique Checklist

	YES	NO
Warm water and soap used	_____	_____
Mechanical friction used	_____	_____
Interlacing fingers technique used	_____	_____
Fingernails cleaned	_____	_____
Paper towels used to turn handles of faucets	_____	_____
Rinse from elbows downward	_____	_____
Hands dried from fingertips toward upper arms	_____	_____

61 Hot and Cold Applications

Overview

Definition

Physical agents applied to an area of the client's body, which bring about a change in tissue temperature, locally or systemically, for a therapeutic purpose. Reactions to heat and cold are modified by mode and duration of application, degree of heat and cold applied, condition of the tissue, and amount of body surface covered by the application. Types of applications include:

DRY APPLICATIONS

Aquamatic (K-matic) pad: A rubber pad of tubular construction that can be filled with distilled water. An electrical control unit heats the water and keeps it at an even temperature. The temperature is set by using a plastic key. This pad permits the maintenance of a constant temperature at the level prescribed by the physician; therefore, it is both safer and more effective than a hot water bottle or electric heating pad.

Frozen bag: A rubberized or plasticized flat bag containing a chemcal substance that is frozen and used as a cold, dry application to the body surface. It must be covered with a protective covering before application.

Heat cradle: A metal cradle in which several electrical sockets are installed for luminous bulbs; a means of providing radiant heat.

Heat lamp: A gooseneck lamp containing a 60-watt bulb, applied 18 in to 24 in from the body site. The heat lamp provides dry-heat radiation.

Ice bag or collar: A rubber or plastic device filled with ice chips and covered with a protective fabric before application to the client's body site. Vasoconstriction of peripheral vessels is caused by cold application. (See Terminology for temperature ranges.)

Ice glove: A rubber glove filled with ice chips, placed in a light covering, and applied to a body surface. It is usually used in a postoperative oral surgery client and for relief of discomfort of the perineum after childbirth.

MOIST APPLICATIONS

Alcohol or cold sponge baths: A means by which reduction of body temperature occurs from evaporation. Cool water or a combination of cool water and alcohol is applied to the skin.

Compresses: Compresses may be either moist (gauze) dressings or washcloths. A compress usually is applied to smaller body areas and must be changed frequently. Compresses may be either hot or cold, sterile or unsterile, as designated by the physician.

1. Hot compresses use the principle of heat conduction and can be sterile or unsterile moist applications. Generally, gauze is soaked in the solution designated by the physician. The excess fluid is wrung out of the gauze to be applied. Sterile precautions are indicated when the compress is to be applied to an open wound or to an organ, such as the eye, to prevent the entrance of microorganisms. An insulating, waterproof cloth is placed over the compress to aid in heat retention. Hot compresses hasten the suppurative process and improve circulation.

2. Cold or ice compresses are usually made of gauze or washcloths. The application of cold to open wounds or to lesions that may rupture requires sterile technique. Cold diminishes the formation and absorption of bacterial toxins. It also causes vasoconstriction, decreased tissue metabolism, and sensory anesthesia. It is used for contusions, sprains, strains, and for controlling hemorrhages. Cold compresses also may be used for an injured eye, headache, tooth extraction, or hemorrhoids. The material used for application is immersed in a basin (clean or sterile, as ordered) that contains pieces of ice and water or ordered solution. If sterile technique is used, the sterile solution bottle is set in the bowl of ice. Compresses should be changed frequently.

Packs: Packs are usually applied to an extensive area of body surface. They may be either cold or hot, sterile or unsterile, as designated in the order. Examples are as follows:

1. Hot pack (fomentation) is a piece of heated, moist towel that is applied to a client's skin to provide superficial heat. The effect of moderate heat is vasodilation, lessened viscosity of the blood, increased tissue metabolism, as well as relief of pain, congestion, inflammation, swelling, and muscle spasms. Application to open wounds or lesions that may rupture should be done using sterile technique. A heating device may be used to keep the pack warm. If the sterile procedure is ordered, the solution, towels, and dry covering must be sterile as well as the gloves or forceps used for wringing them dry.

2. A cool wet pack is composed of bath towels moistened in water cooled with a small amount of ice chips. After wringing, the towels are applied full length to cover the anterior and posterior trunk of the body and each extremity. The temperature of the water is maintained at 75° F. Ice bags may be placed at the axillae, groin, and head. The cool wet pack is used to reduce body tempertaure by evaporation. This procedure may be done under sterile conditions.

3. Ice packs are used occasionally to lower the temperature of a client's limb before surgery or to decrease swelling. It is a method of hypothermia and should be used with caution. Plastic bags of ice, which are covered with a pillowcase or towel, are placed on the specified area. Lower body temperatures are used for checking inflammation and suppuration by decreasing blood supply, slowing cellular metabolism, and inhibiting microbial activity. Extreme cold can destroy tissue if the length of application is excessive, however.

Soaks: A soak usually refers to the immersion of a part of the body, such as a foot or a hand, or may refer to wrapping the part with guaze and saturating it with fluid. The soak may be done under sterile conditions.

Rationale

Heat applications are ordered to

Effect vasodilation.

Soften exudates.

Increase suppuration.

Relax tissue.

Reduce pain.

Increase temperature.

Increase metabolism.

Increase circulation away from the congested area.

Relax muscle spasm.

Cool or cold applications are ordered to withdraw heat from tissue to

Effect vasoconstriction.

Reduce inflammation or edema.

Reduce temperature.

Produce local anesthesia.

Decrease metabolism.

Reduce muscle spasm.

Terminology

Anesthesia: No feeling or sensation

Conduction: The passage of heat from molecule to molecule, as through metal

Congestion: An abnormal accumulation of fluid in a part

Erythema: Redness of the skin from congestion of capillaries

Evaporation: A means by which water leaves the body surface, reducing body heat

Exudate: A substance produced on or in a tissue by a disease or vital process

Hypothermia: The state of lowered body temperature, usually between 78° F to 90° F.

Inflammation: A condition of the tissues in reaction to injury

Insulator: A material or substance that prevents or inhibits conduction, as of heat, for example

Medical asepsis: A condition in which microorganisms are kept within a well-defined area, and any articles or material removed from this area are rendered free of bacteria immediately so that infection will not be transmitted

Metabolism: Activity that takes place within the cells. Metabolism has two phases: *catabolism*, in which the glucose derived from carbohydrates, ketones, and glycerol is broken down into carbon dioxide, water, and energy; and *anabolism*, in which the energy from catabolism is used in the synthesis of enzymes and proteins needed by the body cells.

Microorganisms: A microscopic living body that may or may not be capable of producing disease

Pathogen: An organism capable of producing disease

Radiation: The transfer of heat from warm objects to cool objects in the form of electromagnetic waves

Ranges of temperature: Cool, 65° F to 80° F; cold, 55° F to 65° F; very cold, below 55° F; hot, 105° F to 115° F; warm, 100° F to 105° F; tepid, 80° F to 98° F.

Sterile technique: Absence of any microorganisms. Sterile technique requires using sterile equipment and supplies.

Surgical asepsis: Refers to practices carried out to keep an area free of unnecessary organisms

Suppuration: The formation of pus

Assessment

Pertinent Anatomy and Physiology

1. See Appendix I: *skin.*

2. Beneath the dermis lies the subcutaneous tissue or superficial fascia. The dermis is anchored to the subcutaneous tissue by collagenic fibers; the subcutaneous tissue then attaches the dermis to underlying structures, such as muscles and bones.

3. In youth the skin is extensible and elastic, but as one grows older, certain changes occur. The skin becomes thinner, there are fewer elastic fibers, and fat disappears from the subcutaneous tissue. This combination of events results in skin that is wrinkled in appearance.

4. The major channel of heat loss is the skin. Heat is lost from the body by the physical processes of radiation, conduction, convection, and vaporization.

Radiation is transfer of heat through air from the surface of one object to the surface of another without physical contact. One loses healthy radiation only if surroundings are cooler than the body.

Conduction is the transfer of heat from one object to another by direct physical contact. Humans lose heat by conduction to the air that is in contact with the skin (if it is cooler than the skin), to clothing, to air in the respiratory passages, to food in the alimentary canal, and to cold furniture.

Convection is the movement of air and heat by convection air currents. As heat is conducted to the air surrounding the body, it warms that air. The heated air rises and is replaced by denser, cool air.

Vaporization refers to the loss of heat when water evaporates or changes from the liquid to the vapor state.

5. Heat production is the result of metabolism of foodstuffs. It cannot be decreased below the basal level and cannot be increased to prevent freezing. The activity of the muscles results in a large amount of heat production, which is lowest during sleep and highest during exercise. Glandular activity results in a large amount of heat production in the liver and smaller amounts produced during actions of the other glands. Sympathetic nerve stimulation has a direct effect on metabolic rate. Food intake results in increased smooth muscle activity and increased glandular activity, causing the production of heat to be increased. The body temperature increases with metabolic rate at a rate of 7% for each degree.

6. Temperature regulation is the balance between heat production and heat loss. The center of integration is the hypothalamic thermostat. A cold environment results in vasoconstriction, increased muscle tone, shivering, increased muscular activity, and the urge to seek shelter or clothing. A hot environment results in vasodilation and sweating. If these stimuli continue over a period of time, the basal metabolic rate will be readjusted.

7. Therapeutic applications of heat and cold are dependent on proper duration of treatment to achieve desired effects. Prolonged treatment may have the opposite effect than what was intended. Heat should be applied for a short duration, 15 to 30 minutes. The effects of this type of treatment are vasodilation, increased blood flow to the area, increase in local metabolism, healing, and pain relief. Prolonged heat application (>1 hr) causes reduction of blood flow to the area with deprivation of nutrients and oxygen to the involved tissue. If the heat is removed for 15 to 30 minutes and reapplied, the vasodilation effect is reestablished. Cold should be applied for 15 to 30 minutes to achieve vasoconstriction, reduction of edema, decrease in local tissue metabolism, an increase in the blood supply available for vital centers, and numbness of the nerve endings, resulting in anesthesia of the tissue. Prolonged application of cold (>1 hr) can result in vasodilation, cell dysfunction, and permanent damage to the tissues. People generally become less sensitive to subsequent applications of heat and cold.

Pathophysiological Concepts

TISSUE HEALING AND REPAIR

1. The degree to which body structures return to their normal state after injury depends largely on the body's ability to replace parenchymal cells and to arrange them as they were originally. Repair can be by regeneration or fibrous scar tissue replacement.

2. Wounds can be divided into two types—those in which there is minimal tissue loss, and healing takes place by first intention; and those that have significant tissue loss, and healing takes place by second intention. A sutured surgical incision is an example of healing by first intention. Visible wounds that heal by second intention are burns and decubitus ulcers. When healing by second intention occurs, there is proliferation of granulation tissue into the injured area.

3. Keloid formation is an abnormality in the healing process by scar tissue repair. Keloids involve excessive production of bulging, tumorlike scar tissue masses.

4. There are many factors that influence wound healing: age, nutrition, infection, hormonal influences, blood supply, wound separation, and the presence of foreign bodies.

INFLAMMATION

1. The inflammatory response is closely intermeshed with wound healing and reparative processes. This process acts to neutralize or destory the offending agent, restricts tissue damage to the smallest possible degree, alerts the person to the threat of tissue injury, and prepares the injured area for healing.

2. Common causes of inflammation are trauma, surgery, infection, caustic chemicals, extremes of heat and cold, immune responses, and ischemic damage to body tissues.

3. The inflammatory response is thought to occur in three stages: vascular, exudative, and reparative. The vascular stage is characterized by increased blood supply to the area (hyperemia) causing redness and warmth. The exudative stage involves formation of fluid exudate, made up of the fluid and cells from the blood, damaged tissue cells, and any foreign bodies. When the wound is infected, the exudate, called pus, is described as purulent, and the process is called suppuration. The reparative stage is characterized by replacement of damaged tissue cells, by the regeneration of new cells, or by scar formation.

Assessment of the Client

1. A complete assessment of the client should include history of physical changes from impaired circulation and sensitivity of skin.

2. The appearance of the site for treatment should be assessed, described, and documented accurately.

3. Ascertain if the client is coherent and able to voice concerns if the treatment is too hot or too cold. Determine mobility limitations. If the client is paralyzed, more intensive observations are necessary and time frames for treatment must be altered to meet individual needs.

Plan

Nursing Objectives

Promote healing or reduction of pain and future complications.

Understand and relate the principles of hot and cold applications to the client's prescribed treatment.

Carry out the application with expediency and detailed care.

Reassure and inform the client regarding the application.

Follow safety measures before, during, and after the application.

Client Preparation

1. Prepare the client in advance for the differences in temperature.
2. Bring all equipment to the bedside and offer explanations as the prescribed application is completed.
3. Inform the client of the purpose and expected outcome of the procedure.

Equipment

Client thermometer (to take the client's temperature before beginning the procedure)

Aquamatic pad

Aquamatic pad

Distilled water

Aquamatic pad key

Fabric covering

Frozen bag

Frozen bag

Fabric covering for bag

Heat cradle

Heat cradle with bulbs

Screen (for privacy)

Sheet (for draping)

Heat lamp

Gooseneck lamp

60-watt bulb

Screen (for privacy)

Ice bag, collar, or glove

Ice bag, collar or glove

Protective covering to fit appliance

Ice chips

Basin and scoop

Alcohol or cold sponge bath

Bath themometer

Bath blanket

Basin

Solution (water, with or without alcohol)

Washcloths and towel

Sterile Compresses

Sterile solution, as ordered

Bath thermometer

Sterile gauze squares or sterile washcloths

Sterile basin

Sterile forceps

Sterile gloves

Sterile towels, for covering gauze

Clean Compresses

Solution, as ordered

Bath thermometer

Gauze squares or washcloths

Clean towel for insulation over gauze

Clean gloves for applying compresses

Hot pack or fomentation

Towels

Solution (as ordered)

Basin

Bath blanket

Bath thermometer

Waterproof covering (e.g., plastic)

Dry pack or covering (towels)

Cool wet pack

Bath towels, for moistening

Basin

Ice chips

Towels for dry pack or covering

Waterproof cover (e.g., plastic)

Ice packs

Plastic bags or conventional ice bags

Protective coverings for bags

Ice chips

Bath blanket

Screen (for privacy)

Soaks

Solution as ordered

Basin and towels

Screen (for privacy)

Gauze (if ordered)

Implementation and Interventions

Procedural Aspects

ACTION

RATIONALE

Hot/Warm/Cold/Cool Moist Packs or Compresses

1. Wash hands carefully before beginning application. Wear sterile gloves and use sterile instruments for all sterile procedures.

   Application of heat or cold to open wounds or lesions that may rupture requires sterile technique to prevent contamination.

2. Large, bulky towels may be used for application to larger surfaces. Washcloths or gauze squares are adequate for covering small surfaces.

   Absorbent and loosely woven fibers will hold moisture more successfully. Woolens and flannels absorb liquids more slowly.

3. The solution should be tested before immersion to ensure the correct temperature. A bath thermometer may be used to test the solution by immersing it in the liquid. If the solution is sterile, pour a small amount in a basin and test the temperature of this fluid. The tested fluid is discarded because the bath thermometer is not sterile. All solution touching the client must be sterile.

   Water or solution that is too hot or too cold may cause pain, discomfort, or tissue damage. Once solution has been poured from the sterile container, it may not be poured back or the entire container of solution is considered contaminated.

4. Adequate preparations should be made so that minimal time will be expended in the application of the packs and compresses.

   Exposure to the room air will alter the temperature of the application.

5. Provide adequate support of the area(s) requiring compresses or soaks.

   Weight of the compresses may cause discomfort or strain if the extremity is not supported.

6. Immerse the towel in the solution, wring it out, and wrap it around the site, molding it to the skin (Fig. 61-1).

   Air spaces between the skin and the pack would reduce the effect of the application because air is a poor conductor of heat.

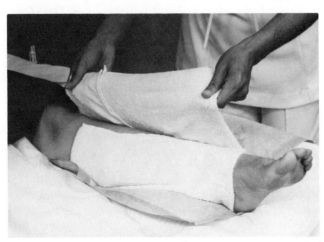

Figure 61.1

ACTION	**RATIONALE**
7. Cover the moist pack with a dry pack and waterproof covering or with a linen protector. If the compresses are sterile, cover with a sterile towel and a waterproof covering. Secure in place with tape or gauze (Fig. 61-2).	The covering will prevent the loss of heat from the moist hot compresses and will prevent soaking the bed linen. Pins are not used to secure a compress because they are excellent conductors of heat and can cause burns.

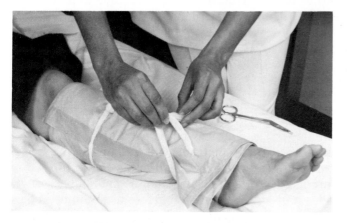

Figure 61.2

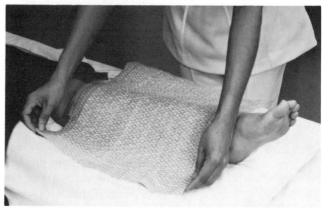

Figure 61.3

ACTION	**RATIONALE**
8. A conductive heat source can be placed over or next to the limb (Fig. 61-3).	The moisture in the towel distributes heat around the limb. The heat source is *never* placed under the limb; this could cause excessive heat buildup, leading to burns.
9. Position the client in proper, near-normal alignment.	Normal positioning promotes comfort. Weight of packs may restrict movement and cause fatigue.

External Application of Heat

ACTION	**RATIONALE**
1. *Aquamatic pad:* Fill the reservoir of the heating device two-thirds full with distilled water.	Distilled water reduces mineral formation, which may lead to eventual malfunction of the moving parts.
2. Tilt the pad end to end after filling the reservoir.	Tilting releases air bubbles that could interfere with even heat conduction.
3. Cover the pad with a soft fabric cover.	The covering should be thick enough to prevent burning the client and yet should be comfortable.
4. Watch carefully for the appearance of erythema or undesirable side-effects.	Skin reactions are the body's way of warning that tissue damage is imminent and must be remedied at once.
1. *Heat lamp:* Be sure that the client's skin is dry, clean, and free of any exudate.	Liquids conduct heat, so dry skin is less likely to be burned. Any exudate present will be hardened by the lamp, thereby increasing discomfort and risk of infection.
2. Place the lamp at a level of 18 in to 24 in away from the area of skin to be treated (Fig. 61-4). The lamp should be placed at an angle rather than over the top of the treatment area. Be certain that the bulb is not more than 60-watt.	A 60-watt bulb produces enough heat to treat the area without the chance of burning that is involved with stronger bulbs. The light should be to the side of the client rather than directly over the area to be treated to prevent the light's falling into the treatment area.

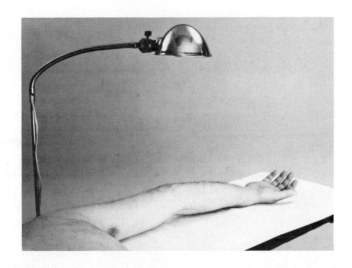

Figure 61.4

ACTION

3. Never place the lamp under the bed linen or allow it to come in contact with bed linens or the client's clothing.

4. Check the client frequently during the treatment (q15min). Recommended duration of treatment is 15 to 20 minutes. Be sure that the client's skin does not get any closer to the bulb than 18 in.

1. *Heat cradle:* The client should be lying in a clean bed. The cradle is placed over the client with the treatment area exposed. Screens may help to ensure the client's privacy while one is setting up the heat cradle.

2. Use the top sheet to cover the cradle. The ends of the sheet should reach to the sides and foot of the bed.

3. The treatment should last for 10 to 15 minutes. The heating element should be no closer to the client than 18 in to 24 in.

External Application of Cold

1. Place the cold application on the treatment area for the time prescribed. Place a protective covering over the application before placing it on the client. In Figure 61-5, a cold source is being applied to a cold moist compress to help maintain the effect of the compress. Check the cold application frequently during the treatment time to ensure that the cold appliance is not in direct contact with the skin.

RATIONALE

The bulb becomes hot and could cause a fire if in contact with fibers.

Reaction to heat treatment varies from client to client. Some people are more sensitive than others. If the skin begins to redden, the treatment should be discontinued.

The heat cradle provides radiant heat. It is less localized than a heat lamp and is used for areas of greater mass.

The top sheet will hold in the heat and prevent cooling by the circulating air. It also protects the client's privacy.

The heat should stimulate circulation and healing; the treatment must not be allowed to burn the client by too much exposure to the heat for too long a period.

Cold produces vasoconstriction and reduces tissue metabolism. Prolonged use of cold will cause prolonged vasoconstriction, which can result in tissue damage. Cold has an anesthetic effect on the skin. This effect may inhibit the body's normal defense mechanisms, such as pain, that alert one when damage is taking place.

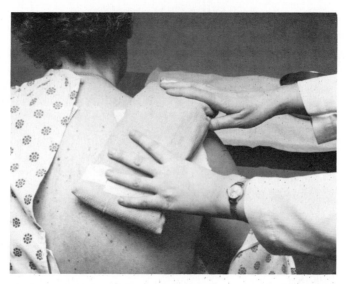

Figure 61.5

2. Cool body soaks usually are performed under sterile conditions. The solution is cooled to the desired temperature by placing the container in ice (Fig. 61-6). (To check the temperature, pour a small amount of the solution into a container and place a bath thermometer in it. This solution is now contaminated and is therefore discarded.) Pour the remaining solution into the sterile basin and assist the client to immerse the affected limb slowly (Fig. 61-7). Use pillows to aid the client in finding a comfortable position. The duration of the treatment is usually 20 minutes. Check the client every 5 minutes.

Soaks often are ordered for treatment of an open wound. The affected area should be immersed slowly to allow time for the skin to acclimatize to the variation in temperature. To avoid fatigue and muscle strain, pillows may be used to prop dependent parts.

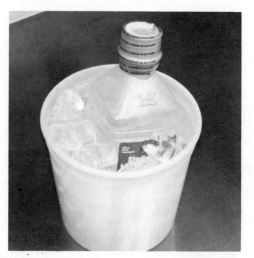

Figure 61.6

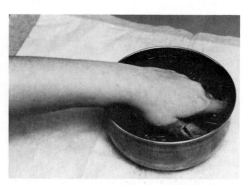

Figure 61.7

Communicative Aspects

OBSERVATIONS

1. Before, during, and after any type of moist or dry application, the client should be observed for signs and symptoms involving the skin and mucous membranes. These should be investigated, evaluated, reported, or treated with appropriate nursing measures. Those clients who are particularly at risk during hot and cold treatments are those

   At the extremes of age;

   Known to have delicate or sensitive skin;

   With impaired circulation;

   Subject to having irritating substances on the skin or mucous membranes (e.g., perspiration, urine, feces, gastrointestinal secretions, exudates);

   Are dependent on others for physical care and protection (e.g., infants and young children, the weak or debilitated, mentally incompetent, unconscious, immobilized, or bedridden);

   Who have an external appliance that is in contact with the mucous membranes or skin (e.g., traction, casts, braces, tubes);

   Who have an injury or disease condition that affects the skin or mucous membranes;

   Who have paralysis of body parts.

2. During hot and cold applications, observe for abnormal circulatory changes such as excessive or prolonged redness, blackness, whiteness, or cyanosis.

3. Verbal statements of discomfort by the client warrant careful observation. If indicated, the treatment should be discontinued and reported appropriately.

CHARTING

Duration	TPR of client before, during, and after treatment
Frequency	Appearance of site
Temperature of solution	Behavior and comments of client
Times	

DATE/TIME	OBSERVATIONS	SIGNATURE
4/8 0800	Warm compresses with K-matic pad at 95° F to right anterior forearm, T98.6°, P80, R24. Skin integrity intact. Moderate swelling of area noted. States he is familiar with treatment. ————————————	G. Ivers RN
0810	States he is comfortable. Skin on right arm appears pink. —————	G. Ivers RN
0820	Compresses removed. Skin appears pink at compress site. T99° F, P84, R18. States that his arm feels better. Range of motion increased since treatments started yesterday. Fluids offered and at bedside. —————	G. Ivers RN

Discharge Planning Aspects

CLIENT AND FAMILY EDUCATION

1. If the client will require hot and cold applications after discharge, teach the client or family the proper technique. Special emphasis must be placed on safety precautions. If the applications are to be sterile, explain the concepts of sterile technique and how to maintain sterility during application. Allow the client and family to demonstrate competency in sterile technique.

2. Teach the client and family about the signs of tissue damage during hot and cold applications. Emphasize the need to keep the heating appliance a specific distance from the treated area. Explain why the cold appliance should be covered and should not be in direct contact with the client's skin. Relate the signs of tissue damage and ask the family and client to assist the health care team in ensuring that the benefits of the treatment are obtained.

Evaluation

Quality Assurance

1. Document the skin area site, duration of treatment, and the condition and appearance of the skin before and after the treatment.
2. The client's response to the heat and cold is important and should be noted. Any untoward reactions to the application should be reflected.
3. Accurately record the type of body soaks, the appearance of the wound or site, and the response of the client.
4. Document any statements of discomfort of the client.
5. Hospital policy should address the application of external sources of hot and cold. The focus should be on client safety. All personnel should be aware of the policies that govern the use of hot and cold application. Yearly in-service programs on these policies as a part of the safety program or quality assurance program may help to ensure consistent application of the policies.

Infection Control

1. Soaks are usually sterile since open wounds are most often involved. Every effort must be made to lessen tissue damage and prevent infection.
2. Wash hands before assembling equipment so that microorganisms will not be transmitted to the client.
3. Clean or disinfect all equipment used for consecutive clients.

Technique Checklist

	YES	NO
Thorough handwashing completed	_____	_____
Procedure explained to client	_____	_____
Appearance, condition, and response of client documented	_____	_____
Packs and Compresses		
Sterile supplies, gloves, and instruments used	_____	_____
Correct size compress applied	_____	_____
Excess moisture squeezed from compress before application	_____	_____
Client positioned in proper alignment	_____	_____
Aquamatic Pad		
Protective covering on pad	_____	_____
Control set on correct setting	_____	_____
Key to control kept in central location accessible to nurses	_____	_____
Heat Lamp or Cradle		
Skin area clean and dry	_____	_____
60-watt bulb used in lamp	_____	_____
Lamp 18 in to 24 in from client	_____	_____
Client checked (q5min)	_____	_____
Heat application left on client the proper length of time	_____	_____
Sheet completely covered cradle	_____	_____
Safety precautions taken to see that client or clothing did not come in contact with bulb	_____	_____
Body Soaks		
Equipment sterile	_____	_____
Sterile technique adherence throughout procedure	_____	_____
Affected part immersed slowly	_____	_____
Client left in comfortable position	_____	_____

62　Incontinent Clients, Care of

Overview

Definition

Care of clients who are unable to control the discharge of urine or feces

Rationale

Prevent secondary problems due to incontinence, such as skin breakdown.

Institute a bladder- or bowel-training program as early as possible to prevent the need for an indwelling catheter.

Terminology

Anal sphincter: The constricting circular muscle that closes the anus

Overflow or paradoxical incontinence: Urine build-up in the bladder until the pressure causes dribbling, which stops when the excess pressure has been relieved

Stress incontinence: Involuntary escape of urine that occurs with straining during heavy lifting, sneezing, or coughing

Total incontinence: Escape of urine when the bladder is unable to store any urine and dribbling is almost constant

Assessment

Pertinent Anatomy and Physiology

See Appendix I: *anus, kidneys, intestine (large), sigmoid colon, rectum, urination.*

Pathophysiological Concepts

1. Pathologic distension of the bladder may occur in both the conscious and unconscious client. Retention of urine may follow an obstruction of the urethra, an enlargement of the prostate gland, or damage to the nerve supply of the bladder. Paralysis of the bladder due to spinal cord injury or disease (neurogenic bladder) may cause retention of urine and produce the same effects as obstruction.

2. A common symptom of abnormalities of the bowel is diarrhea. *Large-volume diarrhea* results from an increase in the water content of the stool, and *small-volume* diarrhea from an increase in the peristaltic action of the bowel. Small-volume diarrhea is usually characterized by cramping and frequent, explosive stools. This form of diarrhea is often associated with intrinsic disease of the colon, such as ulcerative colitis.

3. Another common symptom of pathology of the bowel is impaction. *Fecal impaction* stimulates secretion in the portion of the bowel proximal to the blockage. This results in watery, diarrhealike stools as the body attempts to evacuate the bowel.

4. Other symptoms of bowel problems are abdominal discomfort, hypoactive or hyperactive bowel sounds, and blood in the stool.

5. Cancer may occur in any part of the colon, but it is most commonly found in the rectum. Cancers of the colon and rectum usually are present for a long time before producing any symptoms. Bleeding is a highly significant symptom of colorectal cancer. Other symptoms are changes in bowel habits and a sense of urgency or incomplete emptying of the bowel. Pain is the last symptom to appear.

6. Fecal incontinence is usually related to an impairment of the anal sphincter itself or of the nerves that control it.

Assessment of the Client

1. Assess the client for readiness to begin a bladder- and bowel-training program.

2. Assess the client's skin to detect signs and symptoms of tissue breakdown.

3. Determine the client's emotional status related to the incontinence and efforts to correct it.

Plan

Nursing Objectives

Keep the normal physiologic acts of voiding and defecating intact.

Keep the client as clean and dry as possible to prevent skin complications.

Avoid embarrassing the client.

Assist the family and client to accept the condition and involve them in the retraining program.

Promote a positive self-image for the client.

Client Preparation

1. Any retraining program involving the systems of the body is slow and tedious. The client should understand at the outset what is expected and should participate in the formation of goals. This will enhance cooperation and will promote self-satisfaction when goals are met.

2. Determine the client's fears of dependency on others for care of bodily functions. Meet these fears with patience, understanding, and reassurance.

Equipment

Incontinence pads
Urinal
Bedpan or beside commode

Implementation and Interventions

Procedural Aspects

ACTION	*RATIONALE*
Bladder Incontinence	
1. Keep the skin clean and dry. Place an incontinence pad under the client to absorb the urine. Change the pad as often as necessary to maintain a dry environment and to prevent tissue breakdown (Fig. 62-1). Some clients develop skin reactions to these pads. Careful observation is necessary.	One of the major goals of a bladder-retraining program is prevention of tissue breakdown. The pH of urine is 5.5 to 7.0, making it acidic and capable of causing tissue breakdown. Contact between acidic urine and skin results in a mild chemical reaction or chafing.

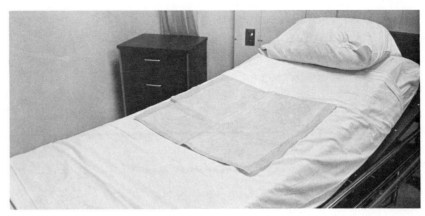

Figure 62.1

ACTION

2. Explain the bladder-training program, using a pleasant, positive approach. Provide privacy for the client during elimination.

3. An indwelling catheter should be used only as a last resort (i.e., when the client is in danger of skin breakdown or when a clean, dry condition is required for wound healing on the buttocks or perineal area).

4. Examples of bladder-training methods include the following:
   a. Offering the bedpan or urinal at regular or preset intervals
   b. Limiting intake of fluids to certain times, followed by an attempt to void
   c. Clamping an indwelling catheter for progressively longer intervals prior to its removal
   d. Forcing fluids for a brief period, waiting 30 minutes to an hour, and then offering the bedpan
   e. Using intermittent catherization to establish a bladder evacuation pattern

5. Keep the client's environment pleasant and odor free. Offer fruit juices to reduce the odor of the urine. Offer acidic juices.

RATIONALE

Speaking to the client in a condescending or criticizing manner impairs the therapeutic nurse–client relationship and may result in decreased cooperation with the bladder-training program.

Catheters are a known major cause of bladder infection. A catheter should be used only for the client's well-being and never for the nurses' convenience.

The objective is to rebuild the bladder musculature slowly by gradually reestablishing normal voiding patterns.

Since attitude is so important in the retraining program, every effort should be made to keep the client in a positive frame of mind. Offering acidic juices decreases urinary infections and increases output.

ACTION	*RATIONALE*
Bowel Incontinence	
1. Create a positive atmosphere from the beginning of the bowel-training program. Show acceptance of the client as a human being. Use of condescending or patronizing speech or manner with the client will hamper the efforts to initiate a successful bowel-training program.	Fecal incontinence is embarrassing and a threat to the client's ego. A therapeutic nurse–client relationship is based on acceptance and trust.
2. Bowel-training methods include the following: a. Using rectal suppositories or enemas to regulate the time of bowel evacuation b. Sitting on the commode in the natural position for elimination c. Ingesting bran and other high-fiber dietary foods at certain times of the day or evening d. Digital rectal stimulation for neurally impaired clients	Regularity and consistency are important aspects of the bowel-training program.

Communicative Aspects

OBSERVATIONS

1. The incontinent client must be diagnosed quickly so that the skin can be kept clean, dry, and intact.
2. Observe the skin frequently for signs of breakdown, such as redness, blisters, and lesions.
3. Watch for early signs of willingness and readiness to begin the training program.

CHARTING

DATE/TIME	OBSERVATIONS	SIGNATURE
3/13 0900	Bowel-training program underway. Incontinent stool. Back and buttocks washed. Backrub given. Skin color pink with no broken areas. 2 cm reddened area on left hip. Turned and positioned in right Sim's position. Bedpan offered every 2 hours with no success. ————————————————	M. Black RN

Discharge Planning Aspects

CLIENT AND FAMILY EDUCATION

1. Bowel- and bladder-training programs require patience and cooperation. The family should be involved from the beginning. Stress must be placed on positive occurrences, and continual encouragement of the client is necessary.
2. If the incontinent client is to go home after discharge, the family should be instructed on how to keep the skin dry and clean. Potential complications should be discussed and strategies planned to avoid them. The family should help set the goals in the retraining program and should be encouraged to maintain these goals after the client's discharge from the hospital.

Evaluation

Quality Assurance

Documentation should be made of measures for keeping the client clean, dry, and comfortable. The condition of the skin, with emphasis on the perineal area, thighs, and buttocks, should be noted. The progress and success of and alterations in the bowel- or bladder-training program should be noted at frequent intervals. Evidence should reflect that continual reassessment of the retraining efforts was made and that the program was readjusted to meet the changing needs and abilities of the client.

Infection Control

1. Lying on wet linens containing the ammonia from decomposing urine can irritate the skin. This condition can progress to ammonia dermatitis and excoriation (tissue breakdown). In this condition, the skin is especially prone to infection.
2. Careful handwashing should be carried out by the nurse and client after each attempt to evacuate the bowel or bladder. Handwashing should also be carried out after any contact with the client, bed linen, or equipment.

Technique Checklist

	YES	NO
Careful handwashing before and after evacuation attempts	_____	_____
Equipment assembled prior to initiation of the procedure	_____	_____
Privacy provided during elimination	_____	_____
Bed linens or pads kept dry	_____	_____
Skin kept clean and dry	_____	_____
Tissue breakdown prevented	_____	_____
Progress of retraining program and condition of skin recorded	_____	_____
Type of retraining method used		
Bladder:		
Preset schedule for offering bedpan	_____	_____
Limiting fluids to specific times, followed by voiding	_____	_____
Clamping catheter progressively	_____	_____
Forcing fluids, followed by voiding	_____	_____
Intermittent catheterization	_____	_____
Bowel:		
Rectal suppositories	_____	_____
Enemas	_____	_____
Digital rectal stimulation	_____	_____
Sitting on commode in natural position	_____	_____
High-fiber food schedule	_____	_____

63 Intake and Output, Recording

Overview

Definition

The accurate measurement of fluids taken into and released from the body; abbreviated "I&O"

Rationale

Determine the general fluid and electrolyte status of the client.

Aid in formulation of a diagnosis.

Assess the need for fluid increase or restriction.

Gain early clues to potentially dangerous physical situations.

Terminology

Diaphoresis: Profuse perspiration

Diuresis: Secretion of urine; often used to indicate increased function of the kidney

Diuretic: A substance that stimulates the flow of urine; some common substances, such as tea, coffee, and water, act as diuretics; a drug prescribed chiefly to rid the body of excess fluid, which accumulates in the tissues and causes swelling

Edema: Abnormal accumulation of a fluid in the intercellular spaces of the body

Electrolyte: A substance that, when dissolved in water, separates into charged particles (ions) capable of conducting an electrical current

Ion: An atom that has an electrical charge. Positive ions are called cations, and negative ions are called anions.

Parenteral fluids: Fluids not taken through the alimentary canal, given instead by the subcutaneous, intradermal, intramuscular, and intravenous routes

Assessment

Pertinent Anatomy and Physiology

1. Water accounts for 50% to 60% of the adult body weight. It acts as an excellent solvent for a great variety of substances and also provides for the ionization of electrolytes. The high specific heat and heat vaporization of water make it especially suitable as a temperature regulator. It also acts as a reagent in many chemical reactions occurring throughout the body.

2. Body fluids are distributed both in the cells and outside the cells. *Extracellular fluid* makes up 20% of the body weight, and *intracellular fluid* accounts for 40% of the body weight. The major cation in extracellular fluid is sodium. The major cation in intracellular fluid is potassium.

3. The body maintains an *acid–base balance* that is compatible with life. The normal pH of blood plasma is 7.35 to 7.45. Blood contains chemical buffers that prevent major changes in the pH from taking place. Mechanisms that help preserve the acid–base balance in the body are the respiratory mechanism, which helps conserve or expel CO_2, and the renal mechanism, which exchanges hydrogen (H^+) ion for sodium (Na^+) and conserves $NaHCO_3$. Alterations in the acid–base balance are called *acidosis* and *alkalosis*.

Pathophysiological Concepts	1. Body fluid levels are dependent on both sodium and water balance. Extracellular fluid volume deficit occurs when there is a reduction in body water. The two main causes are a decrease in the intake of fluids and electrolytes and increased loss of fluid and electrolytes. The extracellular fluid compartment is the source of all body secretions, including sweat, urine, and gastrointestinal (GI) secretions. This means that excessive loss of any of these fluids affords the potential for extracellular fluid deficit. A decrease in body weight is one of the most obvious indications of fluid loss. Measuring I&O affords a second method for assessing fluid balance.
	2. Extracellular fluid excess is generally caused by conditions that favor the retention of sodium and water, such as heart failure, cirrhosis of the liver, and kidney disease. Circulatory overload can occur during administration of intravenous fluids or blood. Development of edema is characteristic of extracellular fluid excess.
Assessment of the Client	1. Ascertain if the client will be able to participate in keeping accurate records of I&O.
	2. Determine if the client understands what is to be done and the reasons for doing it.
	3. Review the client's status, including presence of an indwelling catheter, intravenous infusion, gastric tubes, and other factors affecting I&O.
	4. Assess the client for symptoms of fluid deficit, such as decrease in body weight, thirst, decreased urinary output, weak and thready pulse, loss of skin elasticity, dry or sunken mucous membranes, and elevation of body temperature.

Plan

Nursing Objectives	Record I&O accurately.
	Report discrepancies to the physician.
	Elicit client cooperation in keeping the I&O record.
	Teach the client and family the signs and symptoms of fluid imbalances.
Client Preparation	1. Client cooperation is essential if the I&O record is to be accurate. If the client understands why it is being kept, cooperation is much more likely to be forthcoming. Offer a full explanation in terms the client understands.
	2. If the client can get up to go to the bathroom, a urinal or a receptacle that fits inside the commode to catch the urine should be made available as soon as the client is placed on I&O so that all urine will be saved (Fig. 63-1). If the client has limited mobility, a bedside commode or bedpan may be used.
Equipment	I&O record slip
	Pencil
	Graduated-measurement container

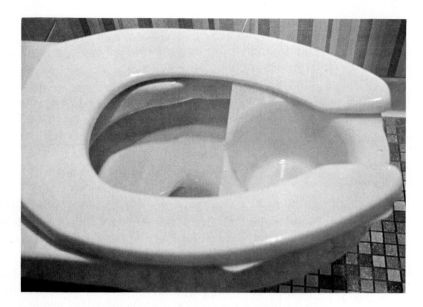

Figure 63.1

Implementation and Interventions

Procedural Aspects

ACTION

1. Give a full explanation to the client.

2. When recording I&O, use as the unit of measurement cc (cubic centimeters) or ml (millilters). Convert household measures as well. A conversion chart should be available on each unit and for each client.

3. Determine if there is an order to force fluids or to restrict the intake of fluids.

4. Check the water pitcher frequently to be certain the client has enough water. This is especially important if the goal is to increase the intake of fluids. Record the amount of water taken (Fig. 63-2). Check the meal tray, as well, and record the amount of fluid taken in the form of beverages, Jello, ice cream, soup, etc. If the client is on a restricted fluid regimen, make water available in quantities that will ensure the maintenance of limitations. Keep an ongoing record of the amount of fluid consumed and ration the amount over 24 hours.

RATIONALE

Cooperation will be enhanced if the client understands the reason for I&O records being kept.

Standardization allows more accurate measurement.

Comprehensive planning for the client should take into account any long-range goals.

Foods that are broken down into fluid in the GI tract are considered fluid intake and must be included in the daily intake measurement.

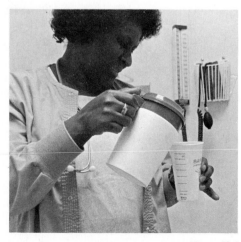

Figure 63.2

ACTION	*RATIONALE*

Plan for more fluid intake in the mornings and afternoon and significantly less during the late evening and night, when the client is sleeping. Be sure that the client understands the reason for and methods of fluid restriction.

Communicative Aspects

OBSERVATIONS

1. Intake includes anything liquid taken by mouth, intravenous (IV) fluids, blood and blood products, gastric feedings and irrigation fluids greater than the amount removed, urinary catheter irrigation greater than the amount removed, and peritoneal dialysis fluid.

2. Output includes emesis, urine, liquid feces, blood loss (approximated), drainage from incisions (approximated), and fluids withdrawn from the body, such as during paracentesis or thoracentesis, in surgical drainage bags, and so on. To approximate, use measures or items that are common knowledge, such as saturated two 4″ × 4″ pads or circle of drainage 4 inches in diameter on dressing.

3. Gross discrepancies between intake and output should be called to the physician's attention.

CHARTING

I&O should be recorded for each shift, as well as for every 24 hours. Discrepancies should be explained in the chart.

DATE/TIME	OBSERVATIONS	SIGNATURE
6/21 1415	Output much reduced from yesterday. 1890 cc yesterday for 24 hours. Has voided only 200 cc in past 8 hours. States she has not been drinking any water or tea since x-rays this morning because of nausea from the barium. Dr. J. notified. IM antiemetic given. ———————————————	F. White RN
1500	Juice and water at bedside. Instructions on proper measurement of fluids. States no more nausea or dizziness. Is taking fluids well now. Has not voided since 1030. ———————————————	F. White RN

Discharge Planning Aspects

CLIENT AND FAMILY EDUCATION

1. Many clients can assist in keeping their own I&O record if they are properly instructed.

2. The client and family should understand the reasons for I&O record keeping.

3. If the client must measure I&O after discharge from the hospital, all family members should be instructed in conversion of household measurements into cc and ml. Conversion charts should be given to the family for ready reference. Be sure that the client and family have the tools needed to measure I&O and have demonstrated reasonable competence in doing so.

Evaluation

Quality Assurance

Measure and record the volumes of fluid ingested or infused, the amount of urine voided, and other sources of output, such as diarrhea or drainage. Any signs of dehydration or overhydration should be documented and reported. Ascertain and document in the care plan the client's fluid likes and dislikes, particularly if fluids are to be forced. Observe and record the color, odor, and clarity of the client's urine. Document any diaphoresis and the number of linen changes necessary. If fluid restriction is ordered, document the maintenance of fluid restriction and the client's level of cooperation. Document an explanation of the I&O measurement procedure to the client and family.

Infection Control

1. If the client is incontinent of urine or extremely diaphoretic, meticulous skin care is essential in addition to measurement of I&O. Abrasions of the skin may become infected.
2. When forcing fluids, take care not to leave at the bedside excess fluid that is in danger of spoiling, such as milk.
3. Wash hands before providing care to the client.
4. If the client has an indwelling urinary catheter and hourly I&O measurement is required, consider the use of a closed urinary drainage system, which facilitates hourly determinations while maintaining the closed system.

Technique Checklist

	YES	NO
All necessary equipment obtained		
I&O forms	_____	_____
Pencils	_____	_____
Measurement container	_____	_____
Bedpan	_____	_____
Urinal	_____	_____
Hands washed before and after assisting client	_____	_____
Procedure explained to client	_____	_____
I&O measured and documented on client's record	_____	_____
Signs of dehydration and overhydration recorded	_____	_____
Fluids forced	_____	_____
Discharge instructions given to client and family on fluid regulation at home	_____	_____

64

Intestinal Decompression, Assisting with

Overview

Definition

The insertion of a tube into the intestinal tract to relieve pressure and aspirate contents. Types of tubes are as follows (Fig. 64-1):

Miller–Abbott tube: A 6- to 10-ft biluminal tube with one lumen for introducing air, water, or mercury to inflate the balloon and another for drainage. A metal tip and balloon are located on the end of the tube. The balloon is inflated after insertion (Fig. 64-2)

Cantor tube: A 10-foot, single-lumen tube with a balloon at the tip of the tube and several holes in the tube at the distal end, near the balloon. Mercury is injected into the balloon before insertion (Fig. 64-3)

Harris tube: A single-lumen tube, which uses a mercury-filled balloon to propel it through the intestinal tract and has a metal tip used for irrigations and suction

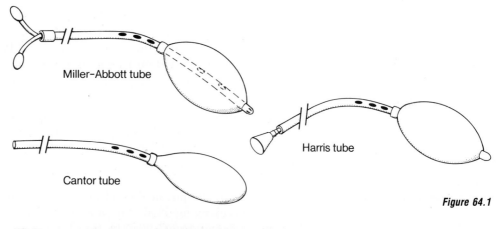

Miller–Abbott tube

Harris tube

Cantor tube

Figure 64.1

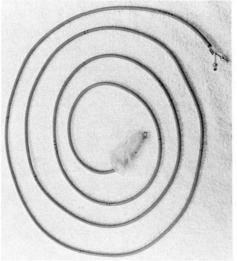

Figure 64.2

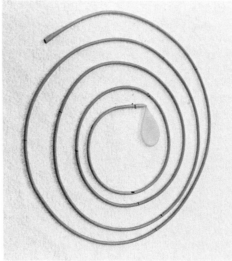

Figure 64.3

Rationale	Remove gas and fluids from the intestinal tract to prevent or treat distension.
	Stimulate natural peristaltic activity.
	Locate and relieve obstruction in the intestine.

Terminology

Atony: Lack of normal muscle tone

Decompression: The removal of pressure, gas, and fluids from the intestinal tract

Distension: The state of being stretched

Peristalsis: A wavelike progression of alternate contraction and relaxation of the muscle fibers of the esophagus and intestines by which contents are propelled along the alimentary tract

Assessment

Pertinent Anatomy and Physiology

1. See Appendix I: *esophagus, stomach, intestine (small), intestine (large), sigmoid colon, rectum, anus.*

2. The lower portion of the stomach joins the small intestine at the pylorus. This opening is surrounded by a muscular ring called the pyloric sphincter or pyloric valve.

3. The ileum forms the distal portion of the small intestine. It is the section that joins the large intestine. A muscular sphincter, the ileocecal valve, surrounds the juncture between the large intestine and small intestine.

Pathophysiological Concepts

1. *Intestinal obstruction* refers to an impairment of movement of contents through the small intestine and large intestine. Mechanical obstruction can result from peritoneal adhesions, hernias, twisting of the bowel (volvulus), telescoping of the bowel (intussusception), fecal impaction, and tumors. Reflex paralysis usually affects the small bowel. Paralytic ileus is seen most commonly following abdominal surgery or trauma.

2. The major effects of intestinal obstruction are intestinal distension and loss of fluids and electrolytes. Bowel obstruction tends to perpetuate itself by causing atony of the bowel and further distension. Distension is also aggravated by accumulation of gases. About 70% of these gases probably result from swallowing air. As the process continues, the distension moves proximally, involving additional segments of the bowel.

Assessment of the Client

1. Assess the client's physical condition, with emphasis on the symptoms that prompted seeking medical attention. Assess the amount of distension and discomfort being experienced by the client. Assess the onset and severity of symptoms. Determine when the client's last bowel movement occurred. Measure vital signs as a baseline for future comparison.

2. Assess the client's knowledge and anxiety level. Determine how much information the client can tolerate when assessing methods suitable for client education.

3. Assess the client's physical characteristics. Determine if the client has ever had nasal surgery, a nasal injury, nasal polyps, or other conditions of the nose that might hinder placement of the tube.

Plan

Nursing Objectives

Allay the client's fears and anxieties.

Assist the physician in inserting the tube.

Ensure proper placement and advancement of the tube.

Maintain patency of the tube to ensure proper function.

Provide for the client's comfort.

Maintain fluid and electrolyte balance.

Observe for signs and symptoms that indicate complications.

Keep accurate records of the amount, color, and type of drainage, intake and output (I&O), and the effects of the treatment.

Assist the client and family in understanding the purpose of the treatment.

Prevent damage to the lining of the gastrointestinal (GI) tract during insertion, suction, and removal of the tube.

Client Preparation

1. If the client seems agreeable, it may help to show the client and family the tube, as well as pictures and/or diagrams about placement and desired results. For some clients, a brief explanation is the only preparation that is wanted or can be tolerated. Determine the client's readiness for information and offer an explanation that meets the individual client's and family's needs.

2. To prevent delays, test all equipment prior to beginning the procedure. Inflate the balloon with air to test patency; then completely deflate the balloon.

Equipment

GI tube, as requested by the physician	Emesis basin
Basin with ice	Wipes
Stethoscope	Suction capability and apparatus
Disposable irrigation set	Adhesive tape (½ in wide)
5 ml to 10 ml of mercury (Hg)	Rubber band
Local anesthetic spray, if ordered	Water-soluble lubricant
Glass of water and straw	Irrigating solution, as ordered

Implementation and Interventions

Procedural Aspects

ACTION	RATIONALE
Miller–Abbott Tube	
1. Inflate the balloon with 20 ml to 50 ml of air to ensure its integrity. Completely deflate the balloon. Label the adaptors ("suction" and "balloon"). Place the tube in a basin of ice for a short time. Lubricate the tube with a small amount of water-soluble lubricant. Proceed as with insertion of a nasogastric tube (see Technique 57, Gastric Intubation).	Be sure that the tube is in proper working order before the insertion is begun. The lubricant decreases friction between the tube and the lining of the GI tract. Chilling the tube makes it less pliable and easier to maneuver during insertion.

ACTION	RATIONALE
2. Be sure that the tube is in the stomach by aspirating gastric content and by auscultating the stomach with a stethoscope while 5 ml of air is pushed through the tube by syringe. Appearance of gastric content and hearing the characteristic rush of air into the stomach help ensure that the tube is indeed in place. Once the tube is in the stomach, 1 ml of mercury may be injected to help the tube through the pyloric valve. Position the client on the right side.	The tube must proceed from the stomach into the intestinal tract. Fluoroscopy may be used to determine when the tube has passed the pyloric valve. Because the valve opens toward the right side, positioning on the right side allows the pull of gravity to facilitate the passage of the tube out of the stomach.
3. Once the tube has passed out of the stomach, inject air into the balloon.	Air in the balloon serves the same function as a bolus of food in the intestinal tract. It stimulates peristalsis and allows the tube to progress through the small intestine to the desired level.
4. Reposition the client every 2 hours. Ambulate the client frequently.	Frequent changes of position facilitate passage of the tube and prevent it from adhering to a segment of the bowel wall.
5. Attach the tube to suction after it clears the pyloric valve. Advance the tube 1 in to 2 in every hour. When the tube reaches the desired level, tape it to the client's nose	The tube should be allowed to advance at a normal peristaltic rate. Taping the tube will secure it at the desired level; however, be certain that the tubing is not placing stress on the client's nose.
6. The tube may be irrigated through the suction lumen. Instill about 20 ml to 50 ml of sterile saline and slowly aspirate intestinal contents from the tube.	Slow instillation and aspiration of contents will prevent cramping and discomfort.
7. Give oral care frequently. Lubricate the client's lips as needed.	Mouth breathing is usually necessary during insertion of an intestinal tube. Mouth breathing causes the lips and tongue to become cracked and dry.

Removal of the Miller–Abbott tube

ACTION	RATIONALE
1. If radiologic examination reveals that the tube has not reached the ileocecal valve, aspriate *all* of the mercury and air from the balloon through the proper lumen. Gradually remove the tube through the nose by gently pulling it out a few inches every 5 to 10 minutes. Administer oral-hygiene care after the tube is removed and at any time during removal, if the client wishes.	Aspiration of all of the contents of the balloon will decrease discomfort as the tube is removed. Gentle removal a few inches at a time will lessen the chance of intussusception, or telescoping the bowel back over itself.

ACTION	*RATIONALE*
2. If the balloon has passed the ileocecal valve, allow it to pass naturally on out of the rectum. Hold the tube out of the rectum firmly and cut the tubing at the nose. Allow the tube to continue out of the rectum by peristaltic action. This may take several days.	The ileocecal valve is a powerful muscular sphincter, which guards the ileum from the backing up of fecal material. Pulling the tube back through this valve would be very painful and could damage the valve.

Cantor or Harris Tube

ACTION	*RATIONALE*
1. Insert the mercury into the tube before tube insertion is begun. Insert the tube through the nose in the manner of a nasogastric tube (see Technique No. 57, Gastric Intubation). Place the tube in a basin of ice before it is inserted. Apply a small amount of lubricant to the tube before insertion.	The weight of the mercury allows gravitational force to pull the tube through the GI tract. The lubricant decreases friction. Chilling the tube makes it less pliable and easier to maneuver during insertion.
2. Frequent position changes are necessary because the tube progresses slowly through the GI tract at the rate of normal peristalsis.	Repositioning prevents the tube from adhering to the side of the bowel or twisting or knotting.
3. The tube may be taped in place as soon as it reaches the desired level. Connect the tube to suction and irrigate with 20 ml to 50 ml of sterile saline as needed.	Secure the tube with tape, but be certain that the tube is not putting strain on the client's nostril.

Removal of Cantor or Harris Tube

ACTION	*RATIONALE*
1. Remove the tube at 6-inch increments by pulling gently.	Because the tube is now going against the normal peristaltic movement, care and patience will be necessary to avoid trauma to the bowel.
2. When the bag of mercury is visible in the back of the throat, withdraw the mercury with a needle and syringe. Continue withdrawing the tube through the nose.	The mercury will have gathered by gravitational pull into a common area at the bottom of the bag. If the bag is removed through the nose with the mercury intact, pulling the large bolus of mercury through the naris will be traumatic. If the mercury is removed, the empty bag will be pulled through the nose with the tube.
3. If the bag of mercury has progressed beyond the ileocecal valve, allow the tube to continue out the rectum by normal peristaltic action.	Trying to pull the bag of mercury backward through the powerful ileocecal valve will cause trauma to the GI tract.

Communicative Aspects

OBSERVATIONS

1. Observe the amount, consistency, and color of the drainage obtained from suction. Note the correlation between the amount of drainage and the amount of input. Note the amount of irrigation fluid used in relation to the amount of drainage returned. Careful I&O recording is necessary.

2. Monitor vital signs throughout the intubation and decompression period. Compare these with baseline measurements.

3. Observe the speed of insertion, or how far the tube is advanced in designated increments (minutes, hours). Record the total amount of time used to insert the tube and to remove it.

4. Note the reaction of the client to the procedure. Note willingness and ability to cooperate. Observe for signs of discomfort and complications, such as pain, bright red drainage, and blockage of the progress of insertion. Note the client's ability to ambulate and turn to facilitate tube insertion and removal.

5. Note the presence of gastric discomfort and measures taken to prevent or alleviate these, such as elevation of the head of the bed.

CHARTING

DATE/TIME	OBSERVATIONS	SIGNATURE
5/27 0900	No.16 Miller–Abbott tube inserted by Dr. K. 1 ml Hg instilled into balloon. Gastric contents aspirated from stomach. To X-ray for fluoroscopy for verification of placement. No pain or discomfort stated thus far. ———	G. Ivers RN
0930	Balloon inflated with 25 ml air. Tube advanced 1 inch as ordered. B/P 122/78, P 82, R 22. Turned to right side. ———	G. Ivers RN

Discharge Planning Aspects

CLIENT AND FAMILY EDUCATION

1. The client and family should understand why it is necessary to pass the tube and what the expected results are.

2. The client may have a sore throat for a few days after removal of the tube. Further irritation of the throat may be minimized by avoiding smoking, coughing, or excessive talking.

3. The client and family should understand why frequent position change during passage of the tube is desirable. Show the family how to ambulate the client, if practical, by securing the remaining amount of tube in a coiled fashion to the gown with a pin and rubber band.

REFERRALS

If obstruction is encountered, surgical intervention may be necessary. If the obstruction is due to cancer, assistance may be sought from the American Cancer Society in the form of counseling or supplies.

Evaluation

Quality Assurance

Documentation should include the condition of the client prior to, during, and after insertion of the tube. A complete description of the drainage should be available. An accurate recording of I&O should be on the chart. The timing and increments of tube advancement should be reflected. The client's reaction to the insertion should be noted. Documentation should reflect that the nurse knew what complications were possible and the measures taken to avoid these complications.

Infection Control

Thorough handwashing before and after insertion and advancement of the tube is necessary. Frequent oral hygiene during tube insertion is necessary to decrease the number of bacteria that may travel to the oral cavity.

Technique Checklist

	YES	NO
Procedure explained to client and family	_____	_____
Equipment assembled prior to beginning procedure	_____	_____
Tube chilled and tip lubricated	_____	_____
Gastric contents aspirated	_____	_____
Auscultation of air in stomach	_____	_____
Fluoroscopy for placement of tube	_____	_____
Tube attached to suction	_____	_____

Approximate rate of intubation

_____ in/min

_____ in/hr

Tube reached desired level at

_____ (time)

Length of time tube left in place

_____

Tube removed per

mouth _____

rectum _____

	YES	NO
All of the air/mercury returned	_____	_____
Complications	_____	_____

_____

65

Intravenous (IV) Infusion Administration

Overview

Definition

The introduction of a solution, blood, or blood derivatives directly into a vein. Types are administration by way of flexible tubes (Angiocath, Intracath) or needles (wingtip, scalp-vein) (Fig. 65-1).

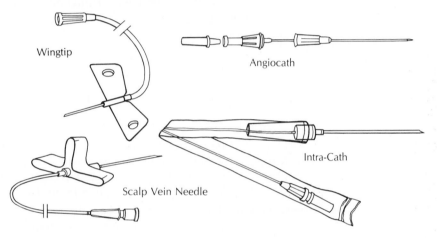

Wingtip

Angiocath

Intra-Cath

Scalp Vein Needle

Figure 65.1

Rationale

Restore or maintain fluid and electrolyte balance.

Provide for basic nutrition.

Provide a vehicle for administering medication.

Transfuse blood or blood derivatives for therapeutic purposes.

Terminology

Agglutination: Clumping of blood cells when incompatible bloods are mixed

Angiocath: A needle within a plastic tubing. The needle is removed after insertion into the vein; the plastic tube remains in the vein for infusion purposes

Antecubital space: The area of the median and basilic veins at the bend of the arm

Bevel of the needle: The slanting or sloping surface of the needle point

Derivatives of blood: Constituent parts of whole blood

Dripmeter: A chamber between the bottle and the tubing allowing observation of the rate of infusion

Edema: Accumulation of fluid in the tissues

Embolus: A foreign mass transported in the bloodstream

Hemolysis: The destruction of red blood cells

Intracath: A large-bore needle with a plastic catheter, which is threaded through it after venipuncture. The needle is withdrawn from the puncture site, and the plastic catheter remains in the vein; a plastic needle guard is placed over the needle and taped to the skin

Ischemia: Interference with the blood flow to an area

Macrodrip chamber: A clear portion of the intravenous (IV) tubing with an enlarged diameter through which the number of drops can be seen and counted to determine the rate at which the IV fluid is dripping; most macrodrips deliver 15 drops to 20 drops/ml; consult the literature accompanying the set

Microdripmeter: A thin needle between the bottle and the tubing, which allows accurate counting of drops; 60 drops equal 1 ml of IV fluid

Plasma: The fluid portion of the blood

Solution: The liquid to be infused; may be a nutrient solution containing some form of carbohydrate (glucose), electrolyte solution containing various amounts of electrolytes usually dissolved in normal saline, or blood volume expanders used to increase the volume of blood after hemorrhage

Thrombus: A blood clot

Unit of blood: 500 ml of blood in a special plastic container that was used to collect the blood directly from the donor

Wingtip needle: A small needle used for unstable veins; the upper portion, which has a butterfly-wing appearance, is used for guidance during insertion and anchoring during infusion

Assessment

Pertinent Anatomy and Physiology

See Appendix I: *blood, blood vessels, skin.*

Pathophysiological Concepts

1. Occlusion of blood flow through a blood vessel can result from the formation of thrombus or the presence of embolus. This interruption in the normal flow of blood interferes with the delivery of oxygen and nutrients to the tissues. Arterial interference results in *ischemia,* and venous obstruction causes *congestion* and *edema.*

2. Compression of the blood vessel occurs when the pressure exerted on the outside of the vessel exceeds that of the blood flow inside. The intravascular pressure is lower in the venous system than in the arterial system; thus the veins are more easily compressed. Application of a restrictive device, such as a tourniquet, can effectively restrict the flow of blood through the vein, causing a pooling in the distal portion of the extremity. This occurs because the arterial system continues to pump blood into the area although the blood is not returning to the heart. This pooling causes distension of the vein and facilitates location and puncture of the vein. It is important to remember that restrictive devices, if applied too tightly, also have the potential for obstructing arterial flow. Great caution must be exercised in the application of tourniquets to ensure that arterial flow is not affected. Too much compression has the potential to cause nerve damage and loss of function. This is from direct compression of the nerve tracts, which often run parallel to the arteries.

3. Pulmonary embolism may result when an obstructive substance blocks the flow of blood into the lung from the right ventricle of the heart. The embolism may consist of a thrombus, air that has accidentally been injected during intravenous infusion, or fat that has been mobilized after a fracture.

Assessment of the Client

1. Assess the client's physical condition in relation to adequate hydration, how long the client has been without fluid, and/or the duration and severity of vomiting. Determine baseline vital signs for later comparison.

2. Assess the condition of the client's veins. Assess the adequacy of the veins to hold the IV needle or catheter, the presence of trauma or previous sites of infusion, and the client's preference for infusion site (for example, if the client is right handed, it may be preferable to start the IV infusion in the left arm or hand).

Plan

Nursing Objectives

Make the client as comfortable as possible.

Prevent infection or complications.

Allay the client's and family's fears and apprehensions.

Observe closely for adverse reactions.

Teach the client and family safety precautions.

Report desired or undesired effects.

Recognize the signs and symptoms of a blood reaction.

Client Preparation

1. Properly identify the client before beginning. Take a card or file with the client's name on it to the room. Match the name to the client's identification band, room number, and bed card before venipuncture is accomplished.

2. Offer adequate explanation to the client to ensure a clear understanding of what will occur and why the infusion is necessary. Have all equipment assembled before entering the room to convey to the client an attitude of confidence and competence.

3. Offer the client the opportunity to go to the bathroom, or offer the bedpan or urinal before beginning. After insertion, the tubing will somewhat restrict the client's mobility.

4. Be sure that the client's gown can be removed after the IV infusion has been started. If not, obtain for the client a hospital gown with snaps.

5. Place a towel or linen protector under the arm to be used for venipuncture so that the linens will not become soiled and complete cleanup will be facilitated.

Equipment

IV solution, as ordered by physician

IV tubing, with accessories as indicated

IV infusion kit or IV tray containing items such as alcohol sponges, antiseptic pads, tourniquet, 2″ × 2″ dressings, and tape

Covered armboard, if needed

IV standard, with wheels if the client will be ambulatory

Needles:

    1-inch needle (gauge determined by the size of the client's veins)

    Wingtip needle

    Scalp-vein needle

    Sterile disposable Angiocath

    Sterile disposable Intracath (small, medium, or large), antiseptic cleaning solution (povidone-iodine), and sterile 4″ × 4″ dressings

Implementation and Interventions

Procedural Aspects

ACTION	RATIONALE
1. Wash hands thoroughly.	Remove as much of the transient flora as possible to prevent introduction of pathogenic organisms into the bloodstream.
2. Prepare the infusion for hanging. Determine the sterility of the solution by being sure that seals have not been broken and that the fluid appears clear. Check the expiration	Cloudiness may indicate contamination and warrants sending solutions back to Central Supply or Pharmacy for replacement.

ACTION

RATIONALE

data on the container. Close the clamp on the tubing and insert the end of the tubing through the rubber stopper into the bottle or bag of fluid. Maintain strict sterility of the contents during opening and insertion.

3. Hang the bag or bottle of fluid with the tubing intact and flush all of the bubbles by allowing the tubing to fill and a small amount to run out the end of the tubing. Fill the drip chamber at least half full. When filling the tubing, maintain the sterility of the end of the tubing. After it is flushed, replace the sterile protective cap over the end of the tubing until the IV tubing is connected to the needle in the client.

Air can cause pulmonary embolism if introduced in sufficient quantity into the bloodstream. Strict adherence to sterile technique reduces the chances of causing infection in the client.

4. Raise the head of the bed until the heart is above the level of the vein selected for venipuncture.

The dependence of the vein below heart level will aid in filling and distending the vein.

5. Apply a tourniquet above the intended site of venipuncture (Fig. 65-2). Be sure that the pulse is still palpable below the site of tourniquet application. The most common sites of venipuncture are located from the antecubital space (median and basilic veins) to the wrist (radial vein). If absolutely necessary, the foot area may be used.

The tourniquet causes constriction of the veins, resulting in engorgement and distension and making the veins more accessible. Care must be taken to ensure that arterial circulation is not impaired. Veins in the upper extremities are considered best for venipuncture because of the possibility of developing phlebitis if the foot or leg veins are used. It is also possible to dislodge plaque in the lower extremities, causing embolus.

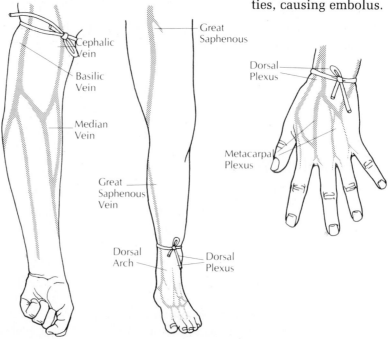

Cephalic Vein
Basilic Vein
Median Vein
Great Saphenous
Great Saphenous Vein
Dorsal Arch
Dorsal Plexus
Dorsal Plexus
Metacarpal Plexus

Figure 65.2

ACTION	RATIONALE
6. If the vein is not distended or easily palpable, lightly pat the area, ask the client to open and close the fist of the involved arm, lower the extremity below the level of the heart, or apply a warm towel to the area. The vein may have a bluish appearance in light-skinned persons. In dark-skinned clients, rely on palpation to determine the location of the vein. Veins should feel bouncy and rubbery, with a slight rebound when lightly pressed. Avoid veins that are thready, reddened, or hard, because phlebitis or arteriosclerotic plaques may be present.	Circulation to a part may be increased by positioning, active and passive exercise, or the application of heat.
7. Cleanse the skin thoroughly with an antiseptic at the anticipated site of venipuncture and in a circular motion outward for several inches (Fig. 65-3). Grasp the skin and retract it over the vein area. Hyperextend the extremity if needed.	Pathogens normally found on the skin may be pathogenic when allowed to enter the bloodstream. Anchoring the skin by retraction and hyperextension of the limb increase the visibility and palpability of the vein.

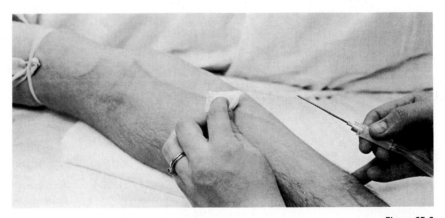

Figure 65.3

ACTION	*RATIONALE*
8. Hold the needle at a 45° angle, bevel up, in line with and beside the vein (Fig. 65-4). Insert the needle through the skin and about ½ in below the intended site of vein puncture (Fig. 65-5).	The pressure needed to pierce the skin is sufficient to force the needle through the vein. Inserting the needle beside the vein prevents accidental trauma to the vein without successful venipuncture.

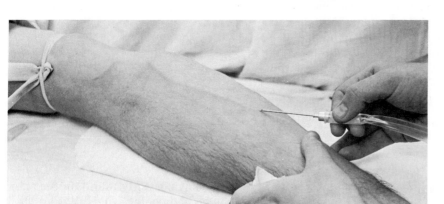

Figure 65.4

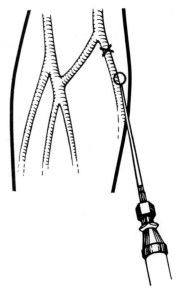

Figure 65.5

ACTION	*RATIONALE*
9. When the needle is through the skin, lower the angle until it is almost parallel to the skin. Gently insert the needle into the vein. Use the free hand to palpate or control and anchor the vein while the needle is being introduced.	Puncturing the vein with the needle at a sharp angle may cause accidental passage through the vein. This may release the pooled blood into the tissue, resulting in hematoma and rendering the vein useless for infusion. Venipuncture will then have to be accomplished in another location.
10. When venous return appears in the needle, continue with catheterization of the vein. If a wingtip or regular needle is used, insert it another ½ in to ¾ in into the vein. Anchor it while connecting the IV tubing. Do not start infusing until the tourniquet is released. Angiocaths or Intracaths are threaded into the vein while it is still distended in the following manners:	The tourniquet causes increased venous pressure, which causes the blood to flow spontaneously back into the needle. This pressure will also keep the vein distended to ease catheterization of the vein.
Angiocath: Thread the catheter into the vein with the stylus still in the sheath, or remove the stylus and thread the sheath only if venipuncture is certain. After the stylus has been removed, it is *never* reinserted. If the sheath will	Threading with the stylus gives more control over the catheter, but it also risks puncture of the vein by the needle tip. If the stylus is removed, the needle cannot be reinserted into the vein if it accidentally slips out during insertion. The stylus is never

ACTION

RATIONALE

not thread after the stylus has been removed, the sheath is removed from the site, and venipuncture is attempted at a new site with a new Angiocath.

Intracath: Thread the long catheter through the center of the needle into the vein. Once the catheter is in the vein, withdraw the stylet from the inside of the catheter. Connect the catheter to the IV tubing. Remove the needle from the skin and cover it with the plastic case to prevent sticking the client again. Tape the case to the client's arm until the catheter is removed.

reinserted into the plastic sheath because of the chance of shearing off part of plastic tubing, causing an embolism.

The catheter threads into the vein. The tourniquet remains tight to encourage backflow of blood through the catheter during the connection of the IV tubing.

11. Release the tourniquet after the tubing is connected. Work quickly but efficiently so that the needle is not accidentally pushed through or pulled from the vein. Open the tubing and allow the fluid to start flowing. Set it at the desired rate.

Releasing the tourniquet relieves the pressure in the vein. Blood will clot in the needle or catheter if not flushed with fluid.

12. Support the needle with a cotton ball or sterile dressing in a position to maximize the flow of the fluid into the vein.

Pressure from the wall of the vein against the needle opening will decrease or stop the flow of the fluid. Determining maximal fluid flow potential allows the opportunity to adjust the flow rate to desired level without fear of positional change increasing the rate and overhydrating the client.

13. Hang the fluid 18 in to 24 in above the site of infusion if the infusion will flow by gravitational pull. If an infusion pump is used, the height of the solution is not relevant to the rate.

Venous pressure normally is greater than atmospheric pressure. IV fluids will flow from an area of greater to lesser pressure. Elevating the bag or bottle of fluid will use gravity to increase the amount of pressure in the tubing.

14. Apply an antiseptic ointment and sterile dressing to the site. Anchor the needle or catheter with tape.

Pathogens normally found on the skin can cause infection. The smooth muscle structure of the vein does not offer resistance to needle movement.

ACTION

RATIONALE

15. Regulate the flow of the IV fluid to the rate specified by the physician. An infusion pump may be applied to monitor the exact rate of infusion (Fig. 65-6). Many different pumps are available; refer to the manufacturer's directions for method of threading tubing through the pump and operating instructions. If a pump is not used, turn the screw clamp or dial to obtain the desired rate of flow (Fig. 65-7).

Three major factors influence the rate of flow: pressure gradient, size of tubing, and viscosity of solution. Regulation of the flow of the fluid helps ensure that the desired amount of fluid is infused over the prescribed length of time.

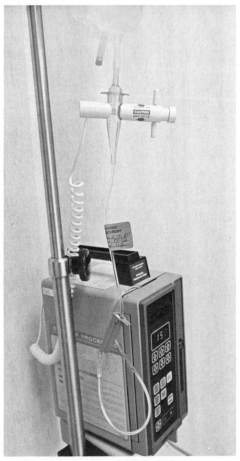

Figure 65.6

16. Restrain the involved arm on an armboard only if the client is unable to hold reasonably still or to hold the arm in the position required to ensure adequate flow rate. Be certain that the restraint is loose enough to avoid interference with the fluid flow or the normal flow of the blood. Angiocaths and intracaths afford the client more mobility. The extremity should be in a position that does not restrict flow of the infusion, but encourages movement.

17. Write the date of insertion, the size of the catheter, and the initials of

Careless movements of the extremity may cause tension on the vein and possibly dislodge the needle or catheter. When the catheter is in the vein, the possibility of accidental dislodgement and penetration of the side of the vein is reduced. Movement is encouraged to prevent stiffness and stasis of the blood in the affected extremity.

ACTION   **RATIONALE**

the nurse inserting the IV needle
or catheter on a piece of tape and
place it on the dressing. Also, add
a piece of tape to the IV tubing
with the date and initials so that it
can be changed every 24 to 72
hours, according to hospital policy
(Fig. 65-8).

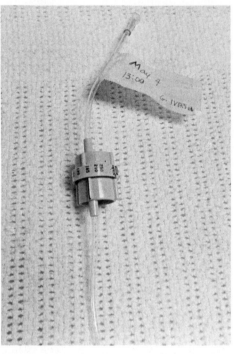

Figure 65.7

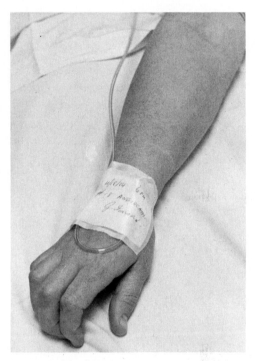

Figure 65.8

18. To discontinue the infusion,
    tighten the clamp to stop the flow
    of fluid. Anchor the needle to pre-
    vent tissue trauma and, with the
    other hand, remove the tape and
    dressings. Gently pull the needle
    or catheter straight out in a steady
    motion. Apply pressure to the
    infusion site with a cotton ball or
    sterile gauze dressing for several
    minutes. Apply a sterile adhesive
    strip or a dressing as indicated by
    the amount of oozing from the site.
    Do not immediately flex the cli-
    ent's arm, since it has been immo-
    bilized for some time.

Tightening the clamp prevents the
fluid from flowing out of the tubing
onto the client after the needle is
removed from the vein, releasing the
counter-pressure. Pressure applied to
the infusion site allows the blood to
clot and prevents bleeding.

Special Modifications

Transfusion of blood

1. Be certain a typing and cross-
   match of blood has been done
   before blood is administered.

Agglutination and hemolysis may
occur as a result of mixing incompatible blood groups.

ACTION	*RATIONALE*
2. Wash hands before and after handling blood.	Prevent cross-contamination and self-contamination.
3. Obtain the blood or blood derivative from the laboratory immediately prior to its administration. Do not keep blood out of proper storage for more than 1 hour.	Improper storage of blood and blood derivatives may cause cell destruction and pathogenic growth.
Proper checking of the blood is absolutely essential to ensure that the right unit is given to the right client. Check the blood identification card against the client's identification band according to hospital policy.	If the wrong blood type is given to a client, a blood reaction may occur. This condition can be life-threatening and must be avoided.
5. Blood is administered through a larger needle or catheter than are other infusions. If it is anticipated that transfusion will be needed, the original venipuncture should be accomplished with a large-bore needle or catheter.	Blood is thick and viscous and requires a larger bore needle for infusion. If the infusion is slowed because of a small needle, the blood may clot.
6. Blood is usually administered through special tubing, which filters the blood as it drips from the bag (Fig. 65-9). A tandem tubing flows into the filter. The first tubing goes to the blood. This tubing is clamped until venous patency of the IV is ensured. The second tubing is attached to a small bottle of normal saline solution. The saline solution is used to prime the tubing and to accomplish venipuncture, if it has not already been done. Once the saline solution is infusing without problems, the saline tubing is clamped off, and the tubing to the unit of blood is unclamped so that the blood may infuse.	The filter removes any small clots and prevents them from entering the vein. The saline solution is used to flush any previously infused fluid from the tubing, since this solution might be incompatible with the blood.

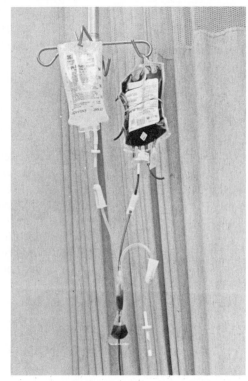

Figure 65.9

ACTION	*RATIONALE*
7. Blood is usually infused at a slow, moderate, or rapid rate, rather than an exact number of ml per hour. Mix the blood frequently by inverting the container during the infusion.	Because of the inconsistency of blood, it cannot be infused at an exactly timed rate. Frequent mixing of the blood helps prevent clumping and clotting.

Communicative Aspects

OBSERVATIONS

1. Check the infusion frequently for proper flow rate. Very rapid infusion is usually contraindicated because of the danger of causing too great a load on the circulatory system. Too slow an infusion rate may result in clotting in the needle or catheter. Flow rate is generally calculated in drops per minute or milliliters per hour.

   a. *Drops per minute:* To calculate, multiply the total amount of infusion (usually 1000 ml) by the number of drops per milliliter (depends on the particular drip chamber; should be available with the literature accompanying the chamber). This is divided by the total number of minutes alloted for the infusion. For example, if 1000 ml is to be infused in 8 hours, the computation would appear as follows:

   $$\frac{1000 \text{ ml} \times 20 \text{ gtt/ml}}{480 \text{ min}} = 41 \text{ gtt/min}$$

   b. *Milliliters per hour:* To calculate, divide the total amount of infusion (usually 1000 ml) by the total time in hours (for example, to be completed in 8 hours). The computation would appear as follows:

   $$\frac{1000 \text{ ml}}{8 \text{ hr}} = 125 \text{ ml/hr}$$

   c. *Microdrip calculations:* The equivalent used for calculating microdrip infusion is 60 microdrops equal 1 ml. To calculate, multiply the number of microdrops in 1 ml by the number of milliliters per hour. For example, when infusing 1000 ml of fluid at 40 ml per hour, the computation would appear as follows:

   40 ml/hr × 60 microgtt/ml = 2400 microgtt/hr or 40 microgtt/min

2. Observe to see that the solution continues to flow into the vein. If the needle or catheter slips out of the vein, the solution will flow into the subcutaneous tissue, causing swelling as the fluid collects. This is referred to as infiltration or extravasation and necessitates discontinuing the IV infusion and restarting it at a different site. If there is a question about whether the needle or catheter is still in the vein, a tourniquet can be applied above the needle, and the IV infusion momentarily stopped. If blood runs into the tubing, the needle or catheter may be assumed to be properly placed. However, if the client experiences pain or burning or if swelling increases, the site should be changed. If an irritating substance, such as a chemotherapeutic agent, is in the fluid, the physician should be notified of the infiltration.

3. Note any signs of redness, tenderness, or pain at the site of injection or path of the vein. This indicates inflammation of the vein, requiring immediate measures to counteract additional complications. The IV infusion is discontinued. The physician may order the application of warm compresses to relieve the discomfort.

4. If more than one bag or bottle of solution is ordered, observe the infusion carefully as it nears completion. The next infusion should be hung before the previous one is completed. This reduces the chance of introducing air into the tubing during the change of solutions. If the infusion is allowed to run dry, a clot may form in the lumen of the needle or catheter. If the infusion is blocked and the blockage cannot be aspirated with a syringe, the site should be changed. Sterile saline solution may be used to irrigate a sluggish infusion; however, never force the fluid in the syringe into the vein to open an occluded infusion because this may dislodge a clot. This clot then becomes an embolus in the client's bloodstream.

5. If any medications are added to the bag or bottle, apply a label to indicate the name of the drug, the dosage, and the time that the medication was added. The date and signature of the person adding medication should also be included. Extreme care must be taken to avoid drug incompatibilities when adding medications to IV infusions. Consult a pharmacology text or a knowledgeable pharmacist before mixing drugs in infusion solutions.

6. At the completion of blood infusion, take the client's vital signs and note the client's condition.

7. Observe the client receiving blood very closely for signs of a blood reaction or other transfusion complications. These include the following:

Fever	Pain
Chills	Dyspnea
Nausea	Shock
Vomiting	Allergic response
Diarrhea	Hematuria

8. If a reaction to the infusion of blood occurs, discontinue infusion of the blood at once. Keep the vein open with normal saline solution until the symptoms can be assessed and the physician is notified. Take the client's vital signs immediately and every 5 to 15 minutes thereafter, depending on the severity of the symptoms and condition of the client. Obtain a urine specimen and send it and the remaining blood or the empty blood bag to the laboratory as soon as possible. All identifying cards and requisitions accompanying the blood should also be sent with the blood bag to the laboratory.

CHARTING

1. Make an entry on the nurses' progress notes about the starting and maintaining of infusions. Vital signs should be taken and charted at the beginning of the infusion to serve as a baseline should any complications occur.

2. Include on the IV record the accurate amount of fluid infused.

Nurses' Progress Notes

DATE/TIME	OBSERVATIONS	SIGNATURE
4/21 0830	1000 ml D5W started via 20-gauge Angiocath in left wrist after povidone-iodine skin preparation. Antiseptic ointment and sterile dressing applied to site. IV infusing at 100 cc/hr with infusion pump. Care of infusion site explained. States he can avoid pulling the tubing and understands the need to ask for help when ambulating to bathroom. B/P 156/80, P 78, R 16. Sleeping at this time. States he will call if any pain, burning, or discomfort is noted in site.	L. James RN

Infusion Record

DATE	INFUSION	TIME START/FINISH	MEDICATIONS	SITE OF INJECTION	RATE
2/3	500 ML whole blood #4258	0930	none	R. forearm #20 angiocath	moderate

Discharge Planning Aspects

CLIENT AND FAMILY EDUCATION

1. Instruct the client and family to report to the nurse any generalized discomfort or pain and swelling at the site of injection.
2. Explain to the client and family the approximate length of time of infusion. Ask them to use the call light when assistance is needed, when the infusion nears completion, if the infusion stops dripping, or if the client experiences any pain.

Evaluation

Quality Assurance

Every hospital should have a formal procedure for administering blood to ensure that adequate precautions are taken to prevent administration of the wrong type of blood. A procedure governing the changing of IV tubing should also be in writing and followed strictly. All hospital policies affecting IV infusion should be based on current Centers for Disease Control recommendations. Documentation of IV infusion should include a description of the site, the process, and the results. Hospital policy should address the consistent changing of the infusion site (e.g., every 48–72 hours) and the frequency of noting on the chart the condition of the IV site (e.g., at least once a shift). The notes should reflect that the nurse understood the possible complications of IV infusion and took precautions to prevent them. The same understanding of complications should be reflected in the administration of blood. Vital signs and indications of blood reaction should be noted. The date and time the venipuncture was made should be documented so that the tubing and site may be changed as mandated by hospital policies. Safety measures and educational efforts undertaken for both the client and family should be documented.

Infection Control

1. Engage in scrupulous handwashing before performing the venipuncture, which is carried out under sterile conditions. Handwashing is necessary after completion of the IV infusion administration technique.
2. Take precautions against accidental contamination by needle stick. Dispose of needles in a designated container that is specially designed and handled to prevent accidents.
3. Prepare the skin by mechanical and chemical cleansing with a bactericidal preparation to render the site of entrance into the vascular system as free as possible from pathogenic organisms.
4. Wash hands before and after handling blood and blood derivatives.
5. The site of the infusion should be changed on a scheduled basis to prevent local or systemic infection. Each hospital should have a policy stating how often tubing, dressings, and sites should be changed. If an IV solution is allowed to hang for longer than 24 horus before infusing, it should be changed because pathogenic organisms will have had a chance to colonize the fluid within that time.
6. Handle blood with extreme care. If personnel are contaminated by blood, report the incident to the employee health department. This is especially important if the blood type is different from that of the employee or if the client had a blood-transmitted disease, such as hepatitis or acquired immune deficiency syndrome (AIDS).

Technique Checklist

	YES	NO
Technique explained to client	_____	_____

Baseline vital signs

   B/P _____ P _____ R _____

Site of infusion _____

Type of needle or catheter

   _____

   Size _____

	YES	NO
Dressing and ointment applied	_____	_____
Desired rate of infusion maintained	_____	_____
Accessory flow control devices used	_____	_____

   Type _____

Duration of infusion _____

Dressing changed how often _____

Site changed how often _____

Tubing changed how often _____

Blood transfused	_____	_____

   # of units _____

   Before beginning transfusion

     Temp _____ B/P _____

     Pulse _____ Resp _____

   After finishing transfusion

     Temp _____ B/P _____

     Pulse _____ Resp _____

Signs of complication noted	_____	_____

66 Isolation Precautions

Overview

Definition

Measures instituted to prevent the spread of microorganisms among hospital clients, staff, and visitors. (The Centers for Disease Control [CDC] in Atlanta, Georgia, recommend two alternatives for implementing isolation precautions. One system relies on the traditional method of established categories of isolation. The other system relies on disease-specific isolation precautions. It is recommended that the hospital infection-control nurse, infection-control committee, epidemiologist, director of nursing service, or a combination of these be familiar with the CDC recommendations and develop guidelines for each individual hospital. The specific techniques used for the categories of isolation precautions will be addressed in this procedure.)

Categories of isolation precautions are as follows:

1. *Strict Isolation:* Designed to prevent transmission of highly contagious or virulent infections that may spread by both droplet and direct contact. Specifications:

   Private Room, with door kept closed, is necessary. The client may share the room with another client with the same diagnosis.

   Masks, gowns, and gloves are essential for all persons entering the room.

   Handwashing is necessary after touching the client or potentially contaminated articles and before taking care of another client.

   Articles contaminated with infective material should be discarded or bagged and labeled before being sent for decontamination and reprocessing.

2. *Contact Isolation:* Designed to prevent transmission of highly transmissible or epidemiologically significant infections. Specifications:

   Private room is needed and may be shared with another client with the same diagnosis.

   Masks are necessary for those in close contact with the client.

   Gowns should be worn if soiling is likely.

   Gloves should be worn for touching infective material.

   Handwashing (same as for strict isolation)

   Articles, contaminated (same as for strict isolation)

3. *Respiratory Isolation:* Designed to prevent transmission of infectious diseases primarily over short distances through air (droplet transmission). Specifications:

   Private room, which may be shared with another client with the same diagnosis, is needed.

   Masks are needed for those who come in close contact with the client.

   Gowns and gloves are not indicated.

   Handwashing (same as for strict isolation)

   Articles, contaminated (same as for strict isolation)

4. *Tuberculosis Isolation (AFB Isolation):* A category for clients with pulmonary tuberculosis (TBF) who have a positive sputum smear or a chest x-ray that strongly suggests active TB. Specifications:

Private room with special ventilation is needed. The door must be kept closed. This client may share the room with another client with the same diagnosis.

Masks are indicated if the client is coughing and does not consistently cover the mouth.

Gowns to prevent gross contamination of clothing are indicated.

Gloves are not indicated.

Handwashing (same as for strict isolation).

Articles are rarely involved in the transmission of TB; however, contaminated articles should be thoroughly cleaned and disinfected or discarded.

5. *Enteric Precautions:* Designed to prevent infections that are transmitted by direct or indirect contact with feces. Specifications:

Private room is indicated if the client's hygiene is inadequate (i.e., the client does not wash hands after touching infective materials, contaminates the environment with infective material, or shares contaminated articles with other clients, as do small children or mentally debilitated clients).

Masks are not indicated.

Gowns are indicated only if soiling is likely.

Gloves are indicated if touching infective material.

Handwashing (same for strict isolation)

Articles, contaminated (same as for strict isolation)

6. *Drainage/Secretions Precautions:* Designed to prevent infections that are transmitted by direct or indirect contact with purulent material or drainage from an infected body site. Specifications:

Private room is not necessary.

Masks are not indicated.

Gowns are necessary if soiling is likely.

Gloves are indicated when touching infective material.

Handwashing is indicated after touching the client or potentially contaminated materials and before taking care of another client.

Articles, contaminated (same as for strict isolation)

7. *Blood/Body Fluid Precautions:* Designed to prevent infections that are transmitted by direct or indirect contact with infective blood or body fluids. Specifications:

Private room is indicated if the client's hygiene is poor (see Enteric Precautions).

Masks are not indicated.

Gowns are indicated if soiling of clothing with blood or body fluids is likely.

Gloves are indicated if touching blood or body fluids.

Hands must be washed immediately if they are or may be contaminated with blood or body fluids and before taking care of another client.

Articles, contaminated (same as for strict isolation)

Care should be taken to avoid needle-stick injuries

Blood spills should be cleaned up promptly with a solution of 5.25% sodium hypochlorite diluted 1:10 with water.

Rationale

Prevent the spread of infectious microorganisms.

Promote an understanding of the infectious process in pursuing rational approaches to containing the organism, using knowledge of the mechanisms of disease transmission.

Promote recovery of the infected or colonized client.

Terminology

Colonization: Presence of microorganisms in or on a host, with growth and multiplication but without tissue invasion or damage; no cellular injury results.

Contamination: The presence of microorganisms on inanimate objects (e.g., clothing, surgical instruments) or in substances (e.g., water, food)

Cross-transmission: A communicable condition superimposed on a person already in the hospital for treatment of a nonrelated condition

Host: The organism from which a parasite receives its nourishment

Infection: The entry and multiplication of an infectious agent in the tissues of the host

Source: The person(s) or thing(s) from which the disease process is emanating; it may be clients, staff, visitors, or contaminated objects in the environment.

Vector: An animal that transmits the causative organisms of disease from infected to noninfected persons

Assessment

Pertinent Anatomy and Physiology

Immunity is a normal, adaptive response. It protects the body from destruction by foreign materials and invasion by microbial agents. *Active immunity* implies that the body has developed or acquired the ability to defend itself against a specific agent. It is achieved by actually having the disease or by immunization. *Passive immunity* is temporary immunity that is borrowed from another source, such as that an infant receives from its mother's milk.

Pathophysiological Concepts

1. Clients' resistance to pathogenic microorganisms varies greatly. Persons with diabetes mellitus, lymphoma, leukemia, neoplasia, granulocytopenia, or uremia and those treated with certain antimicrobials, corticosteroids, irradiation, or immunosuppressive agents may be particularly prone to infection. Age, chronic debilitating disease, shock, coma, traumatic injury, or surgical procedures also make a person more susceptible to infection.

2. Microorganisms are transmitted by various routes. The four main routes of transmission are as follows:

   Contact

   Direct: Direct physical transfer between a susceptible host and an infected or colonized person, such as occurs when personnel turn or bathe clients

   Indirect: Personal contact of the susceptible host with a contaminated intermediate object, usually inanimate, such as instruments and dressings

   Droplet: Infectious agents come in contact with the conjunctivae, nose, or mouth of a susceptible person as a result of an infected person's coughing, sneezing, or talking. Droplets travel no more than 3 feet.

   Vehicle: Applies in diseases transmitted through contaminated food (salmonellosis), water (legionellosis), drugs (bacteremia), and blood products (hepatitis B)

   Airborne: Transmission by dissemination of either droplet residue that remains suspended in the air or dust particles containing the infectious organisms

   Vectorborne: Transmission by vectors is of greater concern in tropical countries (e.g., malaria)

Assessment of the Client

1. Assess the client's and family's level of understanding the infectious process. Determine the knowledge deficits and most effective way to overcome these deficits while gaining the client's and family's compliance in control of the infectious process.

2. Assess the client's physical condition. Determine the level of self-care possible and interventions to promote health. Determine what effects the specific isolation will have on the client and how much compliance can be expected.

3. Assess the infectious process. Determine the proper isolation precautions based on hospital policy and the client's particular condition. Determine specific transmission possibilities and how to prevent contamination of other persons.

Plan

Nursing Objectives

Assist in identifying the infective agent and establishing a diagnosis.

Control and prevent the spread of infection.

Provide physiological support and symptomatic relief.

Teach the client, family, visitors, and ancillary hospital personnel the essentials of infection prevention and control.

Prevent fear and loneliness for the client while adhering to isolation specifications.

Prepare the client in such a way that self-responsibility for infection control will be assumed to the degree possible, based on the client's age, condition, and understanding.

Rationally determine the degree of isolation needed to protect the client and other persons while attempting to keep costs contained and loneliness and embarrassment minimized.

Client Preparation

1. Explain the reasons for the particular isolation precautions. Do not make the client feel guilty or embarrassed about the condition. Present the facts in a straightforward way and inform the client and family of their responsibilities in preventing spread of the infection.

2. Place the client in a private room, if indicated. Explain restrictions on visiting and the client's mobility. Place an isolation card of some type on the door to remind visitors about precautions to be taken.

Equipment

Lined wastebaskets at the bedside, in the bathroom, and at the door

Paper towels and soap dispenser in the bathroom (antiseptic solution for handwashing for highly contagious or virulent microorganisms)

Appropriate isolation card for door

Disposable masks, if specified

Gowns and gloves, if specified

Impervious bags

Implementation and Interventions

Procedural Aspects

ACTION	RATIONALE
1. Determine the proper type of isolation, based on the client's diagnosis and symptoms and identification of the infective organism.	The focus of CDC guidelines is a rational approach to isolation based on common sense and the peculiarities of the particular microorganism. A combination of isolation categories may be used, or one specific category

ACTION	RATIONALE
	may adequately contain the infective agents. Attention should be focused on the reasoning behind the actions rather than on the ritual of the actions themselves.
2. Make frequent visits to the isolation room to check on the client. It is not necessary to go into the room, but simply open the door and check on the client for reassurance.	Loneliness is an unpleasant and much avoided emotional experience, accompanying real or imagined isolation from others. The awareness that one is not alone is basic to psychological homeostasis.
3. Offer diversions, such as television viewing or reading, for the client on isolation precautions. (The pediatric client should have toys that can be terminally cleaned.)	Emotions may be controlled or manipulated by diverting attention from events that cause emotional reactions. Periods of diversion are especially important to isolation clients, who cannot participate in the normal social interaction of the nursing unit.
4. Bathe the client on isolation precautions daily. Give a bed bath if the client's condition prevents bathing in the tub or shower. A private bathroom with bathing facilities should be available to the isolated client. Clean away body discharges quickly and thoroughly.	Cleanliness discourages the growth of microorganisms. Daily bathing provides soothing comfort and relaxation, in addition to retarding the spread of pathogens. It also offers the nurse an opportunity to observe for skin rash, pressure areas, and ancillary problems.
5. Identify the clean and the contaminated areas. Also, identify the discharges considered infective. The goal of isolation is to recognize the substances that contain the infective material and to prevent these substances from coming in contact with other persons. Take whatever measures are necessary to prevent this contact, but take excessive and elaborate measures only if they are indicated and are really necessary to prevent the spread of infective material.	Clean items, surfaces, and areas become contaminated when they come in contact with *infective material*. If the nurse enters a room to ask a question and the infective organism does not travel by the airborne route, wearing a gown and mask is a waste of time and money. However, if the nurse is cleaning up a soiled client who is not known to be infected, wearing a gown would be expedient because of the known flora of the intestinal system.
6. Wearing a gown when entering a room where this precaution is specified should proceed from an understanding of what the nurse is trying to accomplish. Put on the gown with the opening in the back (Fig. 66-1). Overlap the gown in the back and secure it with ties or snaps. To remove the	The goal of gowning is to prevent clothing from coming in contact with infective materials. Take whatever measures are needed to prevent this occurrence. If soiling is heavy, two gowns may be needed. If no contact will be made, wearing a gown may be unnecessary.

ACTION   **RATIONALE**

gown, untie it at the waist and neck (Figs. 66-2, 66-3). Wash the hands thoroughly with soap or an antiseptic and warm running water (Fig. 66-4). Pull off one sleeve by slipping the fingers under the cuff (Fig. 66-5) and pulling the sleeve over the hand. Grasp the other sleeve through the material of the first sleeve and pull it off (Fig. 66-6). Fold the outer contaminated surfaces together (Fig. 66-7) and place the gown in a specified linen hamper (Fig. 66-8). If masks and gloves are specified, they should be of the disposable variety and should be used only once (Figs. 66-9, 66-10).

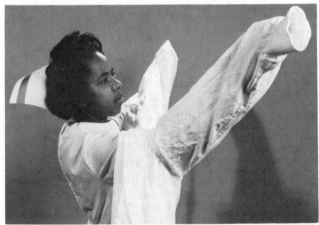

Figure 66.1

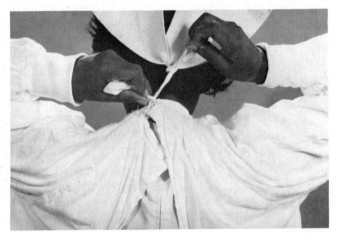

Figure 66.2

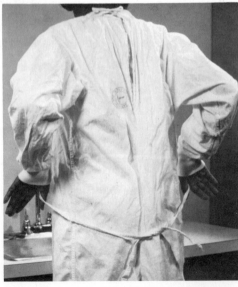

Figure 66.3

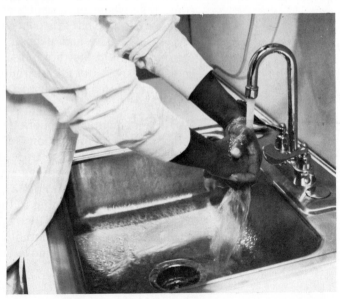

Figure 66.4

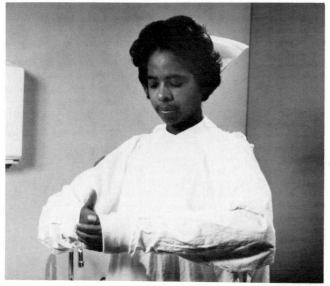

Figure 66.5

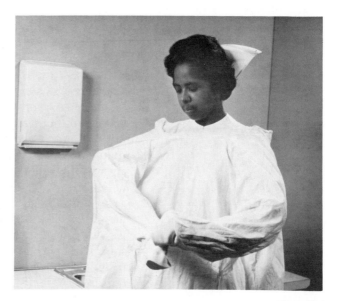

Figure 66.6

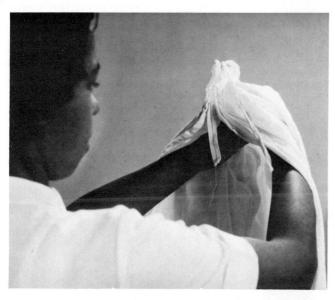

Figure 66.7

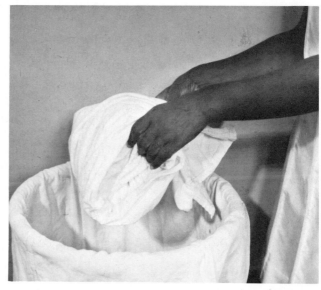

Figure 66.8

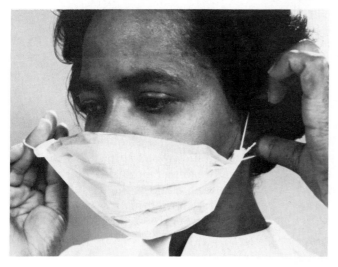

Figure 66.9

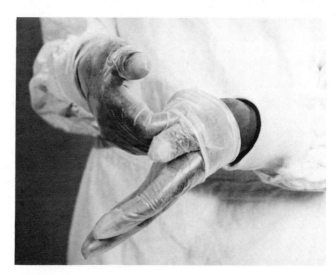

Figure 66.10

ACTION	*RATIONALE*
7. Gather equipment before entering the isolation room to prevent unnecessary trips in and out of the room. The client should have a thermometer for exclusive use. If a digital thermometer is used, take care not to touch any part of the probe except the disposable cover to the client's mucous membranes. If the client cannot control the spread of infective material, as in coughing or sneezing, use a glass thermometer. The same principles apply to the use of stethoscopes and sphygmomanometers. If these items will not come in contact with the infective secretions or materials, they may be used on the isolated client with the same precautions used for all clients.	Organization of equipment and nursing actions minimizes the chance of transfer of infective materials and conserves time and energy.
8. Place contaminated items in a nonpenetrable bag (see the Infection Control section of this technique). To single-bag, simply place the item in the impervious bag, label, and tape shut. To double-bag, place the contaminated item in a bag and close it (Figs. 66-11, 66-12). Another nurse makes a cuff around the top of a second bag and holds it with hands under the cuff. Place the first bag into the second bag, being careful not to touch the outside of the second bag (Fig. 66-13). The second nurse will then securely close the bag by folding, tape it shut, and label it with date, contents, and some type of notation that infective material is contained therein (Fig. 66-14). The bag is then disposed of or transported according to hospital policy.	The goal is to prevent the infective material from coming in contact with anyone or anything else. Use whatever means are necessary to accomplish this. For some items, three or four bags may be needed to contain the infective material adequately and to prevent contamination of other persons. For small items with minimal contamination, a single bag may be adequate.
9. Wash hands thoroughly after contact with the client on isolation precautions. Always use soap. For particularly virulent infectious organisms, washing with an antiseptic may be needed.	Running water mechanically washes away organisms. Soap emulsifies matter and lowers surface tension. Handwashing before and after contact with each client is the most important means of preventing the spread of infection (Fig. 66-15).
10. For a complete list of category-specific isolation precautions, write to the Centers for Disease Control, Atlanta, Georgia.	

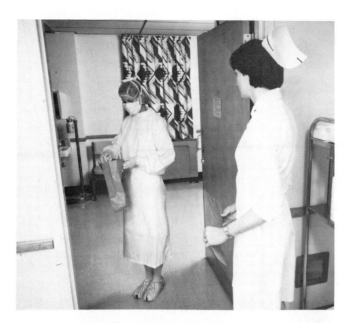

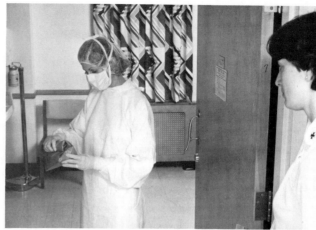

Figure 66.12

Figure 66.11

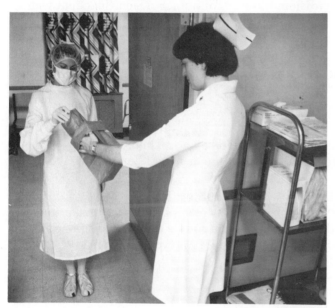

Figure 66.13

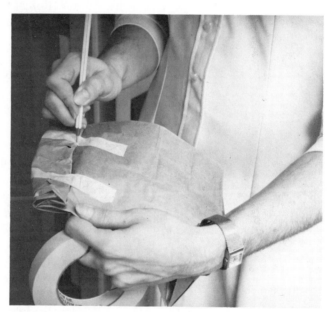

Figure 66.14

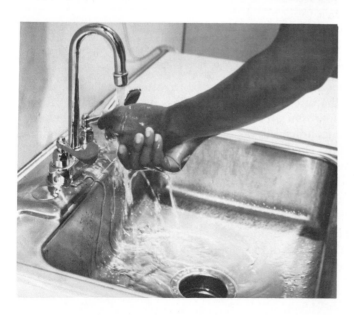

Figure 66.15

ACTION	*RATIONALE*

Special Modifications

> **Severely Compromised Clients**

See Technique 58, Gown and Glove Procedure, Sterile, for details on providing a sterile environment for the client at high risk of becoming infected. When changing a dressing, use of a mask and hair covering may be advisable, in addition to sterile gown and gloves. Keep in mind that the goal is to prevent contamination of the client with substances that might cause infection.	The CDC no longer recognize a specific category such as reverse or protective isolation. They state, "such a regimen does not appear to reduce (the risk to severely compromised patients) any more than strong emphasis on appropriate handwashing during patient care."[1] Therefore, the nurse is advised to take whatever precautions are needed to prevent contaminating the severely compromised client.

Communicative Aspects

OBSERVATIONS

1. Observe the clinical progression of the condition for which the client was admitted, as well as the progress of the infectious condition. Measurement of vital signs and other clinical indicators remains an important part of the care of an isolated client.

2. If the client is experiencing diarrhea, note the frequency, amount, and character of each stool.

3. Inspect the skin for any rash, pressure areas, or other effects of prolonged immobility.

4. Observe the client's emotional response to being isolated. Note the degree of acceptance or rejection of the illness and the degree of compliance with restrictions.

5. If the client is experiencing nausea and vomiting, fever, or diarrhea or is receiving intravenous (IV) feedings, accurate measurement of intake and output (I&O) is needed. If the body fluids are a source of contamination, take adequate precautions when measuring these to prevent the spread of the infectious process.

CHARTING

DATE/TIME	OBSERVATIONS	SIGNATURE
9/10 1430	Enteric precautions maintained. Passive ROM exercises for 15 min. Skin remains clear with no signs of pressure. No more diarrhea since last night.	F. White RN

Discharge Planning Aspects

CLIENT AND FAMILY EDUCATION

1. As much time and energy as necessary should be invested in teaching the client and family about the infectious disease process, how it is transmitted, and how certain precautions can prevent spreading the infection. The client should be allowed and encouraged to take some responsibility for preventing the spread of the infection. The family members should have a clear understanding of their responsibilities to the client, other persons, and themselves in preventing the spread of the infectious process. If the mechanism of infection is understood by the client, the family, and the staff, prevention can be based on knowledgeable use of common sense and established techniques.

2. Teach the family members the techniques specified by the type of isolation (e.g., the gowning technique). Encourage them to ask questions if unsure or anxious about any aspect of care.

3. If the client will go home with the infectious process, explain to the family how to care for the client and how to prevent the spread of the infection after discharge.

REFERRALS

A referral to a visiting health nurse or home health agency may benefit the family that is uneasy about caring for the client at home. Be sure that the referral includes details about the specific infective process for the protection of the nurses and to allow the client to benefit from the referral.

The Centers for Disease Control, Atlanta, Georgia, is an excellent resource for answering questions and providing information about disease prevention and infection control.

Evaluation

Quality Assurance

Documentation of the client's care should reflect monitoring of the clinical progress during hospitalization. The client's vital signs and other pertinent information should be reflected. Attention to the side-effects of isolation, such as emotional problems, should be in evidence. The type of precautions should be noted. The chart should show evidence that the nurse understood the mechanism of transmission of the client's particular infective process and used appropriate means to prevent cross-transmission.

The hospital is responsible for ensuring that clients are placed on appropriate isolation precautions. Each hospital should designate clearly, as a matter of policy, the personnel responsible for placing a client on isolation precautions and the personnel who have the ultimate authority to make decisions about isolation precautions when conflicts arise. Hospital policy should also address proper disposal of infected waste. This is usually done in conjunction with the city's sanitation and sewage departments. The hospital policy manual should offer detailed guidance for proper disposal of needles, care of infected clients, and prevention of cross-transmission.

Infection Control

1. Handwashing is the most important means of preventing the spread of infection. Personnel should always wash their hands, even when gloves are used, after care of a client with an infectious process or one who is colonized with significant microorganisms. Faucet handles, if not foot or knee controlled, should be turned off with a paper towel to prevent recontamination of clean hands. In addition, personnel should wash their hands after touching excretions or secretions, and before touching any client again. Hands should be washed before performing invasive procedures, touching wounds, or touching clients who are particularly susceptible to infection.

2. The use of a private room can reduce the possibility of transmission of infectious agents by separating infected clients from susceptible clients and by reminding personnel to wash their hands, especially if a sink is available at the doorway. However, a private room is not necessary to prevent the spread of many infections. A private room is indicated for clients with highly infectious or virulent infections, for clients with poor hygiene, for clients colonized with significant microorganisms, and for most clients with airborne infections. If infected or colonized persons are not placed in a private room, they should be placed with appropriate roommates (e.g., someone who is not likely to become infected).

3. Masks are recommended to prevent transmission of infectious agents through the air. Masks should cover the nose and mouth. They protect against inhaling droplets and discourage personnel from touching the mucous membranes of their eyes, nose or mouth until after they have washed their hands. Disposable masks are recommended, and they are worn only once.

4. Gowns are recommended to prevent soiling of clothing when caring for clients. Gowns are worn only once and discarded in an appropriate container. Gowns are indicated if the clothing is likely to be soiled with infective secretions or excretions or for highly infectious organisms known to cause epidemiologic problems in hospitals, such as varicella (chicken pox) or disseminated zoster. Clean, freshly laundered gowns or disposable gowns are usually worn. In selected instances, such as when caring for a client with extensive burns, sterile gowns may be worn when changing dressings.

5. There are three reasons to wear gloves: to reduce the possibility of personnel becoming infected, to reduce the possibility of personnel transmitting their own endogenous microbial flora to clients, and to reduce the possibility of personnel being transiently colonized with microorganisms that could be transmitted to other clients. Gloves are needed when touching excretions, secretions, blood, or body fluids that are listed as infective materials. Disposable, single-use gloves should be used. If the gloves come into contact with infective secretions during care, they should be changed before care continues.

6. Bagging of articles is intended to prevent inadvertent exposure of personnel to contaminated articles and to prevent contamination of the environment. Most articles do not need to be bagged unless they are contaminated with infective material. A single bag is probably adequate if it is impervious and sturdy, and the item can be completely enclosed within the bag and placed into the bag without contaminating the outside. Otherwise, double-bagging is indicated. Bags should be labeled or colored to designate that they contain contaminated articles or infective waste.

7. Reusable equipment should be returned to a central processing area to be decontaminated by knowledgeable personnel. It should be bagged and remain bagged until decontaminated. Large items should be disinfected prior to transport.

8. Needles, syringes, and other sharp objects pose a particular threat. Personnel should handle all used needles and syringes cautiously because the extent of potential infection usually is unknown. Used needles should not be recapped. They should be placed in prominently labeled, puncture-resistant containers designated specifically for this purpose. Needles should not be bent or broken by hand because accidental needle puncture may occur. Reusable needles and syringes should be bagged, labeled, and returned for decontamination and reprocessing.

9. Soiled linen should be handled as little as possible with a minimum of agitation to prevent contamination of the air and persons handling the linen. A laundry bag should be in the client's room and should be labeled or of a particular color to denote infection precautions.

10. No special precautions are necessary for dishes unless they are visibly contaminated with infective material. Reusable dishes that are visibly contaminated should be bagged and returned for decontamination.

11. All dressings, paper tissue, and other disposable items soiled with infective material should be bagged, labeled, and disposed of according to hospital policy.

12. Laboratory specimens should be placed in well-constructed containers with secure lids to prevent leaking during transport. Care should be taken when collecting a specimen not to contaminate the outside of the container. Specimens may need to be bagged and labeled to prevent accidental exposure of transportation or receiving personnel.

13. Persons who are infected or colonized with significant microorganisms should leave their rooms only for essential purposes. Appropriate barriers (such as masks and impervious dressings) to prevent transmission should be used by the client and transport personnel. Personnel in the area to which the client is being transported should be notified of the client's arrival and of necessary precautions.

Technique Checklist

	YES	NO
Isolation procedure explained to client and family	_____	_____

Type of isolation maintained

Strict _____

Respiratory _____

Contact _____

AFB _____

Enteric _____

Drainage/secretion _____

Blood/body fluid _____

Other _____

Techniques used

Gowns _____

Masks _____

Gloves _____

Needle Box _____

Biohazard linen hampers _____

Bagging _____

Proper handwashing used	_____	_____
Referral for infectious disease follow-up	_____	_____

Reference

1. Garner J, Simmons B: Guidelines for isolation precautions in hospitals. Infection Control 4(4):325, 1983.

67 Medications, Administration of

Overview

Definition

The process by which prescribed drugs are given to a client. Types include the following:

Oral administration: The process of administering drugs in the liquid or solid state (tablet, capsule) for absorption from the gastrointestinal (GI) tract

Inhalation administration: The process of administering drugs in the gaseous or vapor state for absorption from the respiratory tract

Topical administration: The process of administering drugs in liquid (lotion, liniment), semisolid (ointment, cream), or solid state (lozenges, suppositories) for absorption from the skin or mucous membranes

Parenteral administration: The process of administering drugs in solution or suspension by injection. Types include:

Intradermal: A very small amount of solution (usually 0.1 ml) is injected just below the surface of the skin in the form of a wheal for local rather than systemic effect (e.g., TB skin test, local anesthetic).

Subcutaneous (SC) or hypodermic (H): A small amount (0.5 ml–1.0 ml) of highly soluble medication is injected into the loose connective tissue under the skin for the purpose of administering a drug when the oral route is not feasible (e.g., the drug is destroyed by gastric juices, the client cannot tolerate oral drugs, a more rapid effect than that of oral administration is desired) or a slower, more sustained action is desired than is possible with the intramuscular (IM) route.

Intramuscular (IM): A fairly large amount (up to 5.0 ml)* of solution or suspension is injected into the muscle body when a more rapid absorption is desired than with the SC route or the drug is irritating to the subcutaneous tissues or dangerous if injected intravenously. IM Z-track is a special IM injection in which the SC tissues are pulled aside during injection and allowed to return to normal position after injection, thus sealing off the needle track and preventing irritating or staining drugs (such as dextran iron complex [Imferon]) from leaking into the SC tissues.

Intravenous (IV): Varying volumes of completely soluble solutions are injected directly into the vein for immediate absorption.

Rationale

Aid the body in overcoming illness.

Relieve symptoms of illness.

Promote health and prevent disease.

Aid in diagnosis.

Hydrate the body cells and tissues.

---

*Larger amounts (e.g., 15 ml) of isotonic solutions, such as blood or gamma globulin, occasionally are injected into the gluteus maximus. Amounts of injections may be divided into two doses, even if the total is under 5 ml, if the client is very emaciated.

Terminology

Ampule: A small sealed glass containing sterile solution for injection

Diffusion: The movement of charged and uncharged particles along a concentration gradient

Edema: Accumulation of fluid in the tissues

Meniscus: The convex or concave upper surface of a column of liquid, the curvature of which is caused by surface tension

Placebo: An inactive substance given to satisfy a client's demand for medicine when it is felt that such medication would not be in the best therapeutic interests of the client

Vial: A glass bottle, sealed with a rubber stopper, containing sterile medicine or solution, usually in multi-dose amounts

Assessment

Pertinent Anatomy and Physiology

1. See Appendix I: *skin, blood vessels, skeletal muscles, stomach.*
2. Absorption of oral medications occurs mainly in the small intestine. The intestinal folds greatly increase absorptive ability. Absorption occurs by active transport across the intestinal wall and diffusion.

Pathophysiological Concepts

1. Diminished or impaired circulation may decrease the efficiency with which blood and its nutrients are delivered to the rest of the body. Heart failure results when the heart fails to pump blood in amounts sufficient to meet the metabolic needs of the body. Fluid then accumulates in the tissues, and cardiac output is decreased. Medication in the tissue is poorly absorbed, and desired results are slowed or inhibited altogether. When normal circulation is restored and edema decreases, larger than desired doses of medication may suddenly be released into the vascular system.

2. The kidneys control the concentration of most of the constituents in body fluids, including water and electrolytes. The functional units of the kidneys, the nephrons, filter the blood and selectively reabsorb constituents. Drugs are also filtered through the kidneys. Diminished or altered kidney function can result in undesirable drug build-up. The reabsorption of water by the kidneys is regulated by antidiuretic hormone (ADH), which is formed in the hypothalamus and secreted by the pituitary. Glandular malfunction can result in altered ADH levels and malabsorption of medications. Therapeutic dosages may be rendered useless or toxic.

3. An important function of the liver is the metabolism of hormones and drugs. When the liver is diseased, the plasma-binding ability of drugs is altered because of a decrease in albumin production. There is also a decreased removal of drugs that are metabolized by the liver. Liver disease may greatly alter the action of drugs on the system.

Assessment of the Client

1. Assess the client's physical status as it affects the ability to take oral medications. If nausea and vomiting are present, the IM, IV, or rectal (suppository) route may be preferable.

2. Assess the client's nutritional status. If the client is emaciated, exercise great care in selecting a site for IM injection, being sure that there is adequate muscle mass to contain the dose. It may be necessary to break the dose into smaller amounts and to use shorter needles for injection. In obese clients, be sure that IM injections go into the muscle and not into the fatty tissue. Longer needles may be used, or the injection may be given in the arm or thigh rather than the buttocks.

3. Assess the client's and family's knowledge of drug action, expected results, and possible side-effects. Assess the history of drug use, both prescription and nonprescription.

Plan

Nursing Objectives

Allay the client's fear of and anxiety about the administration of the drug and its expected results.

Administer drugs according to the "Five Rights":

Right drug

Right dose

Right route

Right time

Right client

Observe, report, and record desired therapeutic effects, precautions taken, and untoward reactions of the drug administered.

Client Preparation

1. Before any medication is administered, take a complete drug allergy history. Explain to the client about the drugs being taken and the expected effects. Explain about any anticipated side-effects.

2. Before giving oral medications, be certain that the client has fresh water. If the medication is highly unpalatable, as are many cancer chemotherapeutic drugs and potassium supplements, offer juice or nectar to the client, if not contraindicated because of diet or incompatability.

3. If the drug being given is to have a relaxing, tranquilizing, or sedating effect, ask the client to void, darken the room, and decrease external stimuli before the medication is given.

Equipment

ALL DRUGS

Medication card or file

Medication, as ordered

Tray for carrying groups of medications or cart for transporting medications

ORAL DRUGS

Paper cup or medicine glass

INHALATION DRUGS

Atomizer or inhaler

TOPICAL DRUGS

Glove or applicators for lotions, liniments, and creams

Glove and lubricant for suppositories or special applicator provided with drug

PARENTERAL DRUGS

Alcohol sponge or topical antiseptic

Syringe to accommodate volume of medication

Needle

Intradermal: ½ in, 25-gauge

SC: ½ in to 1 in, 23- to 27-gauge

IM: 1½ in, 20- to 22-gauge, depending on viscosity of solution and muscle size

Tourniquet for IV injection

Implementation and Interventions

Procedural Aspects

	ACTION	RATIONALE

Medication Orders

1. Give all medications, including placebos, only on the order of a licensed physician or other licensed person who is legally allowed to write medication orders according to state law.

   Prescription of medications is a legal privilege granted by state law. These laws differ from state to state.

2. Be sure that every order includes the name of the drug, dose, route, time(s) to be given, and signature of licensed person.

   These parameters are considered the minimum information required for safe administration of medications.

Preparation of Medications

1. Review drug literature carefully for any unfamiliar medication, including usual dose, route, and precautions or possible side-effects. If in doubt about any drug ordered, consult the charge nurse, pharmacist, physician, or nurse practitioner until all doubts are resolved.

   It is the professional nurse's responsibility to be familiar with every drug he or she administers.

2. Check the medication label three times:
   (a) When the container is removed from the storage area (Fig. 67-1)
   (b) When pouring or measuring the medication (Fig. 67-2) or when comparing the prepackaged medication with the Kardex
   (c) Immediately before returning the container to the storage area (Fig. 67-3) or before discarding the package

   Triple-checking helps reduce the chance of medication error.

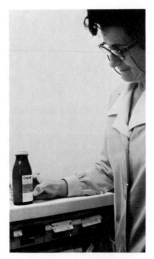 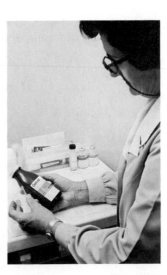 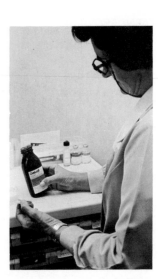

Figure 67.1 *Figure 67.2* *Figure 67.3*

ACTION	*RATIONALE*
3. Solid stable dosage forms may be prepared up to 1 hour before administration. Check any contra-indications (e.g., the need for refrigeration).	Stable forms, such as tablets and cap-sules, will not decompose while standing.
4. *Tablets, capsules preparation:* Pour desired number into cap of bottle and from there into medicine cup (Fig. 67-4). *Do not* touch medica-tions with fingers or return medications to container from cup. If the medication is individually packaged in unit-dose form, take it to the client unopened. In the cli-ent's room, open the dose and pour directly into the client's hand or mouth. *Do not* touch the medication unless the client needs assistance. Wash hands before assisting the client with taking the medication.	Avoidance of touching the medication reduces the chance of cross-contamination. Handwashing further reduces the chance of spreading infection.

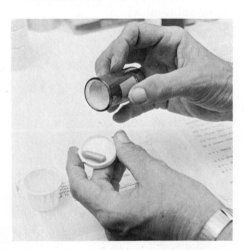

Figure 67.4

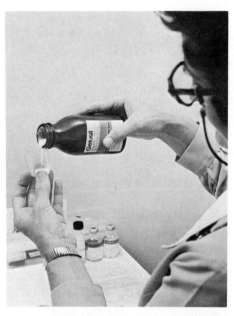

Figure 67.5

5. *Liquids, preparation:* Shake the bottle thoroughly, unless specifi-cally contraindicated by notation on the bottle or label. Pour the medication with the cup at eye level and with the bottle label in view (Fig. 67-5). Pour until the level of the medication is even with the mark on the measuring cup, designating the ordered quan-tity of medication. Wipe the edge of the bottle before replacing the cap. Many liquid preparations are also prepackaged. Read the label to see if the individual dose should be shaken to mix before administering.	Particles held in suspension can be evenly dispersed throughout the medication by shaking the bottle. Exact dosage must be given to obtain maximal therapeutic effect. Many drugs contain sugar or its derivatives to enhance palatability. If not wiped clean, the cap may stick to the bottle.

ACTION	**RATIONALE**
6. *Topical and inhalation medications preparation:* Prepare according to label.	Preparations vary and should be prepared according to the individual manufacturer's directions.
7. *Parenteral preparations:* Most injections are prepackaged. Be sure that the right dose is in the syringe and inject according to the manufacturer's directions. If the medications is in a vial, clean the stopper thoroughly with an alcohol sponge (Fig. 67-6). Inject air into the vial in an amount equal to the amount of solution to be withdrawn (Fig. 67-7). Aspirate the amount of medication needed and remove the needle from the vial (Fig. 67-8). The vial should be upright when the air is injected into the vial, and the needle should not be within the medication itself. The vial should then be turned upside down, and the needle should be located within the solution when the medication is withdrawn.	Prepackaging ensures the sterility of the drug, decreases the chance of contamination, and provides easier storage and distribution. Cleansing the stopper reduces the chance of introducing microorganisms into the sterile container. If air is not injected to replace the fluid being removed, a negative pressure is created, causing difficulty in aspirating the medication from the vial. The needle is not placed in the medication when the air is injected because of the chance of creating air bubbles within the medication. The needle must be within the medication for withdrawal to avoid filling the syringe with the previously injected air.

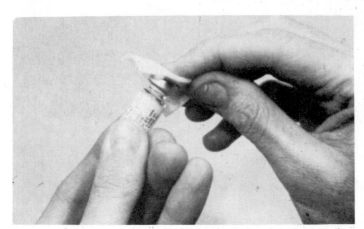

Figure 67.6

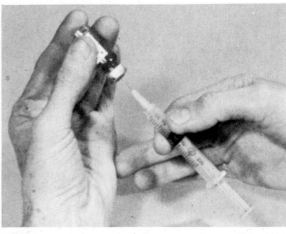

Figure 67.7

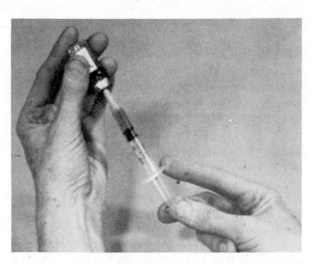

Figure 67.8

ACTION

If the medication is in an ampule, file one side of the indented neck (Fig. 67-9). With the filed side in view, break off the top of the ampule with a pushing movement. Hold the top of the ampule with a sponge (Fig. 67-10). If the ampule has a colored line around the neck, there is no need to file it (Fig. 67-11). Place the needle into the ampule and invert it to withdraw the medication (Figs. 67-12, 67-13).

RATIONALE

Care must be taken to avoid injury breaking off the top of the ampule. Using a pad or sponge will protect the fingers from the edges of the ampule.

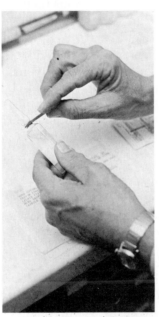

Figure 67.9

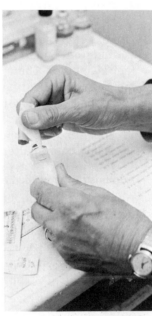

Figure 67.10

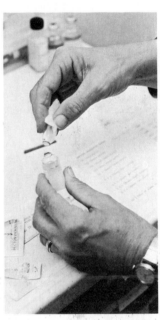

Figure 67.11

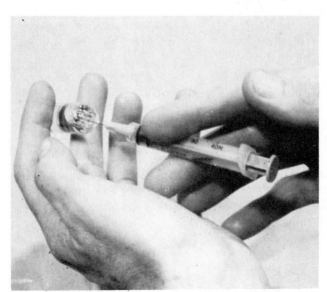

Figure 67.12

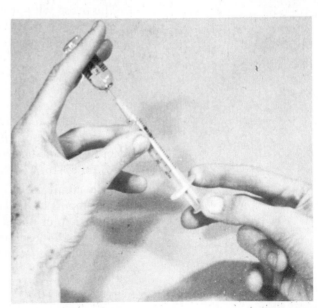

Figure 67.13

ACTION	*RATIONALE*
8. Do not give drugs that have changed color, consistency, or odor. Do not give medications from unlabeled containers or containers whose labels are unreadable. Only a pharmacist may legally fill or relabel bottles in most states.	Changes in medications may mean that they are no longer stable and cannot be depended upon to produce desired results. The primary concern is to protect the client from mistakes and errors.
9. Exercise caution when mixing medications. Do not give medications if they change color or form a precipitate when mixed. Check a compatibility chart *before* mixing.	Some drugs react with each other when mixed and undergo chemical changes, as evidenced by the color change or precipitate. This means that they may no longer be the medications that were ordered and may, in fact, be harmful.
10. Use extreme caution when converting from one measurement system to another. There are several methods of converting units, but all depend on knowing the basic equivalents. See conversion tables in Appendix 3 for common conversions and computation techniques.	When possible, exact measurements should be made. In conversions, approximation is sometimes necessary. If in doubt, check with the pharmacist, physician or nurse practitioner. Keep the client's safety uppermost in mind.

Administration of Medications

ACTION	*RATIONALE*
1. Administer routine medications within 30 minutes of the designated time. Certain medications, such as antibiotics and chemotherapeutic agents, must be administered at the designated time.	Certain drugs depend on maintenance of a constant blood level for maximal benefit.
2. Stat and preoperative medication orders must be given exactly on time.	The purpose of a stat order is to control the timing of administration.
3. The nurse who prepares the medications must be the one who administers and charts it. Before administering any drug, identify the client by checking the medication card or file against the bed card and the client's identification band. Ask the client's name and wait for a response before administering the medication. (Figs. 67-14, 67-15, 67-16, 67-17).	This precaution protects the client and the nurse from mistakes.
4. If the client refuses the medication, report to the charge nurse, physician, or nurse practitioner. Discard the dose down the sink and chart the reason for refusal.	Documentation and communication help ensure that informed and knowledgeable care is given.

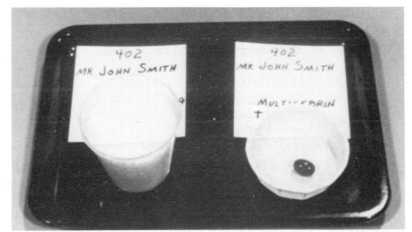

Figure 67.14

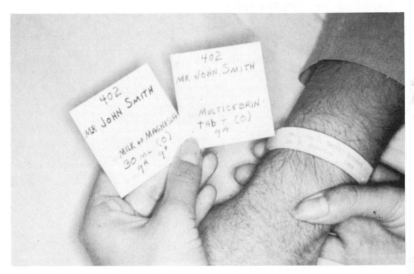

Figure 67.15

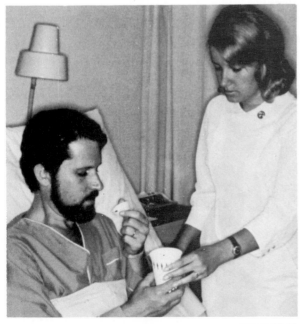

Figure 67.16

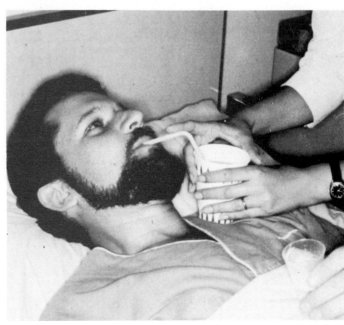

Figure 67.17

ACTION	**RATIONALE**
5. If the client vomits soon after administration of oral medications, attempt to identify the medications. Report the incident, and *do not* repeat the medications until requested to do so.	It is difficult to determine the exact amount of medication absorbed by the client.

Special Precautions for Special Drugs

1. *Digitalis preparations:* Note the radial pulse rate before administering (Fig. 67-18). If the pulse is below 60 beats/minute, evaluate and notify the appropriate person before administering digitalis preparations.	Digitalis increases the force and strength of ventricular contraction; however, it also slows the heart rate by decreasing conduction through the A-V node.

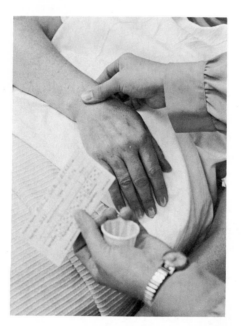

Figure 67.18

2. *Heparin:* Inject heparin into the SC tissues of the abdomen or iliac crest. Inject 0.1 ml of air following the heparin. Draw up this amount of air when drawing up the injection. Do not draw back on the plunger of the syringe to check vein insertion. Never massage the site after an injection of heparin.	These SC routes are desirable because they are distant from major muscle groups, and their use reduces the possibility of hematoma. Aspiration is avoided because of the possibility of causing hematoma by shaking the needle. The air injected after the heparin prevents leakage and hemorrhage into intradermal layers. Massaging can also cause dispersal of the medication, resulting in hematoma.

ACTION	RATIONALE
3. *Insulin:* Rotate the sites of insulin injection in a consistent manner according to a definite plan (Fig. 67-19). When mixing regular and long-acting insulins, draw up the regular insulin first. Clean the tops of both vials of insulin with an alcohol sponge. Inject the amount of air into the vial that is equal to the amount of insulin to be withdrawn (Fig. 67-20). Invert the insulin and withdraw the desired amount (Fig. 67-21).	Rotation of sites is necessary because of the frequency of insulin injection and the chance of tissue breakdown. Regular insulin should be kept free of contamination with the insoluble long-acting insulins because regular insulin may be given by IV route in an emergency.

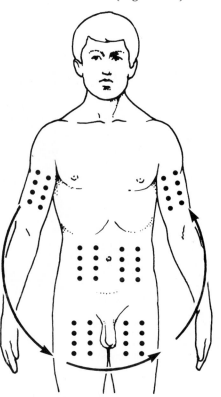

Figure 67.19

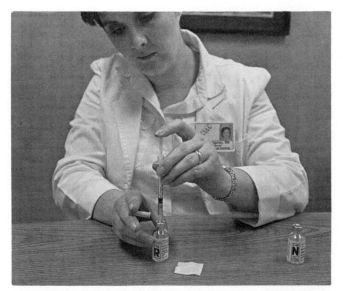

Figure 67.20

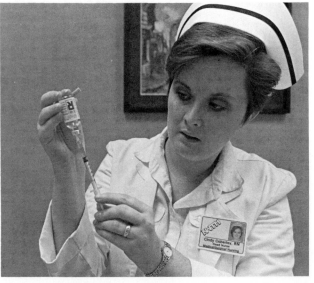

Figure 67.21

ACTION	RATIONALE
Remove the needle from the vial. With the needle uppermost, aspirate an amount of air equal to the amount of the second insulin to be withdrawn (Fig. 67-22). Invert the second insulin and inject the air into the vial. Be careful not to inject any of the first insulin (Fig. 67-23). Withdraw the prescribed amount of the second insulin (Fig. 67-24). Withdraw the needle from the second vial before turning the vial upright (Fig. 67-25).	

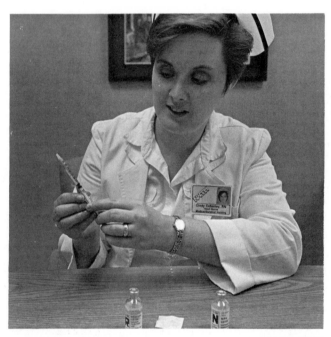

Figure 67.22

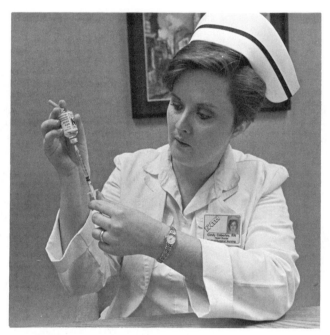

Figure 67.23

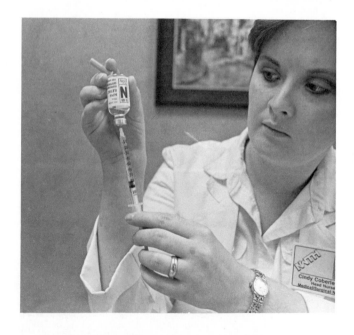

Figure 67.24

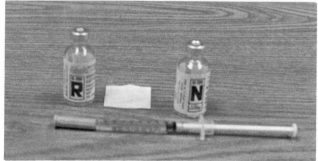

Figure 67.25

ACTION	RATIONALE
4. *Narcotics*: Assess the respiration rate before giving narcotics. A respiratory rate below 12 is considered a contraindication to administering a narcotic without physician approval. Also assess the pulse rate.	Most narcotics have a selective depressant action on the respiratory center. The pulse rate may be used as an indicator of pain (e.g., pain and discomfort are often accompanied by an increase in the normal pulse rate).
5. Paraldehyde is always given with a glass syringe.	Paraldehyde, an extremely potent sedative, reacts chemically with plastic.
6. PRN medications are ordered to be used as needed by the client at the nurse's discretion. Check the client record to ensure that sufficient time has elapsed since the last dose. Chart the dose immediately after administration and record the reason for giving the medication.	Current recording of the times and amounts of PRN medication are essential to prevent accidental duplication of doses.

Oral Drugs—Solids

ACTION	RATIONALE
1. Avoid handling oral medication. Introduce it into the client's mouth directly from the medication container or package.	This reduces the chance of cross-infection and side-effects to the nurse, who can absorb some medications through contact with the skin.
2. If the client has difficulty swallowing the oral drug, place it as far back in the throat as possible.	Stimulation of the back of the tongue elicits the swallowing reflex.
3. Offer the client a drink of water with the medication if not contraindicated.	Fluids administered with a drug facilitate swallowing and hasten absorption from the GI tract.

Oral Drugs—Liquids

ACTION	RATIONALE
1. Liquid drugs, except cough syrups, oils, and antacids, may be diluted with ½ oz of water or juice.	Dilution of a drug hastens its absorption.
2. Corrosive drugs (e.g., hydrochloric acid) and staining drugs (e.g., liquid iron preparations) should be given through a straw.	Corrosive and staining drugs are harmful to tooth enamel.

Topical Drugs—Ophthalmic

ACTION	RATIONALE
1. Position the client either supine or sitting with the head back. Cleanse the eyelid of secretions prior to administering the eye medication.	The dependent position aids gravitational flow of the drops into the eye. If not removed, debris on the eyelid might be washed into the eye.
2. Instruct the client to look upward with the eye open normally. Hold the eyelids open with gentle pressure on the bony prominences above and below the eye.	Pressure on the eyeball itself may cause damage and discomfort.

ACTION

RATIONALE

3. Direct the medication into the lower conjunctiva rather than directly onto the corneal surface (Fig. 67-26).

The cornea is very sensitive and easily damaged. Placing the drop directly onto the cornea will stimulate the blinking reflex.

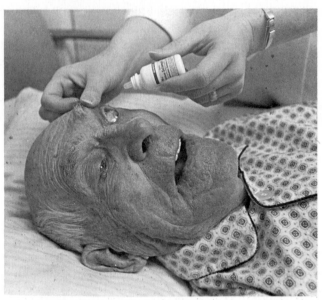

Figure 67.26

4. Using a sterile cotton ball, gently press over the inner canthus or wipe from the inner canthus outward. This will prevent the medication from draining down through the lacrimal duct.

Absorption of excess drug by way of the nose or pharynx may lead to toxic symptoms.

5. Once the medication bottle is opened, it is not sterile. Be careful not to touch any part of the eye with the applicator. If both eyes are to receive medication, a separate container of medication will be used for each eye. Label each container clearly to prevent confusion.

Take precautions not to spread infection. Cross-contamination between the client's own eyes can be prevented by using separate containers to medicate each eye.

Topical Drugs—Otic

1. Position the client in the recumbent position on the unaffected side.

Use the force of gravity to help disperse medication throughout the ear canal.

2. Gently pull the adult's ear up and back to allow the drops to fall to the side of the canal (Fig. 67-27).

This action straightens the ear canal.

3. Ask the client to remain lying quietly on the unaffected side for several minutes after administration.

It takes a few minutes for the medication to reach the inner aspects of the ear canal.

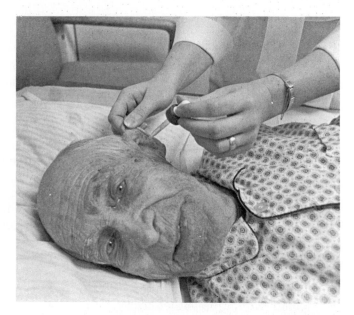

Figure 67.27

ACTION	**RATIONALE**
Topical Drugs—Nasal	
1. Position the client in the supine position with head hyperextended.	This position facilitates access to the nostrils and allows the drops to flow with gravitational pull.
2. Instill the drops into the nose without touching the dropper to the client's skin. Gently raise the tip of the nostril to insert the medication (Fig. 67-28).	Microorganisms can be spread by direct contact with the client's skin.

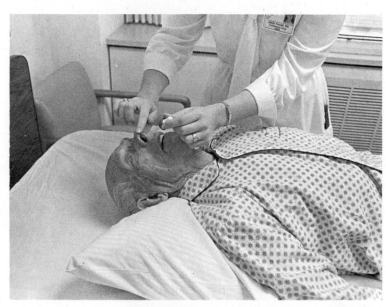

Figure 67.28

ACTION

RATIONALE

Topical Drugs—Sublingual

Place sublingual tablets under the client's tongue to dissolve.

The rich blood supply under the tongue creates an avenue for rapid absorption of drugs.

Topical Drugs—Suppositories

1. *Vaginal suppository:* Place the client in the lithotomy position with the hips slightly elevated. Don clean gloves if insertion is to be done manually. Many suppositories come with a special applicator for insertion. Lubricate the suppository with a water-soluble gel and insert it into the vagina as far as possible. Ask the client to remain with hips elevated for 5 minutes. Provide the client with a perineal pad.

The vagina has no sphincter muscle to prevent the suppository from running out. It requires about 5 minutes for the coating of the suppository to melt from body heat and for the medicine to be dispersed.

2. *Rectal suppository:* Place the client in Sim's position on the left side. Don clean gloves. Lubricate the suppository with a water-soluble gel. Spread the client's buttocks and insert the suppository about 2 inches into the rectum (Figs. 67-29, 67-30). Ask the client to hold the suppository for 10 minutes.

The anal canal of an adult is about 1 inch long. Insertion of the suppository 2 inches into the rectum ensures passing the internal sphincter and facilitates retention. It takes about 10 minutes for the coating of the suppository to melt so that the medication can be dispersed.

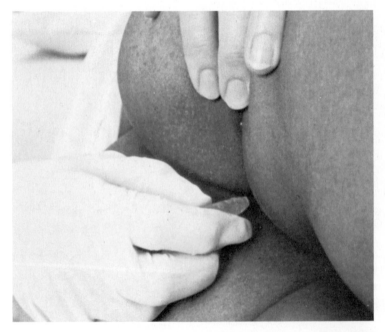

Figure 67.29

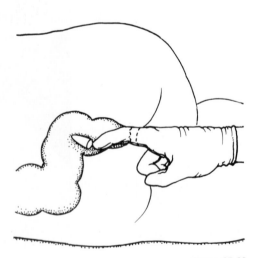

Figure 67.30

ACTION | **RATIONALE**

Parenteral Drugs, Intradermal Injection

Cleanse the skin on the medial forearm with an alcohol sponge, using firm circular motions moving from the center outward. Insert the needle, bevel up, at a 15° angle until just the tip is under the outer layer of skin (Figs. 67-31, 67-32). Aspirate to ensure that the needle is not in a vein. Inject the solution, causing formation of a small blister or bleb.

The medial forearm provides good visualization of the response to the testing media.

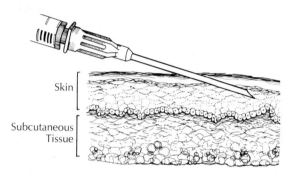

Figure 67.31

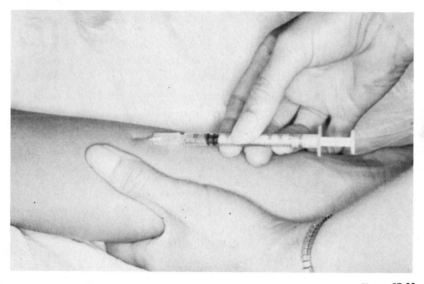

Figure 67.32

ACTION   **RATIONALE**

Parenteral Drugs, SC Injection

(Consult previous cautions about insulin and heparin.)

1. Select a site containing loose connective tissue free from large blood vessels and nerves. Rotation of sites lessens irritation and improves absorption (Fig. 67-33).

Usual sites are outer thighs. These areas are poorly supplied with sensory nerves, and injection here causes less pain than in other sites.

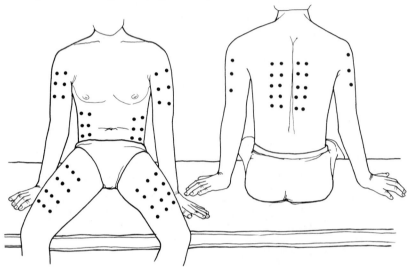

Figure 67.33

2. Cleanse the area with an alcohol sponge in a circular motion from the center outward.

This reduces the presence of microorganisms on the skin prior to puncture.

3. Elevate the subcutaneous tissue by squeezing it gently upward in cushion fashion.

Elevating the tissue helps prevent the needle from entering the muscle. SC tissue is abundant in well-nourished persons and sparse in emaciated or dehydrated persons.

4. Insert the needle at an angle between 30° and 90°, depending on the amount and turgor of the tissue (Figs. 67-34, 67-35). Once the needle is inserted, release the grip of the tissue.

Injection of solutions into compressed tissue causes pressure against the nerve endings and pain.

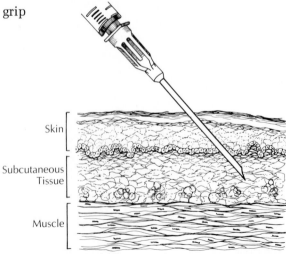

Skin

Subcutaneous Tissue

Muscle

Figure 67.34

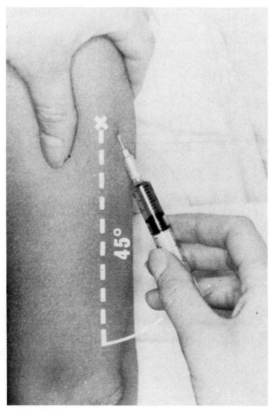

Figure 67.35

ACTION

5. Gently pull back the plunger of the syringe to determine if the needle is in a blood vessel (consult previous cautions about the administration of heparin). If blood appears, withdraw the needle and apply pressure to the area until bleeding stops. Apply a sterile adhesive strip. Obtain a new syringe of medication and reinject it in a different place. Again, check to see if the syringe is in a blood vessel. If no blood appears, inject the solution slowly.

6. Quickly withdraw the needle. Rub the area gently with an alcohol sponge.

Parenteral Drugs, IM Injection

1. Draw approximately 0.2 ml to 0.3 ml of air into the syringe after the medication has been drawn up. The lighter air bubble rises to the top of the solution and is injected last.

RATIONALE

Substances injected into a blood vessel are absorbed immediately. The rationale for administering SC injection is usually the desire to have the medication absorbed slowly.

Quick withdrawal prevents pulling the tissue and causing pain. Rubbing aids in dispersion and absorption of the medication.

The injection of an air bubble after the medication cleanses the needle and prevents leakage of irritating solution back into the SC tissue as the needle is withdrawn.

ACTION

RATIONALE

2. Assist the client into a comfortable position. Ask the client to take a deep breath prior to needle insertion. Select a site in a large muscle away from large vessels and nerves. Usual sites include the dorsogluteal and ventrogluteal (upper and outer buttocks) (Fig. 67-36) and the vastus lateralis (anterolateral thigh) in adults. The deltoid (upper arm) and anterior thigh may also be used.

Being in a comfortable position and drawing in a deep breath may help the client relax. Injection into a tense muscle causes pain.

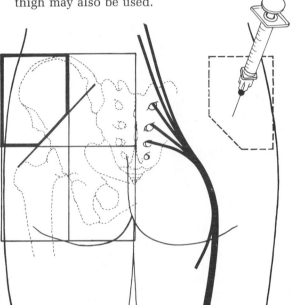

Figure 67.36

3. Cleanse the skin site with an alcohol sponge in a circular motion from the center outward.

4. Firmly insert the needle at a 90° angle directly into the muscle (Figs. 67-37, 67-38). Pull back the plunger on the syringe. If blood appears, the needle has entered a vein, and restarting is necessary (see previous section, SC Injection, step 5). Inject the medication slowly and remove the needle quickly. Massage the area for a few seconds. If slight bleeding occurs, apply direct pressure with the sponge for 15 to 30 seconds.

Microorganisms normally found on the skin may be pathogenic if introduced into the body.

Muscle tissue is vascular. IM injection placed accidentally into the vein could endanger the client. Quick removal of the needle minimizes pain and trauma. Massaging aids in dispersion and absorption of the medication.

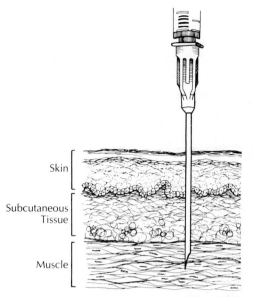

Skin

Subcutaneous Tissue

Muscle

Figure 67.37

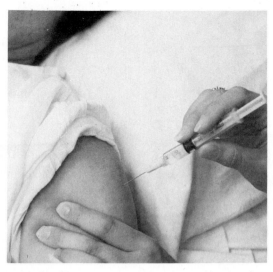

Figure 67.38

ACTION	**RATIONALE**

Parenteral Drugs, IM Z-track Injection

Use the same precedure as for IM injection with the following exceptions:

1. Use only the upper outer aspect of the gluteus maximus (buttocks) for Z-track injection.	The gluteus maximus is large enough to absorb the irritating medication.
2. Compress the SC tissue. Displace the SC tissue laterally before injection. Insert the needle straight into muscle while the skin is still displaced laterally (Fig. 67-39). Inject the medication.	Compression of the SC tissue helps ensure that the medication does indeed enter muscle tissue. When the tissue is released, the needle track is sealed off.

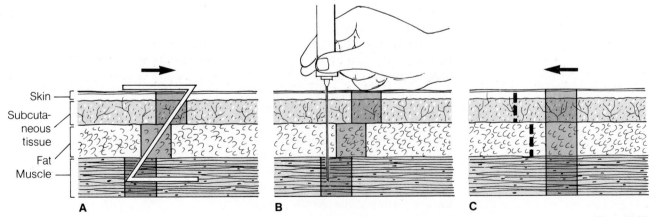

Skin

Subcutaneous tissue

Fat

Muscle

A   B   C

Figure 67.39

ACTION	RATIONALE

3. Before releasing the tissue, wait about 10 seconds after the needle has been withdrawn.

This delay and the 0.3-ml air bubble help seal off the injected fluid and prevent leakage back into SC tissue.

4. *Do not massage* the injection site.

Tissue compression from massage could force the solution back along the needle path.

Parenteral Drugs, IV Injection
(See also Technique No. 65, Intravenous Infusion)

1. Refer to the literature for the drug and review carefully the suitability of the drug for IV administration, dilution requirements, and a safe rate of administration.

Absorption by way of the vascular system is immediate.

2. Dilute the medication as directed, using a sterile, previously unopened vial of diluent.

Diluent used for previous injection may have been accidentally contaminated.

3. When a patent IV infusion is running, cleanse the port for injection with an alcohol sponge. Clamp the IV tubing above the site of injection and insert the 21-gauge needle through the self-sealing double wall. Inject the medication according to the manufacturer's or physician's recommendations. Remove the needle and unclamp the tubing, thus reestablishing patency to the infusion.

Pathogens present on the IV tubing may be forced slowly into the bloodstream if not removed. Some medications are injected slowly so that the client will not be overwhelmed by the sudden effect. Some medications must be administered quickly so that they will not bind with serum proteins.

4. Direct IV injection requires caution and skill. Consult the hospital policy manual to determine who may perform this procedure. For direct IV injection, cleanse the skin carefully with alcohol or an antiseptic cleanser. Accomplish venipuncture (see Technique No. 65, Intravenous Infusion). Be sure by aspiration of blood that the needle is in the vein. Release the tourniquet. Inject the medication slowly, with frequent aspirations to ensure that the needle is still in the vein. When the injection is completed, withdraw the needle and apply direct pressure to the injection site until bleeding stops. Apply a sterile adhesive strip.

Direct injection into the venous system usually requires a specially trained nurse or physician. To prevent the introduction of pathogenic microorganisms directly into the bloodstream, scrupulous cleansing is necessary. If the tourniquet is not released, the medication will pool and cause increased pressure in the vein. If the medication is injected too rapidly, toxic reactions or shock may occur. Inject at the rate recommended in the literature.

Communicative Aspects

OBSERVATIONS

1. After administration of any drug, the client should be observed for desired results, such as reduction of pain or fever; expected side-effects, such as dryness of mouth and vertigo; and untoward reactions, such as anaphylactic shock.

2. Monitor vital signs frequently during hospitalization. Observe fluctuations in vital signs in relation to medication administration.

CHARTING

1. All medications given must be charted somewhere on the client's legal record. There is usually a medication record for this purpose. PRN doses are also explained in the Nurses' Progress Notes.

2. Chart any reactions, as well as pulse and respirations, in the Nurses' Progress Notes.

3. If, for any reason, a scheduled dose is omitted, record an explanation in the Nurses' Progress Notes.

DATE/TIME	OBSERVATIONS	SIGNATURE
6/20 1000	Demerol 50 mg. given IM in gluteus maximus for lower back pain. P 88, R 26.	P. Dillon RN
1025	Sleeping quietly now. R 14. Traction on.	P. Dillon RN

DATE/TIME	OBSERVATIONS	SIGNATURE
8/14 0900	Digitoxin 0.1 mg po withheld due to pulse of 52 beats per min. Dr. G notified. ECG done as ordered. States no chest pain. No dyspnea or cyanosis noted. Resting in semi-Fowler's position with oxygen at 3 liters.	P. Dillon RN

Discharge Planning Aspects

CLIENT AND FAMILY EDUCATION

1. The client has a right to know about the medications being taken during hospitalization. If the medications are to be taken after discharge, it is beneficial to call the client's attention to the dosage schedule used in the hospital, with special suggestions about drugs to be taken after a meal because of potential damage to the lining of the stomach, drugs to be taken with a liquid other than water, drugs to be taken around the clock because they depend on continual exposure to the bloodstream, and so on.

2. Give thorough and complete directions about any medications sent home with the client. Explain to the client and family member the name of each medication, the reason the medication is to be taken, the expected results, when and how to take the medicine, and how long to continue administration. The client and family should also know the normal side-effects and any potential problems involved with each specific medication. They should be told of any special storage requirements, such as refrigeration or storage out of light. If there are several medications, it may be beneficial for the family to have these instructions put in writing for future reference. Clients and family members should be taught how to administer any drugs requiring special technique, such as rectal or vaginal suppositories, insulin, or inhalants. Ensure adequate understanding by assessment of a return demonstration.

3. Use this opportunity to caution the client and family members about the indiscriminate use of over-the-counter drugs for minor symptoms. Drugs should be taken only if absolutely necessary. Important symptoms may be masked by overusage of medications. Most medications should be taken only on the advice of a physician or licensed practitioner.

4. If the client has an allergic reaction to a drug while in the hospital, tell the client the name of the drug (both the generic and trade names). Caution the client to inform all medical personnel about this allergy any time medical attention is sought in the future.

Evaluation

Quality Assurance

Initial documentation should include an assessment of the client's allergy history, with emphasis on previous allergic reactions to drugs. All drugs taken during hospitalization, the names, amounts, times, and any untoward reactions should be documented. The symptoms that prompted the client to seek hospitalization should be noted in relation to the effects of the drug regimen (i.e., if the client was admitted for hypertension, note whether the antihypertensive medication relieved the symptoms). All teaching should be documented with emphasis on the instructions about home administration of medications prior to discharge.

Infection Control

Handwashing should be done after caring for each client. In the administration of oral and topical medications, handwashing is important to prevent the spread of infection from one client to another. In the administration of parenteral medications, careful handwashing is important because the natural defensive barrier of the client, the skin, is broken. The potential for cross-infection is increased. It is also important to remove from the client's skin as many pathogens as possible before administering parenteral medications.

Technique Checklist

	YES	NO
Client and family understood why the medications were given	_____	_____
All orders for medications were followed correctly	_____	_____
Complete written record of medications received is on the client's chart	_____	_____
Unexpected reactions are documented fully in the Nurses' Progress Notes	_____	_____
Complete instructions given before discharge about take-home drugs	_____	_____
Oral _____		
Written _____		
Allergies to medications experienced	_____	_____

68   Neurologic Signs

Overview

Definition

Evaluation of the neurologic status of the client by obtaining objective and subjective data through a series of tests and evaluation techniques

Rationale

Aid in the recognition of increased intracranial pressure.

Aim for early prevention of increased intracranial pressure and its effects.

Aid in determining the degree of paralysis.

Determine the level of conciousness.

Terminology

Decerebrate posturing: The posture assumed because of a brain lesion in the diencephalon, pons, or midbrain; the legs are extended with plantar flexion, and the arms are held rigidly at the side with the palms turned outward (Fig. 68-1)

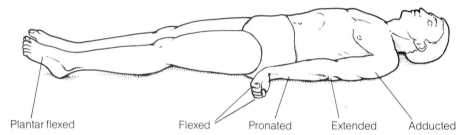

Plantar flexed   Flexed   Pronated   Extended   Adducted

Figure 68.1

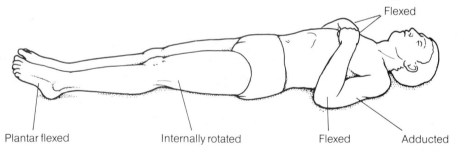

Flexed

Plantar flexed   Internally rotated   Flexed   Adducted

Figure 68.2

Decorticate posturing: The posture assumed because of a lesion of the corticospinal tract near the cerebral hemisphere; the legs are extended, the feet are extended with plantar flexion, and the arms are internally rotated and flexed on the chest (Fig. 68-2)

Flaccid posturing: The posture assumed because of brain damage to the motor area of the brain; there is no muscular control of the body

Hypoxia: Varying degrees of lack of oxygen

Intracranial pressure: Pressure within the cranium

Pulse pressure: The difference between systolic and diastolic blood pressures

Vital signs: See Technique 92, Vital Signs

Assessment

**Pertinent Anatomy
and Physiology**

See Appendix I: *brain.*

**Pathophysiological
Concepts**

1. Unconsciousness may be due to many causes. Metabolic coma occurs when metabolism of the cerebral cortex and brain stem is disrupted by toxins, drugs, anoxia, or hypoglycemia. The most common cause of coma is a mass directly involving the brain stem. The mass may be the result of edema, brain tumor, or blood clot. The mass expands, creating increased pressure and displacing the cerebral tissue away from the mass toward a less dense area. This herniating tissue may compress the third cranial nerve, causing unilateral pupil dilatation. Continued herniation may lead to infarct and irreversible brain damage.

2. Disruptions in the brain cause a predictable pattern of change in the level of consciousness. Symptoms progress from decreased concentration and lethargy to unresponsiveness. Yawning and sighing are signs of changes in the level of consciousness. Pupils may respond to light briskly. As the coma progresses, respirations increase and then stop momentarily (Cheyne–Stokes). The pupils become fixed at midpoint and are unresponsive to light. Decerebrate posturing becomes more and more pronounced. Apnea and flaccidity occur in the final stages of coma preceding brain death.

3. Pressure on vital centers in the brain causes an increase in pulse, pulse pressure, and variable respirations. There is usually associated hypoxia. Pressure on the hypothalamus may increase or decrease temperature.

Assessment of the Client

1. Assess the ability of the client to comply with verbal directions. This is a part of the assessment of the neurologic status.

2. Assess the ability of the client to withstand a thorough neurologic assessment. If medical crisis is present, the complete neurologic assessment may have to be postponed until the client is more stable.

3. Assess vital signs before beginning the neurologic assessment to provide a means of comparison.

Plan

Nursing Objectives

Protect the client from further neurologic damage.

Allay the fear and anxiety of the family and client.

Record and report observations accurately.

Gain data on which to base medical diagnosis involving the medication and treatment regimens.

Client Preparation

1. Explain to the conscious client why the neurologic signs are being measured. Even if the client is unconscious, explain when and why the light is being directed into the client's eyes, since the degree of perception, even when the client is apparently unconscious, cannot be accurately determined.

2. Tell the client and family why neurologic signs are checked frequently. Before beginning, gather all equipment to avoid delays and client anxiety.

Equipment

Flashlight	Applicator
Stethoscope	Pen
Sphygmomanometer	Safety pin
Thermometer	Glasgow Coma Scale
Tongue blade	

Implementation and Interventions

Procedural Aspects

ACTION

1. Assess the level of consciousness by approaching and speaking to the client. Direct the client to perform simple tasks, such as moving an extremity or grasping the nurse's hand, which will also demonstrate any hemispheric weakness. Measure the client's eye, motor, and verbal responses by using the Glasgow Coma Scale (see Charting section of this technique). Explain that an assessment of the client's nervous system is to be carried out and elicit the client's cooperation.

2. Exert pressure on the nailbed to see if the client responds to pain. A safety pin may be used to stroke the client's skin with first the sharp side and then the dull side to determine the client's ability to distinguish between sharp and dull.

3. Assess the pupils by noting their size (they should be equal at about 1.5 cm–6 cm round, in the middle of the eye (Fig. 68-3A); and their reaction to light (they should constrict promptly when a light is shown into the eye; Fig. 68-3B).

RATIONALE

The center of conciousness, the pons, may be damaged by direct trauma or associated pressure, resulting in a change in the level of consciousness. Eye movement, speaking, and comprehension are measurable indicators of the client's level of consciousness.

Suppression of the pain response is indicative of decreased consciousness.

Edema of the pupillary muscle may result in an abnormal pupil size or a fixed pupil. Dissimilarity of the pupils may indicate neurologic damage.

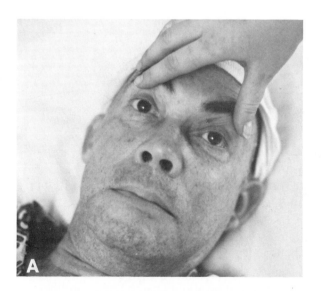 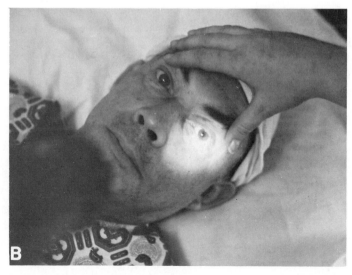

Figure 68.3

ACTION	*RATIONALE*
4. Assess muscle strength by asking the client to grip both hands and squeeze the nurse's fingers. Note any weakness on either or both sides. Ask the client to push or pull the nurse's hand to ascertain equality of response.	Hemiplegia, paraplegia, or quadriplegia may be indicated by absence of motor function.
5. Assess reflexes to determine possible nerve damage. Assess the blink reflex by lightly brushing the client's eyelashes while holding the client's eyes open. Test the gag reflex by holding the client's tongue down with a tongue blade and touching the back of the pharynx with an applicator. This should make the client gag. Check the plantar response, or Babinski reflex, by running a pen along the outer lateral aspect of the foot from the heel to the little toe and continuing across the ball of the foot toward the great toe (Fig. 68-4). Flexion of the toes indicates the normal response or a negative Babinski. A positive Babinski is evidenced by fanning of the toes (Fig. 68-5).	Absence of the blinking reflex may indicate damage to the 5th or 7th cranial nerve. Depression of the gag reflex occurs when there is involvement of the 9th or tenth cranial nerve. A positive Babinski may indicate upper motor neuron lesion.

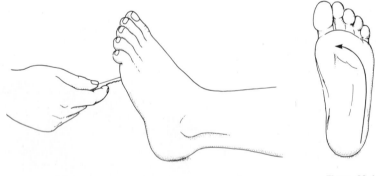

Figure 68.4

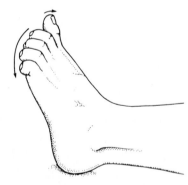

Figure 68.5

Communicative Aspects

OBSERVATIONS

1. Report any change in pulse rate, pulse pressure, temperature, or respiratory rate in the neurologically compromised client.

2. Observe the neurologic signs as first assessed and then in relation to previous assessment. Depression of neurologic response may indicate deepening coma. Improvement of neurologic response may indicate reduction in edema of the brain.

3. Report to the physician any changes in the level of consciousness and/or motor response.

4. Prepared scales produce a numerical rating of the client's neurologic status. The Glasgow Coma Scale is an example.

CHARTING

Notation of neurologic assessment should appear frequently in the nursing progress notes according to the policy and form advocated by the agency or institution. The following is an example of charting:

DATE/TIME	B/P	P	R	PUPILS	GRIP	REFLEX
3/21 0900	112/78	88	22	=&reac	none	pos Babinski
0915	92/44	72	14	fixed	none	

0915 Dr. J notified of worsening condition.
Unresponsive at this time. ———————————————————— J. White RN

The Glasgow Coma Scale is used extensively as a means of assessing and recording the level of consciousness. An example of charting with the Glasgow Coma Scale is shown in Fig. 68-6.

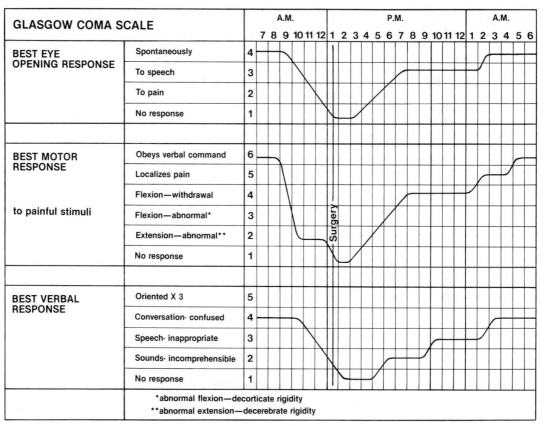

Figure 68.6

Glasgow Coma Scale. How to Score Reponses:

Scoring of Eye Opening: **4** = If the patient opens his eyes spontaneously when the nurse approaches; **3** = If the patient opens his eyes in response to speech (spoken or shouted); **2** = If the patient opens his eyes only in response to painful stimuli such as digital squeezing around nail beds of fingers; **1** = if the patient does not open his eyes in response to painful stimuli.

Scoring of Best Motor Response: **6** = If the patient can obey a simple command such as "Lift your left hand off the bed."; **5** = if the patient moves a limb to locate the painful stimuli applied to the head or trunk and attempts to remove the source; **4** = if the patient attempts to withdraw from the source of pain; **3** = if the patient flexes only his arms at the elbows and wrist in response to painful stimuli to the nail beds (decorticate rigidity); **2** = if the patient extends his arms (straightens his elbows) in response to painful stimuli (decerebrate rigidity); **1** = if the patient has no motor response to pain on any limb.

Scoring of Best Verbal Response: **5** = If the patient is oriented to time, place, and person; **4** = if the patient is able to converse although not oriented to time, place, or person (e.g., "Where am I?"); **3** = if the patient speaks only in words or phrases that make little or no sense (e.g., "B—H, N—K."); **2** = if the patient responds with incomprehensible sounds such as groans; **1** = if the patient does not respond verbally at all.

Discharge Planning Aspects

CLIENT AND FAMILY EDUCATION

1. Explain to the family why the client's neurologic signs are checked frequently.
2. Request the family to tell the nursing staff of any noticeable differences observed about the client. Their assistance is valuable, not only because they know the client well and are more attuned to normal responses, but also because this action can help them to feel that they are a part of the client's recuperation process.
3. Encourage the family to ask questions about the client's condition and progress.

Evaluation

Quality Assurance

Documentation should reflect an ongoing assessment of the client's neurologic condition. Drastic alteration in neurologic status should be accompanied by documentation of physician notification, implementation of physician orders, and outcomes of prescribed therapies. The documentation should reflect that the nurse was aware of the possible complications of neurologic degeneration and knew how to assess and evaluate the client's condition. In addition, evidence should show that the nurse recognized alterations from normal and was able to correct or report them in an efficient and effective manner.

Infection Control

1. Assessment of the client should be preceded and followed by handwashing.
2. Equipment used for consecutive clients should be cleaned and disinfected between uses.
3. Care must be taken during neurologic assessment not to break the client's skin. The skin serves as the body's first line of defense. Any break in the integrity of the skin is a potential source of infection.

Technique Checklist

	YES	NO
Procedure explained to client and family	_____	_____
Client able to speak	_____	_____
Client aware of time and place	_____	_____
Responsive to painful stimuli	_____	_____
Pupils equal and reactive	_____	_____
Muscle strength similar bilaterally	_____	_____
Reflexes intact		
Blinking reflex	_____	_____
Gag Reflex	_____	_____
Babinski Neg _____ Pos _____		
Neurologic status		
Improved _____		
Worsened _____		
Vital signs monitored in conjunction with neurologic signs	_____	_____
Frequency of readings _____		
Documentation on chart		
Neurologic assessment	_____	_____
Glasgow Coma Scale	_____	_____
Vital signs	_____	_____

69 Oral Hygiene

Overview

Definition

The process of cleansing and freshening the teeth, gums, and mouth

Rationale

Keep the teeth, gums, and mouth in good condition.
Freshen the mouth and relieve offensive odors.
Prevent sores and infections.
Provide a sense of well-being and comfort.

Terminology

Dentures: Artificially constructed teeth
Glossitis: Inflammation of the tongue
Halitosis: Offensive breath odor
Stomatitis: Inflammation of the mucosa of the mouth

Assessment

Pertinent Anatomy and Physiology

1. See Appendix I: *mouth, teeth.*
2. The *lips* are composed of connective tissue and striated muscles. The outer surface is covered with skin, and the inner surface is lined with mucous membrane.
3. The *tongue* is an accessory organ composed of interlacing bundles of striated muscle fibers. The mucous membrane on the undersurface is thin and forms a fold called the frenulum linguae, which extends from near the tip of the tongue to the floor of the mouth. The top of the tongue is covered with nipple-shaped projections called papillae, some of which contain nerve endings sensitive to touch. The receptors of taste are the taste buds, which are also located in the papillae of the tongue. At the top of each bud is an opening through which substances enter in order to stimulate receptors.
4. *Saliva* is an important mechanical and chemical cleanser of the mouth. It combines with food particles to aid in digestion.

Pathophysiological Concepts

1. Malocclusion of the teeth occurs when the upper and lower teeth do not fit together when the mouth is closed. It may be hereditary or a result of injury or radical surgery. The result is an inability to chew properly.
2. Dental caries are localized destruction of tooth tissue by bacterial action. Demineralization of the surface enamel ultimately causes destruction of the dentin and pulp of the tooth. Caries are actually caused by the acid produced by the bacteria, which form a colony on the tooth surface.
3. The major cause of tooth loss in adults over 35 years of age is gum disease.

Assessment of the Client

1. Assess the condition of the client's mouth. Determine whether or not the client has artificial dentures. Inspect the gums for swelling or inflammation. Note whether the gums seem puffy, protude down into the spaces between the teeth, bleed easily, or are discolored. Inspect the mouth for loose teeth or untreated dental caries. Note foul-smelling breath, which may indicate infection in the mouth.

2. Assess the client's usual hygienic habits related to tooth care: frequency of brushing the teeth, frequency of flossing the teeth, and frequency of visits to a dentist. Assess the client's knowledge of proper methods of caring for the mouth and teeth.

3. Assess the physical condition of the client in relation to ability to participate in own care. If the client has impairment of the upper extremities, assistance with oral care may be required.

4. Assess factors that would increase the need for oral care (such as chemotherapy, antibiotics, vomiting, nutritional deficiencies, immunologic deficiencies, and herpes).

Plan

Nursing Objectives

Carry out individualized oral-hygiene measures appropriate to the assessed needs of the client as often as necessary to maintain a healthy, fresh mouth.

Observe the teeth, gums, and mucous membranes carefully for early signs of soreness and infection.

Teach the client and family proper oral-hygiene technique and preventive care.

Client Preparation

1. Oral care is usually done by the client during the morning bath and at bedtime. If the client is able to go to the bathroom, self-care is probably possible. Assist with assembling equipment, if needed, and monitor the client whose condition warrants.

2. Explain to the client who cannot do self-care, as well as to the family, how the oral-hygiene procedure will be done and why it is important. Proper oral care is a matter of developing good habits. Encourage the client to engage in preventive dental care every day.

3. Determine the client's usual method of caring for the mouth and teeth and provide the needed equipment. If the client cannot sit up, the side-lying position will facilitate oral care. Place equipment within reach.

Equipment

Toothbrush and toothpaste

Curved basin

Dental floss

Towel

Cool water and cup

Mouthwash

Lip lubricant

Medicated swabs, if needed

Bulb syringe, if needed

Gloves, if needed

Tongue blades, if needed

Implementation and Interventions

Procedural Aspects

ACTION

Bedridden Client Who Is Alert

1. Wash hands before giving oral care. Perform oral-hygiene measures when needed or desired by the client. Oral care is usually done with the daily bath. However, it should be done as often as the client needs it to maintain comfort and a sense of well-being.

2. If the client must use the side-lying position, place a towel and curved basin under the chin.

3. Use a toothbrush with soft bristles. Rinse the toothbrush with cool water and apply a strip of toothpaste.

4. Brush in the direction of tooth growth. Do one section at a time. Place the bristles parallel to the tooth surface, free edges up and extending beyond the gum line. Turn the bristles toward the teeth with one sweeping stroke and bring tips of the bristles firmly over the gum tissue and the tooth surface (Figs. 69-1 to 69-3). Repeat

RATIONALE

The oral cavity is the site of many normal bacteria, which may be pathogenic if introduced to susceptible persons. Handwashing will eliminate most of these bacteria. Clients with acute infections or chronic illnesses will need more frequent mouth care.

The side-lying position will allow the rinse water to return by the flow of gravity and will lessen the chance of accidental choking from the water flowing down the throat.

Firm bristles may cause abrasion to the sensitive gums. Water softens the bristles.

The oral cavity contains a balanced biological system of microorganisms. Oral care should be designed to remove retained food debris, rather than to remove all microorganisms from the mouth. Brushing in the direction of the tooth will facilitate removal of food particles as well as stimulating the gums.

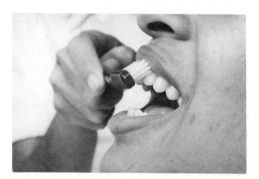

Figure 69.1

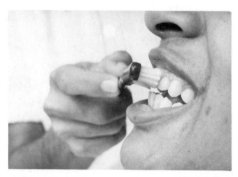

Figure 69.2

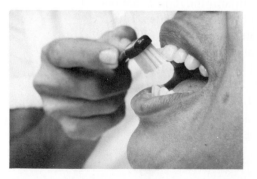

Figure 69.3

ACTION   **RATIONALE**

this stroke 5 times over each section of the mouth, on the outer
surfaces (Fig. 69-4), inner surfaces
(Fig. 69-5), and biting surfaces
(Fig. 69-6).

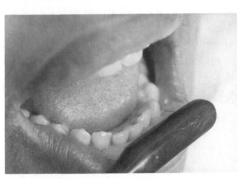

Figure 69.4

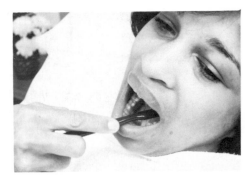

Figure 69.5

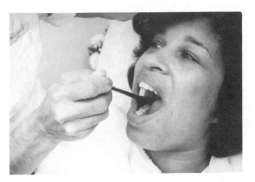

Figure 69.6

5. Do not exert undue force over the
   gum surface.

   Gum tissue is sensitive and will bleed
   if too much pressure is used. However, gums that bleed very easily may
   indicate pathology.

6. Assist in flossing the teeth, if the
   client cannot do so. Place the client in the semi-Fowler's position.
   Wrap the dental floss around the
   middle finger of each hand and
   loop several times to stabilize
   (Fig. 69-7). Use the index fingers to
   stretch the floss (Fig. 69-8). Insert
   the floss between each of the client's teeth and move in a sawing
   manner to clean the sides, back,
   and front of each tooth, (Fig. 69-9).
   To remove the floss, release it from
   the backmost finger and pull it
   through the teeth.

   Plaque is a build-up on the teeth,
   which forms continually. If left in
   place, plaque can lead to gum and
   tooth disease. Flossing helps remove
   plaque. Care must be taken not to
   floss too roughly, causing the gums to
   bleed.

7. Allow the client to rinse the mouth
   and gums with cool water and
   mouthwash (Fig. 69-10).

   Thorough rinsing after flossing will
   rinse the dislodged bacteria and
   plaque from the mouth.

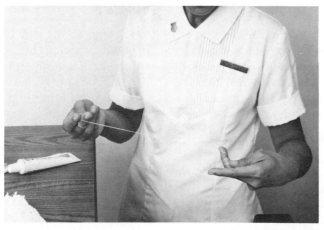

Figure 69.7

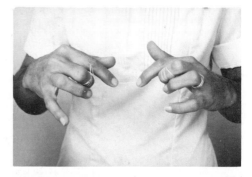

Figure 69.8

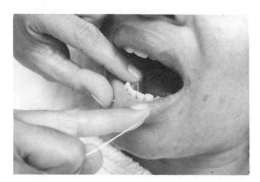

Figure 69.9

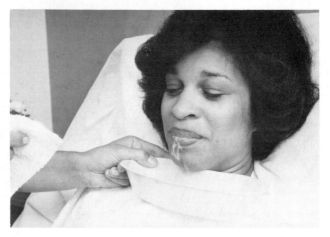

Figure 69.10

ACTION	RATIONALE
Unconscious Client	
1. Turn the client's head well to the side. Place a linen protector under the chin (Fig. 69-11).	Aspiration may occur if body alignment is not altered to facilitate drainage.
2. Brush the client's teeth gently in the previously described manner. Use a padded tongue blade to gently separate the upper and lower teeth.	The oral cavity of an unconscious person is not exposed to the normal stimulation and cleaning from eating. Meticulous oral hygiene is needed to prevent tooth and gum complications.

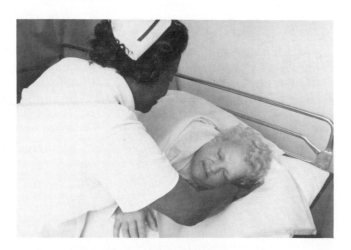

Figure 69.11

ACTION

RATIONALE

3. Careful irrigation of the mouth with a bulb syringe and a small amount of water will help remove debris (Figs. 69-12, 69-13). Follow insertion of water with immediate and complete suction of all irrigation fluid to prevent aspiration (Fig. 69-14). Take care that none of the fluid is allowed into the trachea. Use a medicated swab to freshen the client's mouth.

Medicated swabs may be used to freshen the mouth but are *not* a substitute for brushing and rinsing. Water in the trachea may cause choking or aspiration into the lung.

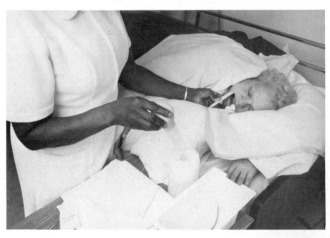

Figure 69.12

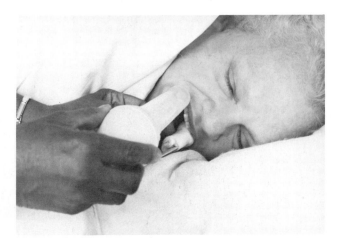

Figure 69.13

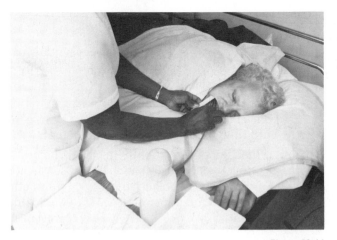

Figure 69.14

4. Administer complete oral-hygiene at least twice a day to the unconscious client. In addition, clean and refresh the mouth with swabs or rinsing every hour or two. Lubricate the client's lips with some type of lubricant.

Mucous membranes tend to dry quickly when oral fluids are not being consumed, when the client is mouth-breathing, or when the client is receiving inhalation gases (such as oxygen). Frequent mouth care is vital for these clients.

ACTION	RATIONALE
Special Modifications	
1. For care of artificial dentures, see Technique No. 46, Dentures, Care of.	
2. Clients on chemotherapy frequently use saltwater rinses instead of teeth brushing, to accomplish oral care. Place ½ tsp salt in 1 cup of warm tap water (or sterile water if the client has open sores in the mouth). Allow the client to rinse the inside of the mouth thoroughly with the water.	Chemotherapy predisposes the client to hemotologic complications such as bleeding gums. Brushing may traumatize the gums and cause bleeding. Mouth care is still important to reduce pathogens and add to a sense of comfort and well-being.

Communicative Aspects

OBSERVATIONS

1. Note the condition of the teeth and gums.

2. Assess the effectiveness of the oral hygiene.

3. Note signs of infections or irritated areas, as well as the presence of halitosis. Note bleeding of the gums and what caused it.

CHARTING

DATE/TIME	OBSERVATIONS	SIGNATURE
5/2 0845	Oral care given, teeth brushed gently, and mouthwash used. Gums are less swollen than yesterday. No bleeding. Eating well without discomfort. ————	G. Williams RN

Discharge Planning Aspects

CLIENT AND FAMILY EDUCATION

1. If the client's teeth or mouth need dental attention, inquire about method and frequency of oral care at home. Enlist the suggestions and cooperation of significant family members as recommendations for improvement in oral-hygiene habits are made. If young children are in the home, stress the importance of acquiring good dental-care habits early in life. Stress the importance of preventive dentistry.

2. If the client's mouth is in obvious need of immediate attention, notify the physician if the condition may affect the outcome of the current hospital stay. Otherwise, recommend to the client and/or family that a dentist be consulted as soon as possible after leaving the hospital. Stress the importance of regular dental care.

3. If the family will assist the client in dental care after discharge, demonstrate how to care for another person's teeth and gums with emphasis on safety precautions (prevention of aspiration, prevention of traumatizing the gums). Allow the family member to demonstrate competence in administering oral care to the client.

Evaluation

Quality Assurance

Document the initial assessment of the client's dental condition. The notes should reflect any complications of dental hygiene, including bleeding of gums or pain. Document the presence of loose teeth, especially if the client will undergo surgery. It is important that the anesthetist or anesthesiologist be aware of any loose teeth before surgical intubation. Notation of the frequency of oral hygiene and the results should also be made.

Infection Control

1. Strains of the bacterium *Streptococcus mutans* are the most frequent cause of tooth decay. The primary metabolic food of this group is sucrose. Carbohydrate in a typical diet is composed of 30% to 50% sucrose; therefore, the bacteria have ideal conditions for destruction of enamel of the teeth. Oral-hygiene measures help reduce the amount of bacteria in the mouth and prevent tooth decay and infections.

2. Proper mouth care can help prevent stomatitis and gingivitis.

3. Cracked lips and bleeding gums provide an entry for pathogenic organisms into the body.

4. Meticulous handwashing before and after administering oral hygiene is necessary. Transmission of pathogenic microorganisms can be greatly minimized by handwashing.

Technique Checklist

	YES	NO
Procedure explained to client before beginning	_____	_____
Condition of client		
Conscious _____		
Unconscious _____		
Condition of teeth and gums noted	_____	_____
Loose teeth _____		
Dentures or partial plate _____		
Swollen gums _____		
Bleeding of gums _____		
Gums discolored _____		
Missing teeth _____		
Location _____		
Type of oral care administered		
Brushing _____		
Flossing _____		
Swabbing _____		
Saline rinse _____		
Oral care done by_____		
Oral care given _____ (how often)		
Client and family taught proper preventive dentistry techniques and procedures	_____	_____

70

Paracentesis (Abdominal and Thoracic), Assisting With

Overview

Definition

Abdominal paracentesis: Aspiration of fluid from the peritoneal cavity

Thoracic paracentesis (thoracentesis): Aspiration of fluid or air from the pleural cavity

Rationale

Reduce pressure on vital organs.

Aid the physician in diagnosis.

Terminology

Adhesions: Fibrous, scar-tissue bands

Ascites: Accumulation of serous fluid in the peritoneal cavity

Peritoneal cavity: A potential space between the visceral peritoneum and the abdominal wall peritoneum

Pleural cavity: A potential space between the visceral pleura covering the lung and the parietal pleura lining the rib cage

Pneumothorax: A collection of air in the pleural cavity

Syncope: Fainting; a transient loss of consciousness

Transudate: Fluid that passes through the pores of a membrane, especially that which passes through capillary walls

Assessment

Pertinent Anatomy and Physiology

1. The *peritoneum* is the largest serous membrane in the body. It consists of a double-walled sac. The outer layer of the sac is the *parietal peritoneum* which lines the abdominal cavity. This peritoneum bends back over the abdominal viscera, forming the *visceral peritoneum*. The potential space between these layers is called the peritoneal cavity. The only fluid normally located in this space is the small amount secreted from the serous cells. The peritoneal cavity is lined with serous membranes. The cells in the surface layer secrete a slippery serous fluid, which protects against friction when organs rub against the body wall or glide over one another. The female peritoneum is not a closed sac, since the free ends of the uterine tubes open directly into the peritoneal cavity.

2. The *thoracic cavity* is the space above the diaphragm within the walls of the thorax. The lungs are located within the thorax. The lungs are multilobed organs used for gaseous exchange of oxygen and carbon dioxide. Each lung is contained within a transparent, serous membrane called the pleura. This closed sac consists of two layers: the visceral pleura, which adheres to the surface of the lung, and the parietal pleura, which lines the inner surface of the chest wall. The potential space between these two layers is called the pleural cavity and contains the small amount of fluid secreted by the serous membranes. As the lungs expand with air, the layers glide against each other with a minimum of friction.

Pathophysiological Concepts

1. If the squamous cell layer of the peritoneum is injured by surgery or inflammation, there is a danger of adhesions forming and causing the sections of the viscera to grow together. This may alter the position and movement of the abdominal viscera.

2. *Ascites* is an abnormal accumulation of fluid within the peritoneal cavity. This fluid is a transudate of plasma and is continually being exchanged with vascular fluid. When the venous flow through the liver is obstructed, as in cirrhosis, there is increased production of lymph. Pressure fluctuations cause fluid to leak out of the capillaries in the visceral circulation. A rise in aldosterone levels also causes the retention of sodium and water.

3. The pleural cavity is a potential space in which serous fluid or inflammatory exudate can accumulate. *Pleural effusion* is an abnormal collection of excess fluid or exudate in the pleural cavity. Tumors adjacent to the visceral pleura often insidiously provoke pleural effusion.

Assessment of the Client

1. In ascites, measure the size of the abdomen at the largest part with a fabric tape measure. Determine the onset of symptoms and previous history of fluid in the abdomen. Weigh the client and take vital signs for baseline measurement. Determine the effect of the ascites on the respiratory sufficiency of the client by checking for unusual diaphragmatic movement.

2. For the client with fluid in the lungs, determine the amount of respiratory impairment. Measure respiratory rate and auscultate the lungs. Assess the onset of symptoms and previous history of respiratory problems. Determine if the client smokes and how much. Assess the thoracic expansion to see if it is what would be expected for a person of this weight and height.

3. Determine how much the client knows about the procedure. Determine readiness to learn when deciding how much information to give about the technique and when education should be offered. Assess the client's and family's level of acceptance of the condition, their understanding of the prognosis, and the extent of their support group.

4. Assess the client's allergy history. A topical anesthetic is often used. Determine if the client has ever had an allergic reaction to any medication, in particular to the medications used by dentists when teeth are pulled.

Plan

Nursing Objectives

Allay the client's and family's fears by adequate preparation.

Prevent or reduce infection.

Observe and record any adverse effects during or after the procedure.

Record the site of puncture, characteristics of drainage, and amount of fluid obtained.

Maintain fluid and electrolyte balance.

Offer assistance to the physician and support to the client during the procedure.

Client Preparation

1. Since the site of needle insertion is in close proximity to vital organs, it is essential that the client remain quiet and immobile during the procedure, especially during the insertion phase. Offer a thorough explanation of what will occur. Explain that physical support will be available from the nurse during the procedure.

2. Determine the hospital policy on signing consent forms for invasive procedures.

3. The urinary bladder is subject to rupture if damaged while distended. Ask the client to void before beginning paracentesis.

4. Pathogens on the skin and hair could be introduced into the body cavity through the puncture site. Prepare the skin around the site with an antiseptic and shaving, if necessary. Instruments must be sterile. Maintain aseptic conditions throughout the procedure to reduce the possibility of infection.

Equipment

Thoracentesis or paracentesis tray (with needles, knife handles and blades, trocar and cannula, rubber or plastic tubing, syringes, basins, and sterile linen)

Topical anesthetic of physician's choice

Large basin, sterile

Sterile specimen holders

Antiseptic preparation solution

Sterile 2″ × 2″ gauze bandage or small adhesive strip

Tape

Sterile gloves

Laboratory requisition, if indicated

Large catheter (at physician's request)

Intravenous tubing (at physician's request)

3-Way stopcock

Drainage system, if needed

Implementation and Interventions

Procedural Aspects

ACTION	RATIONALE
Abdominal Paracentesis	
1. Position the client in the semi-Fowler's position. Remove gown and provide a sheet for the female client's upper body to protect modesty.	The semi-reclining position encourages pooling of the fluid in the lower portion of the peritoneal cavity facilitating insertion of the needle or trocar. It also facilitates respiration and reduces pressure on the aorta.
2. After the area has been prepared, the physician will place sterile drapes around the puncture site. A small amount of local anesthetic may be injected at the site. The usual site of puncture is midway between the symphysis pubis and the umbilicus in the center of the abdomen. A small incision is made, through which the trocar and cannula are passed. When the trocar is removed from inside the cannula, the fluid can flow through the cannula, which is connected to the tubing. The open end of the tubing is connected to a drainage system if the cannula is to be left in place. The physician may slowly aspirate the desired quantity of the fluid and remove the cannula without attaching the system to drainage.	Local anesthetic may reduce discomfort when the cannula and trocar are inserted. The trocar plugging the cannula initially not only facilitates insertion into the peritoneal cavity, but allows for controlled drainage of the fluid. The reason for abdominal paracentesis often is to obtain a specimen for laboratory analysis, not to drain all of the fluid.

ACTION	*RATIONALE*
3. Keep in physical contact with the client during the procedure. Place a hand on the client's wrist or shoulders. Offer encouragement to the client throughout the procedure. Speak in low, soft tones in a confident and reassuring manner.	A sudden or unexpected movement by the client during the procedure could cause trauma to vital organs. A hand on the client can have a calming and reassuring effect, as well as serve as a physical restraint.
4. After removal of the cannula, apply a padded sterile dressing to the site. Watch the dressing for drainage and change as needed.	The site may continue to drain until it seals itself.

Thoracentesis

ACTION	*RATIONALE*
1. Position the client in an upright position, sitting on the side of the bed with the bulk of the body weight supported on an overbed table (Fig. 70-1). The client should be leaning slightly forward and may lean on the nurse, if necessary, for restraint purposes.	Because of the pull of gravity, fluid tends to localize in the base of the body cavity. The upright position facilitates the removal of fluid.

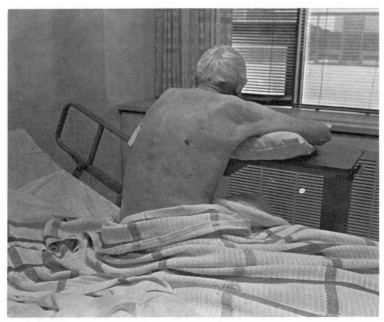

Figure 70.1

ACTION	*RATIONALE*
2. Warn the client not to cough or move suddenly during this procedure.	Sudden movement might cause injury to vital organs.

ACTION

3. Preparation is the same as for an abdominal paracentesis. The physician may percuss or auscultate the client's chest. The thoracentesis needle is inserted between the intercostal space into the pleural cavity (Fig. 70-2). The fluid is withdrawn by direct aspiration with a syringe. A 3-way stopcock is used to remove the fluid from the syringe and still keep the system airtight. The needle may be connected to a negative-pressure drainage setup if ordered.

RATIONALE

Percussion and auscultation help determine where the fluid is located. The expansion of the lungs depends on the presence of a vacuum and negative pressure in the lungs.

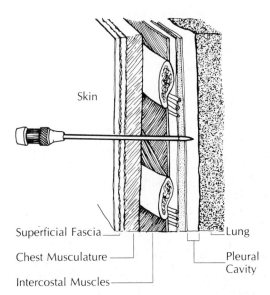

Skin

Superficial Fascia

Chest Musculature

Intercostal Muscles

Lung

Pleural Cavity

Figure 70.2

4. Apply direct pressure and a dressing or adhesive strip after the needle is withdrawn.

Pressure should be applied to allow the site seal itself.

5. Place the client on the unaffected side after thoracentesis.

This prevents seepage caused by coughing or gravitational pull.

Communicative Aspects

OBSERVATIONS

Abdominal Paracentesis

1. During the procedure and after, note the client's physical status, pulse, respirations, and skin color.

2. Observe the client for untoward reactions associated with electrolyte imbalance.

3. Record the amount, color, odor, and viscosity of the fluid aspirated or drained.

4. After the tube is removed, check the dressings frequently. If fluid continues to drain, change the dressings, clothing, and bed linen as often as necessary to keep the client clean and dry.

Thoracentesis

1. Evaluate at frequent intervals the presence or development of dizziness, fainting, tightness in the chest, uncontrollable cough, blood-tinged, frothy mucus, and rapid pulse. Pneumothorax and tension may result from thoracentesis. Pulmonary edema and cardiac distress can be produced by a sudden shift in mediastinal contents when large amounts of fluid are aspirated.

2. Record the amount, color, odor, and viscosity of the fluid withdrawn.

3. Observe the reaction to the actual procedure, degree of tolerance and apprehension, and feelings of relief after the procedure ended.

CHARTING

DATE/TIME	OBSERVATIONS	SIGNATURE
7/26 0900	Left thoracentesis done by Dr. K. Procedure explained to Mr. S and his wife before beginning. Permit signed and both voiced understanding of explanations. T 98.8° F, B/P 146/88, P 88, R 26.	G. Ivers RN
0930	Left side of chest prepared with Betadine. 5 ml of Xylocaine 1% injected into the left side of chest by Dr. K. P 90, R 26. Trocar introduced using sterile technique. Sterile specimen obtained; 250 ml clear, odorless fluid obtained. Pressure dressing applied to puncture site. Specimen stat to lab. Remains alert. P 82, R 18.	G. Ivers RN
0945	Placed on right side. Pillow to back. B/P 150/80, P 72, R 16. Resting quietly. States feeling no pain now. Able to breathe much better. Lung sounds heard bilaterally. Respirations less labored.	G. Ivers RN
1100	Remained on right side for 1 hour; no seepage from puncture site. P 80, R 16.	G. Ivers RN

Discharge Planning Aspects

CLIENT AND FAMILY EDUCATION

1. Instruct the client to remain on the unaffected side for at least 1 hour after thoracentesis.

2. Instruct the client and family about any anticipated side-effects. Tell them to report any problems to the nurse at once.

3. If the client having abdominal paracentesis is subject to recurrence of ascites, prepare the client and family for this possibility. Tell them to measure the abdomen daily and to notify the physician when the ascites begin to build up. Fluid restriction may decrease the amount and frequency of ascites. If the ascites is due to alcoholic cirrhosis, it is imperative that the client not continue to drink alcohol.

REFERRALS

The alcoholic client and the family may benefit from a referral to Alcoholics Anonymous or related support groups such as Al-Anon. The client having a thoracentesis may benefit from some of the services available from the American Lung Association or the American Cancer Society.

Evaluation

Quality Assurance

Documentation of paracentesis of the abdomen or thoracic area should include an assessment of the client's physical condition on admission. Presenting symptoms should be described and exact measurements given for later comparison. Explanations of the procedure should be documented, along with client and family response. Note the client's reaction to the procedure. Descriptions of the fluid returned and the client's condition, vital signs, and alterations in physical and mental condition after the procedure should be reflected. Follow-up care should be documented. The record should reflect anticipated side-effects and measures taken to prevent or control each.

Infection Control

1. Thorough handwashing must precede the paracentesis procedure.

2. Great care must be taken not to introduce pathogenic organisms into the closed sacs of the pleural and peritoneal cavities. These procedures are done under sterile conditions.

3. Meticulous handwashing should be done before and after caring for the client who is undergoing paracentesis. Handling of dressings and drainage should be done carefully. If an infectious process is suspected, the dressings should be disposed of in the proper method consistent with wound and skin isolation.

Technique Checklist

	YES	NO
Procedure explained to client and family	_____	_____
Permit signed	_____	_____
Abdominal Paracentesis		
Size of abdomen		
Before procedure _____		
After procedure _____		
Respiratory difficulty		
Before procedure _____		
After procedure _____		
Drainage tube left in place	_____	_____
Drainage aspirated and cannula removed	_____	_____
Total amount of drainage	_____	_____
Dressings changed × _____		
Complications _____		
Thoracentesis		
Respiratory difficulty		
Before procedure	_____	_____
After procedure	_____	_____
Pulse and respiratory rate		
Before procedure _____		
After procedure _____		
Amount of drainage removed	_____	_____
Drainage to laboratory	_____	_____
Time _____		
Pressure to site for _____ min		
Dressing to site	_____	_____
Adverse reactions		
Difficulty breathing _____		
Rapid pulse _____		
Blood-tinged mucus _____		
Coughing _____		
Tightness in chest _____		
Dizziness or fainting _____		

71 Pediculosis, Nursing Care

Overview

Definition An infestation with lice

Rationale
Relieve itching and scratching.
Destroy lice and their eggs (nits).
Sterilize infested clothing.
Give hygienic care and prevent spread of condition.

Terminology

Body louse: A parasite that lives chiefly in the seams of undergarments, to which it clings. Its bite causes characteristic minute hemorrhagic points and much itching.

Nits: Lice eggs; on hair shafts they are white or light gray and look like dandruff, but they cannot be brushed or shaken off the hair (Fig. 71-1)

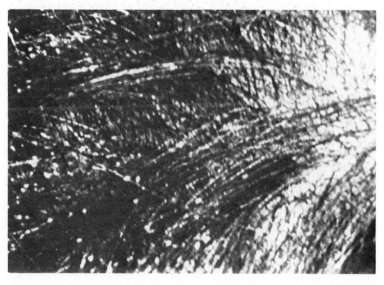

Figure 71.1

Pediculicides: Preparations for the treatment of pediculosis, designed to kill the lice, inactive nits, and relieve the generalized discomfort

Pediculus humanus, var. capitis: Variety of lice that infests the hair and scalp

Pediculus humanus, var. corporis: Variety of lice that infests the body

Phthirus pubis: Variety of lice that infests the shorter hairs on the body, usually the pubic and axillary hair

Assessment

Pertinent Anatomy and Physiology

See Appendix I: *hair, skin.*

Pathophysiological Concepts

1. Lice that are parasitic on humans are head lice, body lice, and pubic lice. Pubic lice, also called crab lice, live in the pubic and axillary hair and in the eyebrows and lashes.
2. Lice live on human blood that is obtained by biting the skin.
3. Head lice hatch eggs in silvery, oval envelopes that attach to the shafts of the hair. The eggs, called nits, can be removed only by using a fine-tooth comb.

Assessment of the Client

1. Assess the extent of the lice infestation on the client. Determine which areas of the body are infested and the duration of the problem.
2. Assess the entire family for lice infestation. If one member of the family has lice, it is expected that others will also.
3. Assess the client for any infected areas by observing for scratching of the skin.

Plan

Nursing Objectives

Reassure the client and family about the use of the pediculicide applications.

Relieve the physical and emotional manifestations of the client's condition.

Prevent the spread of pediculosis to other persons.

Client Preparation

1. The problem of pediculosis can be greatly reduced by client and family education. This education should begin during the preparation phase of treatment with thorough explanations about the spread and prevention of pediculosis. As the equipment is brought to the room, the client and/or family member should be told how the procedure is done so that it can be repeated at home if necessary.
2. Chances of spreading the condition can be reduced if all equipment is gathered before the procedure is begun. This will eliminate the need to leave the room or have other personnel enter during treatment.

Equipment

Pediculicides, as ordered by the physician

Shampoo

Comb and brush

Bath towels

Safety pins

Gauze, to protect eyes

Gloves, gown, and cap

Bland ointment for skin, if ordered by physician

Implementation and Interventions

Procedural Aspects

ACTION	*RATIONALE*
1. Take precautions to minimize the chance of spreading the infestation by wearing a gown, gloves, and cap when treating the client.	Pediculosis can spread directly by contact with infected areas, or indirectly through clothing, bed linen, combs, and brushes.
2. Cover the client's eyes with gauze pads prior to treatment with a pediculicide.	Pediculicides may be irritating to the delicate eye tissue.
3. Application techniques vary for different medications. Follow manufacturer's directions or those of the physician for application.	Medicines usually are applied to the entire scalp.
4. Use clean towels to cover the head area after the application of the pediculicide. Leave the face exposed. The medication usually is left in place for 15 minutes. Refer to the manufacturer's directions.	The lice are more thoroughly destroyed if the area is covered and left for a short time. The face is not covered so that the client can breathe more freely.
5. Dispose of all linen and towels in a specially marked linen isolation hamper.	The lice may be spread by direct contact to linen room personnel if they are not warned.
6. The lice and nits should be dead and removable after 15 minutes. Comb the hair with a fine-tooth comb; many commercial preparations include these with the pediculicide.	The adult louse lays eggs, which she glues to the hair shaft with a tenacious material applied near the root of the hair. The pediculicide will kill the nits and lice, but removal of the nits from the hair may require brisk combing and brushing.
7. After application of the medication, the client's hair should be washed with shampoo and warm water, being careful not to get it in the eyes or ears.	Shampooing will cleanse the dead pediculi from the hair and scalp. It also will leave the hair fresh.
8. The client should put on a clean gown and sit in a clean chair as the bed is changed. Remove the linen carefully from the bed and place in the special hamper. The gown, gloves, and cap are also placed in the isolation hamper.	Shaking or fanning the linen in the air may spread the lice to others.

Special Modifications

Axillary and Pubic Regions

1. Place a towel under the hips and shoulders. Drape the client.	Protect the client's modesty and self-image as much as possible.

ACTION	*RATIONALE*
2. Apply the pediculicide as ordered or recommended by the manufacturer. Leave in place for 15 minutes or as long as indicated. Thoroughly cover the hair in the pubic region and axillae. When finished, clean the medicated area with soap and warm water.	Allow time for all lice and nits to be killed; then the preparation must be removed to prevent skin irritation.

Communicative Aspects

OBSERVATIONS

1. Gain the full cooperation of the client by careful explanations and allowing time for questions and expression of feeling. Observe how the client feels about the condition.

2. Observe and chart what the client looks like, the appearance of the pediculosis and nits, amount and location of scratching by the client, any broken skin areas, and how the client reacts to the treatment.

3. Watch for secondary complications, such as impetigo and eczema.

CHARTING

DATE/TIME	OBSERVATIONS	SIGNATURE
7/29 1000	Pediculosis treatment with prescribed shampoo. Entire scalp wet with Rx and allowed to remain in place for full 10 minutes. Rinsed and shampooed. No live lice found. Nits removed with fine comb. Bed linen changed and clothing sent home with family to be washed in hot water. Use of Rx explained to family and methods of eliminating the infestation discussed. Referred to public health department for follow-up.	F. White RN

Discharge Planning Aspects

CLIENT AND FAMILY EDUCATION

1. Head lice infestation can happen to anyone; it should not be considered a sign of being dirty. Emphasize to the client and family that head lice problems do not respect class or social level.

2. Instruct the family members about how to rid their clothing and home of pediculi. They should understand that pediculosis can be spread directly or indirectly through clothing, bed linens, brushes, and combs.

3. Teach the family members that linen and personal care items of the infested person need separate and careful handling to prevent spreading the condition to others. Infected items, such as combs and brushes, should be boiled to kill the lice. Pediculicidal sprays are also available.

4. Adequate instruction must be given on how to avoid reinfection.

REFERRAL

A public health referral may expedite the elimination of the infestation in the home. If there are school-age children in the home, the school nurse should be notified of the problem so that steps can be taken to prevent the spread of lice throughout the school.

Evaluation

Quality Assurance

1. Document how the client looks and feels about the condition of pediculosis.
2. Any broken areas of the skin from scratching or any other cause must be recorded and treated to prevent infection of the areas.
3. The overall cleanliness of the individual should be noted and recorded throughout care.
4. The presence of nits on the client's hair should be recorded on the chart. Also record how the client tolerated the treatment and the apparent level of success. Subsequent reassessment of the success of the treatment should be noted throughout the hospitalization.

Infection Control

1. Certain precautions are indicated if the client has pediculosis while in the hospital. The following hospital precautions are recommended: client in a private room; masks not necessary; gowns, gloves, and caps should be worn for close contact during treatment for removal of the lice infestation.
2. Precautions in the hospital should be applied for 24 hours after the start of effective therapy.
3. Body lice are vectors for rickettsial disease, trench fever, epidemic typhus, and relapsing fever. The causative organism may be in the gastrointestinal tract of the insect and excreted on the skin surface.
4. The bite of the louse causes intense itching, and resulting scratching may lead to complications. Infectious complications of head lice infestation are pyoderma (pus-forming infections of the skin) and dermatitis. The complications are usually treated with systemic antibiotics and topical corticosteroids.

Technique Checklist

	YES	NO
Treatment explained to client and family	_____	_____
Nurse wore cap, gown, and gloves during treatment	_____	_____
Client's eyes protected during treatment	_____	_____
Linen disposed of in clearly marked isolation hamper	_____	_____
Lice and nits eliminated	_____	_____
Infestation of family members found	_____	_____
Treatment demonstrated to family	_____	_____

72 Perineal Irrigation

Overview

Definition

Cleansing of external genitalia after surgical incision. This is a sterile procedure, unlike routine perineal care, which is done for hygienic cleansing of the female perineum.

Rationale

Increase local circulation to the perineal area.

Keep the perineal area clean.

Minimize offensive odors.

Prevent infection.

Decrease discomfort from tenderness and edema due to operative trauma.

Terminology

External genitalia (vulva): In the female, consists of the mons pubis, labia majora, labia minora, clitoris, vestibule of the vagina, vulvovaginal glands, and bulb of the vestibule

Labia majora: The hairy fold of skin on either side of the vulva

Labia minora: The small fold of skin of either side, between the labia majora and the opening of the vagina

Mons pubis: A rounded eminence located anterior to the symphysis pubis of the bony pelvis. The mons is a fat pad covered with skin and hair.

Perineum: The area between the vulva and the anus in a female and the area between the scrotum and the anus in a male

Assessment

Pertinent Anatomy and Physiology

See Appendix I: *anus, genitalia (female), genitourinary system (male), vagina.*

Pathophysiological Concepts

1. The skin of the mons pubis, which is abundant in sebaceous glands, may become infected because of changes in dietary habits, normal variations, or poor hygiene. The mons pubis is usually the site of pubic lice infestation.

2. Between the hymenal opening and posterior joining of the labia minora are located the ducts of the Bartholin's glands. Bacterial infection of the Batholin's ducts may cause bilateral or unilateral swelling and pain that may become so severe that ambulation is inhibited. Purulent discharge is suggestive of gonococcal infection, but a culture is necessary for accurate determination. Infection may progress to abscess formation, which requires excision and drainage.

3. Inflammations, including infections of the lower genitourinary tract (vulva, vagina, and cervix) are relatively common, since this area is readily accessible to infectious organisms. The moisture and warmth of these tissues provide an excellent environment for growth of pathogens.

Assessment of the Client

1. Assess the client's understanding of the reasons for perineal care and how it relates to health and well-being.

2. Assess the client's sense of embarrassment in relation to how much information to offer about the procedure.

3. Assess the need for the procedure, the condition of the client's perineum, and the amount of teaching needed. Assess the incision for normal healing, the condition of the sutures, and the presence of potential problems.

Plan

Nursing Objectives

Cleanse the perineal area to provide a satisfactory environment for healing.

Reduce the client's anxiety during an embarrassing treatment.

Provide for the client's comfort and privacy.

Observe the condition of the genitoperineal area.

Report the physical and emotional effects of the treatment.

Teach the client self-care.

Client Preparation

1. Procedures dealing with the reproductive organs may be a source of embarrassment. Place the client in a dorsal recumbent position with triangular draping to avoid unnecessary exposure (Fig. 72-1)

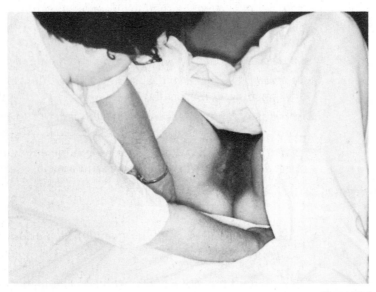

Figure 72.1

2. An explanation of the reason for this procedure, as well as a matter-of-fact attitude on the part of the nurse, may greatly enhance the client's comfort and well-being.

Equipment

Bedpan

Drape sheet

Tray containing sterile gloves, sterile cotton balls, sterile forceps, and sterile solution, as ordered

Sterile irrigating container and tubing

Sterile irrigating solution, usually sterile saline

Bath thermometer

Implementation and Interventions

Procedural Aspects

ACTION	*RATIONALE*
1. After perineal surgery, dressings are usually not applied. The perineum should be irrigated with warm, sterile, saline solution or as ordered by the physician. Irrigation usually takes place several times a day, after each voiding and bowel movement.	Due to the location of the perineum, it is difficult to secure a bandage to the area. Cleansing after elimination helps prevent infection. Gentle irrigation will lessen tension on the suture line and minimize discomfort. Since the integrity of the skin has been compromised by the incision, all equipment coming in contact with the perineal area should be sterile.
2. Wash hands thoroughly before beginning procedure.	Attempt to decrease the chance of cross-contamination.
3. Assemble necessary supplies and equipment.	Prevent the need to interrupt the procedure by having all equipment on hand.
4. The irrigation solution should be warm (105° F). To warm and check the solution without contaminating it, place the bottle in a container of hot water for 5 to 7 minutes. Pour a small amount into a bowl and check it with the bath thermometer. If it is the proper temperature, discard the test solution and continue the procedure.	Temperatures above 105° F may injure the delicate perineal tissue.
5. Position the client by elevating the head of the bed slightly, with the client in the supine position, knees flexed. Place a bath blanket over the client and fanfold the covers to the foot of the bed. Position the client on a bedpan or fracture pan to catch the irrigation solution. If this is too uncomfortable, pad the area beneath the buttocks to catch the solution.	The force of gravity will aid in the flow of the solution onto the perineal area. The position of the client should be one of comfort and facilitation of the procedure.
6. Maintain a sterile field and exert a minimum of pressure during irrigation. Don sterile gloves.	Every effort must be made to prevent pathogenic organisms from contaminating the incision.
7. Expel air from the tubing and hold the irrigating container 6 inches above the perineal area.	If the container is held higher, there will be greater pressure, since the higher the column, the greater the force.
8. With the nozzle at the level of the anterior labia or scrotal base, allow the solution to flow downward over the perineum into the bedpan or padding.	Rinse the perineum area. The area above the perineum is considered clean and the area below is contaminated.

ACTION	*RATIONALE*
9. *Female perineum:* The gloves should still be sterile. Grasp the sterile forceps in one hand and with the other gently spread the labia, if needed, to expose the surgical area. Use the forceps to secure the sterile cotton balls. With a cotton ball, cleanse the right side of the vulvoperineal area with a downward stroke from front to back. Clean the left side and middle in a similar manner using a new sterile cotton ball each time. *Male perineum:* Maintaining sterile technique, grasp a cotton ball with the forceps and cleanse the perineal area with single downward strokes. Use a new cotton ball for each stroke until the area is cleansed.	Cotton balls must be used in a downward motion in cleansing to prevent moving from an area of contamination into an area not contaminated and increasing the risk of infection.
10. The anus and buttocks should be dried with a towel.	Wetness causes irritation and bacterial growth.
11. Dispose of all linen in an appropriate hamper. Place all disposable equipment in a paperbag and dispose of properly.	Precautions must be taken not to spread infection.

Communicative Aspects

OBSERVATIONS

1. Note any foul odor or discharge, as well as signs, symptoms, behavior and complications.

2. Note the condition of the suture line, the presence of sutures or staples, any drainage, and any breaks or openings.

3. Observe for signs of infection, such as drainage, pus, inflammation, or discoloration.

CHARTING

DATE/TIME	OBSERVATIONS	SIGNATURE
3/12 0930	Sterile perineal irrigation to incision area after bilateral orchidectomy. Suture line clear, sutures remain in place with no drainage. Slight redness of area. Area cleaned with sterile saline solution. ———————————	G. Ivers RN

Discharge Planning Aspects

CLIENT AND FAMILY EDUCATION

1. If the perineal irrigation is ordered for postdischarge care, instructions should be given to the client and/or family on sterile technique, preparation of solution, height of container, position to assume during irrigation, and care and storage of equipment. Be sure that the client and family have the equipment needed and have demonstrated knowledge of proper technique.

2. This procedure affords an excellent opportunity to emphasize the importance of cleansing from front to back in the perineal area.

3. Stress the importance of securely wrapping all of the soiled material before disposing of it to prevent cross-infection of other persons.

Evaluation

Quality Assurance

Document the position of the client and tolerance of the procedure. Document the condition of the perineum before and after the treatment. Note the type of solution used for irrigation, the duration of the treatment, and any untoward reactions. Note the condition of the incision and any drainage.

Infection Control

1. After perineal surgery, the objective of perineal care is to prevent infection. Sterile technique should be used.
2. Cleansing the skin and drying it thoroughly helps prevent infection. The normal flora on the skin may be pathogenic if allowed to enter the bloodstream.
3. Handwashing and gloves should be used to avoid the chance of cross-infection between clients.

Technique Checklist

	YES	NO
Procedure explained to client	_____	_____
Equipment assembled before beginning	_____	_____
Draping used to protect privacy	_____	_____
Temperature of irrigation solution was 105° F.	_____	_____
Sterile technique maintained	_____	_____
Cleansing completed properly and as ordered	_____	_____
Infection avoided	_____	_____
Procedure(s) recorded	_____	_____

73 Peritoneal Dialysis

Overview

Definition

Instillation of a solution and its subsequent removal from the peritoneal cavity for the purpose of removing metabolic waste or correcting chemical imbalance

Rationale

Remove organic substances resulting from metabolism, when the kidneys are not functioning properly.

Remove toxic substances from the body.

Remove excess fluid build-up in the body, which the kidneys would normally remove if functioning properly.

Correct electrolyte imbalance.

Decrease edema.

Terminology

Atelectasis: An airless state resulting in collapse of lung tissue

Dialysate: The solution used to irrigate the peritoneal cavity

Hyperkalemia: Abnormally high potassium level in blood plasma

Paracentesis: Withdrawal of fluid through a needle or small tube from the peritoneal cavity

Assessment

Pertinent Anatomy and Physiology

1. See Appendix I: *kidneys.*
2. Serous membranes line the closed cavities of the body and cover the organs contained within these cavities. Cells in the surface layer secrete a slippery serous fluid, which protects against friction when these organs move against each other. The peritoneum lines the abdominal cavity and covers the abdominal viscera. There is a difference between the peritoneum of the female and the male in regard to the concept of a closed cavity. Although the peritoneum is a serous membrane in both the male and female, unlike the male peritoneum, the female peritoneum is not a closed sac, since the free end of the uterine tubes open directly into the peritoneal cavity. This means that there is communication with the external environment by way of the uterus and vagina.

Pathophysiological Concepts

1. The peritoneum may be used as the dialyzing membrane and substitutes for kidney function during reversible kidney failure. Peritoneal dialysis is done on a temporary basis to maintain stability of the body's fluid system during such crises as decreased cardiac output (due to myocardial infarction, cardiac arrhythmias, and cardiac tamponade) and altered peripheral vascular resistance (due to congestive heart failure). The principles on which peritoneal dialysis is based are diffusion and osmosis. The peritoneal membrane has two surfaces. The visceral surface covers the abdominal organs, and the parietal surface lines the abdominal cavity. The dialysate is instilled between these two surfaces. Fluids and solutes can cross this membrane by the process of osmosis, diffusion, and filtration. Impurities and dissolved particles

can be filtered from the system to compensate for the failure of the damaged kidneys to perform this function.

2. Peritoneal dialysis depends on the integrity of the abdominal wall and the peritoneal layers to fulfill the filtration function. This method cannot be used for clients who have peritonitis or severe adhesions or who have recently undergone abdominal surgery. This technique is not recommended for clients who are awaiting renal transplant.

Assessment of the Client

1. Obtain baseline assessments for comparisons to determine the effectiveness or possible complications during treatment. Measure the client's vital signs, especially blood pressure. Another important measurement is weight.

2. Assess the presence of edema. Check the client's extremities for signs of swelling. Assess the condition of the skin. Note color and presence of exudate, which might indicate removal of waste through the skin to compensate for failure of the kidneys to filter the blood properly.

3. Renal function testing is usually done to determine the effectiveness of kidney activity. Peritoneal dialysis is a short-term therapy. Large doses of diuretics are given to determine if urinary output can be significantly increased. If the client is in irreversible kidney failure, peritoneal dialysis is not considered a viable option.

4. Assess the client's abdominal area for signs of infection or distension. Assess the presence of scars and determine their origin and time of occurrence. Measure the client's abdominal girth for later comparison.

5. Assess the client's breath sounds. Determine the presence of fluid in the lungs or atelectasis.

Plan

Nursing Objectives

Keep an accurate record of the client's weight and vital signs.

Accurately monitor and record intake and output.

Observe carefully for signs of complications, such as change in the level of consciousness, hallucinations, tachycardia, and severe abdominal pain.

Comply with prescribed orders for solutions to be used, number of cycles, and timing of inflow, diffusion, and outflow.

Encourage the client to adhere to dietary restrictions before and during treatment.

Maintain sterile technique.

Client Preparation

1. Baseline vital signs from which physiologic changes can be measured must be taken before initiating the procedure. Accurately measure weight, temperature, pulse, respirations, and blood pressure.

2. Explain to the client and family exactly what will take place and why. Explain that there will be initial discomfort when the paracentesis is done; however, after this period, the client should not experience any pain. There may be some pressure when the fluid is instilled with slight shortness of breath due to the displacement of abdominal viscera upward to impinge on the diaphragm. However, this is usually relieved by raising the head of the bed slightly.

3. Check the hospital policy on consents. This is an invasive procedure and should require signed evidence of informed consent to treatment.

4. Dietary preparation may include a low-protein diet several days prior to dialysis to reduce the amount of metabolic waste in the circulating blood. During dialysis, protein restriction is not usually necessary. The diet is usually high in calories, with sodium and potassium restricted.

5. Seizures are a possible side-effect of peritoneal dialysis. Pad the siderails and make arrangements for the close observation of the client during and after the procedure.

6. A full bladder increases the risk of bladder perforation during insertion of the peritoneal catheter. Ask the client to void before the procedure.

Equipment

Paracentesis setup (see Technique 70, Paracentesis, Abdominal and Thoracic.)

Two bags of dialysate (usually 1 liter each)

Two bags for drainage (usually 1 liter each)

Sterile sutures and dressings

Implementation and Interventions

Procedural Aspects

ACTION

RATIONALE

1. Explain the procedure to the client. Before beginning, be certain to weigh the client on the same scale to be used daily to determine weight. Assist the physician with insertion of the tubing into the peritoneal area by paracentesis. The tubing is usually sutured into place.

The client's cooperation is needed during paracentesis and during dialysis, since mobility will be inhibited and frequent repositioning may be needed. Fluid loss and reduction of edema are usually reflected in weight loss. Consistent monitoring of weight on the same scale is necessary. Suturing the tubing in place helps prevent accidental removal.

2. Allow the dialysate to warm to room temperature before administering to the client.

Wide temperature variations may shock the nervous system.

3. Identify the dialysate. *Be careful not to use IV fluids accidentally.* Connect two bags or bottles of dialysate to a Y-connector, which is attached to the tubing from the client's abdomen (Fig. 73-1).

Proper identification of dialysate is critical. Diffusion can occur in both directions through the peritoneal membranes. It is essential to use hypertonic solution to dialyze the client. Isotonic or hypotonic solutions will cross the peritoneal membrane, further compromising the client's condition by adding fluid to the already overloaded system. When the dialysate runs into the client's peritoneal area, the abdominal viscera are displaced upward and may compress the lungs, causing shortness of breath. Raising the client to the sitting position may facilitate breathing.

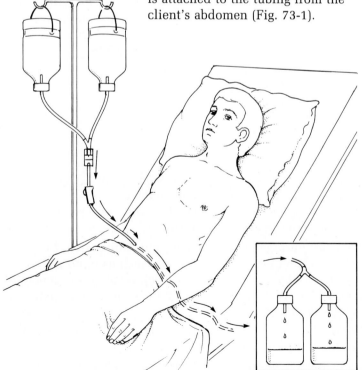

Figure 73.1

ACTION	RATIONALE
Release the clamps between the dialysate and the client. Be sure that the tubing between the client and the drainage bags or bottles is clamped. Allow the prescribed amount of dialysate to run into the client. Monitor the client to see that shortness of breath does not occur. Inspect the abdominal insertion site for leaking. Clamp the tube and leave the dialysate in the client for the prescribed time, usually 20 minutes.	
4. At the end of the prescribed time, place the client in the semi-Fowler's position with the bed raised to its highest position. Open the clamps between the client and the drainage system. Allow the dialysate to drain by gravity for the prescribed time, usually 30 to 40 minutes. Reposition the client at intervals.	Gravity will promote drainage of the fluid from the client's peritoneal cavity. Drainage may be enhanced by position changes or by elevating the head of the bed to different angles.
5. Measure the client's blood pressure, pulse, and respirations every 15 minutes during the first dialysis, then hourly. Output may exceed input; however, if the excess is more than 200 ml, notify the physician.	The filtered impurities and fluids will occupy some space; however, large discrepancies may indicate abnormal fluid loss. Analysis of vital signs may provide warning of possible complications.
6. Keep the site clean and dry. A sterile dressing should be applied over the insertion site. If the dressing becomes saturated, it should be changed, using sterile technique.	Any break in the skin offers a potential entry point for pathogenic organisms. The area around the insertion site should be kept as free of pathogens as possible.
7. Apply a dressing to the abdomen after the tube has been removed. If the dressing becomes saturated, apply a dry dressing.	Residual fluid may remain after the drainage tube has been removed. It may leak out through the insertion site.

Communicative Aspects

OBSERVATIONS

1. Observe the hydration status of the client. Monitor intake and output. Weigh the client daily on the same scale. Calculate the amount of drainage in relation to the amount of dialysate instilled. The difference reflects the amount of fluid retained or the amount filtered from the system.

2. Observe the client during dialysis for signs of complication. Measure the abdominal girth. Watch for signs of bleeding, such as rapid pulse, bleeding at the catheter site, or blood in the urine or stool. Be alert for increased abdominal pressure, which may cause rapid, shallow respirations, restlessness, or rales. Evaluate electrolyte balance. Imbalance may be indicated by leg cramping or diarrhea (from hyperkalemia). Monitor the vital signs carefully. Be alert for seizure activity.

3. Hourly urine excretion should be recorded. Any change in the appearance of the output should be noted.

CHARTING

Peritoneal Dialysis Record

DATE	TIME	SOLUTION	WEIGHT	OUTPUT PERITONEAL	URINE	B/P
7/5	0800	1000 ml	61 kg (136 lb)			126/60
	0815					130/70
	0830					128/70

Nurses' Progress Record

DATE/TIME	OBSERVATIONS	SIGNATURE
7/5 1030	Peritoneal dialysis completed. VS have remained stable. Alert and awake with no statements of pain or discomfort. 1000 ml instilled; 1040 ml returned. Weight now 61 kg (136 lb). Urine output steady, 16 to 24 ml/hr. Dark yellow with sediment. Sensorium intact. Skin turgor good. Paracentesis tube removed and sterile dressing applied. ———————	F. White RN

Discharge Planning Aspects

CLIENT AND FAMILY EDUCATION

1. Explain the procedure to the client and family. Explain how the dialysis will be done and what restrictions of mobility and diet will be required. Answer any questions and reinforce previous teaching.

2. Tell the client to notify the nurse if shortness of breath or abdominal pain occurs. Explain to the family the symptoms to watch for and ask for their cooperation in notifying the nursing staff of any possible complications.

3. Caution the client about excessive movement in bed after insertion of the tube, which might cause the tube to dislodge from the intended site.

Evaluation

Quality Assurance

Different institutions may have standard forms for recording the amount of dialysate, the return, and other meaningful parameters, such as weight and vital signs. An ongoing narrative of the client's reaction and nursing actions should also appear in the nurses' progress notes. Evidence that the nurse understood what complications to watch for and took precautions to avoid them should be reflected. Evidence of the effectiveness or ineffectiveness of the treatment should be reflected in the charting following the procedure. Safety measures to ensure that only dialysate is infused into the peritoneum should be reflected in the hospital policy manual and/or inservice programs.

Infection Control

1. Peritoneal dialysis is carried out using sterile technique. The site of puncture should be cleansed with an antiseptic cleanser prior to insertion of the catheter and tubing. The dressing around the site should be sterile. If the dressing should become saturated, it is considered contaminated and must be changed, using sterile technique. The tubing and bags or bottles should not be contaminated during hanging or changing.

2. Strict handwashing should be carried out before and after peritoneal dialysis. Wear sterile gloves when handling any equipment that will come in contact with the site of insertion or the fluid to be instilled.

3. Daily cultures of the return drainage may be ordered to detect signs of peritonitis, which is a common side-effect of repeated dialysis.

Technique Checklist

	YES	NO
Procedure explained to client and family	———	———
Amount infused and returned charted	———	———
Abnormal discrepancies reported to physician	———	———

Complications arose:

Shallow or labored breathing ———

Cardiac arrhythmias ———

    Abdominal rigidity ———

    Abdominal pain ———

    Bleeding ———

        Site ———

        Urine ———

        Stool ———

Leg cramping ———

Diarrhea ———

Fever ———

Seizure activity ———

	YES	NO
Daily vital sign notation	———	———
Daily weight, same scale	———	———
Time weighing occurred	———	———

74   Phlebotomy

Overview

Definition

A venisection to remove a quantity of the circulating blood

Rationale

Decrease the venous return of the heart, thereby causing a decline in the right ventricular output.

Decrease the volume of circulating red blood cells.

Terminology

Pathogens: Disease-producing organisms

Syncope: Fainting

Venisection: Opening a vein for blood extraction

Assessment

Pertinent Anatomy and Physiology

1. See Appendix I: *blood, blood vessels, heart, skin*
2. The mature red blood cell is called an erythrocyte. The production of red blood cells is determined, for the most part, by tissue oxygen needs. A glycoprotein, erythropoietin, is released, and in several days, red blood cells are released by bone marrow. Red blood cells have a life span of about 4 months.

Pathophysiological Concepts

1. Anemia results when the total number of circulating red blood cells is abnormally low or the hemoglobin is below 13 g to 14 g/100 ml in males and below 11 g to 12 g/100 ml in females. Anemia may be due to excessive loss or destruction of red blood cells or to deficiences in the production of the red blood cells.
2. *Polycythemia* is an abnormally high total red blood cell mass. Relative polycythemia is due to loss of blood volume without corresponding decreases in the red cells. Primary polycythemia is a proliferating disease of the bone marrow in which there is great increase in the total red blood cell mass and volume. Secondary polycythemia results from an increase in the level of erythropoietin. The goal of treating primary polycythemia is to relieve pulmonary hypertension and reduce blood viscosity; this may be done in part by phlebotomy.

Assessment of the Client

1. Assess the client for signs and symptoms of polycythemia that may have prompted seeking medical attention: headaches, night sweating, weight loss, poor memory, hearing impairment, respiratory difficulty, mental changes (level of consciousness), flushing of face, and cyanosis of face and extremities.
2. Assess the client's familiarity with this procedure. Ask if the client has ever donated blood at a local blood bank.
3. Assess baseline vital signs, including temperature, pulse, respirations, and blood pressure.
4. Assess the client's past history to determine if the client has ever had hepatitis.

Plan

Nursing Objectives

Promote the client's comfort.

Prevent infection.

Maintain fluid and electrolyte balance.

Alleviate the client's apprehension and fears.

Client Preparation

1. Explain how and why the phlebotomy will be done. Answer any questions in a truthful and straightforward manner.

2. Pathogens are normally present on the client's skin. Preparation of the skin with an antiseptic solution should precede venipuncture.

Equipment

Phlebotomy tray, including needle, tubing, bag or bottle for blood, and gauze pads

Tourniquet or blood pressure cuff

Alcohol sponges

Labels, if needed

Antiseptic solution

Implementation and Interventions

Procedural Aspects

ACTION

1. Place the client in the reclining or semireclining position. Apply a tournique and accomplish venipuncture. A blood pressure cuff inflated to 100 mm to 120 mm Hg will accomplish the same effect (Fig. 74-1).

RATIONALE

Constriction of the vessels by the tourniquet will cause pooling of the blood in the distal extremities. This facilitates location and puncture of the veins.

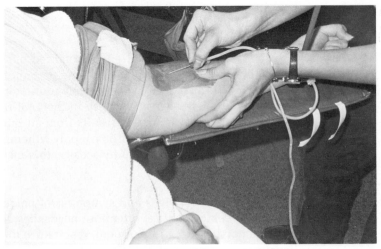

Figure 74.1

2. Apply labels to the blood if it is to be saved. Attach the tubing from the collection bag or bottle to the needle. Place the collection receptacle in a position below the level of the extremity.

Proper labeling is essential for accuracy in testing. Gravitational pull and vacuum in the bag or bottle will aid in the flow of the blood into the container.

ACTION	RATIONALE
3. Ask the client to open and close the fist of the involved arm (Fig. 74-2).	Slow, rhythmic exercise of the extremity will hasten venous blood flow and accumulation.

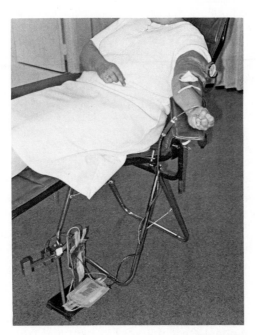

Figure 74.2

ACTION	RATIONALE
4. Remove only the amount of blood ordered by the physician. This amount is usually 500 ml. Observe the client closely for complications during phlebotomy. When the desired amount is drawn, clamp the tubing and withdraw the needle. The blood is usually sent to the laboratory for disposition. Be sure that it is labeled with the client's name and other identifying data required by the hospital.	Adverse effects may result if too much blood is removed. Monitor vital signs and note color and breathing patterns.
5. Cleanse the venipuncture site with an alcohol sponge and apply direct pressure for 2 minutes.	Bleeding may occur at the puncture site until clotting occurs.
6. Have the client remain in bed for at least 1 hour following venisection.	A sudden decrease in circulating blood volume may cause syncope. After 1 hour, the circulatory system has had time to adjust to the decreased blood volume.

Communicative Aspects

OBSERVATIONS

1. Observe for signs and symptoms of polycythemia, including cyanosis, hypertension, itching and pain in the fingers and toes, headache, difficulty concentrating, and problems with hearing.
2. Observe the client during and after the procedure for signs of shock.

CHARTING

DATE/TIME	OBSERVATIONS	SIGNATURE
3/5 2000	Expressing difficulty catching his breath. R 32. Red face and overt cyanosis. B/P 200/98, P 94. Dr. J. notified. ——————————	G. Ivers RN
2130	Phlebotomy done as ordered by Dr. J. 500 ml blood removed from left ante- cubital space. Very drowsy and still cyanotic. Oxygen continously at 6 liters. T 98.2°, B/P 170/94, R 28, P 92. States he has had this procedure done many times before. Siderails up and bed left in low position. ——————	G. Ivers RN
2245	B/P 188/84, P 90, R 24 and less labored. Still drowsy. Color improved slightly in face and nailbeds less cyanotic. No further bleeding from site of venipuncture. Up to bathroom with help with difficulty. Call light left at bed- side. Wife in attendance. Blood labeled and sent to laboratory as ordered. —	G. Ivers RN

Discharge Planning Aspects

CLIENT AND FAMILY EDUCATION

1. Reinforce explanations to the family and the client about why the phlebotomy was done. Answer questions as candidly as possible.

2. Offer liquids frequently after phlebotomy, unless contraindicated. Explain to the family why it is necessary to force fluids and elicit their cooperation.

3. Instruct the client and family to call for the nurse during the 1-hour period of bed rest after phlebotomy if anything is needed or complications arise.

Evaluation

Quality Assurance

Documentation should include the symptoms noted that support the removal of blood from the client. Teaching of the client and family and the response to education efforts should be noted. The site of the venipuncture and amount of blood removed should be noted, as well as the disposition of this blood. Any untoward side-effects and the measures taken to counteract them should be noted. The nurses' progress notes should indicate that the nurse knew what complications to watch for and took appropriate measures to protect the client.

Infection Control

1. Phlebotomy is an invasion of the circulatory system. Microorganisms that are normally present on the skin may be pathogenic when introduced into the circulation system. The skin must be cleansed with an antiseptic solution prior to venipuncture.

2. Strict handwashing must be carried out before accomplishing venisection. Hands should also be washed after finishing the procedure.

Technique Checklist

	YES	NO
Procedure explained to client and family	———	———
Venipuncture accomplished without problem	———	———
Location ———————		
Amount of blood removed ———————		
Complications		
Dizziness/fainting ———		
Headache ———		
Shock ———		
Hemorrhage ———		
Client remained in bed for 1 hour after venisection	———	———

75 Physical Examination of an Adult, General Considerations

Overview

Definition

A systematic review of the body systems and structures of an adult. (A description of the complete physical examination is beyond the scope of this text. The reader is referred to Bates B: *A Guide to Physical Examination*, 3rd ed. Philadelphia, JB Lippincott, 1983.)

The four methods of examination are:

Inspection: Visual observation of the body part

Palpation: Examination of the body part by the use of touch

Ausculation: The process of listening for sounds produced within the body

Percussion: Assessment of the body by tapping with the fingers

Rationale

Observe, examine, and assess the client before determining nursing priorities in planning care.

Terminology

Ophthalmoscope: Instrument used for detailed examination of the eye

Otoscope: Instrument used to inspect the ears

Percussion hammer: Instrument shaped like a hammer, with a head often made of hard rubber or plastic

Speculum: Funnel-shaped instrument for widening the orifices or canals of the body for examination (e.g. vaginal speculum, nasal speculum)

Sphygmomanometer: Instrument used to measure blood pressure

Stethoscope: Instrument used to transmit sounds from the client's body to the examiner's ears

Assessment

Pertinent Anatomy and Physiology

1. See Appendix I: *all systems are important during a physical examination.*

Assessment of the Client

1. Assess the ability of the client to comply with positional changes required during the physical examination. In some conditions, such as those affecting the bones, respiratory system, and nervous system, some positions are impossible to assume and even a small change may result in pain and discomfort.

2. Assess the level of anxiety about the illness or the examination itself. Determine if the client has ever had a thorough physical examination.

3. Assess the client during the examination for signs of fatigue or discomfort.

4. Assess baseline vital and neurologic sign measurements for later comparison.

Plan

Nursing Objectives

Facilitate the examination to prevent fatigue and discomfort of the client.

Drape and position the client to provide optimal visualization with minimal discomfort and embarrassment.

Develop a sound basis for nursing actions by thorough examination of all systems.

Offer adequate explanation to the client to ensure cooperation.

Protect the safety of the client.

Client Preparation

1. Offer a brief explanation of what will occur during the examination to help alleviate anxiety.

2. Ask the client to void before the examination. Bladder musculature responds to pressure stimulation and relaxation, which might result in involuntary emptying of urine during the examination.

3. Take the client to the treatment room or examination room for the physical examination or hang a sign on the client's door to prevent unauthorized persons entering during the procedure. The procedure requires privacy and is best conducted in a well-lighted area with little noise.

Equipment

Towel	Tongue depressor
Bath blanket or sheet	Disposable examining gloves
Stethoscope	Brown paper bag or plastic bag
Sphygmomanometer	Adjustable lamp
Flashlight	Vaginal speculum, if needed
Otoscope	Rectal endoscope, if needed
Ophthalmoscope	Lubricant
Percussion hammer	

Implementation and Interventions

Procedural Aspects

ACTION	RATIONALE
1. Do not leave the client unattended on a narrow examining table.	Consideration must be given to the safety of the client first.
2. Screen and drape the client to protect modesty and preserve privacy. Ask the male client to remove all clothing. Place a towel over his genitalia and a sheet over his entire body. Ask the female client to undress, placing a towel over her breasts and a sheet over her entire body or allow her to wear a hospital gown with the opening in the front. Do not tuck the sheets in at the bottom of the bed or table.	The client is entitled to privacy. Some of the positions required in physical examination and some of the techniques necessary may embarrass the client. Maintenance of a matter-of-fact attitude can lessen anxiety.

ACTION

3. Gather all equipment before beginning the examination and check it to see that it is in proper working order. All actions during the examination should be deliberate, coordinated, and smooth.

4. Ask the client to assume the position that facilitates visualization of the system being examined. Positions include the following: *supine*—lying flat on the back (Fig. 75-1); *Sim's position*—on the right side, tilted forward with the left knee slightly flexed over the top of the right knee, the right arm is to the back and the left arm to the front of the body (Fig. 75-2);

RATIONALE

When the staff seems capable and in control, the client may sense the confidence and be less anxious.

Proper positioning can greatly enhance the ability to assess fully the system being examined.

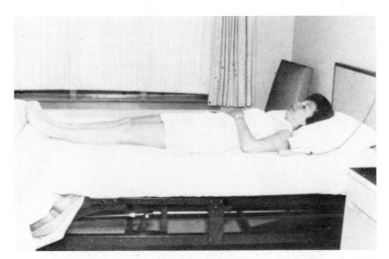

Figure 75.1

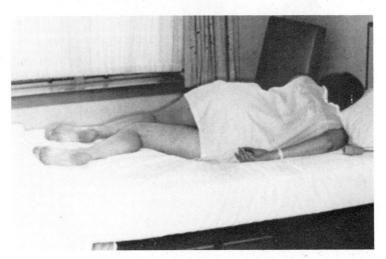

Figure 75.2

ACTION   **RATIONALE**

lithotomy—on the back with knees
flexed, slightly apart, and the feet
secured in stirrups in an elevated
position or on the level of the body
plane; the hands are folded across
the body (Fig. 75-3); *modified
lithotomy*—on the back with the
knees flexed and the heels touching (Fig. 75-4); *Knee–chest*—on the
stomach with the buttocks elevated, the knees pulled up to touch
the chest, the head turned to one
side and resting on the folded
arms (Fig. 75-5).

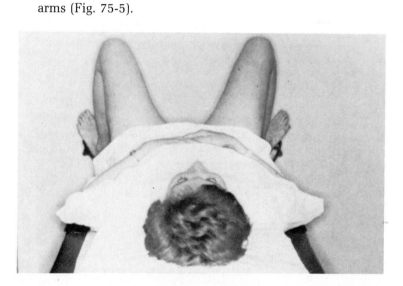

Figure 75.3

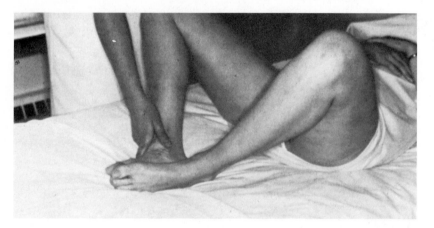

Figure 75.4

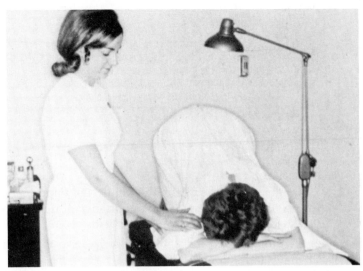

Figure 75.5

ACTION

RATIONALE

5. After the examination, return the client to the room. Clean off any lubricant from the body and leave the client in a comfortable environment.

The physical examination can be very tiring. Leave the client in an environment conducive to getting some rest.

Communicative Aspects

OBSERVATIONS

1. The actual examination usually proceeds from head to foot, including a general review of body systems. The genitalia and rectum are generally done last to avoid prolonging any embarrassment the client might feel and to prevent introducing microorganisms to other parts of the body. The following is a synopsis of the observations made during the examination:

   Head: Cuts, bumps, pediculosis

   Eyes: Pupil reaction, cataracts, and hemorrhages of the internal eye (ophthalmoscopic examination)

   Ear: Excessive wax, foreign objects, lacerations, and intact eardrum (otoscopic examination)

   Chest and lungs: Rales, breath sounds, congestion, rib abnormalities, and scars (stethoscopic examination)

   Extremities: Reflexes, range of motion, dexterity, and abnormalities (percussion hammer)

   Back and spine: Alignment, ability to move freely, and abnormalities

   Nervous system: Equilibrium and steadiness

   Genitalia: Abnormalities, tumors, infection, drainage, and enlarged prostate (male)

   Rectum: Hemorrhoids, polyps, tumor, bleeding and fissures (glove and lubricant)

2. Observe the client during the examination for signs of fatigue and discomfort. Observe the overall response to the examination.

3. Note the client's ability to resposition and to follow the instructions.

CHARTING	DATE/TIME	OBSERVATIONS	SIGNATURE
	1/10 1100	Physical examination done by Mrs. J, Family Nurse Practitioner. To treatment room by wheelchair. Full explanation of procedure given. Seemed relaxed and compliant with requests to turn. No problem noted with assuming positions for examination. Skin intact. Returned to room in 35 min. by wheelchair. B/P 146/72, P 88, R 16. Resting quietly at this time. ————————	B. Lake RN

Discharge Planning Aspects

CLIENT AND FAMILY EDUCATION

1. Emphasize to the client and family the importance of periodic physical examinations. Discuss the importance of reporting symptoms to the physician as early as possible to enhance care.
2. Reinforce or explain information given to the client by the examiner during the examination.

Evaluation

Quality Assurance

Documentation should include the explanation given to the client before the examination and the client's reaction to the physical examination. Document any abnormal findings. The ability of the client to assist and comply with instructions should be reflected.

Infection Control

Equipment used for consecutive clients should be cleaned thoroughly after each use. Handwashing should precede and follow the physical examination. Any swabs, pads, or dressings used in the examination should be disposed of in a paper or plastic bag.

Technique Checklist

	YES	NO
Procedure explained to the client	_____	_____
Client able to attain all positions requested	_____	_____
Abnormalities or problems noted during physical examination	_____	_____
Client left in clean and comfortable environment	_____	_____

76

Position, Change of (Manually and Mechanically)

Overview

Definition

Turning, moving, or lifting the client in bed, from the bed to a chair, and from the bed to a stretcher, either manually or using a mechanical lifting device

Rationale

Prevent complications related to prolonged bedrest.

Promote optimal comfort.

Ensure safety of both the client and the nurse.

Facilitate transportation of the client.

Terminology

Abduction: Lateral movement of the limbs away from the median plane of the body

Adduction: Movement of a limb toward the median plane of the body

Atrophy: A wasting due to lack of nutrition

Contracture: A permanent shortening of a muscle, resulting in abnormal position of the body part

Decubitus ulcer: Pressure sore; an ulcer of the skin generally over a bony prominence, resulting from pressure on the area

Fowler's position: On the back in bed with the bed raised to the normal sitting position

Lateral position: Side-lying in bed

Prone position: Lying on the abdomen with the face turned to one side

Recumbent: Lying down

Supine position: Lying on the back

Assessment

Pertinent Anatomy and Physiology

See Appendix I: *skeletal muscles, skeletal system, skin, vertebral column.*

Pathophysiological Concepts

1. The muscles of the body are meant to work. Movement stimulates the muscles, promotes tone, and adds to general well-being. When immobility is forced upon a person, inactivity causes the muscles to atrophy and decrease in size and strength. With disuse, the joints become stiff and immobile.

2. Immobility may predispose to pressure over certain areas of the body, especially the bony prominences. With extended pressure, tissue breakdown may result. (See Technique 78, Pressure Sore).

Assessment of the Client

1. Assess the ability of the client to participate in the moving and repositioning process. Determine client mobility, physical limitations, and desired results.

2. Evaluate the client's knowledge of the principles of proper body mechanics. Assess deficits and determine the best time to teach the client and family about proper lifting and moving techniques.

3. Assess the presence of drains, tubes, and other equipment that might impede or alter positioning techniques.

4. Assess the presence of decubiti, surgical incisions, fractures, or bruises, which might cause pain if not handled carefully.

Plan

Nursing Objectives

Facilitate safe client transfer, preventing injury to the client and to personnel.

Allay the client's fear of and anxiety about repositioning.

Determine the reactions and tolerances of clients being moved.

Teach the client to assist in moving or lifting as much as possible within physical limitations.

Maintain proper body alignment.

Adhere to proper body mechanics principles.

Facilitate the comfort of the client.

Client Preparation

1. If the client understands what is expected and is told how to assist in the moving procedure, cooperation is more likely. Explain in advance the goal of the activity and its importance to the client.

2. If the client is helpless, place a draw sheet or soft pad under the hips to be used for turning during the bath.

3. If a mechanical lifting device is used, check it before the client is placed in it to be sure of proper working conditions and to prevent accidents.

Equipment

Inflatable turning device, sheepskin, soft pad, or draw sheet

Hydraulic lift, if necessary

Stretcher

Pillows for support

Chair

Implementation and Interventions

Procedural Aspects

ACTION	RATIONALE
Moving the Client up in Bed	
1. The client can assist in the procedure by grasping the top of the flat bed, if able. Place one arm under the client's shoulders and the other arm under the hips. Ask the client to pull at the same time as the nurse moves forward toward the top of the bed on a prearranged signal. Also, ask the client to bend the knees and push against the mattress with the heels for the feet to provide momentum for the move. If the client is unable to assist, two nurses will be needed for	Pulling or pushing the client on a smooth surface requires less force than lifting. The bed should be in a flat position so that the client will not be moving uphill, which requires more energy. When the client and nurse move at the same time, optimal use of the energy of both is obtained.

ACTION   **RATIONALE**

the moving procedure. Two nurses
place their hands under the client's hips and shoulders, and both
pull up at a given signal, using
proper body mechanics (Fig. 76-1).

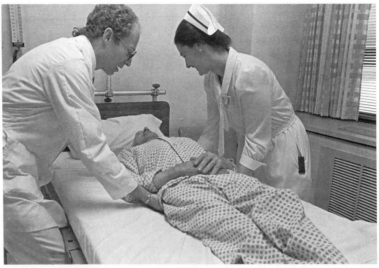

Figure 76.1

Turning the Client to the Side

1. To turn onto the left side, first
   move the client over to the right
   side of the bed (Fig. 76-2), crossing
   the right leg over the left. The left
   arm is placed in abduction and
   external rotation with the elbow
   flexed; the right arm is placed in
   abduction and flexion over the
   chest. Stand on the side of the bed
   to which the client is being turned.

A minimum of energy is required to
turn an object by rolling it.

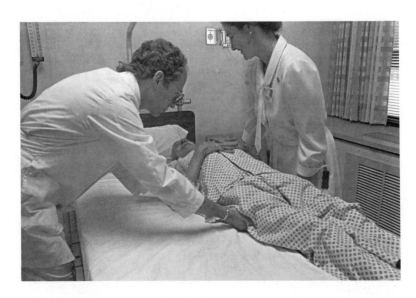

Figure 76.2

ACTION	*RATIONALE*

Place one hand on the client's right hip and the other hand on the right shoulder. Pull the client over onto the left side (Fig. 76-3).

2. Be aware of safety precautions for both the client and the nurse. Place the siderails up on the side of the bed opposite the nurse when one person is turning the client. Use proper body mechanics.

If the siderail is up on the side of the bed opposite the nurse, the client may be prevented from accidentally falling from the unattended side of the bed.

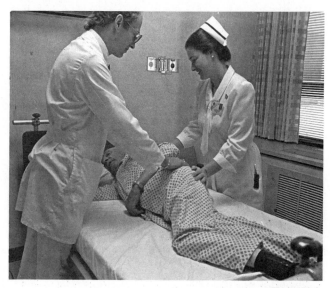

Figure 76.3

Logrolling the Client

1. Place the client's arms across the chest (Fig. 76-4) and place a pillow between the knees. Tell the client that the whole body must be kept rigid, with the exception of the legs.

For the client with spinal injury, flexion of the back may cause further injury to the spinal column.

2. Move the client's entire body to the side of the bed, maintaining the spinal column in straight alignment. Keep the spinal column rigid by keeping the turn sheet taut (Fig. 76-5). Turn the client by grasping the rolled edges of the turn sheet and rolling the client to the side (Fig. 76-6). Prop the client in the desired position with a pillow to the back (Fig. 76-7).

Using the turn sheet, or draw sheet, the client's back can be kept straight by holding the sheet taut. Propping should maintain straight alignment of the spinal column.

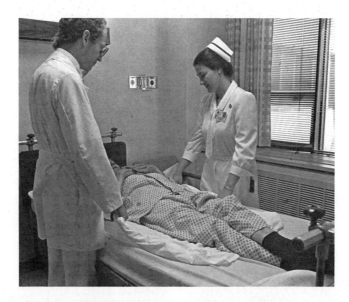

Figure 76.4

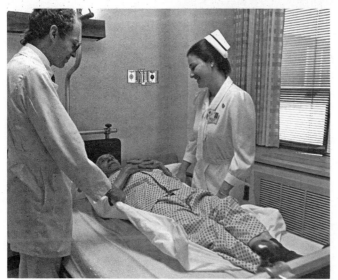

Figure 76.5

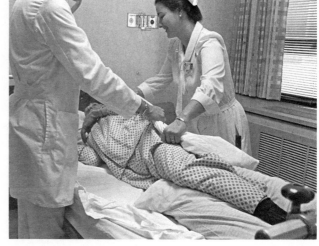

Figure 76.6

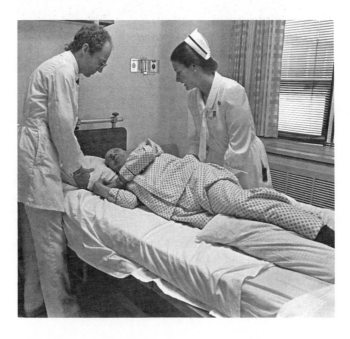

Figure 76.7

ACTION	*RATIONALE*
Moving a Client from Bed to Stretcher	
1. Pull the client from the bed to the stretcher by using two to six persons, as indicated by the client's condition and size (Figs. 76-8, 76-9). Buckle the client on the stretcher with the safety belt (Fig. 76-10).	Sliding rather than lifting an object on a flat surface conserves energy and prevents strain. Belts on the stretcher may help prevent falls.

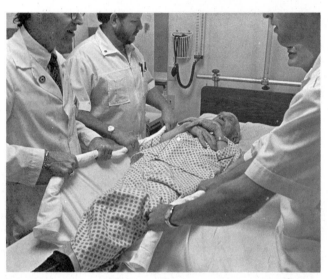

Figure 76.8

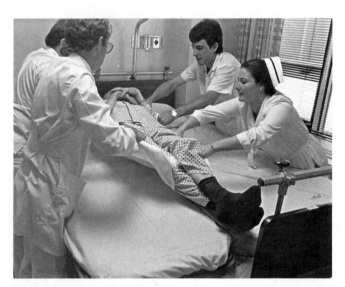

Figure 76.9

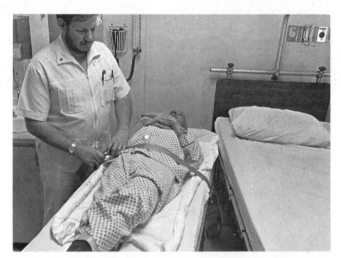

Figure 76.10

2. The three-person lift may be used. Three persons stand on the same side of the client, placing their arms well under the client along the body bulk with emphasis at the points of greatest weight, the chest and hip areas. At a given signal, the client is lifted to the chests of the personnel and carried	Holding an object closest to its center of gravity will conserve energy. The three-person lift offers more of a chance for client falls and staff injury. It should be used only if absolutely necessary.

ACTION

to the cart, using proper body mechanics principles. Use this technique only if there is no way to get the cart next to the bed to slide the client onto the cart.

Moving a Client From the Bed to a Chair

1. Place the chair parallel to the bed at a point nearest the client's hips.

2. Assist the client into the sitting position on the side of the bed. With one hand under each of the client's axillae (Fig. 76-11), assist the client into the standing position in front of the chair. Allow the client to become stable. Then, still supporting the client, slowly assist the client to turn, with a pivoting motion, until in position to sit in the chair (Fig. 76-12). The

RATIONALE

The shorter the distance an object is lifted, the less energy required.

Sitting momentarily on the side of the bed allows the client to regain a sense of equilibrium in the altered position. The client must be supported during the entire procedure to prevent falls.

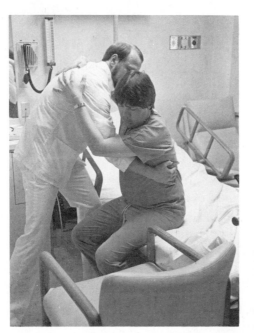

Figure 76.11

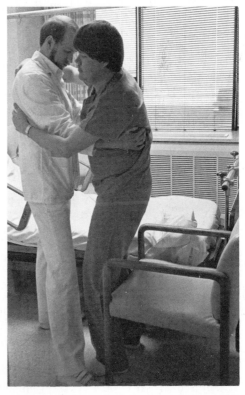

Figure 76.12

ACTION

RATIONALE

client may assist in lowering into the chair, if able, but the nurse should maintain support until the client is safely seated (Fig. 76-13). Be sure that the chair is steady and will not move as the client is lowered into it. If the client is unsteady, two nurses should assist.

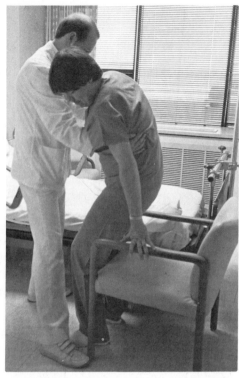

Figure 76.13

Moving the Client With a Hydraulic Lift

1. Place the sling under the client by rolling from side to side while the client is flat in bed. Attach the sling to the lifter and carefully lift the client from the bed.

The use of a mechanical lifting device conserves energy and reduces the possibility of unnecessary injury.

2. A locked wheelchair should be ready to receive the client. Slowly lower the client into the chair. When the client is safely settled in the chair, release the lifter.

It is important to proceed slowly to ensure the client's safety.

Positioning the Client After Turning or Moving

1. For the client in the supine position, take care to prevent footdrop (See Technique No. 56, Foot Care). Place a footboard on the bed to alleviate this problem. A firm mattress will provide the back support the client needs. Place the pillow well under the client's shoulders. Handrolls may be placed in the client's hands.

Placement of a pillow under the head only can cause neck strain from the unnatural position of the pillow tilting the head forward. Handrolls help maintain the normal functional appearance of the hands and prevent a clawlike appearance. A pillow under the knees may inhibit circulation and predispose to clotting and venous stasis in the legs.

ACTION

2. For the lateral recumbent position, place a pillow under the head and neck. A pillow to the back will offer added support (Fig. 76-14). Support the upper arm and the uppermost leg with a pillow (Figs. 76-15, 76-16). Flex both the hips and the knees.

RATIONALE

Maintain normal cervical alignment. Breathing is easier with the upper arm supported rather than resting its full weight on the chest area. A pillow under the leg maintains lumbosacral alignment.

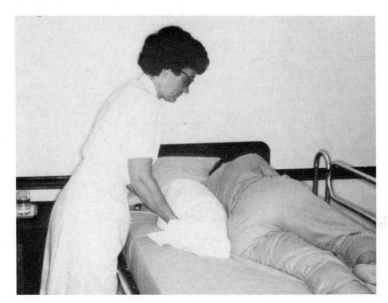

Figure 76.14

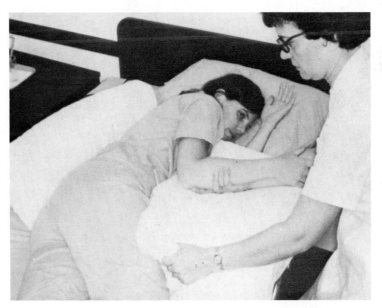

Figure 76.15

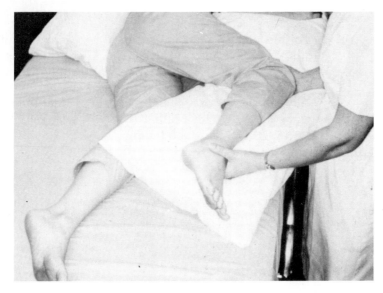

Figure 76.16

ACTION	RATIONALE
3. When the client is sitting in a chair, place a pillow behind the lumbosacral area. Any dependent limbs should be supported in the position of normal function. Apply restraints, if necessary, to prevent falling.	Supporting dependent areas relieves the pull of the weight of these areas and enhances comfort.

Communicative Aspects

OBSERVATIONS

1. Observe the client's appearance and vital signs before moving and lifting. These may offer contraindications to moving at the time. Observe the client during the move to assess tolerance and ability to assist.

2. If the client is prone to fainting, lying flat in bed will usually relieve this problem. Protect the client from injury.

3. Turn the helpless client every 2 hours to prevent complications or the sequelae of immobility. This includes the postoperative client.

4. Observe the condition of the client's skin during turning. Massage pressure areas.

CHARTING

DATE/TIME	OBSERVATIONS	SIGNATURE
5/7 1000	Moved to the side of the bed with no difficulty. Sat on the bedside for 2 minutes with no signs of dizziness. Seems to have good body control. Up in chair for 10 minutes. P 82, R 22, B/P 150/88. ————————	L. Davis LVN

Discharge Planning Aspects

CLIENT AND FAMILY EDUCATION

1. Instruct the client and family in moving and lifting techniques, detailing all safety precautions for the client, as well as for the persons doing the moving. Allow the client and family to demonstrate proficiency in the moving and lifting techniques before discharge.

2. If the client will be dependent over a long period of time, stress the importance of being as cooperative as possible in helping with the moving process.

3. Illustrate and demonstrate the principles of good body mechanics.

REFERRALS

If the client is to be referred to an extended-care facility, inform the persons who will be doing daily care about the usual daily schedule and the most effective turning methods. If the client will require care at home, a referral to a home health agency may be appropriate.

Evaluation

Quality Assurance

Documentation should reflect the turning and repositioning schedule of the client during hospitalization. Attention to the turning or repositioning technique should be in evidence at least every 8 hours. The condition of the skin should be reflected in the nurses' progress notes. Cooperation of the client should be noted. Instructions for turning the client at home should be noted.

Infection Control

Handwashing should be done before and after attending each client. Ensure that cross-infections is minimized by thorough handwashing technique.

Technique Checklist

	YES	NO
Positioning procedure explained to the client and family	_____	_____
Client's position changed at least every 2 hours	_____	_____
Technique demonstrated to family	_____	_____
Falls prevented	_____	_____
Complications of immobility prevented	_____	_____

77 Preoperative, Perioperative, and Postoperative Care

Overview

Definition

Preoperative: The period of psychological and physical preparation, determined by the needs of the individual client, from the time of hospital admission to the actual surgical operation

Perioperative: The period of time in the surgical cycle during which the surgical operation takes place

Postoperative: The period of recovery, beginning when the client is removed from the surgical table, incorporating a series of activities aimed at meeting the client's physical and psychological needs

Rationale

Preoperative Period

Prepare the client physically and emotionally for the surgical procedure.

Decrease the possibility of postoperative infection.

Prevent avoidable complications.

Perioperative Period

Ensure safe, proper positioning of the client before, during, and after surgery.

Safeguard sterility to prevent postoperative infection.

Observe and provide intensive physical and psychological support (if local anesthetic is used).

Offer information and support to the family.

Postoperative Period

Restore the client to the highest level of function possible.

Meet the individual needs of the client on return to the unit, and thereafter until discharge from the hospital.

Inform, support, and comfort the family.

Terminology

PREOPERATIVE PERIOD

Allay: To subdue or reduce in intensity

Nonverbal fear: A concern that is not expressed verbally but may be expressed overtly by some action or behavior (e.g., a facial grimace or clenched fists)

Operative permit or consent: Written, informed permission given by the client or legal representative for the operative procedure to be done; different hospitals have various regulations about who obtains and witnesses consents. The purpose is to ensure that the client understands the proposed surgery, anesthetic, and risks of complications or sequelae; in addition, the consent protects the physician and hospital against claims of unauthorized surgery.

Pathogen: An organism or material capable of producing disease

Rapport: A relationship marked by accord or affinity

Surgical preparation: Preoperative preparation of the skin on and around the surgical site to render it as free as possible of microorganisms without damage to the physical or physiologic integrity of the site

PERIOPERATIVE PERIOD

Anesthesia: Loss of sensation or feeling; the types are

Local: Anesthesia confined to a limited or small localized area of the body
Examples:

Infiltration: Anesthesia produced by the injection of the anesthetic solution directly into the tissues

Topical: Application of a local anesthetic directly to the involved area

Regional: Insensibility caused by interruption of the sensory nerve conductivity of any region of the body.
Examples:

Nerve block: Anesthesia produced by blocking the transmission of impulses through a nerve

Spinal: Anesthesia produced by injection of the agent beneath the membranes of the spinal column

General: A state of unconsciousness and insusceptibility to pain produced by an anesthetic agent
Examples:

Endotracheal: Anesthesia produced by introducing an anesthetic agent through a tube inserted into the trachea

Inhalation: Anesthesia produced by the respiration of a volatile liquid or gaseous anesthetic agent

Hypothermia (induced): A deliberate reduction of temperature of part or all of the body; sometimes used as an adjunct to anesthesia in surgical cases involving a limb. Induced hypothermia also is used as a protective measure in cardiac and neurologic surgery. Local hypothermia refers to lowering of the temperature of only a part of the body, such as a limb. General hypothermia refers to the reduction of body temperature below normal to reduce oxygen and metabolic requirements.

Positions Used for Surgery

Lateral positions: Several versions of the side-lying position used for surgery on the kidney and the chest. The kidney position places pressure on the lower leg and arm, and pools blood in these areas.

Lithotomy positions: The client is in the supine position with the buttocks at the break in the operating table. The thighs and legs are flexed at right angles, and the feet are in stirrups elevated above the table. After the client is properly positioned, the bottom section of the table is lowered. This position is used for perineal, rectal and vaginal surgery.

Prone position: The client lies abdomen downward with face turned to one side and arms at the sides; the palms are pronated (turned downward) and the fingers extended. This position is used for back, spinal, and some rectal surgery.

Reverse Trendelenburg position: The client lies supine with head elevated and feet lowered. This position permits better visualization of the biliary tract during surgery.

Supine position: The client lies flat, back downward and abdomen upward, arms at the sides, palms down with fingers extended and free to rest on the table, legs straight with feet slightly separated. This is the position most commonly used for surgical procedures.

Trendelenburg position: The client lies supine; the head and body are lowered into the head-down position, and the knees are flexed by breaking (bending at a predetermined position) the table. This position is used for lower abdominal and pelvic surgery. Because the upward position of the viscera decreases diaphragmatic movement and thus interferes with breathing, this position is not maintained any longer than necessary.

Stages of Anesthesia

Stage I: Extends from the beginning of the administration of an anesthetic to the beginning of the loss of consciousness

Stage II (stage of excitement or delirium): Extends from the loss of consciousness to the loss of eyelid reflexes

Stage III (stage of surgical anesthesia): Extends from the loss of the eyelid reflex to cessation of respiratory effort. At this stage, the client is unconscious, muscles are relaxed, and most reflexes have been abolished.

Stage IV (stage of danger or overdose): An undesired stage that is complicated by respiratory and circulatory failure, whereupon death follows unless the anesthetic is discontinued immediately and artificial respiration is performed

POSTOPERATIVE PERIOD

Dehiscence: Literally means "bursting forth"; after surgery, refers to the spontaneous release of sutures or suture line after healing has begun

Evisceration: The spontaneous protrusion of viscera through a surgical incision

Positions Frequently Used after Surgery

Dorsal position: The client lies supine without elevation of the head. The head is turned to one side to facilitate evacuation of secretions.

Fowler's position: The client lies supine with the head of the bed elevated at least 45° into a sitting position.

Sims' position or lateral position (semiprone): The client lies on either side, with the upper arm forward, the under leg slightly flexed at the thigh, and the head turned to one side to facilitate the evacuation of secretions and prevent aspiration. A pillow is placed at the back for support.

Surgical aseptic technique: The practices that aim at eliminating pathogenic agents during surgery

Assessment

Pertinent Anatomy and Physiology

1. Fluid and electrolyte balance must be maintained before, during, and after surgery. An *electrolyte* (sometimes called a salt or mineral) is a substance in the body capable of developing electrical charges when dissolved in water. Fluids are present in two body spaces, outside the cells (extracellular fluid, such as plasma), and inside the cells (intracellular [interstitial] fluid, in which tissues and cells are bathed). The fluid and electrolyte balances must be in equilibrium to promote homeostasis in the body.

2. Metabolic activity is described in terms of the basal metabolic rate (BMR). The BMR is the amount of heat produced by the body cells when they are as close to being at rest as is possible during life.

3. Hair grows over the entire surface of the body except the lips, palms, soles of the feet, and parts of the genitalia. Microorganisms are normally present in the hair on the body. Removal of the hair helps to reduce the amount of microbial activity on and around the operative site.

Pathophysiological Concepts

1. When a blood clot becomes dislodged from its original site, it may be carried to the heart. If it survives the coronary circulation to reach the right ventricle, it may be forced into the pulmonary artery, where it can block the main artery or one of its branches. Symptoms are sharp, stabbing pain in the chest, dilated pupils, and rapid, irregular pulse. This condition is often fatal.

2. Respiratory complications from surgical procedures are always a risk. Pneumonia often is due to the presence of microorganisms (e.g., *Staphylococcus aureus*). Hypostatic pneumonia is inadequate aeration of the lungs, often due to immobility. Atelectasis may be due to blocking of the bronchial passageways due to mucous plugs.

3. Hemorrhage is uncontrolled loss of blood from the incision area or from some other part of the body. It may or may not be due to the surgical procedure. The escaped blood may appear on the dressing or may remain pooled inside the client.

4. Urinary retention occurs frequently after surgery. Anesthesia, especially spinal anesthesia, decreases the bladder tone. If the client cannot urinate when desired or if urination is frequent and in very small amounts, measures may have to be taken to correct the urinary problem.

Assessment of the Client

1. Preoperatively, assess the client's physical condition. Clients who are debilitated before surgery may have a longer postoperative period. Assess nutritional status in relation to the ability of the tissue to regenerate after surgery. Assess the knowledge level of the client about the pending surgical procedure. Assess the level of apprehension and misunderstanding about the surgical procedure. Explore various teaching methods to decide which is best for this client. Determine the presence of any symptoms with a full description so that determinations can be made postoperatively about which symptoms are related to the surgery and which were already present. Assess baseline vital signs. Determine the effect that the surgery will have on the client's body image, and identify methods to assist the client to handle these changes.

2. Perioperatively, assess the stability of the client. Assess any reactions to the anesthesia and any fluctuations in vital signs. Be alert for any complications that may arise. Assess the client for any special positional limitations or needs that may complicate positioning for the surgical procedure.

POSTOPERATIVE ASSESSMENT

Immediate Postoperative Period: Frequent assessment during the stage of recovery from anesthesia is imperative. During this critical period, assess the vital signs at least every 15 minutes. Rectal temperature should be taken every hour. Assess the length of time required for the client to arouse and to awaken fully. Constant attendance is required during the waking period. Assess the client's readiness to return to the hospital room by stability of vital signs and return to consciousness (indicated by the return of the reflexes, such as gag, blink, swallow, and cough).

Extended Postoperative Period: Assess the client immediately on return to the unit. Assess the patency of drain tubes, infusions, vital signs, and level of consciousness. Determine the presence of pain and assess the advisability of administering pain medication. During the postoperative period, assess the return of normal function, any fluctuations in vital signs, relief of symptoms for which the surgery was performed, and progress of the client recovering from surgery. Determine compliance of the client and assess the need for additional teaching to assist in recovery. Determine if the family needs support or assistance in dealing with surgical outcomes and with the client's current condition. Frequent assessment of vital signs, including temperature (at least every 4 hours), should be done so that any complications can be treated as early as possible.

Plan

Nursing Objectives

PREOPERATIVE PERIOD

Promote early assessment of the psychological and physical needs of the preoperative client.

Implement a plan of nursing care that meets the client's individual needs by using a series of educational and supportive activities to prepare the client and family for surgery.

PERIOPERATIVE PERIOD	Maintain the safety of the client during surgery.

Assist with procedures and techniques during surgery to decrease anesthesia time and safeguard the client's well-being.

Obtain, label, and send specimens to the proper departments to aid in diagnosis.

Carefully document the progress of the operation on the operating room (OR) sheet to provide a legal record for reference.

POSTOPERATIVE PERIOD

Assess and meet the physical needs of the postoperative client

Offer psychological support to the client and family during the recuperation process.

Implement a plan of personalized nursing care that relates to individual client needs.

Assist the client to an effective and efficient postoperative period.

Client Preparation

PREOPERATIVE PERIOD

1. The preoperative client is subject to many emotions regarding preoperative procedures. Offer a clear and calm explanation of what to expect. Consider the client's level of education, experience, and willingness to learn when explanations are offered.

2. Reassure and support the family so that they will know what to expect during the surgical and recuperation period. Offer an explanation about procedures and hospital routines and begin discharge planning activities at this time.

3. Prepare and assist the client during the preoperative period when diagnostic study may be done to determine the extent of the problem or amount of surgical intervention needed. Know normal values of tests and report significant deviations to the physician.

4. Act as the client's advocate in obtaining answers to questions about the surgery, risks, expected outcomes, and any other questions the client may have. Ensure that the consent form is signed and that the client understood what the form said and what the consent involved.

5. Place the client in a hospital gown before going to surgery. If the surgical procedure is on the head, face, or mouth, the client may be able to wear pajama bottoms or surgical pants. Physicians usually have preferences in this regard. Ask the family to take all jewelry and valuables while the client is in surgery. If the client has artificial dentures or a partial plate, ask that these be removed before the client goes to the surgical suite. Assist the client to perform oral care. A mouthwash may be used and the teeth may be brushed; however, caution the client not to swallow any of the liquid.

PERIOPERATIVE PERIOD

Carefully identify the client, the procedure to be done, and the limb, breast, or area involved. It is essential to identify the exact area of pathology properly to ensure that the client receives the proper surgical intervention. If the surgical procedure will be performed with the client under local anesthesia, explain during the procedure what is happening in a calm and confident voice to soothe and reassure the client. Answer questions slowly, clearly, and loudly enough to be heard easily. If the client is having a general anesthetic, provide support and reassurance during the intubation phase and during the recovery phase. Handle the client gently during transport-and-transfer activities and during preparations for the surgical procedure.

POSTOPERATIVE PERIOD

Knowledge that the surgery is completed may reduce the client's anxiety and enhance cooperation. As the client regains consciousness, explain that the operation is over, relate where the client is, and remind the client of the presence of tubes and drains. Repetition and clarification may be necessary.

EQUIPMENT

Preoperative Period

Operative consent form (see manual on hospital policy)

Preoperative checklist

Hospital gown

Personal hygiene requisites

Denture cup (if needed)

Surgical shaving preparation tray or kit

Perioperative Period

Operating room supplies (as needed)

Postoperative Period

Siderails

IV standard

Emesis basin

Tissues

Blanket

Stethoscope

Sphygmomanometer

Thermometer

Any special equipment

Implementation and Interventions

Procedural Aspects

ACTION

Preoperative Period

1. Surgical preparation may involve shaving the operative area (Figs. 77-1 to 77-5). Moisten the skin and lather with soap or cream preparation. Use a very sharp razor to remove all hair in and around the operative site. Be careful not to scratch the area because this would be a possible source of infection. Rinse the area thoroughly and dry.

RATIONALE

Surgical skin preparation is done to remove as many organisms as possible without injuring the natural skin barrier. The integrity of the skin must be maintained.

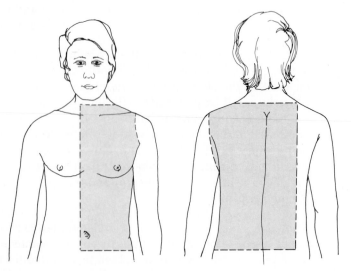

Figure 77.1

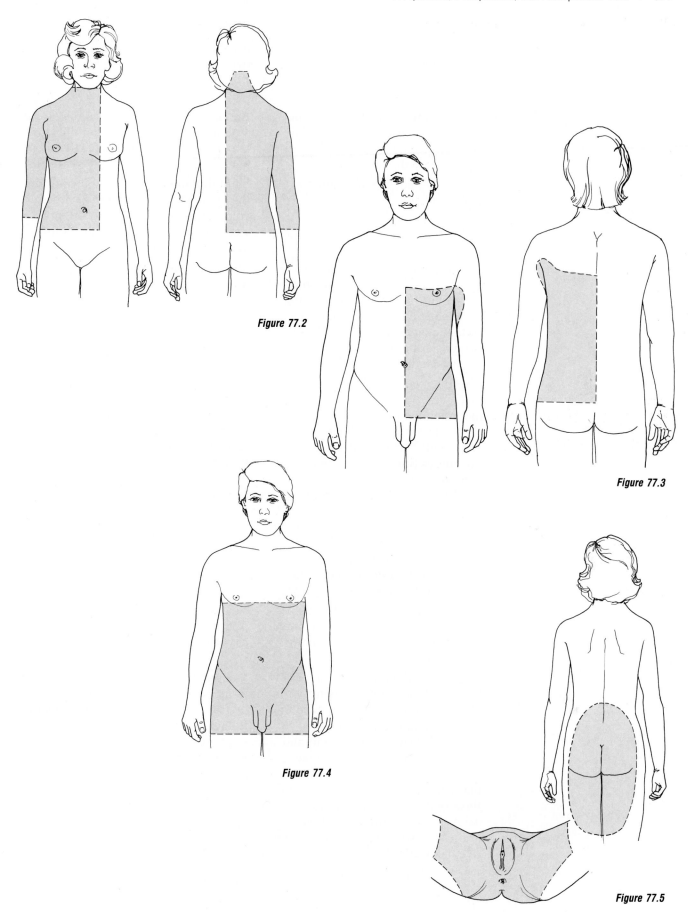

Figure 77.2

Figure 77.3

Figure 77.4

Figure 77.5

ACTION	RATIONALE
2. Administer preparatory medications as ordered. A preopertive sedative may be ordered the night before surgery.	A calm and rested client is anesthetized more easily.
3. Be certain that the client does not receive food or fluids during the preoperative period for the time specified by the physician.	An empty stomach reduces the danger of distension and aspiration during the anesthesia and post-anesthesia periods.
4. Administer enemas if ordered preoperatively	Emptying the intestines will prevent the contents from being discharged involuntarily and will aid in the prevention of post-operative distention, gas, and impaction.
5. Check to see that the client has been prepared properly and that the permit is signed before giving the preoperative medication. Ascertain allergies, if unsure, before administering preoperative medication. Have the client void.	The preoperative medication may alter the client's physical as well as psychological state.
6. Give the client's personal articles to a family member or place them in a safe place. Safety precautions should be taken. Ask the client to remove all hairpins, hairpieces, prostheses (including artificial dentures and partial plates, artificial limbs), and jewelry before surgery. If the clients does not wish to remove the wedding band, it may be taped in place. If there is a chance the client's fingers will swell after surgery, however, the ring should be removed.	Protect the client's personal property during surgery. Any personal item that might cause a spark during anesthesia should be removed before surgery because the gases used in surgery are highly volatile. Hair clips that might cause scalp pressure must be removed also.
7. Measure the client's vital signs before administering the preoperative medication and before the client leaves for surgery.	Vital signs aid in determining the physical status of the client and serve as early indicators of complications.
8. Administer the ordered preoperative injection. Properly identify the client. After the injection, raise the siderails and caution the client to remain in bed. Tell the client and family that the medication may make the client sleepy and unstable when walking without support. Be sure that the bed is in the lowest position. Caution the client against smoking after the preoperative medication.	Preoperative medication may be given to reduce reflex irritabilities caused by fear and pain, to assist in smooth induction of anesthesia, to minimize secretions, and to protect the cardiovascular system by depressing the vagus nerve.

ACTION	RATIONALE
9. A plan of care should have been started on admission. Follow the care plan with emphasis on timing and thoroughness of preoperative teaching.	Effective preoperative teaching promotes faster recuperation, less frequent need for drugs, fewer complications, and possibly a shortened stay.
10. Show consideration of the feelings and fears of the family. Tell relatives where to wait during the operative procedure and answer any questions that they may have.	A surgical procedure causes apprehension for the family as well as the client. Sympathetic attention and understanding can greatly allay fears.

Perioperative Period

(Please note that perioperative nursing is an extremely skilled art and requires experience and specialized knowledge; a complete description is beyond the scope of this text. What follows are general considerations for care during the surgical procedure. Please refer to an operating room text book for a complete discussion of the nurse's responsibilities.)

ACTION	RATIONALE
1. Set up the room with sterile supplies and equipment before the arrival of the client. Maintain sterile technique when opening packs and preparing for the surgery.	Limiting the amount of time needed to begin the operation will decrease the nervousness and anxiety of the client.
2. Greet the client by name in a friendly and positive manner. Establish the surgical procedure to be performed and the name of the client's physician. Check the name of the client with the name band and the chart. Ensure the proper identification of the client and the proper surgical procedure to be done.	It is imperative to safeguard the client by assuring that the right surgery is done on the right client. Being friendly and positive is reassuring to the nervous client.
3. Assist the client onto the surgical table. Obtain as much assistance as is needed to ensure the client's safety. Secure safety straps to prevent the client from falling from the table. The client may be drowsy from the preoperative medication and may require more assistance than under usual circumstances.	Preoperative medications often produce drowsiness. The client will not have the usual control over muscles and coordination. Assistance and careful monitoring are necessary to prevent accidents.
4. Remain next to the client during the induction phase of anesthesia. Report any complications to the anesthesiologist.	Offering reassurance and constant observation of the client may prevent complications or allow early detection so that measures may be taken to alleviate them.

ACTION	*RATIONALE*
5. Carefully document the progress of the operation, noting the condition of the client and any special procedures, such as catheterization, nasogastric intubation.	The OR record is a legal document. All occurrences during the operation must be noted.
6. Observe during the operation to ensure that sterile technique is maintained. Be prepared to ensure continued sterile technique by having extra gowns and gloves ready in case they are needed.	Any break in sterile technique necessitates changing of the gown and gloves to prevent the possibility of contaminating the client or compromising the sterile field.
7. Monitor the sponge count as well as blood and fluid loss during the surgery. Weigh the sponges for an accurate estimate of blood loss. Keep the surgical team informed of the amount of blood loss during surgery. Make sure that the number of sponges counted at the end of the procedure matches exactly the number of sponges counted at the beginning of surgery. Account for all sponges opened.	During the intensity of surgery, it is important that the physical condition of the client be monitored. Attention to the amount of blood lost is an excellent indicator of how the client is progressing. Because sponges are used to pack the incision during surgery to decrease bleeding into the operative field, it is imperative that no sponges accidentally be left in the incision. Accurate counting will decrease this possibility.
8. Move the client carefully from the surgical table onto a cart. Obtain adequate assistance to prevent accidents to the client or to the staff. Escort the client to the recovery area and give a complete report to the receiving nurse.	Usually, the client will be unable to assist with the removal from the surgical table; adequate help is therefore essential to prevent falls, injuries, or unnecessary strain on the suture line. A complete report will enable the receiving nurse to give more comprehensive and individualized care.

Postoperative Period

1. Have the bed ready to receive the client after surgery. The sheets should be fanfolded (see Technique No. 30, Bedmaking). All necessary equipment should be available: IV pole, emesis basin, siderails, vital sign monitoring equipment, suction equipment, and any other equipment specific to the surgical procedure performed.	The move from the Recovery Room will be uncomfortable for the client. It should be done as quickly and safely as possible.
2. Move the client gently and carefully from the cart to the bed. Lock the wheels of the cart during transfer to the bed.	Many surgical wounds are closed under considerable tension. Care should be taken not to disturb the suture line or injure the client by a fall.

ACTION	**RATIONALE**
3. Exercise extreme caution in maintain a patent airway during the immediate postoperative period. Prevent obstruction by the insertion of an airway (Fig. 77-6). Remove secretions from the throat by suction. If permitted, turn the client's head to one side. While the client regains consciousness, encourage deep breathing and coughing to bring up secretions.	The most common cause of obstruction is the tongue falling back against the throat from relaxation induced by the anesthesia.

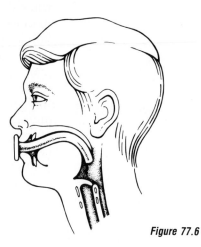

Figure 77.6

4. Monitor the client's vital signs at least every 15 minutes during the period of emerging from anesthesia. Vital signs include temperature, pulse, respiration, blood pressure, and level of consciousness. Measure the intake and output (I&O) as well.	Temperature elevation may indicate infection or brain damage. Pulse rate change may indicate inadequate oxygenation of the blood. The level of consciousness should progress from unconsciousness to alert. Any lapse (i.e., from a waking to a disoriented state) must be evaluated for possible causes.
5. Accurately assess and record intake and output during the early postoperative period. Most clients will be receiving IV fluids, which must be assessed for proper speed of delivery, type of fluid, and amount of fluid. The first voiding is very important and should be measured and recorded accurately. Tubes and drains must be patent, and all drainage must be recorded accurately.	Fluid balance is an indicator that the body is returning to normal after anesthesia. Urinary output is especially important because some forms of anesthesia can cause urinary retention or suppression. Fluid buildup near the suture line may cause undesirable tension and discomfort.
6. Use aseptic technique to check the dressings for complications from the surgery. Check pulse rate frequently.	Early signs of complication, such as hemorrhage and wound problems, may be detected by inspecting dressings and watching for increased pulse rate.

ACTION	*RATIONALE*
7. Encourage the client to engage in deep breathing at regular, frequent intervals. Assist the client to splint the operative area with a pillow when deep breathing (Fig. 77-7). Ask the client to expand the lungs fully, hold the breath for a second or two, then release. (Coughing may be ordered to help relieve lung congestion, although the routine use of this procedure has diminished in popularity. Splint the operative area and instruct the client to cough as deeply as possible to bring up any phlegm or obstructive material.)	Frequent position changes help relieve general discomfort, increase circulation, and aid in the prevention of pulmonary congestion. Splinting the operative area prevents undue stress and tension from the strenuous activity.

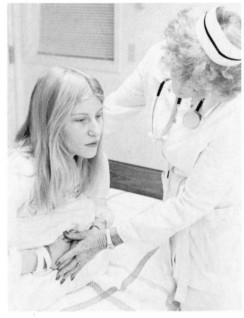

Figure 77.7

8. Consider the feelings of the family during the postoperative period. They should be involved as soon as possible in the recuperation process. Allow them to visit as soon as the client is fully reactive. Answer questions and offer support. Tell the family to let the client awaken slowly, and to avoid shaking or shouting in an effort to hasten the awakening process.	The feelings of comfort and security are enhanced by involvement in the care. Not knowing what is happening is a fear-producing state. Anxiety can be reduced and rapport increased by involving the client and family in postoperative care as soon as possible.
9. Ambulate the client as soon as the physician allows. Two persons should be in attendance during the first few ambulation attempts. Begin slowly. If the client feels dizzy or light-headed, pause for a few seconds of rest. Deep breathing and looking ahead instead of down at the floor may help.	Early ambulation has been associated with quicker recovery. Because of weakness, the client may fall if not fully supported on both sides. Looking straight ahead instead of down decreases dizziness and facilitates ambulation.

ACTION	**RATIONALE**
10. Assess the pain experienced by the client in relation to origin, duration, and amount of relief received by administration of pain medications. Gas pains are common after surgery and may be relieved by ambulation or by insertion of a rectal tube (see Technique No. 6, Enema and Rectal Tube). Antiemetics may relieve nausea.	Certain discomforts are expected during the postoperative period. Pain after surgery is usually relieved by narcotics and analgesics. It is important to assess whether the pain is a result of the surgery or some complication, such as pulmonary embolus or pneumothorax.
11. *Legal aspects:* Refer to the hospital policy and procedure manual(s) to determine the legal aspects of treating postoperative clients in each individual hospital.	Laws vary from state to state.

General Guidelines

Send the client's chart to surgery and to the recovery room. All preoperative orders are generally canceled after surgery.	The chart is a written record of the client's hospital stay and should include all aspects of care.
Hot water bottles are *not* left in the bed of a postoperative client.	In the depressed state common after anesthesia, the client may receive severe burns from hot water bottles.
Recovery room personnel usually will come to the unit to give the nurse caring for the client a review of the client's progress during and since the operation.	Continuity of care is essential if the client is to receive professional nursing care.
The chart usually includes a completed sheet from anesthesia personnel and from the circulating nurse and recovery room personnel.	Written records provide historical reference and aid in continuity of care.

Special Modifications

1. In preoperative preparation of children, it is important to note the presence of any loose teeth. These should be called to the attention of the anesthesiologist or anesthetist.	The muscles of the throat relax during anesthesia and if a loose tooth is accidentally knocked out, it could fall into the throat and be aspirated.
2. Emergency surgery often will eliminate the possibility of adequate preparation of the client and family, especially in relation to preoperative teaching. This does not mean that this area should be forgotten entirely. When it is appropriate, teaching should be done during the postoperative period. Emergency surgery will also be a very stressful situation; sensitivity to the plight of the family and frequent dissemination of information are absolutely essential. Some of	Emergencies are high-stress occurrences. Treat the client and family as you would want to be treated in the same situation.

ACTION	***RATIONALE***

the information that is needed before performing emergency surgery includes the time and amount of last food consumption, allergies, and time and amount of any drugs or medication taken before the surgery. This information may have to come from the family. It should be elicited in a calm, concerned, and reassuring way.

Communicative Aspects

OBSERVATIONS

Preoperative Period

1. Note and record vital signs, symptoms, behavior, and complications of treatment.

2. Observe preoperative test results and report any discrepencies to the physician.

3. The aging process may affect reactions to injury (*i.e.,* the reactions are often less pronounced and slower to appear in the older adult). Certain drugs, such as scopolamine, morphine, and barbiturates, may be poorly tolerated in the older client and may cause confusion and disorientation. Observe the elderly in particular, and all clients generally, for drug reactions.

4. Observe vital signs in evaluation of the client's physical condition before surgery. Observe and report temperature elevation, pulse irregularities, respiratory difficulties, or blood pressure discrepancies. Any undue cough or congestion of which the physician is unaware should be reported because it may indicate postoperative problems.

5. Encourage the preoperative client to have a positive attitude toward surgery. Provide opportunities for expression of fears. The client's recovery may be influenced by expectations of the surgical procedure. Report any client concern to the physician.

6. Observe renal function before surgery. If the client has problems, the necessity of the operative procedure will have to be weighed against the possibility of complications after surgery. In clients with limited renal reserve, measurement of I&O and comparisons are vital. Dehydration and malnutrition are common conditions that can seriously affect the preoperative client. Observe and record I&O, eating habits, and general physical condition.

Perioperative Period

1. Know the interactions of drugs used in preanesthetic preparation of the client. Be aware of desired effects and possible side-effects. Determine which drugs are used for anesthesia in an effort to provide more informed and comprehensive care after surgery during both the induction and arousal phases of anesthesia.

2. Be aware of and assist in positioning the client.

3. Observe the client's mental and emotional outlook regarding the surgery. If the client expresses concern about surviving the surgery or reservations about going through with the surgical procedure, notify the physician.

4. Observe the client's condition during surgery. Monitor the amount of blood loss as well as the removal of any fluid or tissue.

Postoperative Period

1. Be alert to early signs of complications. Ensure patency of the client's airway. Respiratory depression may occur in the form of shallow respirations due to anesthesia, sedatives, or opiates given for pain. Surgical shock is indicated by the character of the pulse, respirations, and blood pressure. Report a weak, thready pulse, shallow respirations, and a falling or low blood pressure. There may also be symptoms of sighing respirations, air hunger, ringing in the ears, cold, pallor, and restlessness.

2. Pulmonary embolism may be evidenced by a sharp pain in the chest area.

3. Evaluate the condition of the wound site and drainage. Note whether the wound is intact and any evidence of dehiscnece or evisceration.

4. To ensure fluid and electrolyte balance, note the client's ability to take fluids orally when allowed. If fluids are administered by infusion, observe how the infusion is tolerated, as well as the condition of the infusion site and tubing. Any vomiting should be recorded (i.e., amount and appearance). The client's ability to void is important as well as the character and amount of urine. If the client has a urinary catheter, note patency of the tube and the appearance of the urine.

5. Watch for abdominal distension, which may indicate intestinal obstruction, gas, or other complications.

6. Observe the condition of the skin in relation to adequate nutrition and hydration. Note the readiness of the client to resume normal eating habits and diet.

7. Note any circulatory complications and signs of clot formation in the legs. Obesity, debility, advanced age, and muscular inactivity may precipitate clotting. Fever accompanying inflammation of the veins may indicate thrombophlebitis.

8. Note the ability, readiness, and willingness of the client to ambulate. Observe and compare progress made from one attempt to the next. Ambulation should improve progressively until the client is able and anxious to ambulate frequently with a minimum of assistance.

9. The occurrence of the first stool after surgery is important since this indicates a return to normal bowel function. Appearance of the stool is important to indicate the possibility of internal bleeding or passage of preoperative barium.

10. Note the client's ability and willingness to comply with the preoperative teaching regimen. Determine deficits and reinforce teaching when necessary.

11. Note postoperative laboratory measurements and report any discrepencies form expected results immediately.

12. Infection (respiratory, wound, or other) may be indicated by increased temperature or erythema. Respiratory infection also may be manifested by difficult breathing, pain in the chest, and coughing.

13. Continued observation of vital signs will offer early indications of complications.

CHARTING

Preoperative Period

1. Include the following in the charting before the client is taken to the surgical area:

Client's appearance, behavior, and pertinent conversation

Current temperature, pulse, respiration, and blood pressure

Artificial dentures (full or partial), presence and disposition

Preoperative medication (include time given)

Significant observations relating to physical or psychological status

Amount of urine voided before surgery

Time of departure to surgery and mode of transportation

All precautions taken to preserve the client's safety

Information given to the client and family regarding the surgery

DATE/TIME	OBSERVATIONS	SIGNATURE
2/15 0830	Bathed and gowned for surgery. Voided 250 ml, no problems. Preoperative medication given IM, BP 126/78, P 76, R 18 T 98.2 F. Instructed not to smoke, drink any water, or get up without help. Siderails up. Wife in room. Both appear calm. Jewelry given to wife. No dentures. States, "I am ready to get this over with." Operative permit signed and on chart. ——————	F. White RN
0910	To surgery by stretcher. ——————	F. White RN

Perioperative Period

Consult the individual hospital Operating Room/Surgical Suite for specific charting forms and procedures.

Postoperative Period

1. Chart the client's appearance, behavior, vital signs, presence and condition of dressings, tubes, casts, or any appliance or equipment that was not present when the client went to surgery.

2. Chart the level of consciousness when the client is returned to the unit from the recovery room, as well as any problems or statements of pain or discomfort.

3. Charting during the recuperation phase should include a synopsis of the postsurgical recovery process at least every 8 hours. This should cover the condition of the client, vital signs in relation to tissue repair, condition and presence of dressings and tubes, condition and appearance of suture line, progress of the client in ambulation, nutritional status including continuation of intravenous infusion and ability to tolerate liquid and solid foods, acceptance of limitations imposed by the surgery, and understanding of the client and family about the surgical procedure and recovery period.

DATE/TIME	OBSERVATIONS	SIGNATURE
4/2 1100	Returned from surgery by stretcher. Responding to verbal stimuli. Dressing on lower right abdomen contains area (3 cm circumference) of dark drainage, reinforced. Color of skin pink. BP 136/88, P 92, R 24, T 97.6° F. Pulse is strong and regular. Respirations shallow. Turned to left side and encouraged to take five deep breaths. Incision area supported with pillow. IV in left wrist, infusing at 100 ml/hr. Wife in attendance. Siderails up and instructions given about calling for a nurse to get up to go to the bathroom. States no pain at this time. Is due to void. Blinking and swallowing reflexes noted. Ice chips given per order Dr. B. ——————	F. White RN

Discharge Planning Aspects

CLIENT AND FAMILY EDUCATION

Preoperative Period

1. Reinforce the explanation given by the physician regarding the operative procedure and the recovery periods. Be available to answer any questions the client and family may have.

2. Explain oxygen, drainage tubes, intravenous fluids, and specific reasons for the presence of these items. Offer explanations within the tolerance of the client and family. Some people want to know everything; for some, this only heightens anxiety.

3. Offer preoperative instruction in deep-breathing techniques. If ventilatory assistance devices will be used after surgery, show them to the client before surgery and explain how and why they are used. Explain that deep breathing expands the lungs and helps to prevent complications such as pneumonia.

4. Inform the client about the frequency of vital sign measurement after surgery and the reasons.

5. Explain the preparations for surgery, including enemas, shaving the operative site, sedation, withholding of fluids, and any other specific preparations that will occur.

6. If there is a probability that the client will stay in the intensive care area for a period after surgery, explain why and the differences between that area and the nursing unit. If the client and family have some warning about this possibility, anxiety and alarm will be decreased when it occurs.

7. Before abdominal surgery, show the client how to turn from side to side and how to assume Sims' position. Encourage a turning routine every 2 hours for the first 24 hours after surgery to stimulate circulation, maintain muscle tone, and prevent respiratory and circulatory complications.

8. Demonstrate active and passive exercises that may be done during the recuperation period. Show the client how to move the feet, one at a time, in a circle and how to flex the legs alternately while lying in bed. These actions will help to lessen abdominal gas pain, facilitate moving from side to side, aid in adjustment to sitting, standing, and ambulating, and increase circulation in the legs to minimize thrombus formation.

9. Explain the medication routine. Tell the client and family that the purpose of the preoperative medication is to relax the client and possibly to decrease secretions. This will result in feelings of dry mouth and thirst. Following surgery, medications will be available to decrease the pain.

10. Explain the reasons for and method of recording all I&O after surgery. Enlist the participation of the family and client in keeping this accurate.

11. Give specific instructions to the family about where to wait during the surgery and where and when they may see the physician. Tell the family that they will be kept informed about the client's condition and progress during the surgical procedure.

12. Explain the recovery room experience to the client and family so they will not be alarmed by the amount of time between the end of surgery and the return to the room. Tell the client to expect to wake up in the recovery room.

13. If the client will be awake during surgery, explain that the preoperative medication will have a relaxing effect. If a local anesthetic will be used, explain this to the client with a brief description of what will happen. Assess the ability of the client to assimilate this information and the client's willingness and desire to hear when determining how much detail to include. Answer any questions as truthfully and completely as possible.

14. If the client appears nervous, ask a nurse from the surgical suite to make a preoperative visit so the client will see a familiar face when transported to the surgical suite.

Perioperative Period

Some hospitals provide a liaison nurse to keep the families informed of the progress of the client during surgery. This is imperative if the surgery is excessively long, that is, over 2 or 3 hours, or if complications arise.

Postoperative Period

1. Reinforce the physician's explanation of the surgical procedure and limitations on activities. Answer questions if possible, or refer the client and family's questions to the physician.

2. Implement the preoperative teaching techniques regarding breathing, exercise, and ambulation. Reinforcement of the need to turn and do the exercises may be needed.

3. Institute a plan of teaching for the client's individual needs in relation to the surgery performed and the client's current condition. Emphasize techniques that will have to be continued after discharge. Involve the family in these techniques. Be sure that the family and client feel confident about home care. Answer any questions and demonstrate techniques such as dressing change until the family or client feels comfortable about doing them.

REFERRALS

Visits from a home health nurse may benefit the client whose postoperative recuperation will be lengthy and who is discharged with dressings, tubes, drains, or any equipment requiring nursing expertise and guidance. If the surgical procedure involves an alteration to self-image that will require an adjustment period (e.g., amputation of a limb, mastectomy, reconstructive surgery), referral to the appropriate support organization (e.g., the American Cancer Society, American Diabetic Association, Reach for Recovery, etc) may provide the client and family with needed support, financial assistance, equipment provision, or information needed to cope with the physical and emotional problems.

Evaluation

Quality Assurance

1. *Preoperatively,* the record should reflect symptoms that substantiate the condition requiring surgical intervention. There should be evidence of the client's understanding of the procedure, the need for the procedure, risks, and sequelae. If questions were raised, the nature of the questions as well as the responses offered should be noted. A complete record of allergies should be noted. Previous experience with surgery should be reflected as well as any complications or unusual events involved. Baseline vital sign and laboratory data should be available for later comparisons. A complete record of explanations and teaching to the client and family should be reflected, as well as an assessment of the level of understanding. Compliance with the physician's preoperative orders should be reflected, including notes and observations about the client's tolerance and understanding of procedures.

2. *Perioperatively,* records should be available relating to the progress of anesthesia and the client's vital signs and reactions to the anesthetic. An ongoing record of the progress of the surgery should be included in the client record as well as the presence and handling of any complications or breaks in sterile technique. Any specimens taken should be noted as well as the disposition of each.

3. *Postoperatively,* the record should reflect detailed progress of the client during the recuperation phase. During the recovery from anesthesia, recording of vital signs at frequent intervals, usually every 15 minutes, should be reflected. Transport to the unit, condition of the client, and safety measures taken should be noted. Monitoring of the client during the postoperative pe-

riod should reflect a progressive pattern from dependence to independence. Measures taken to promote independence should be noted. Of special interest are all safety precautions taken to ensure a safe recovery period. Raising siderails, placing the call light within reach, alerting the family to remain with the client, any type of restraint, and all measures taken to ensure safety should be noted on the chart. Measurement of vital signs, including temperature, should be noted at regular intervals (usually every 4 hours). Concerns voiced by the client or family should be noted, as well as attempts to allay these concerns. Discharge teaching should be reflected. The condition of the client, measures taken to prevent complications after discharge, and feelings expressed by the client and family about discharge should be noted.

Infection Control

1. Surgical procedures are carried out under the strictest sterile conditions. Preoperative scrubs and shave preparations are attempts to render the operative site as free as possible from bacteria and pathogens that might invade the system and cause infection.

2. Surgical scrub handwashing technique varies from 3 to 10 minutes depending on hospital policy. Mechanical scrubbing with running water and a bactericidal soap is effective in removing most of the pathogenic organisms on the hands (see Technique No. 60, Handwashing).

3. Sterile gown and gloves are worn during surgery (see Technique No. 58, Gown and Glove Procedure, Sterile). Any break in sterile technique during surgery warrants immediate attention and reapplication of new sterile scrub clothing and drapes.

4. After surgery, the incision site is considered a sterile area. When dressings are changed, use sterile technique. Any soaks or applications to the incision must be sterile (see Technique No. 61, Hot and Cold Applications).

5. Strict handwashing before and after caring for the surgical client is essential. Dressings should be discarded in plastic bags that are taped shut to prevent accidental contamination of others.

Technique Checklist

	YES	NO
PREOPERATIVE PERIOD		
Client and family understand what the surgery will include and why it is necessary	_____	_____
Physical assessment and history complete	_____	_____
Consent form signed	_____	_____
Identification band on client	_____	_____
Laboratory results on chart	_____	_____
Preoperative procedures carried out		
Enema _____ (no.)	_____	_____
Shave prep	_____	_____
Bath or shower with bactericidal preparations	_____	_____
Bedtime sedation	_____	_____
NPO at midnight	_____	_____
Preoperative medication	_____	_____
_____		
Artificial dentures removed	_____	_____
Hairpins and jewelry removed	_____	_____
Valuables to family	_____	_____
Siderails up on bed		

Technique Checklist

		YES	NO
PERIOPERATIVE PERIOD	Room set up before operation	_____	_____
	Sterility of equipment maintained	_____	_____
	Client greeted on arrival to OR	_____	_____
	Identity of client ensured by checking		
	Identification band	_____	_____
	Chart	_____	_____
	Location of surgery assured by		
	Asking client	_____	_____
	Checking operative consent	_____	_____
	Other _____		
	Continuous monitoring of vital signs	_____	_____
	Transferred without injury to client	_____	_____
	Transferred without injury to staff	_____	_____
	Positioning accomplished	_____	_____
	Complete recording of surgical progress	_____	_____
	Sterile technique maintained throughout surgical procedure	_____	_____
	Sponge count correct	_____	_____
	Amount of blood loss charted	_____	_____
	Specimen(s) transported to laboratory	_____	_____
	Type _____		
	Report given to recovery nurse regarding client's condition	_____	_____
POSTOPERATIVE PERIOD	Transported safely to unit from surgical or recovery area	_____	_____
	Pain controlled by medication	_____	_____
	Nausea or vomiting	_____	_____
	Tubes and drains patent	_____	_____
	Catheter_____		
	IV_____		
	Incisional drain_____		
	Nasogastric tube_____		
	Other_____		
	Breathing exercises done (how often) _____		
	Turned every_____ hours		
	Ambulation		
	Date sat up _____		
	Date ambulated _____		
	Complications_____	_____	_____
	Condition of incision satisfactory	_____	_____
	Sutures removed	_____	_____
	Discharge teaching done	_____	_____
	Family and client feel confident about ability to provide home care	_____	_____
	Client knows when to return for follow-up visit to physician	_____	_____

78

Pressure Sore (Decubitus Ulcer), Prevention and Treatment

Overview

Definition

A pressure sore, also called a decubitus ulcer or bed sore, is a circumscribed area in which cutaneous tissue has been destroyed. The destruction is caused by restriction of blood flow to the area owing to excessive or prolonged pressure; pressure sores may occur in many areas with progressive destruction of the underlying tissue (Fig. 78-1). Most common sites of pressure sores:

Over bony prominences: Coccyx, hip (greater trochanter and ischial prominences), elbow, heel, shoulder blade (scapula), knee (patella), ankle prominence (malleolus), back of head (occiput), and ear

Between folds of flesh in obese clients: Under breasts, under buttocks, and on abdomen

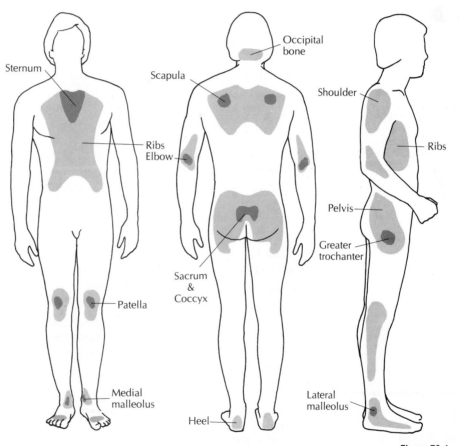

Figure 78.1

Rationale

Prevent pressure on any one area of the body for excessive lengths of time.

Ensure the client's comfort.

Prevent the spread of pathogenic microorganisms.

Alleviate the client's fear and anxiety regarding the pressure sore that has already developed.

Terminology

Excoriation: Loss of superficial layers of the skin

Maceration: The process of softening a solid by steeping in a fluid

Assessment

Pertinent Anatomy and Physiology

See Appendix I: *blood, blood vessels, skin.*

Pathophysiological Concepts

1. The stages of decubitus ulcer formation are
   Stage I: Reddening of the skin not relieved by massage or by relief of the pressure believed to have caused it

   Stage II: Superficial tissue damage involving skin breakdown

   Stage III: Ulceration involving the dermis, which may or may not include the subcutaneous tissue; stage that produces serosanguineous drainage

   Stage IV: Ulceration into the deep structures with invasion of the deep tissue or structures such as fascia, connective tissue, muscle, or bone

2. Decubitus ulcers are a potential problem of the immobile. Those particularly at risk are the elderly, the obese, the emaciated, and the paralyzed, whose mobility is impaired. Contributing factors to decubitus ulcer formation are continuous exposure of the skin to moisture, circulatory impairment, a break in the skin, inadequate nutrition, dehydration, inhibited sensory reception, and a lack of natural adipose tissue, which normally pads bony prominences.

Assessment of the Client

1. Assess the general condition of the client. Note nutritional status, ability of the client to eat (presence of natural or artificial dentures), ability of the client to chew food thoroughly, and amount of adipose (fat) tissue. Also note the mobility of the client, circulatory status in extremities, urinary and bowel continence, sensory perception in extremities and trunk, and level of hydration.

2. Assess the condition of the pressure sore. Note the stage or amount of tissue destruction. Assess the kind of care or treatment the area has received before hospitalization and the effectiveness of this care.

3. Assess the client's entire body to determine if other pressure sores are evolving. Assess the presence of other pressure areas, the degree of redness, or lack of sensation. Check all bony prominences, folds of skin, and any area that might have received pressure due to the presence of tubing or drains (e.g., the penis, vulva, nasal cavity).

Plan

Nursing Objectives

Maintain clean, dry skin.

Examine bony prominences, cartilaginous areas, and skin folds regularly.

Observe and note factors that may interfere with the healing process.

Prevent or reduce infection and promote healing.

Identify areas of risk and prevent additional sores.

Client Preparation

1. Explain to the client why frequent turning will be done and how best to participate in the turning process to make it as easy and as painless as possible.

2. Tell the client what is involved in decubitus care. If special padding is to be used, gather it before beginning care and explain its use to the client.

Equipment

Cleansing solution (e.g., hydrogen peroxide)

Normal saline solution

Heat lamp (if ordered)

Medicated ointment (as ordered)

Disinfectant solution, as ordered

Dressings (as necessary)

Irrigation kit (if necessary)

Implementation and Interventions

Procedural Aspects

ACTION

1. Pressure sores are caused by prolonged pressure, which restricts blood flow to the area resulting in tissue breakdown. (Fig. 78-2). The desirable aspect in the treatment of pressure sores is prevention. Frequent turning, relief of pressure, and encouragement of circulation to the skin overlying bony prominences are essential to prevention and early detection. Turn the client at least every 2 hours or as ordered. Each time the client is turned, check the skin closely for signs of pressure areas. Gently massage bony prominences with lotion. Place the client in a variety of positions, including prone. Be

RATIONALE

Massage will promote the circulation to the area bringing needed nutrition to the cells and preventing destruction of skin cells owing to lack of adequate blood supply. Lying in the prone position is an excellent means of relieving pressure on the bony structure of the back. Each alteration of position causes a shift in the area receiving pressure. Evenly distributing pressure over the body will prevent excess pressure on one area, resulting in a pressure sore. Rolled pads form a harder surface than do flattened pads and because their use is highly localized, may cause pressure sores themselves. Use padding judiciously. Pillows are the best form of padding.

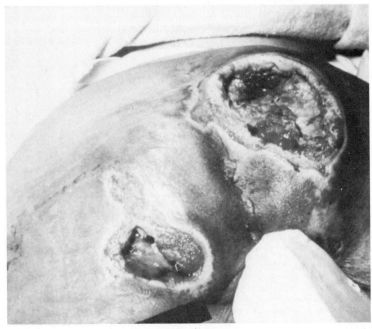

Figure 78.2

ACTION	**RATIONALE**
sure that the client's breathing is not restricted and that the client is comfortable. Sitting is also a desirable means of shifting weight and pressure, if the client is able and the time is not prolonged. Use rolled pads to keep body parts in alignment, but be certain that the pads themselves do not cause pressure.	
2. Wash hands carefully before and after caring for the client's pressure sore. There are a variety of methods for cleansing a pressure sore. Use the physician's preference or the method prescribed in the hospital procedure manual. One method is to cleanse the area thoroughly with hydrogen peroxide followed by cleansing with normal saline. Apply a heat lamp for 20 minutes, placed at a distance of 45 cm to 50 cm (18 in–20 in) from the client. Monitor the lamp and progress of the treatment at very frequent intervals (see Technique No. 61, Hot and Cold Applications).	Handwashing has been shown to remove the majority of the pathogenic organisms present on the skin. The application of a heat lamp to a person whose sensitivity to external stimuli is already decreased, as evidenced by the formation of the pressure area, warrants very careful monitoring. Use extreme caution to see that the lamp is no closer than the prescribed distance and that the bulb is no more than 60 watts. Monitor at least every 5 minutes and discontinue at the first sign of problems.
3. The use of rubber or other protective materials may cause the client to perspire. The more desirable bed covering is a sheepskin, air mattress, flotation pad, eggcrate mattress, or other coverings designed to decrease pressure and enhance circulation. The use of these devices does *not* eliminate the need for turning the client or massaging the pressure areas (Fig. 78-3).	Perspiration causes moisture buildup and further predisposes tissue breakdown. Special mattresses are designed to evenly distribute the body weight so that one area does not receive greater pressure than others.

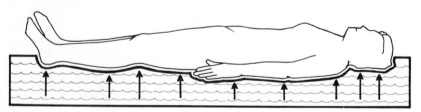

Figure 78.3

ACTION	**RATIONALE**
4. Encourage bowel and bladder control if the client is able to cooperate. Offer the bedpan and urinal frequently. Change linen and give skin care as often as necessary to keep the client dry.	Moisture from incontinence causes maceration of the skin.
5. Encourage the intake of a high-protein diet. Between-meal feedings may help to ensure an adequate intake.	A deficient nutritional status is detrimental to the healing process.

Communicative Aspects

OBSERVATIONS

1. Promptly report any reddened or whitened area, either of which may indicate irritation. Give special attention to these areas by massage, turning to keep the client from lying on these areas, and continued observation to see that further damage does not occur.

2. Observe for systemic conditions that may encourage the formation of pressure areas: impaired circulation, fever, alteration of cell function. Observe for adequate intake of food and fluid to meet systemic needs.

3. Check the client frequently for environmental factors that encourage the formation of pressure areas: wrinkled bed linen, objects in the bed, top bed linen applied tightly enough to restrict movement, and pressure or irritation from casts, adhesive, tubing, braces, traction, and other equipment.

4. Observe any drainage from an open pressure sore. Note the type of drainage, amount, and frequency of appearance. If persistent, culture and sensitivity tests may be needed to determine causative agents and effective means to destroy them.

5. The prescribed treatment of pressure sores is the responsibility of the physician. Preventive measures should be planned, implemented, and evaluated by the nursing staff.

CHARTING

DATE/TIME	OBSERVATIONS	SIGNATURE
6/19 0945	Small, reddened area 5 cm in diameter located on coccyx. Cleansed with hydrogen peroxide and saline. Heat lamp applied for 15 min. Slight redness noted in surrounding area after 15 min. No drainage. Turned to left side. Skin over bony prominences massaged with lotion. 60 ml water taken orally. Resting quietly at this time. ———————————————————	G. Ivers RN

Discharge Planning Aspects

CLIENT AND FAMILY EDUCATION

1. Instruct the client and family about the importance of frequent turning and repositioning.

2. Instruct the client and family about methods to avoid pressure, early signs of impending tissue breakdown, and the most likely sites of breakdown.

3. Tell the family to keep the client clean and dry and to keep the bed free of wrinkles and objects that might cause pressure.

4. Teach the family decubitus care. Ensure understanding of the procedure and adequate skill in performance by observing a return demonstration. If dressings are used, teach sterile technique and method of application to the family.

5. Be certain that the family has adequate materials at home to continue decubitus care. These may include an irrigation set, heat lamp, hydrogen peroxide, and dressings.

REFERRALS

If the client is to be cared for at home by a family member, referral to a visiting nurse agency or home health care agency may provide the family with the encouragement and assistance needed to accomplish the difficult tasks required. The knowledge that they will not be completely severed from professional counsel and advice after the client is discharged is a great comfort to families. If the client is referred to an extended care facility for continued care, include a written plan of care, including the turning schedule to which the client is accustomed.

Evaluation

Quality Assurance

The presence of a pressure sore is a challenge to all nurses. The goal of treatment is healing the sore and returning the skin to previous condition. The greater challenge is prevention of further excoriation of the skin and the formation of additional pressure sores. Quality nursing care must be reflected in the record with regard to frequency of turning, care of the pressure area, and prevention of further complications.

Infection Control

Pathogenic infestation of the pressure area causes further breakdown and progressive invasion deeper and deeper into the skin and underlying tissue. Dressings from the pressure sore must be handled as with any infectious process. Meticulous handwashing before and after caring for the wound is essential. During the bath, clean the areas near the pressure sore and on all bony prominences well with soap and water.

Technique Checklist

	YES	NO
Location and size of pressure sore _____		
Client and family understand how a pressure sore forms and methods to prevent further deterioration at present site and formation of additional pressure areas	_____	_____
Care of the pressure sore		
How often _____		
Medication used _____		
Condition of pressure sore improved with care	_____	_____
Client turned q _____ hr	_____	_____
Client will be dismissed to		
Home _____		
Extended care facility_____		
Family taught turning technique	_____	_____
Family taught care of pressure sore	_____	_____
Referral form compiled for extended care facility to foster continuity of care	_____	_____

79

Radiation Therapy, Nursing Care

Overview

Definition

The therapeutic use of radium, radon, radioactive gold, and other radioactive substances, to kill malignant cells

Rationale

Prolong life by destroying malignant cells.

Aid in the client's comfort.

Cause partial or complete remission of the malignant process.

Terminology

Alopecia: Loss of the hair

Anorexia: Loss of appetite

Malaise: Feelings of tiredness and fatigue

Radioactive: The ability of a substance to emit alpha, beta, or gamma rays from its nucleus

Radium: A metallic radioactive element found in pitchblende that exists in a continuous state of disintegration; useful in treating disease because it kills cells, especially young, immature, actively growing, abnormal cells (e.g., cancer and leukemia cells)

Radon: A radioactive gas that is a by-product of radium disintegration

Shielding: Sealing off radioactive materials

Assessment

Pertinent Anatomy and Physiology

1. The smallest units of structure capable of carrying on vital functions are the cells. The nucleus is the control center of the cell as well as the storehouse for genetic information found in chromosomes and genes. Cells divide according to a prearrange design, which is governed by the genetic material.

2. Radiation therapy consists of two types of energy: ultraviolet radiation (sunlight) and ionizing radiation (x-rays and gamma rays). All cells are susceptible to ionizing radiation, especially the rapidly dividing cells of the gastrointestinal (GI) epithelium and the bone marrow.

Pathophysiological Concepts

1. Normally, cell division proceeds at an orderly pace, rapidly enough to ensure proper growth and repair of tissues. Occasionally certain cells may begin to divide with abnormal rapidity, with no regard for the needs of the body. These abnormal cells crowd out the surrounding normal cells, robbing them of their nourishment and resulting in a malignant neoplasm that is called a cancer. The genetic makeup of certain cancer cells is different from that of normal cells.

2. Radiation acts at the cellular level, causing cell death as particles of radioactive energy disrupt the normal genetic makeup of the cell and interfere with activity and mitosis (cell division). Radiation exerts its greatest effect during certain phases of the cell cycle. Radiation is injurious to all cells, but is most harmful to rapidly proliferating cells of cancerous tissue. Normal tis-

sue appears able to recover more quickly from the effects of radiation than does cancer tissue.

3. During pregnancy, heavy doses of ionizing radiation have been shown to cause microcephaly, skeletal malformations, and mental retardation.

Assessment of the Client

1. Assess the history of the client in relation to the condition for which the radiation treatment is being done. Determine the onset of symptoms and the progress of the condition. Assess current symptoms.

2. Clients with cancer are usually frightened and often depressed. Assess the emotional and psychological outlook of the client. Assess the previous exposure of the client to the diagnosis of cancer. Determine factual information from distortions on the part of the client and family. Decide how much education is needed and the best approach for this particular client and family.

3. Cancer is a family problem. Although only one person may be affected with the cancer itself, all of the family is involved. Assess the psychological status of the family.

4. Assess the client's knowledge level about radiation therapy. Determine the presence of pregnant women who might wish to visit and any others who are particularly at risk to the hazards of radiation therapy (e.g., children).

Plan

Nursing Objectives

Maintain a calm and reassuring manner.

Prepare the client adequately for the impressive size of the machinery used in cobalt therapy and for the possible side-effects.

Maintain an optimistic outlook.

Treat side-effects and minimize discomfort.

Take adequate precautions to protect staff, visitors, and other clients from the harmful effects of radiation.

CLIENT PREPARATION

1. The machinery used to administer radiation therapy, such as the linear accelerator, is massive and may frighten the client (Fig. 79-1). For their own protection, personnel stand behind a lead screen or wall during treatments. For

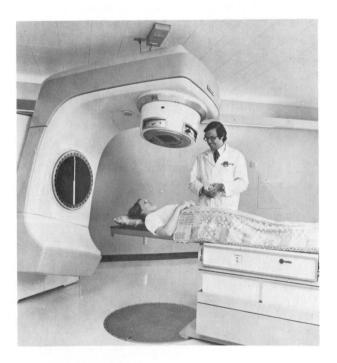

Figure 79.1
(Courtesy, Varian)

these reasons, the client may be frightened of the first treatment if not adequately prepared. Let the client know about how, where, and when the treatments will be done. Explain that there is no pain involved. Prior positive preparation can do much to help the client accept these treatments.

2. Explain the reason for and expected effects of the therapy before beginning. Before receiving the radioactive materials, the client should understand fully the care that will be rendered, visitor limitations, and restrictions on the client. Radiation therapy frequently causes nausea. This should be presented to the client in a matter-of-fact way so that if nausea and vomiting do occur, the client will not view these symptoms as a set-back but as a normal progression of the therapy. Other expected side-effects are hair loss and discoloration of the skin.

3. Tell the client that the action of the radiation is painless. There may be some discomfort from surgical implantation; however, there is no sensation involved in radiation action.

Equipment

Radiation signs for the hospital room door
Lead aprons

Implementation and Interventions

Procedural Aspects

ACTION

1. Be aware of the three methods of self-protection against radiation. All staff members should know these.

   Time: Personnel should spend the least amount of time possible in one span with the radiation therapy client. Work quickly and return at intervals to check the client.

   Distance: The farther away from the implant the personnel stand, the less is the chance for contamination. Keep as far from the source of radiation as is possible. Keep as much bulk between the nurse and the source as possible.

   Shielding: Personnel who spend extended time with the client, (> 15 min) should wear lead aprons (Fig. 79-2). The client may also be screened with lead screens or be placed in a lead-lined room. The client should be in a private room with the area of implant pointing toward an outside wall if a lead-lined room is available.

RATIONALE

Radiation interferes with normal cell division to kill cells. Because cancer cells are more rapidly proliferating, they are more susceptible to radiation than are normal cells. Normal cells can be affected however, and for this reason adequate precautions should be taken to safeguard staff and family members from the harmful effects of radiation.

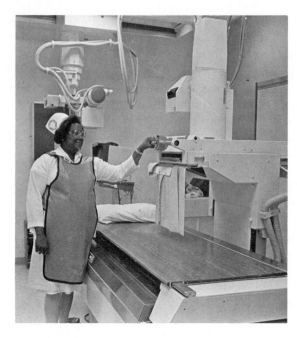

Figure 79.2

ACTION	*RATIONALE*
2. Limit visiting privileges to the radiation client. Young children and any adult female who might possibly be pregnant should not visit. Visitors should remain at least 3 ft away from the client. Hang a sign on the door indicating that radiation is being used in this area. Explain carefully to the client the reasons for these restrictions to alleviate any feelings of resentment or abandonment. Check on the client frequently to combat feelings of loneliness and fear. It is not necessary to remain with the client for a long time. It is not even necessary to enter the room every time, merely let the client know that someone cares and is interested.	Young children and developing fetuses have very rapidly proliferating cells within their bodies. These cells are more susceptible to destruction by radiation than are normal adult cells. Radiation cells exposure can be decreased by distance.
3. Radium and radon seeds can become dislodged from the body cavity in which they are implanted. If any unusual metallic-appearing needles, seeds, capsules, or tubes are ever found in or near the radiation client's room, *do not touch*. Ask the radiologist or other trained personnel from the radiation therapy department to come to the unit and pick up the item. They will use long-handled lead forceps and can safely handle the materials. Check all dressings and linen before they leave the room to be sure	Radioactivity is determined with a Geiger counter by an experienced technician or radiologist. Touching the radioactive material exposes the person to great doses of radiation and is very harmful. It must therefore be done by experienced personnel.

ACTION	RATIONALE

none of the radioactive material has become dislodged accidently. If the implant is in the bladder, all urine must be collected and visually examined for radioactive materials. If systemic radioactive isotope therapy is being carried out, save all body waste, including emesis, until it is positively deemed nonradioactive. Save the body waste in a metal emesis basin or bedpan and do not touch it.

4. Handle the client on radium therapy with great care so that the radium remains in the exact location desired by the radiologist. Measures to guard against dislodging the radium include bed rest, use of an indwelling catheter, minimal movement in bed, and the administration of sedatives and antiemetics. Physical care should be kept to a minimum until the implant is removed.

The radium is implanted so that maximum exposure is given to the cancerous cells. This is accomplished to a great extent by positioning. If the radium is dislodged, the carcinogenic effects will not occur in the area necessary to kill the neoplasm.

Communicative Aspects

OBSERVATIONS

1. Observe for usual side-effects, including nausea, vomiting, anorexia, skin reactions, malaise, and alopecia.
2. Observe for any reactions to therapy so that early treatment can be started. A bland cream may help local skin reaction; discourage vigorous rubbing. Antiemetics may help to curb nausea.
3. Observe the client's level of acceptance of the clinical diagnosis of cancer.
4. Observe the client's environment for any signs of dislodged radioactive materials.

CHARTING

DATE/TIME	OBSERVATIONS	SIGNATURE
5/3 0950	Returned from OR after radium implant in cervix. B/P 136/60, P 82, R 16, T 97.6° F. Flat in bed at this time. Foley catheter patent, draining yellow urine. Cautioned to remain in bed. Fruit juice offered, refused. No nausea at this time.	G. Ivers RN

Discharge Planning Aspects

CLIENT AND FAMILY EDUCATION

1. Side-effects of radiation therapy are fairly common among all clients. Tell the client about the side-effects so that they will not be viewed as a set-back. Avoid such statements as "People always get nauseated from radiation treatments", however. The goal is to decrease the client's fear and anxiety if the side-effects do occur, not to increase the chances of their occurring by the power of suggestion. If skin reactions occur, they must *never* be referred to as "radiation burns" since this implies carelessness. Refer to this discoloration as dermatitis or skin reactions.
2. Explain the visitor restrictions to the client, family, and friends in a patient and sympathetic manner. This may seem unusually painful for the family who is already stunned by the news that their loved one has cancer. Answer

questions honestly and support the feelings of the family. Do not alarm the family unduly, but offer an explanation of the visiting regulations so that compliance will be enhanced without guilt or resentment.

REFERRALS

The American Cancer Society may assist the client in obtaining supplies for posthospital care (e.g., wheelchairs, dressings, ambulatory assistance equipment). If transportation assistance is needed to and from the radiation treatment facility, volunteer organizations such as service clubs, religious groups, and others are often willing to provide rides.

Evaluation

Quality Assurance

Each hospital procedure manual should have guidelines for the care of clients undergoing radiation therapy. The rooms to be used, the proper person to call in case of accidental dislodging of the radiation devices, and visitor regulations, should all be addressed. Documentation should include the location, the type, and the length of time that the radiation implant remained in place. Any problems should be noted. The side-effects of the radiation treatment should be noted with the steps taken to alleviate them. Documentation should reflect that the nurse knew possible side-effects and complications from this type of treatment and took steps to prevent or control them. A summary of the client's condition and vital signs should be noted at frequent intervals (at least every 8 hours). Documentation of teaching of the client and family should be made with an assessment of the client and family's acceptance.

Infection Control

The implant will be placed into the client during a surgical procedure under sterile conditions. Handwashing should be done before and after caring for the radiation client, to prevent cross-infection; however, washing has no effect on the amount of radiation received. It is important that the client be protected from infectious processes because the radiation therapy tends to be debilitating from the side-effects.

Technique Checklist

	YES	NO
Client and family understood the reason for and expected outcomes of therapy	_____	_____
Type of radiation therapy		
Linear accelerator _____		
Radium implant _____		
Radon seeds _____		
Other _____		
Location of implant _____		
Visitor restrictions explained to client and family	_____	_____
Side-effects of treatment		
Nausea _____		
Vomiting _____		
Skin reactions _____		
Anorexia _____		
Alopecia _____		
Malaise _____		
Other _____		
Implant removed on _____ (date)		
Client and family informed of possible side-effects after dismissal	_____	_____

80 Range-of-Motion Exercises

Overview

Definition

Range of motion (ROM) is the maximum amount of movement that is possible in any particular joint.

Rationale

Provide optimal activity and functioning of the musculoskeletal system throughout all stages of life.

Prevent loss of function that can result from prolonged inactivity of any joint or muscle.

Provide regular exercise, which is essential to optimal functioning and affects all systems of the body.

Prevent bone decalcification.

Increase circulation and waste removal.

Prevent complications during periods of illness when regular body movement and function are limited, because every body area may be subject to dysfunction in cases of prolonged immobilization.

Provide maintenance regimens for degenerative and rheumatoid arthritis.

Terminology

Abduction: Movement away from the body midline

Active exercise: Exercise performed by the person

Adduction: Movement toward the body midline

Anklylosis: Fixation or immobilization of a joint from disease, injury, or surgery

Atony: Absence of muscle tone

Atrophy: Wasting of muscle

Circumduction: Movement that combines flexion, extension, abduction, and adduction, in which the distal end of the part forms a circle and the shaft of the part describes the surface of a cone (Fig. 80-1A to D)

Contractures: Conditions of fixed, high resistance to passive stretch of muscles resulting from fibrosis of the tissues supporting the muscles or joints, or from disorders of the muscle fibers

Edema: An accumulation of fluid in the tissues (swelling)

Extension: Movement increasing the angle of the joint

Flexion: Movement decreasing the angle of the joint, *Dorsiflexion* is backward flexion or bending of the hand or foot (Fig. 80-2); *plantar flexion* is bending or stretching of the foot in the direction of the sole (Fig. 80-3)

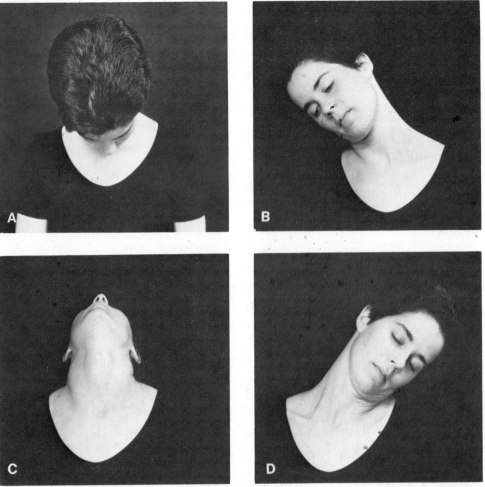

Figure 80.1 A , B , C , and D

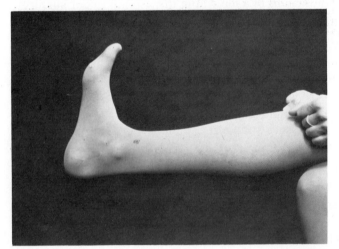

Figure 80.2

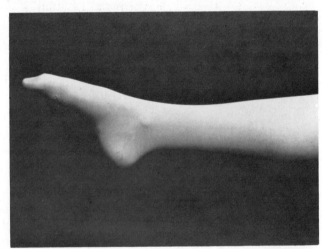

Figure 80.3

Hyperextension: State of exaggerated extension

Isometric exercise: Movement involving a muscular contraction

Isotonic exercise: Rhythmic movement, involving muscle contractions, resulting in a change in muscle length, such as extension of a limb

Lateral rotation: Away from the midline of the body

Medial rotation: Toward the midline of the body

Osteoporosis: Loss of calcium, nitrogen, and phosphorus from the bone

Passive exercise: Movement of the client's body by another person

Resistive exercise: External resistant force used in active exercise, such as equipment that is pushed forward with the lower leg to strengthen the thigh and calf muscles

Rotation: The twisting of a part of the body around the longitudinal axis of that area (Fig. 80-4)

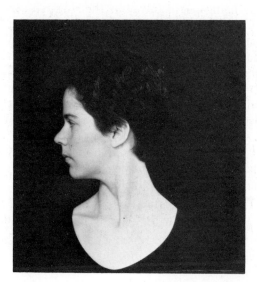 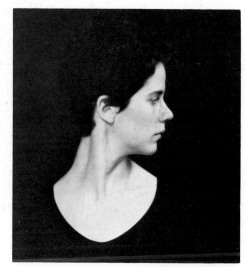

Figure 80.4

Supination: Movement that causes the palm or foot to be upward

Thrombus: A blood clot in a vein

Assessment

Pertinent Anatomy and Physiology

1. See Appendix I. *skeletal system, skeletal muscles, vertebral column.*

2. Exercise has many positive effects on the cardiopulmonary system. The heart rate increases. Blood flow is redirected from nonexercising tissues to those areas of greater need, the heart and muscles. This redirection of blood increases the cardiac output and stimulates the heart muscle. Ventilation also increases promoting removal of secretions from the bronchial area.

3. Metabolism includes all of the physical and chemical activity occurring in the body. The basal metabolic rate is the amount of energy used by the cells when the body is as much at rest as is possible during life. Exercise increases the metabolic rate according to the degree of exertion.

Pathophysiological Concepts

1. Immobility can initiate a series of problems for the musculoskeletal system. Lack of stimulation from the stress of bearing weight during normal physical activity can result in demineralization of the bone, or osteoporosis. The bones become spongy and eventually may become deformed from fractures. With continued disuse, muscles tend to atrophy. When normal tone of the muscles no longer is able to keep the bones in proper alignment, the stronger muscles dominate and cause unusual deformities called *contractures*. This condition involves the joints, ligaments, and tendons and is irreversible without surgical intervention. Formation of pressure sores also accompanies immobility.

2. Multisystem problems may result from prolonged inactivity and immobility. Respiratory activity is decreased with a resulting buildup or pooling of secretions, which can result in pneumonia. Cardiovascular problems occur because of the gravitational pull on the body in the supine position. Blood pools in the veins. This causes an increase of fluid in the tissue because blood is not being carried away by the sluggish cardiovascular system. Edema is the result. A common threat from slowed venous activity is the formation of a clot, or thrombus. Normally, the blood flows through the veins so quickly that clots do not have time to form unless there is a disruption in the integrity of the vein that catches the cells. When the blood flows more slowly, it is easier to pool and clot. Stasis and pooling of urine is a problem in the kidneys that may result in the formation of stones or infection. Lack of activity also decreases peristalsis and results in constipation and impaction.

Assessment of the Client

1. Assess the physical condition of the client in relation to ability to perform full ROM exercises. Determine any joint limitations and possible causes. Assess the gait and manual dexterity of the client.

2. Assess the level of understanding of the client and family regarding the purpose of ROM exercises, why they are important and expected results.

3. Assess the client's age and life-style. Consider the goals for this client, noting that not every client will require the same level or program of exercise.

Plan

Nursing Objectives

Promote optimal motor function by establishing proper body alignment and a regular exercise regime.

Prevent disability and deformity.

Initiate active and passive exercise as soon as possible.

Use mechanical aids as indicated (e.g., walker, crutches, cane, Foster frame, overbed trapeze).

Increase circulatory function.

Prevent complications such as phlebitis and thrombi.

Client Preparation

1. Explain to the client and family the importance of and need for exercise. This is the basis for treatment. Instructions must be clear and easily understood.

2. The client should be dressed in nonrestrictive clothing. Provide for privacy by adequate screening and draping.

3. Emphasize the responsibility of the client as the instructions on range of motion are given. This is the key to effective results. Assist the client in understanding that nurses and therapists are the teachers and helpers in ROM therapy; progress and participation are the responsibilities of the client. The partially or totally immobilized client must develop an acceptance of the body and feelings of self-control.

4. Allow the client to rest after strenuous daily routines, such as ambulation and breathing exercises, before beginning ROM exercises. If the client is physically able, ROM exercises may be done during the bath.

PRINCIPLES OF EXERCISE

1. Active exercise is preferable to passive exercise.

2. Each joint of the body has a normal range of motion.

3. ROM exercises are planned for each client according to age group, body build, and condition.

4. ROM is affected by the client's genetic makeup, physical condition, and disease process.

5. Techniques to treat and reverse specific conditions must be planned individually by a qualified therapist or physician.

Equipment

Depends on the client's needs, restrictions, and abilities

Implementation and Interventions

Procedural Aspects

ACTION

RATIONALE

Active ROM Exercises

1. Active exercises are performed by the client with supervision and encouragement by the nurse. Exercises may be done while the client is in bed, standing, or during daily activities. Each motion should be repeated three times or as tolerated by the client.

More strength is required for the client to do the exercises; the result is increased muscle tone and feelings of self-esteem.

2. The neck should be placed in the following positions: flexion, in which the head moves forward with the chin on the chest; extension, in which the head is in the normal upright position, and hyperextension, with the head tilted as far back as possible; lateral flexion in which the head is tilted toward each shoulder; and rotation, with head moving in a circular motion to the right, back, left, and front.

ACTION   **RATIONALE**

3. The shoulder should be placed in the following positions: flexion, in which the arm is raised from the side, forward to a position above the head; extension, which moves the arm from the upward position back to the side of the body; hyperextension, when the arm is moved behind the client's body (Fig. 80-5); abduction, in which the arm is moved from the side outward and upward with the palm facing down; adduction moves the arm back to the side with the palm down (Fig. 80-6); internal rotation, in which the arm is out from the body with the elbow bent and the hand and forearm are brought from the straight-up position forward to the straight-down position; external rotation, which brings the hand and forearm back to the upward position with the elbow flexed (Fig. 80-7); and circumduction, in which the arm is moved in a full circle alongside the body (Fig. 80-8).

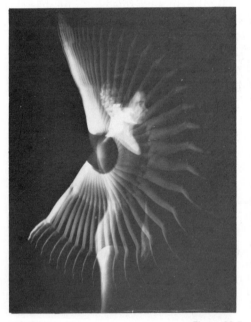

Figure 80.5

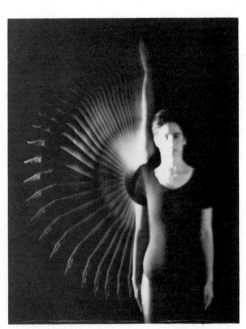

Figure 80.6

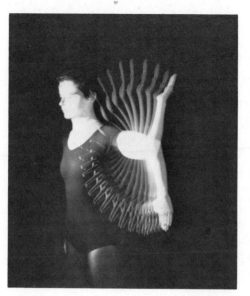
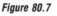

Figure 80.7

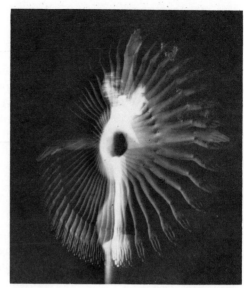

Figure 80.8

ACTION	RATIONALE

4. The elbow should be placed in the following positions: flexion, in which the arm is stretched outward in front of the body and the elbow is bent, bringing the palm upward toward the face, and extension, which straightens the elbow back to the outstretched position.

5. The forearm should be placed in the following positions: supination, in which the forearm is rotated until the palm is facing upward; pronation, in which the palm is rotated to a downward position.

6. The wrist should be placed in the following positions: flexion, in which the hand is stretched forward with the palm approaching the forearm; extension, with the back of the hand brought upward on an even plane with the forearm; hyperextension, which moves the back of the hand toward the top of the forearm. Abduction bends the hand away from the thumb side and adduction bends the hand toward the thumb side.

ACTION

RATIONALE

7. The fingers and thumb should be placed in the following positions: flexion, which results in the formation of a fist; extension, which moves the fingers out to an even plane with the forearm; hyperextension, which moves the fingers as far backward as possible; abduction, in which the fingers are spread apart, and adduction, in which the spaces between the extended fingers are closed.

8. The hip should be placed in the following positions: flexion, moving the leg forward and upward; extension, returning the leg back to normal standing position; hyperextension, moving the leg backward (Fig. 80-9); abduction, moving the leg outward to the side from the body; adduction, returning it to normal standing position; internal rotation, turning the foot inward with the toes pointed toward the other foot; external rotation, turning the foot outward with the heel pointed toward the other foot; and circumduction, which moves the foot in a circular movement with the knee straight, to the side of the body.

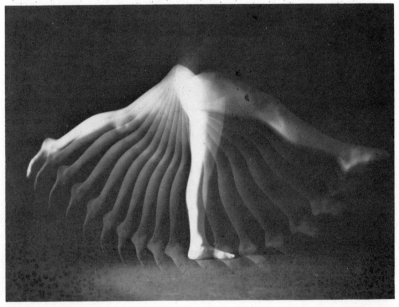

Figure 80.9

ACTION

9. The knee is placed in the following positions: flexion, in which the knee is bent with the heel lifted upward off the floor; extension, in which the foot is returned to the floor (Fig. 80-10); and circumduction, in which the foot is lifted from the floor and the lower leg is moved in a circular movement.

10. The foot and ankle should be placed in the following positions: flexion, in which the toes are bent downward; extension, when the toes are returned to normal position; hyperextension, when the toes lifted into the air; plantar extension, when the foot is moved as far downward as possible; dorsal flexion, when the foot is moved as far upward as possible; adduction, in which the toes are separated as far from each other as possible; adduction, when the toes are squeezed together; eversion, in which the side of the foot is lifted outward; and inversion, in which the inner aspect of the foot is lifted upward and inward.

11. The trunk should be placed in the following positions: flexion, in which the trunk is bent forward at the waist; extension, when the trunk is raised back to the natural standing position; hyperextension, in which the back is bent backward beyond the normal standing plane; lateral flexion, with the trunk bent toward the side; and circumduction, in which the trunk is moved in a circle from the waist.

Passive ROM Exercises

1. Passive exercises are performed by the nurse or therapist on the client who is unable to perform them alone. The same movement of joints as was explained in active ROM exercise is desired, but because of limitations of position and condition, full range usually is not obtained. As much range as possible is the goal. Perform each movement three times or as tolerated by the client. Use proper body mechanics.

RATIONALE

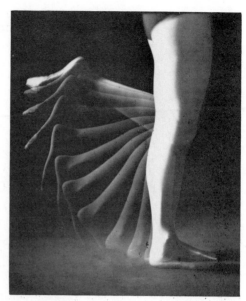

Figure 80.10

Proper body mechanics will ensure that the nurse or therapist is not injured or strained during exercises.

ACTION	RATIONALE

2. The head should be flexed (Fig. 80-11), extended, hyperextended, and laterally extended to each side.

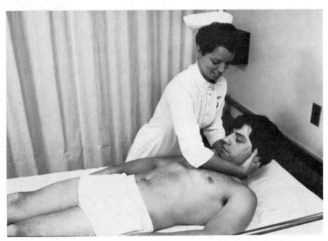

Figure 80.11

3. The shoulder should be flexed, extended (Fig. 80-12), abducted (Fig. 80-13) and adducted, and then rotated externally (Fig. 80-14) and internally (Fig. 80-15).

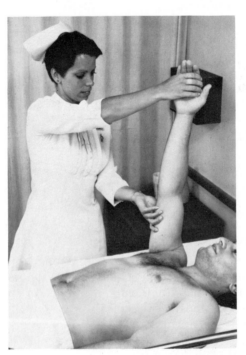

Figure 80.12

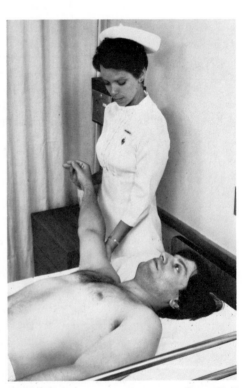

Figure 80.13

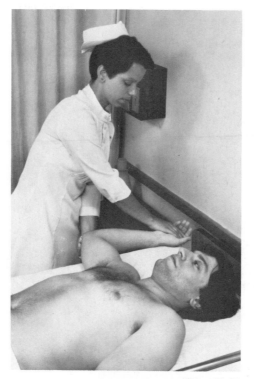

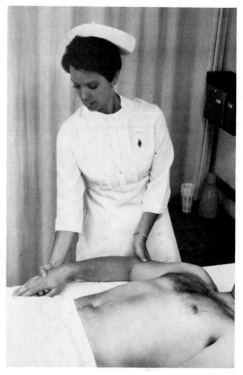

Figure 80.14

Figure 80.15

ACTION

RATIONALE

4. The elbow and forearm should be
   flexed (Fig. 80-16), then extended,
   supinated, and pronated.

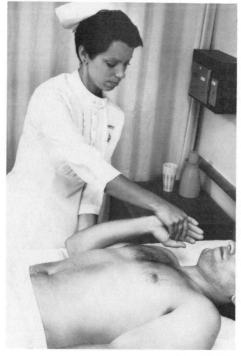

Figure 80.16

ACTION   **RATIONALE**

5. The wrist and hand should be
   flexed (Fig. 80-17) and hyperextended (Fig. 80-18); the fingers
   may be flexed at the same time; abduction and adduction of the wrist
   may be performed as the fingers
   are spread and closed.

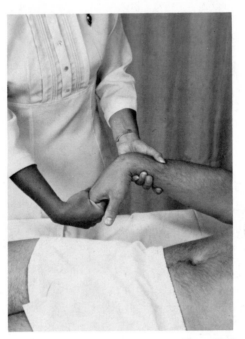
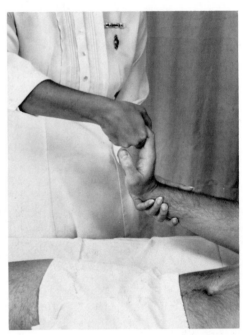

Figure 80.17   *Figure 80.18*

6. The leg and hip should be flexed
   (Fig. 80-19), externally (Fig. 80-20)
   and internally (Fig. 80-21) rotated,
   and abducted (Fig. 80-22) and adducted (Fig. 80-23). The ankle
   should be dorsal flexed, inverted,
   and everted. The ankle also should
   be plantar flexed. The toes should
   be flexed and hyperextended.

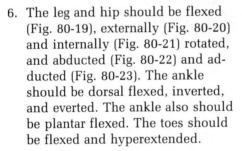

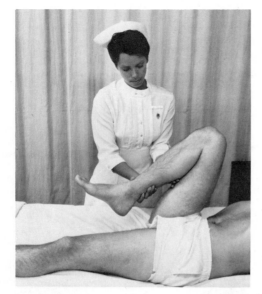

Figure 80.19

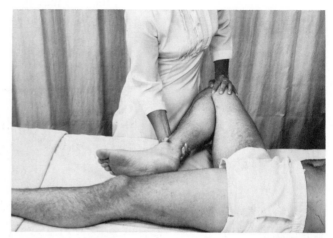

Figure 80.20

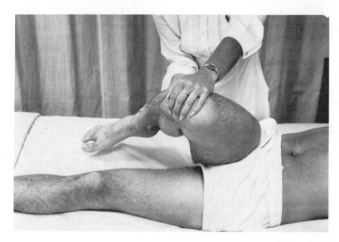

Figure 80.21

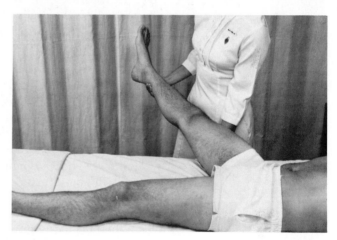

Figure 80.22

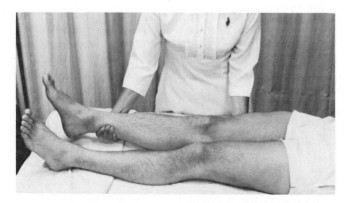

Figure 80.23

ACTION   *RATIONALE*

7. With the client in the prone position, the arm may be hyperextended (Fig. 80-24). The hip then may be hyperextended (Fig. 80-25).

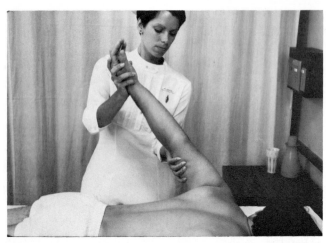

Figure 80.24

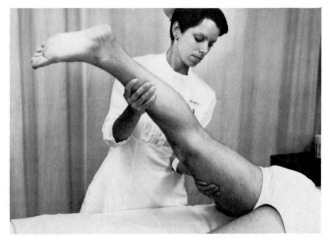

Figure 80.25

Special Modifications

If the client has debilities or restrictions due to illness or injury, ROM should be as inclusive as possible but should not jeopardize present mobility. If allowed, heat to the joints may facilitate the performance of ROM exercises. A physician's order may be needed for the application of heat; check the hospital policy.

Client comfort is important; however, ROM exercises may be uncomfortable or painful. If the client knows why these exercises must be done, cooperation may be enhanced.

Communicative Aspects

OBSERVATIONS

1. Observe the client's ability to perform ROM exercises. When passive ROM exercises are performed, observe for pain, discomfort, and change in the client's ability to assist in performing the exercises. Observe for increases in the client's range of motion of both the affected and unaffected extremities.

2. Observe for pressure areas, especially over the bony prominences, which may be indicated by redness, whiteness, or a break in the skin.

3. Observe for edema, which may interfere with the supply of nutrients to the body.

CHARTING

DATE/TIME	OBSERVATIONS	SIGNATURE
5/10 0930	Passive ROM exercises. Able to move left leg and arm with more control than in previous sessions. Slight increase in the range tolerated in the left shoulder noted. Skin clear, no signs of pressure. Turned to left side. ———	G. Ivers RN

Discharge Planning Aspects

CLIENT AND FAMILY EDUCATION

1. If the client will be discharged home and will continue to need passive ROM exercises, the family should be shown how to perform these exercises in a safe and effective manner. Emphasize proper body mechanics and full ROM of all joints. Allow the client to perform a return demonstration to assess technique and understanding of principles.

2. The client and family should understand why the exercises are important as well as the goal of the program.

REFERRALS

The client and family may benefit from a referral to a resource in the community, such as a physical therapist, or a state vocational rehabilitation agency if long-term care is needed.

Evaluation

Quality Assurance

Documentation should include a record of observations, preventive measures, and intervention methods used to alleviate immobilization of any part of the body. The progress and effectiveness of treatment also should be documented. The time and pertinent observations should be made every time the exercise program is carried out. Safety measures taken during exercises should be noted.

Infection Control

Handwashing should be done before and after contact with any client to prevent cross-contamination.

Technique Checklist

	YES	NO
Procedure explained to client and family	_____	_____
Active ROM exercises by client	_____	_____
Passive ROM exercises performed on client	_____	_____
ROM exercises demonstrated to family	_____	_____
Development of pressure area	_____	_____
Location _____		

81

Rectal (Digital) Examination

Overview

Definition

A diagnostic procedure in which a gloved finger is inserted into the rectum for examination

Rationale

Detect changes in the anatomy of the rectum or of the organs or tissues palpable through the wall of the rectum.

Detect the presence of pathology in surrounding organs (> 50% of cancerous lesions of the large intestine are within reach of the examiner's finger).

Determine the presence of a fecal impaction.

Obtain specimens for diagnostic testing.

Terminology

Knee–chest position: A position in which the client lies on the stomach with the buttocks elevated, the knees pulled up to touch the chest, the head turned to one side and resting on the folded arms

Sims' position: A semiprone position in which the client lies on the left side, right knee and thigh drawn well up above the left, left arm behind the back and right arm on the bed or table; the chest is inclined forward

Sphincter: A circular muscle constricting an orifice or opening

Assessment

Pertinent Anatomy and Physiology

See Appendix I. *anus, intestine (large), rectum, sigmoid colon.*

Pathophysiological Concepts

1. Most colorectal cancer does not produce symptoms until late in the course of the disease. Bleeding is a highly significant early symptom. Others include change in bowel habits, diarrhea, constipation, and pain (a very late symptom).

2. Inflammatory bowel disease results in irritation of the bowel. Ulcerative colitis tends to be a continuous inflammatory process, whereas Crohn's disease skips areas of the colon. Both diseases form lesions that are prone to hemorrhage. Care must be exercised when doing a rectal examination on a client with a known or suspected inflammatory bowel disease.

Assessment of the Client

1. Assess the onset of symptoms that prompted the client to seek health care assistance. Determine if the client has had any bowel problems or changes, rectal bleeding, or pain.

2. Assess the usual pattern of bowel habits. Assess nutritional patterns in relation to amount of bulk and fluid taken orally each day.

3. Assess the physical condition of the client in regard to ability to assume positioning to enhance rectal examination. Determine the presence of other symptoms that might interfere with rectal examination, for example, nausea, seizures, pain, hemorrhoids, or rectal bleeding.

Plan

Nursing Objectives

Allay fear and anxiety of the client regarding pain, discomfort, and the findings of the examination.

Provide for the client's comfort and safety.

Maintain the client's dignity and privacy by minimizing the amount of exposure by draping and screening.

Assist in obtaining tissue specimens, if indicated.

Teach the client and family the importance of early detection and treatment.

Assist in adequate preparation of the client.

Client Preparation

1. Ask the client to void before the examination because emptying the bladder reduces the pressure within the abdominal and pelvic cavities and allows the rectum to be examined in its usual anatomic position with greater comfort for the client.

2. Explain to the client what will take place during the rectal examination and why the examination must be done. A matter-of-fact attitude may reduce the client's anxiety.

Equipment

Clean glove

Lubricating, water-soluble jelly

Drape sheet and screen

Specimen container (if needed)

Implementation and Interventions

Procedural Aspects

ACTION	RATIONALE
1. Provide privacy and increase the client's ability to relax by adequate screening and draping. Ask the client to breathe deeply during the examination. Remind the client that regular breathing promotes relaxation and reduces discomfort.	Modesty and training inhibit relaxation of the voluntary muscles. The contracted external anal sphincter will cause discomfort when it is irritated mechanically during insertion of the examiner's finger into the rectum.
2. Place the client in either Sims' or the knee–chest position.	The area to be examined can be more readily reached for accurate determination of findings by proper positioning.
3. Fanfold the top linens to the foot of the bed. Drape the client's legs with one drape and use another drape or blanket to cover the trunk (Fig. 81-1).	Warmth and privacy facilitate relaxation and cooperation.

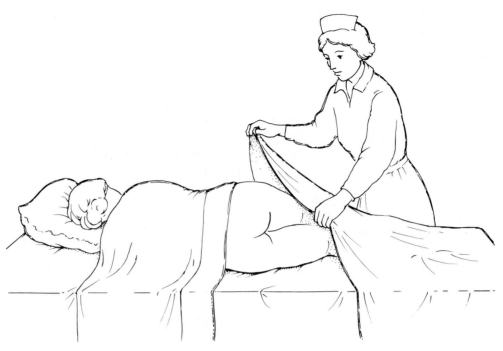

Figure 81.1

ACTION

4. Apply the glove to the examination hand. Drop several drops of lubricant onto the index finger of the gloved hand.

5. Using the ungloved hand, lift and separate the buttocks. Inspect the area for lumps, rashes, as well as signs of inflammation and bleeding. Ask the client to strain, unless the client has a known or suspected cardiac problem. Look for signs of hemorrhoids or breaks in the skin around the anus. Place the index finger against the anus, and, as the client relaxes, gently insert the fingertip into the anal canal. Instruct the client to relax and progress the finger as far as possible. Palpate the walls of the rectum feeling for nodules or irregularities. Note the tone of the sphincter muscle, and any tenderness or bleeding. Ask the client to strain and note any lesions that might be out of reach otherwise. In men the prostate may be palpated; in women the cervix is usually felt.

RATIONALE

Avoid contaminating the tube of lubricant by touching it with the gloved hand. Form the habit of dropping the lubricant onto the hand without touching the tube.

Straining causes contraction of the muscles of the rectal area and may enable the examiner to palpate tumors. The client should be allowed to relax after initial insertion and palpation to avoid fatigue.

ACTION	*RATIONALE*
Gently withdraw the finger and examine for any fecal material or blood. If a specimen is taken, place it in a clean container (in a sterile container if the stool specimen is for culture). Transport the specimen to the lab at once.	
6. After the examination, cleanse the rectal area with a warm, moist cloth. Leave the client in a clean, comfortable environment.	Removal of the lubricating jelly and any stool that may have escaped after the examination will make the client feel cleaner and more comfortable.

Communicative Aspects

OBSERVATIONS

1. Observe the anal area for any abnormalities.
2. Observe the drainage that appears following the examination to determine the presence of blood or abnormal stool.
3. Observe the client during the examination for discomfort, ability to assume the desired position, and anxiety about findings.

CHARTING

DATE/TIME	OBSERVATIONS	SIGNATURE
7/27 1400	Rectal examination done. No abnormalities palpated. Small hemorrhoid noted at anal entrance with no signs of bleeding. Fecal material semisoft, brown. Client continues to voice fears of having cancer; schedule for barium enema in AM————————————	B. JOHNSON RN, ANP

Discharge Planning Aspects

CLIENT AND FAMILY EDUCATION

1. Discuss positive aspects of early detection of abnormalities. Stress yearly physical examinations for high-risk groups, especially women and men over age 50 and those who have a family history of cancer.
2. Inform the client and family that rectal bleeding at any time warrants immediate attention and should be checked by a physician.
3. Stress the importance of good bowel and nutritional habits. Use this opportunity to encourage the judicious use of over-the-counter laxatives. Remind the client that "normal" is what is normal for each person and does not necessarily mean that the bowels must move every day.

Evaluation

Quality Assurance

Documentation should reflect that the nurse knew how to perform the examination and what expected results were. Any deviation from normal should be noted, and evidence that the physician was notified of the abnormalities should be reflected in the chart. Any symptoms should be noted. The reaction of the client to the procedure also should be reflected. The record should show that the nurse knew about possible complications and took measures to prevent them.

Infection Control

Careful handwashing before and after this procedure is essential. The rectal area is considered contaminated. It is not necessary to carry out this procedure under sterile conditions; however, rectal microorganisms can be pathogenic if allowed to invade the other body systems. Handwashing is an effective means of removing the bacteria.

Technique Checklist

	YES	NO
Procedure explained to client	_____	_____
Client able to assume desired position	_____	_____
Sims' _____		
Knee–chest _____		
Rectal abnormalities noted		
Lesions _____		
Hemorrhoids _____		
Bleeding _____		
Lumps in rectum _____		
Abnormalities reported to physician	_____	_____
Client left in clean environment	_____	_____
Client understood the results of the examination	_____	_____

82

Respiratory Care

Overview

Definition

The administration of medications and therapeutic gases into the respiratory tract

Rationale

Assist in oxygenation of the client's blood by providing a readily usable source of pure oxygen.

Improve breathing by the administration of bronchodilators, mucolytics, and other drugs directly into the lungs by means of aerosol instillation.

Increase vital capacity by forcing gases under pressure into the client's lungs in a controlled situation.

Assist the client in critical condition in the maintenance of the basic life function of breathing until the client is physically able to breathe unassisted.

Maintain an atmosphere of high humidity in an effort to break up secretions and aid the client in coughing to remove them from the respiratory tract.

Terminology

Anoxia: Oxygen deprivation, which if severe enough may cause cell death in as short a time as 30 seconds

Atomization: Production of large droplets from a solution

Bronchodilators: Drugs that enlarge the passageways of the lungs

Dyspnea: Difficulty breathing

Mucolytics: Drugs that liquefy secretions and facilitate expectoration

Nebulization: Production of a fine mist from a solution

Uvula: Small, soft structure hanging from the free edge of the soft palate in the midline above the root of the tongue

Assessment

Pertinent Anatomy and Physiology

1. See Appendix I. *bronchial tree, trachea.*

2. The lobules are the functional units of the lungs in which gas exchange takes place. The gas exchange structures consist of a bronchiole and the alveolar sacs and ducts. Blood enters the lobule through the pulmonary artery and returns to the heart by means of the pulmonary vein. The alveolar sacs are cup-shaped, thin-walled structures that intercommunicate.

3. Ventilation is the mechanical process of taking in and releasing air from the lungs. Inspiration involves the downward movement of the diaphragm to increase the size and volume of the lungs. This results in a decrease in the pressure within the airways of the lungs below that of the atmosphere, and air moves into the lungs. Expiration involves a passive reflex action of the lung structures, causing lung volume to decrease so that pressure in the lungs is greater than that in the atmosphere, and air moves out of the lungs.

4. The act of breathing is normally effortless and not controlled by the conscious will. Increases in exercise and metabolism result in an increase in the respiratory rate. Respiratory movements are normally smooth, with equal expansion of both sides of the chest.

Pathophysiological Concepts

1. *Pneumonia* is an inflammation of the lungs, in particular the alveoli and bronchioles. It may be caused by infectious and noninfectious agents. Agents that cause pneumonia usually are inhaled into the normally sterile lung. Lobar pneumonia involves a large portion or an entire lobe of the lung. Usually, it occurs in otherwise healthy adults. Bronchopneumonia may be caused by any pathogenic organism. Hospitalized clients are particularly susceptible to the bacteria present in their environment. Bronchopneumonia is common among the very young and very old as well as the debilitated. Bronchopneumonia is characterized by slow onset and low-grade fever, with cough and expiratory rales. Viral pneumonias usually follow a viral infection such as chicken pox.

2. Normal lung expansion depends on maintenance of a negative pressure in the lungs and an unobstructed airway. *Pneumothorax* is collapse of the lung that occurs when air gets into the pleural spaces. Lung reexpansion usually is accomplished by insertion of a closed system in to the pleural space to reestablish proper pressure gradients. *Atelectasis* is the incomplete expansion of a part of the lung because of airway obstruction or lack of the lubricating substance in the lungs that keeps the alveoli expanded. Atelectasis means collapse of the alveoli. Coughing and deep breathing are important to preventing atelectasis.

3. Emphysema causes trapping of air in the alveoli. The work of breathing is greatly increased. Air is taken into the lungs with relative ease, however, the act of expiration is markedly difficult. Hyperinflation of the lungs causes an increase in the anteroposterior dimensions of the chest resulting in the typical barrel-chest phenomenon.

4. Asthma is one of the most common chronic conditions of children under age 17. In addition, many adults are afflicted with the respiratory problem. This disease is characterized by bronchospasm in response to various stimuli. It also causes edema of the mucosal surface of the bronchioles and increased mucus production. Wheezing and dyspnea are a result of the airway obstruction. Bronchodilators and smooth muscle relaxants are used to treat the condition. Preventive measures include avoidance of the triggering allergens.

Assessment of the Client

1. Assess the respiratory patterns of the client. Determine rate, ease of inspiration and expiration, presence of cyanosis, and breath sounds.

2. Assess the client's history of respiratory problems. Determine previous occurrences of pneumonia, asthma and other allergies, shortness of breath, tuberculosis, and other breathing difficulties. Asses the history of the client in relation to type of tobacco used, duration, and frequency.

Plan

Nursing Objectives

Ensure that the client receives the right gases at the right rate.

Observe for signs of inadequate oxygenation.

Evaluate the client's reaction and tolerance to positive-pressure treatments and notify the physician if problems occur.

Maintain patency of breathing equipment.

Assist the family in handling their feelings when assisted ventilation is used to prolong life.

Maintain continuous high humidity by keeping vaporizers filled and the room closed.

Provide the prescribed respiratory assistance in a safe and therapeutic manner.

Client Preparation

1. When an externally applied device will be used to administer oxygen, show the client the device and explain its purpose before it is applied, if possible. This is especially true of the face mask because it covers such a large area and can be very frightening.

2. Positive-pressure treatments can be frightening to the client who is unprepared for the sudden influx of air. Many think that their lungs are going to "burst." Offer an explanation that will allow the client to be prepared for this sensation in order to gain greater compliance. If positive-pressure or other breathing enhancers are to be used postoperatively, allow the client to see and to test them before surgery, if practical.

3. The success of a high-humidity atmosphere depends greatly on keeping the system closed to the greatest degree possible. Explain the goals of this type of therapy to the family and client and ask for their help in providing optimal conditions.

Equipment

Oxygen source

Cannula, catheter, or face mask

Medication and nebulizer

Positive-pressure machine or apparatus

Steam inhalator or vaporizer

Implementation and Interventions

Procedural Aspects

ACTION	RATIONALE
1. Protect the client in the high oxygen atmosphere from the hazard of fires. Place "no smoking" signs in visible places and enforce them. Electrical equipment must be used with extreme care and should be checked by a qualified biomedical technician to ensure that it is safe to use in the presence of oxygen. Explain to the client and family about smoking restrictions.	Oxygen is a basic necessity of life. Without it, cells die, and life cannot be sustained. When oxygen is being administered, remember that it is highly suppportive of combustion. Take every precaution to prevent accidents.
2. Oxygen may be administered to the client in a variety of ways.	Oxygen is not stored in large quantities in the body and so must be supplied continuously.
Catheter: A small plastic tube that is inserted into the nose, through the nasal passage, and into the oropharynx. To approximate the distance of insertion, measure in a horizontal line from tip of nose to the earlobe (Fig. 82-1). Insert the catheter to this length. After insertion, check the client's mouth; the tip of the catheter should be visible at the level of the uvula. Connect the end of the catheter to the oxygen tubing and adjust the rate as ordered, (usually between 5 and 8 liter/min). Tape the catheter in place changing it every 8 hours (Fig. 82-2).	If the catheter is inserted too far, it may stimulate the gag reflex or pass into the esophagus, causing inflation of the stomach.

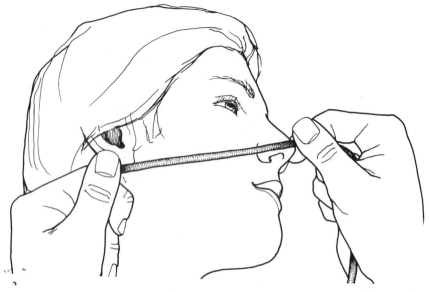

Figure 82.1

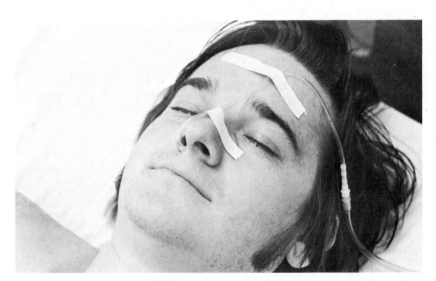

Figure 82.2

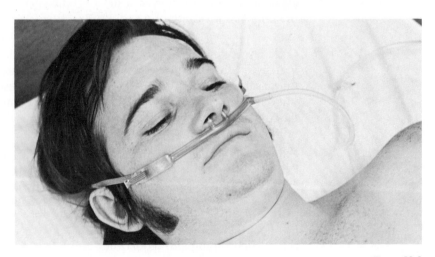

Figure 82.3

ACTION

Cannula: A plastic tube with two protruding outlets that fit into the nose. It is held in place by an elastic band around the head (Fig. 82-3). Instruct the client to breath through the nose with the mouth closed.

Face mask: A means of administering oxygen when the percentage of oxygen must be very high (near 100%) or when the client is mouth breathing. Place the face mask over the client's nose and mouth (Fig. 82-4). Offer frequent reassurance.

RATIONALE

Mouth breathing prevents the oxygen from benefiting the client.

The face mask may cause a suffocating sensation due to the area covered. The client needs repeated reassurance during this type of therapy.

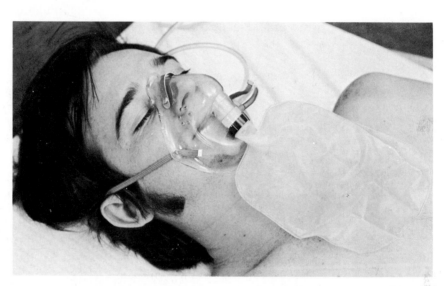

Figure 82.4

3. Affix a distilled water source to the oxygen source before the oxygen is allowed to go to the client. Keep the bottle two-thirds full. Set the flow meter at the desired rate. Give frequent oral hygiene during oxygen administration. Place the client in a comfortable position, usually semi-Fowlers, or the semi-sitting position to facilitate breathing.

Oxygen causes a drying effect on the delicate mucous membranes. To prevent drying, oxygen usually is administered after being run through a water source to provide some degree of humidification. Flow meters usually are set to measure liters per minute. Because the mucous membranes may become dried, frequent rinsing of the mouth and oral hygiene will promote the client's comfort.

4. Positive-pressure treatments help inflate the lungs, expand vital capacity, and aid in medication administration by direct inhalation. A special machine may be used to force the pressurized air into the client's lungs. Because of the hazards involved, these treatments should be administered by someone with considerable knowledge

Positive-pressure machines cause increased pressure during inspiration. The pressure of the gases is usually 10 to 20 lb/in.

ACTION

RATIONALE

and training in the use of this type of specialized equipment. However, the nurse has the responsibility to be alert to signs indicating that the client needs a treatment; to signs indicating its effectiveness; to know its expected therapeutic results; and to be able to recognize untoward effects that warrant attention of indicated complications.

5. Breathing enhancement after surgery may be encouraged by using small, hand-held devices into which the client breathes. Some resistance may be offered by the machine (Fig. 82-5).

These breathing assistance apparatus usually are not attached to external pressure or gas sources. They are often brightly colored and offer visual stimulation and challenge to the client to breathe deeply.

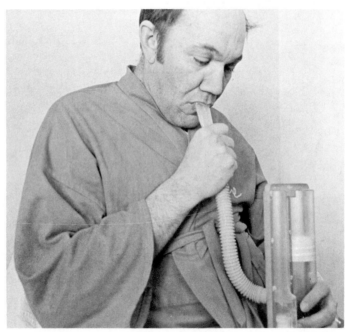

Figure 82.5

6. Highly humidified environments often are ordered, especially in the pediatric area. This may be accomplished by use of a tent-type apparatus to make a localized humidified atmosphere or it may be allowed to distribute throughout the room. The boundary of the humidified environment must be kept closed as much as possible. The humidity may be either warm (steam) or cool (cool mist). If the administration is by tent, the edges must be kept folded under the mattress. If the room is the boundary, the doors and windows must be kept closed.

Humidified environments are desirable in the presence of conditions causing considerable pulmonary congestion. The humidity helps to liquefy the mucus and secretions to facilitate expectoration. Humidity also helps to relieve the discomfort of dry mucous membranes.

Communicative Aspects

OBSERVATIONS

1. Watch all clients for signs of inadequate oxygenation of the blood, such as cyanosis, restlessness, dyspnea, confusion, or an abrupt change in mental acuity.

2. Observe humidifier bottles to make certain that they do not run dry. This could result in nonhumidified oxygen being administered, which can cause great discomfort.

3. Evaluate the patency of oxygen tubing. Kinks and knots will cause stoppage of the oxygen delivery.

4. During positive-pressure treatments, observe the client for gastric distension, which means air is being forced into the stomach rather than into the lungs.

5. Observe for severe chest pain, rapid pulse, and dyspnea, which may indicate pneumothorax.

6. If the client has a nasal cannula, observe for mouth breathing, which negates the benefit of oxygen. Watch to see that the client breathes through the nose.

CHARTING

DATE/TIME	OBSERVATIONS	SIGNATURE
4/19 1430	Oxygen by cannula. Relaxed. No difficulties noted with breathing O_2 at 4 liter/min, P 76, R 14.	F. White RN

Discharge Planning Aspects

CLIENT AND FAMILY EDUCATION

1. Reassure the client and family that there is no pain involved in oxygen administration. Prepare the client for some drying of the mouth and nose and encourage the intake of fluids, if not contraindicated by condition.

REFERRALS

If the client is to be discharged with oxygen at home, instruct the family where and how to obtain oxygen and how to use the equipment. If positive-pressure treatments are to be done at home, refer the client to a home health or visiting nurse association for assistance in learning how to do the treatments and how to care for the equipment at home. If the hospital has a respiratory care service, assistance in home care may be obtained before discharge. Assistance in paying for services and equipment may be available from the American Lung Association.

Evaluation

Quality Assurance

Documentation should include the symptoms exhibited for which the respiratory therapy was ordered. History of respiratory problems and allergies should be noted. Evidence of explanations to the client and family should be reflected. Any medications given by the inhalatory route should be noted. The reaction of the client to the therapy and any complications should be noted. The nurse should show evidence that consideration was given to the potential side-effects and complications possible with respiratory therapy and that preventive measures were taken. Any untoward effects should be reported to the physician and should be documented with disposition of the problem. The hospital should have a standard policy for caring for equipment used by successive clients. In addition, the administration of advanced respiratory care by qualified persons should be addressed in the hospital policy. Evidence that the treatments were carried out by qualified personnel designated by hospital policy should be on the chart.

Infection Control

1. Equipment used for oxygen administration should be disposable, if possible. It should not be used for more than one client. Equipment that will be used for multiple clients must be effectively cleaned to disinfect and render it free from all infectious organisms that might infect other susceptible persons.

2. Bronchopneumonia is often a hospital-acquired infection which is preventable by proper handwashing and decontamination of inhalation equipment. Respiratory infections could prove fatal to persons with chronic obstructive lung disease. These persons should avoid exposure to others with known respiratory tract infections. Hospital personnel with respiratory infections should not care for sick clients.

3. Handwashing is essential before and after any treatment or care of clients with respiratory problems.

4. Persons with bronchopneumonia or other respiratory infections should be encouraged to cover the mouth with a tissue when coughing and to cover the nose when sneezing. Teach client's to wash their hands frequently to prevent the transfer of microorganisms.

Technique Checklist

	YES	NO
Procedure explained to client and family	_____	_____
Type of oxygen administration apparatus used		
Catheter _____		
Cannula _____		
Face mask _____		
Rate _____ liter/min		
Oxygen humidification source kept full	_____	_____
Humidified environment ordered	_____	_____
Steam _____		
Cool mist _____		
Tent type _____		
Room type _____		
Positive pressure treatments	_____	_____
How often _____		
Breathing enhancements	_____	_____
How often _____		
Complications _____		
Client and family understand home care	_____	_____

83   Restraints, Adult

Overview

Definition

A physical method of restricting movement or confining an adult client to the bed or chair

Rationale

Prevent the client from falling out of the bed or chair.

Prevent injury to the client or others.

Immobilize the client to promote the healing process or aid in therapy.

Terminology

Clove hitch knot: A knot used in restraints that allows the client some movement. It is loose so that circulation of the part is not restricted (Figs. 83-1, 83-2).

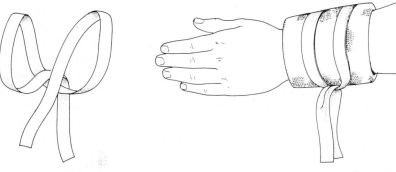

Figure 83.1   *Figure 83.2*

Posey belt: A restraint belt that is placed around the client's chest or waist to prevent falls from the bed or chair.

Square knot: A knot used in restraints most often to secure a tie to the bed frame or back of a wheelchair, used because it will not slip (Figs. 83-3, 83-4).

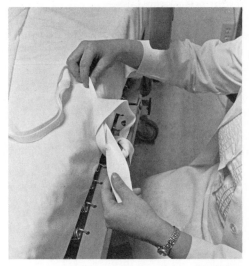
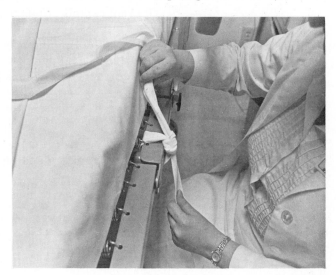

Figure 83.3   *Figure 83.4*

Assessment

Pertinent Anatomy and Physiology

See Technique No. 80, Range-of-Motion Exercises

Pathophysiological Considerations

See Technique No. 80, Range-of-Motion Exercises

Assessment of the Client

1. If the client already has some type of restraints applied, assess the immediate need for restraint.
2. Ascertain if the client is very restless or has delicate skin. Additional padding may be necessary.
3. Determine how rational the client is and explain the procedure accordingly. Determine whether the client has a history of falls or has problems with disorientation or dizziness.
4. Choose a restraint for the client that best meets the needs of the client and fulfills the desired results while providing as much freedom of movement as can be allowed safely.
5. Assess the need for the restraint. All avenues should be exhausted before restraints are used on a client. A geriatric chair or wheelchair with waist restraint may be an alternative. Asking family members or professional sitters to remain with the client to prevent falls is another possibility. Consider the possibility of reality orientation, less sedation, administration of oxygen (if allowed), change of setting, reducing external stimuli, establishing daily routines, increasing self-care modes, use of full bedrails, or music therapy. Another strategy might be to determine the high-risk periods of the day or night for this client based on accurate and thorough history taking. There is continuing focus by the legal profession on the indiscriminate use of restraints. Be certain that restraint is the only way to protect the client before implementation.

Plan

Nursing Objectives

Attempt to gain compliance by giving the client a careful explanation before applying the restraints.

Use restraints only when *absolutely* necessary.

Prevent complications that might arise from falls.

Client Preparation

The use of restraints may have negative connotations for the client and family. Give a careful and adequate explanation in a kind and nonjudgmental way before the restraints are applied.

Equipment

Posey belt, to prevent the client from falling from a chair or out of bed. The three types of Posey belts are 1) locked chest, 2) unlocked chest, and 3) unlocked waist.

Wrist and ankle restraints (may be made of cloth, stockinette, leather, or foam rubber)

Implementation and Interventions

Procedural Aspects

ACTION

RATIONALE

Posey belt

1. Use a belt that fits the client.

These belts can be obtained in small, medium, and large sizes.

2. Place the belt under the client's waist. If the chest style is used, slip the arms of the client through the shoulder straps with the opening in the back (Fig. 83-5).

Positioning the belt in this manner will facilitate securing the restraint on the client.

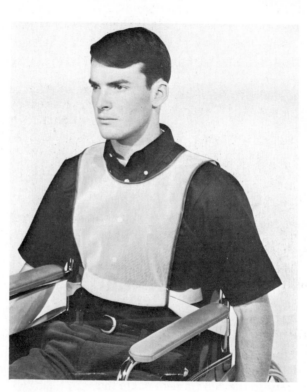

Figure 83.5

3. Position the buckles in the front of the client.

This position will make it easier to secure and loosen the restraint. This is especially important in the event of an emergency when the client must be removed quickly from the restraints.

ACTION	*RATIONALE*
4. Secure the belt by placing the end of the belt through the loops. Secure the long straps of the belt to a chair or the bed frame (Fig. 83-6). The belt should fit snugly but not tightly.	The goal is to limit the movement of the client, but care must be taken not to cause discomfort. Be careful to fasten the restraints to the bed frame rather than to the bedrail which could cause respiratory problems or pain if the rails were lowered.

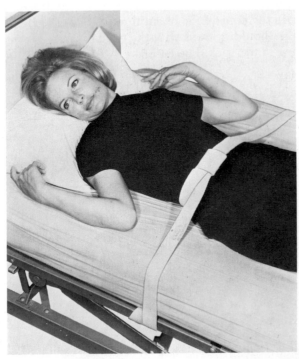

Figure 83.6

5. If a locked belt is used, center the belt with the padded side under the client's back. Secure the long straps to the bed frame; buckle the short straps around the client's waist. Fasten the buckle with a key. Be sure the key is in an easily accessible location. *Every health-care provider on the unit should know where the key is kept.*	Quick access to the key is essential in case of an emergency in which the belt must be removed quickly.

Wrist and Ankle Restraints

1. Place the client in a comfortable position in proper body alignment. Pad the bony portion of the wrist or ankle.	The possibility of abrasions caused by friction are decreased over areas of bony prominences. Proper body alignment also decreases discomfort from immobility.
2. Use the clove hitch knot to apply wrist-type restraints to an extremity.	This knot will not impair circulation to the extremity and does permit some mobility.
3. If leather restraints are used, pad the extremity well.	The leather can cut into the client's skin and impede circulation.

ACTION	RATIONALE
4. Check for sensation and circulation to the affected part before leaving the client. Check the immobilized extremity every hour.	The client may twist or pull against the restraint, thereby tightening it and impairing circulation to the extremity.
5. Do not place restraints on both extremities on the same side of the client.	The client could fall out of bed and be suspended from the restraints. Restraining opposite extremities (i.e., right leg and left arm) increases mobility without creating a safety hazard.
6. Remove the restraint(s) at specific intervals under appropriate supervision of nurse or family.	Skin care and range-of-motion (ROM) exercises should be performed unless contraindicated.
7. Turn the client every 2 hours and reposition.	Immobility causes pulmonary stasis and impaired circulation to the skin and body tissues.
8. Periodically reevaluate the need for restraints.	Restraints should be used for the safety and welfare of the client. When sensorium returns the client may no longer need the restraints.
9. Always leave the client in a comfortable position with the bed in low position and the siderails up.	Provide every safety precaution possible.

Communicative Aspects

OBSERVATIONS

1. Restraints that are too tight will impair circulation. Improperly applied restraints may cause irritation to the skin and impair circulation. Check restraints and extremities every hour. To prevent skin irritation, place sufficient padding over bony prominences such as ankles and wrists. Check these areas to ensure that the padding is in the proper place and is not adding to discomfort or tightness of restraints.

2. Remove the restraint at specified intervals to allow movement of the extremity. When restraints are removed, observe the extremity carefully for any sign of redness, edema, or bruising. Observe the unrestrained client carefully to be sure that falls do not occur.

CHARTING

DATE/TIME	OBSERVATIONS	SIGNATURE
6/29 0830	Posey belt to waist. Attempting to climb over siderails. Seems more confused than yesterday. Waist restraint does not seem to bother or upset him. Siderails up, bed in low position. Dozing at this time. Dr. K. notified of increased confusion. ————————	F. White RN

Discharge Planning Aspects

CLIENT AND FAMILY EDUCATION

1. Instruct the client and family of the purpose and necessity of the restraint.
2. Explain to the client that repositioning will occur at intervals and that the restraint will be reapplied as often as necessary to ensure comfort.
3. If the client should need restraints at home, demonstrate to the family members the proper methods of restraint and safety precautions to take.
4. While the client and family are in the hospital, ask them to alert the nurse if a restraint is causing discomfort or is improperly secured.

Evaluation

Quality Assurance

Document the frequency of checking the restraints (e.g., every hour). Note and record the behavior and mental status of the client while restrained. Special attention given to the skin areas around the restraints should be noted in the chart. Circulation in the extremity must be noted, as well as any signs of impairment and the measures taken to prevent complications. Document the reason for the restraints and any other alternatives that were tried, with a summary of results. Note which extremities were restrained and the method of restraint. Document the explanation to the family and the nurse's assessment of their level of understanding and acceptance.

Infection Control

1. If cloth restraints are used, it is important to use clean restraints to prevent any cross-infection, particularly if the client has any open lesions.
2. If bony prominences, such as wrists or ankles, are not padded before applying a restraint, the skin may become broken owing to the friction of the restraint. If proper precautions are not taken, these broken areas may become infected.

Technique Checklist

	YES	NO
Need for restraints assessed and alternatives explored	_____	_____
Technique explained to the client and family (purpose and method of restraint)	_____	_____
Restraints properly applied	_____	_____
Key in central place with location known to all co-workers	_____	_____
Comfort of client maintained during restraint period	_____	_____
Padding applied to bony prominences as needed	_____	_____
Skin integrity maintained	_____	_____
Circulation of extremities checked every hour and documented on the chart	_____	_____
Procedure explained and demonstrated to family with emphasis on safety precautions	_____	_____

84 Shaving the Client

Overview

Definition

Removal of facial hair (whiskers) from the male client or removal of hair by mechanical means in preparation for surgery

Rationale

Whiskers tend to itch and irritate the skin after 2 or 3 days growth.

The unshaven client may have a poor self-image owing to an unkempt appearance.

Hair on the body harbors microorganisms that may invade the body during surgery.

Assessment

Pertinent Anatomy and Physiology

See Appendix I. *hair, skin.*

Assessment of the Client

1. Assess the area to be shaved for any reddened or broken areas. Determine the presence of bony prominences that will require caution when shaving over and around these areas. Assess the presence of moles, small skin lesions, or any skin appendage protruding from the smooth line of the face, which may get cut or nicked when shaving.

2. Assess the amount of assistance the client needs. Allow the client to participate as much as possible.

3. Assess the client's usual shaving habits. Determine the time of day the client usually shaves, type of razor used, type of lotion used after the shave, and any allergies to soap or shaving creams. Ask the client how he usually shaves, which area first, and how he stretches the facial skin to prevent cuts and reach all areas easily.

Plan

Nursing Objectives

Promote optimal physical comfort by keeping the client clean-shaven.

Prevent trauma to the tissues by using proper technique.

Reassure the family and friends by the well-groomed appearance of the client.

Provide a pathogen-free surface for surgical incision.

Client Preparation

1. Explain what will happen to the client before beginning. Even the comatose client should receive some explanation because the actual depth of perception cannot be measured.

2. Gather all equipment and bring it into the room before beginning the procedure to avoid unnecessary delays.

Equipment

Razor and blade

Shaving lather or soap

Basin with hot water

Bath towel, face towels, and washcloth

After-shave lotion, powder, antiseptic solution

Electric razor (if client prefers)

Bactericidal cream or lotion

Dressings, if ordered, to cover surgical preparation area

Implementation and Interventions

Procedural Aspects

ACTION	*RATIONALE*
1. Determine the policy of the hospital regarding who may shave clients and which clients may be shaved (*i.e.*, diabetics). Allow the client to assist in facial shaving as much as possible.	Some hospitals contract with barber services, and nurses are allowed to shave only in cases of extremely critical or highly infectious clients. Participation in care enhances self-esteem
2. Protect the client's linen by placing a dry towel around the area to be shaved. For the face, place the towel around the client's shoulders.	Wet or soiled linens may produce chilling or discomfort.
3. Steam the area to be shaved with a hot towel for 5 minutes to soften the facial beard before continuing. Be careful not to burn the client. Apply soap or lather to the area to be shaved.	Heat, moisture, and lather help to reduce surface tension and soften the beard on the face. Lather and moisture are usually adequate preparation for other body surfaces.
4. To shave the face, shave in the direction in which the hair grows. For facial hair that grows in a downward direction, begin along the sideburns with short downward strokes of about 2 ½ cm (1 in). There are many irregular surfaces on the face. Around the nose, mouth, and neck areas, pull the skin taut and be especially careful, taking very short strokes (Fig. 84-1).	Shaving in the direction that the hair grows prevents nicks and scraping the skin.

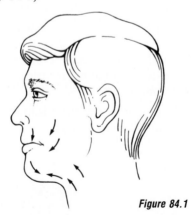

Figure 84.1

ACTION	**RATIONALE**
5. To shave other body areas, long strokes are effective over large, flat body surfaces. If the area is marked by curves and contours, use smaller strokes. Remove all of the hair in the designated area. (See Technique No. 77, Preoperative, Perioperative, and Postoperative Care for areas to be shaved for different surgeries.) If a sterile preparation is ordered, cleanse the area with a bactericidal solution, and apply a sterile dressing using sterile technique.	Minimize trauma to the skin by taking gentle but even strokes, avoiding erratic pressure, which might cause nicks or cuts.
6. After washing off the soap or lather and drying the face, apply a lotion with the palms of the hands. Leave the client in a clean and dry environment.	After-shave lotion or other astringent lotions (check hospital policy) act to close the facial pores.

Special Modifications

1. Many women shave the axillae area and legs as part of their normal hygiene. If this is requested, shave these areas as explained in surgical preparation above. Longer strokes are effective on the legs; however, care must be taken around the ankle and knee area. A cream lotion is usually preferable for the legs. Wait for several minutes before applying deodorant to the female axillae after shaving.	Every effort should be made to promote the client's feelings of self-esteem and comfort. Take care not to nick or cut the skin.
2. If the client prefers, shave with an electric razor. Shave in both directions to ensure complete removal of the hair shaft. Observe safety precautions when using electrical equipment; namely, the razor should be checked and approved as safe by the biomedical department, and electric razors are not used in the presence of oxygen or near water (in the tub or shower).	Electric razors are less likely to cause nicks and cuts. Many people feel they do not shave as closely as a razor blade, however.
3. For some clients who have a bleeding disorder, depilatories are often used. A physician's order is necessary for the use of such a product in many hospitals.	A depilatory is a cream that loosens the hair or whisker so that it can be washed off with a washcloth without using a razor.

Communicative Aspects

OBSERVATIONS

1. Note the client's tolerance of the procedure.
2. Observe for any nicks or cuts inflicted with the razor.

CHARTING

DATE/TIME	OBSERVATIONS	SIGNATURE
12/3 0930	Shaved by nurse with no difficulty. Small abrased area noted on left jaw. Stated this was from the accident. Right arm remains in cast, elevated on pillows. Fingers blanch and move well. Did not seem to tire during procedure.	G. Ivers RN

Discharge Planning Aspects

CLIENT AND FAMILY EDUCATION

1. If the client will not be able to shave himself after discharge, demonstrate for the family how to shave someone in bed. This may be particularly frightening or mysterious to those who have never shaved another person.
2. Explain to the client and family why such a large area must be shaved in preparation for surgery. Explain that the entire area will be rendered as pathogen-free as possible to decrease the chance of infection.

Evaluation

Quality Assurance

Documentation should include notation that the shaving was done, how the client tolerated the procedure, and any complications or problems. Document the area shaved in preoperative preparation. Any additional measures to make the area germ-free should be noted, such as application of a sterile dressing.

Infection Control

1. Any break in the skin is a potential entry for pathogenic organisms. Take extreme care not to cut or nick the client during the shave.
2. Wash hands before and after shaving the client.
3. The purpose of the surgical shave preparation is to remove as many pathogens as possible and to remove hair in which these pathogens reside. Remove as much of the hair as possible. Use a bactericidal solution to further remove microorganisms.

Technique Checklist

	YES	NO
Procedure explained to client	_____	_____
Client indicated understanding of what was to occur	_____	_____
Face shaved	_____	_____
Cuts or nicks _____ (location)		
Astringent applied	_____	_____
Surgical skin preparation	_____	_____
Area _____		
Family understands how to shave client after dismissal	_____	_____
Explanation _____		
Demonstration _____		

85 Subclavian Catheterization, Assisting With

Overview

Definition

Introduction of a polyethylene or Teflon catheter into one of the large veins connecting to the superior vena cava

Rationale

Monitor central venous pressure (see Technique No. 40, Central Venous Pressure [CVP]).

Administer intravenous fluids when peripheral veins have proven inadequate.

Provide a route for prolonged intravenous therapy.

Provide a route for the insertion of a temporary pacemaker electrode.

Provide a safe route for the administration of hyperalimentation fluid.

Assessment

Pertinent Anatomy and Physiology

1. See Appendix I: *blood vessels*.
2. The subclavian vein is considered a vein of the upper arm because it is at the end of the venous system of the upper extremity. It extends to the sternal end of the clavicle, where it unites with the internal jugular vein, which leads into the superior vena cava (Fig. 85-1).

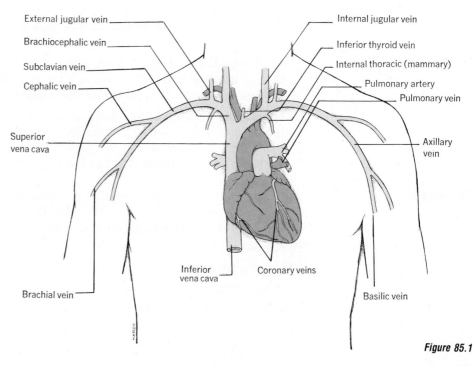

External jugular vein

Brachiocephalic vein

Subclavian vein

Cephalic vein

Superior vena cava

Internal jugular vein

Inferior thyroid vein

Internal thoracic (mammary)

Pulmonary artery

Pulmonary vein

Axillary vein

Brachial vein

Inferior vena cava

Coronary veins

Basilic vein

Figure 85.1

Pathophysiological Concepts

Valsalva maneuver occurs when the client inhales deeply and then bears down as if straining at stool. This results in an increase in intrathoracic pressure and impedes venous return to the heart. This maneuver also causes peripheral resistance and an immediate shift of blood volume from the heart and chest to the leg veins. A danger associated with this act is the mobilization of clots in the legs.

Assessment of the Client

1. Assess the familiarity of the client with the procedure and with basic anatomy regarding the heart and veins. Assess whether the client understands the need for the subclavian infusion. Determine if the client and family understand both the potential hazards and benefits of subclavian infusion.

2. Assess baseline vital signs of the client before the technique is performed to have an adequate comparison after insertion of the subclavian catheter. Assess the physical condition of the client. If the subclavian infusion is for the purpose of nutrition, measure the client's weight on a scale that can be used daily.

3. Assess the allergies of the client. Betadine, which contains iodine, often is used to cleanse the skin. A topical anesthetic, such as procain HCl (novocain) or Xylocaine may be used to anesthetize the area of needle insertion.

Plan

Nursing Objectives

Assist with the insertion of the subclavian catheter.

Ensure continued patency of the subclavian catheter.

Allay the anxieties of the client and family.

Secure the tubing to prevent complications such as premature removal.

Prevent infection by careful attention to dressing change and sterile technique.

Assist the client in proper breathing technique during catheter insertion and dressing changes to prevent air embolus.

Adequately hydrate or nourish the client.

Client Preparation

1. Offer a thorough explanation of the procedure to the client and family. Be sure that they understand why the procedure is necessary and the expected outcomes. Answer any questions they may have or refer them to the physician or practitioner.

2. Teach the client Valsalva's maneuver, which involves deep inspiration, then bearing down as when straining at stool. Explain that this will be used during insertion and when the tubing is changed.

3. Prepare the infusion setup before catheter insertion is accomplished. The tubing should be inserted into the infusion and primed. Take care that all air is removed from the tubing. An infusion pump or fluid regulator usually is connected to all tubings attached to subclavian intravenous catheters.

Equipment

Subclavian tray containing several large Intracaths, an antiseptic cleansing solution (such as povidone-iodine [Betadine]), tape, gauze pads, and a 5-ml or 10-ml syringe with a plain tip

Fluids (as prescribed)

Venous pressure setup (if prescribed)

Infusion pump or fluid controller

2-ml to 3-ml syringes, needles, and topical anesthetic (if requested)

Implementation and Interventions

Procedural Aspects

ACTION

RATIONALE

1. Cleanse the puncture site thoroughly with an antiseptic cleanser, such as povidone-iodine (Betadine), or alcohol for those clients allergic to iodine. The entire procedure is performed using sterile technique.

Pathogens found on the skin may be transferred by needle puncture directly into the client's vascular system.

2. The client should be in Trendelenburg position with a rolled towel or pillow under the shoulder to be punctured. Turn the client's head to the side opposite the needle insertion site (Fig. 85-2).

This position not only encourages filling and distension of the veins in the upper extremities, but it also provides for clear visualization of the field by the person inserting the catheter.

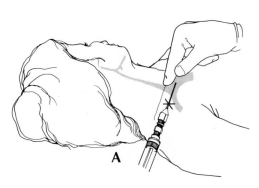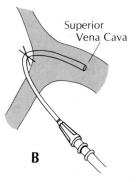

Figure 85.2

3. The physician or practitioner will puncture the vein, thread the catheter, and remove the stylet from the catheter. The tubing is then attached and the solution is allowed to infuse very slowly. The needle will be removed from the skin and a guard placed over it. This guard is taped to the skin.

Infusion of dangerous fluids (e.g., hyperalimentation), or of large quantities usually is postponed until radiologic confirmation of the location of the catheter. The guard prevents the needle from sticking the client during movement after insertion.

4. Ask the client to perform the Valsalva maneuver as the stylet is removed from the catheter and during the attachment of intravenous tubing.

The Valsalva maneuver increases peripheral resistance and decreases the chance of introducing air into the subclavian vein and the superior vena cava.

5. An antibiotic ointment usually is placed over the insertion site. A sterile 4 × 4 gauze pad may be placed over the site and taped securely in place.

The antibiotic ointment and sterile dressing help to prevent cross-contamination of the wound.

ACTION	*RATIONALE*
6. Change the dressings according to hospital and Centers for Disease Control standards. The usual frequency for dressing change is every 24 to 48 hours. Intravenous tubing, filter, and infusion pumps should be changed every 24 hours. Generally speaking, infusion bottles should be changed every 24 hours unless they contain dextrose, in which case they should be changed every 12 hours.	Because of the proximity of the puncture site to the heart, extreme caution must be exercised against contamination with pathogens. Dextrose solutions are particularly susceptible to the growth of pathogens.

Communicative Aspects

OBSERVATIONS

1. Observe for signs of air embolism, which include sharp pains in the chest and cyanosis. Observe for subcutaneous bleeding or pneumothorax. Observe the client for signs of sepsis, including high temperatures, malaise, and confusion.

2. Observe the subclavian infusion at least every hour, even if an infusion regulator is used. Overhydration is a distinct possibility owing to the large diameter of the vena cava and the proximity of the heart.

3. Observe the patency of the catheter and the integrity of the dressing. If the dressing becomes wet, the tubing may be leaking or the IV may be clogged. Observe the catheter for kinking when it is folded back for dressing.

4. Observe the site for signs of bleeding.

CHARTING

DATE/TIME	OBSERVATIONS	SIGNATURE
7/13 0800	R. subclavian catheterization with large intracath by Dr. L. Valsalva maneuver explained and demonstrated. Performed maneuver satisfactorily during removal of stylet and connection of IV tubing. Normal saline infusing at keep-open rate. To Radiology for confirmation of catheter placement. Sterile dressing in place with no evidence of bleeding. ————	G. Ivers RN

Discharge Planning Aspects

CLIENT AND FAMILY EDUCATION

1. Explain to the client and family about the need to keep the dressing area free of infective organisms. Tell them that sterile technique will be used to change the dressing, and that they should avoid touching the dressing or site.

2. Explain to the client that turning and movement are important to prevent pulmonary problems. However, the client must be careful not to dislodge the catheter accidentally. Explain any mobility limitations. Show the client how much tubing is available and assist in initial turning efforts so that the client will feel comfortable about the infusion.

3. Instruct the client about the Valsalva maneuver. Explain that this maneuver will be used during infusion tubing change. Tell the client that the nurse will say when to bear down and when to relax so that the maneuver will be effective and the client will not tire from needless straining.

Evaluation

Quality Assurance

Documentation should include instructions and explanations given to the client and family before the procedure, and an assessment of their understanding afterwards. The size of the catheter used should be noted. Documentation should note which subclavian vein was catheterized and any problems with insertion or infusion. If the catheter was radiologically assessed for placement, the report should be accessible before the administration of any fluids that require subclavian administration for safety. Documentation of tubing and dressings changes should appear in the chart. In addition, use of the Valsalva maneuver for safety during tubing changes should be noted. The chart should contain evidence that the nurse understood the dynamics behind subclavian infusion and possible side-effects, and any actions taken to prevent contamination or complications.

Infection Control

1. Maintenance of sterile technique is essential when inserting or handling a subclavian infusion. The heart is very near the insertion site, and contamination with pathogenic organisms could lead to severe complications. Bactericidal ointments often are placed over the site to discourage infection.

2. Thorough handwashing should precede any care given to the client with a subclavian infusion.

3. The dressing and tubing must be changed on a regular schedule. Dextrose solutions should not be left hanging for more than 12 hours owing to the chance of bacterial growth.

Technique Checklist

	YES	NO
Technique explained to client and family	_____	_____

Site _____

Type of infusion _____

| Radiologic confirmation of catheter placement | _____ | _____ |

Dressing changed q _____ hr

Tubing changed q _____ hr

Vital signs monitored q _____ hr

Complications _____

_____

Duration of subclavian catheter therapy _____

86   Suction, Oral and Nasal

Overview

Definition

Aspiration of secretions by a rubber or polyethylene catheter (14 F–18 F) connected to a suction source

Rationale

Maintain a patent airway through the mouth or nose to the trachea.

Obtain secretions for diagnostic purposes.

Terminology

Asphyxiation: A decrease in the amount of oxygen and an increase in the amount of carbon dioxide because of interference with respiration

Hypoxia: Varying degrees of lack of oxygen

Patent: Open; unobstructed

Polyp: A small tumor commonly found on mucous membranes

Assessment

Pertinent Anatomy and Physiology

1. See Appendix I: *bronchial tree, trachea.*
2. The nose consists of the external portion that protrudes from the face and the internal portion that projects into the skull over the top of the mouth backward opening into the throat. A narrow vertical partition, the nasal septum, separates the nose into two cavities. The surface of the nasal mucosa is lined with mucus. Small, hairy projections called cilia also line the nasal tract. These cells push dust and particles backward to the throat for elimination by the gastrointestinal (GI) system. The nose warms and cools inspired air, accumulates moisture, and cleans the air before it gets to the lungs. The nose is also the organ of smell.
3. Immobility often leads to complications that may be preventable by diligent nursing interventions. When the client lies in the supine position for extended periods, secretions tend to pool in the lungs, bronchial tree, and trachea. If these secretions are not removed, they may cause asphyxiation. Normally these secretions are removed by coughing or swallowing.

Pathophysiological Concepts

1. The nasal cavities are formed by the nasal septum. In some persons, the septum is markedly displaced to one side or the other. This condition, called *deviated septum,* can cause problems in suctioning. Other conditions that may cause problems in the nose are the presence of polyps, or hypertension, which may cause frequent nosebleeds.
2. Pneumonia is an inflammation of the lungs. Pathogens flourish in a moist, warm environment. Allowing secretions to pool in the throat and lungs can predispose the client to pneumonia.

Assessment of the Client

1. Assess the ability of the client to remove secretions by coughing and swallowing. Determine how mobile the client is, ability to turn and move in bed, and ability to remove the secretions from the mouth. In addition, determine the client's awareness of the importance of removing secretions.

2. Assess the ability of the client to understand the suctioning technique. Assess previous experience with suctioning and the amount of fear or anxiety being experienced by the client.

3. Assess the respiratory sufficiency of the client, the rate and quality of respiration, and any difficulty the client may be having with breathing. Note the color of the client's skin and any signs of cyanosis.

Plan

Nursing Objectives

Maintain a patent airway to facilitate the exchange of gases.

Obtain secretions for diagnostic purposes.

Stimulate coughing and deep breathing.

Client Preparation

1. Tell the client what will occur, even if the client is semiconscious and does not appear to understand what is happening. Explain to the client and family that the purpose of the procedure is to stimulate coughing and keep the airway from becoming obstructed.

2. Position the client to facilitate drainage of secretions from the pharynx and to prevent aspiration (e.g., head elevated and turned to one side). Place a towel across the client to protect the bed linens.

3. Prepare the suction equipment. The amount of suction will depend on the age of the client and the thickness of secretions. The usual amount of suction is 110 to 150 mm Hg for adults, 90 to 100 mm Hg for children, and 50 to 90 mm Hg for infants. Open the end of the catheter package, but do not remove or contaminate the catheter at this time.

Equipment

Suction source (wall mount or portable)

Tubing and Y-connector or suction air vent

Sterile rubber or polyethylene suction catheter (14 F to 18 F)

Sterile water and sterile basin

Plastic bag (to hold contaminated catheters)

Sterile gloves

Sterile pad and clean towel

Implementation and Interventions

Procedural Aspects

ACTION	RATIONALE
1. Wash hands thoroughly before beginning. Open the sterile suction catheter package. Don one sterile glove. Grasp the end of the catheter with the sterile hand and the suction tubing with the other hand. Attach the catheter to suction. Remove the catheter from the package without contaminating it (Fig. 86-1).	Prevent the spread of microorganisms by mechanical and barrier methods. The oral and nasal passages are not sterile; however, it is recommended that suctioning be considered a sterile procedure.

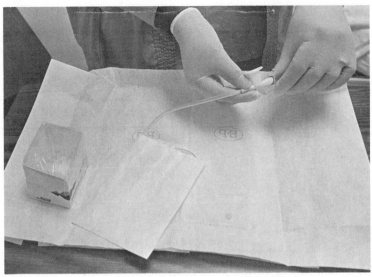

Figure 86.1

ACTION

2. Dip the catheter tip in the sterile water or saline which has been poured into the sterile container (Fig. 86-2).

RATIONALE

Moistening the catheter reduces friction and eases insertion.

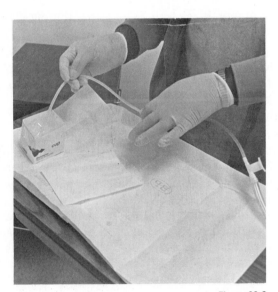

Figure 86.2

3. Insert the catheter through the mouth or a nostril. Never force the catheter nor apply suction during insertion.

Insertion into the mouth may stimulate the gag or cough reflex and aid the client in bringing up the secretions. Forcing the catheter or using suction as the tube is inserted may cause trauma to the delicate mucous membranes that line the nasal and oral tract.

ACTION

RATIONALE

4. Withdraw the catheter with a gentle rotating motion while suction is obtained by placing one finger over the Y-connector or suction air vent. (Fig. 86-3). Do not suction for more than 15 seconds at a time. Suction for 3 to 5 seconds, allow the client to breathe, then continue suctioning for another 3 to 5 seconds, for no more than 15 seconds.

A partial vacuum is created by continuous suction. Rotating the catheter and intermittent suction prevents tissue trauma from occurring when the mucosa is drawn into the catheter during prolonged suction in one area.

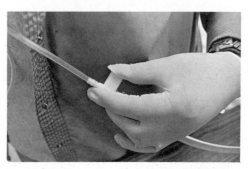

Figure 86.3

5. Apply suction for no more than 15 seconds at one time.

The airway is obstructed during suctioning and hypoxia is intensified.

6. Remove the catheter and wipe the end with the sterile pad. Flush the tube by aspirating some of the sterile water through it; repeat the suctioning maneuver until the passageway is cleared of secretions.

Thick secretions tend to clog the catheter. Periodic flushing will help to keep the tube patent and will add to the success of the suctioning procedure.

7. Discard used disposable catheters in a lined waste container. If the catheters are reusable, place them in a plastic bag, tape the top shut and label with name of contents and date. Place specimens in a sterile specimen container for transport to the laboratory. Label with client's name and the area from which the secretions came. Gently clean the client's nose and mouth area. Administer oral care. Leave the client in a clean and comfortable environment.

Pathogens are transmissible on contaminated equipment. Proper labeling and disposal can prevent contaminating co-workers and other clients and also prevents errors in reporting results. Secretions may adhere to the face and cause discomfort. Removal is usually possible with a warm washcloth.

8. Use extreme caution in suctioning clients who have had nasopharyngeal surgery. The pharyngeal cavity should not be suctioned in postoperative tonsillectomy clients because this may dislodge the clots and cause hemorrhage.

Clotting is the mechanism by which abnormal and dangerous blood loss is prevented. If the clot is dislodged, bleeding may occur until a new clot is formed. This is extremely dangerous for the client who has had surgery on the nose and throat area.

ACTION	RATIONALE
Special Modifications	
For suctioning children, use a suction catheter size 8 F to 18 F depending on the size of the child and the thickness of the secretions. Children are often oxygenated before the suctioning procedure. This hyperinsufflation technique involves administering five rapid breaths through a bag and mask (or a ventilator) with a high oxygen concentration (100%). Suctioning then is completed.	The small child's nose cannot accommodate a large catheter without trauma to the nasal mucosa. Hyperinsufflation enriches the oxygen content of the child's blood for the short period during which oxygen deprivation will occur as the child is suctioned.

Communicative Aspects

OBSERVATIONS

1. Note the amount of secretion and the consistency, color, and odor. Observe how much sterile water was used for flushing the tubing so that an accurate measure of the secretion that was suctioned can be obtained.
2. Observe the reaction of the client to the procedure. Note signs of apnea, hypoxia, or pain in the chest area.

CHARTING

DATE/TIME	OBSERVATIONS	SIGNATURE
9/28 1210	Bilateral nasal suctioning done. Positioned on left side with head elevated about 30°. 30 ml of thick purulent yellowish secretions obtained. States she felt like she was choking during procedure. States she can breathe much easier now. Turned to right side with pillow to back. R 18, P 82. Resting. —	F. White RN

Discharge Planning Aspects

CLIENT AND FAMILY EDUCATION

1. Instruct the client to expectorate secretions into a tissue when possible.
2. Explain to the client and family that the purpose of using sterile catheters and gloves is to prevent cross-contamination. Explain the role of good handwashing in that respect as well.
3. Instruct the client and family to call for assistance if the client experiences any respiratory difficulty. Instruct in using the call light.

Evaluation

Quality Assurance

Documentation should include a description of the secretions returned from the suctioning procedure. The procedure itself should be described, as well as the amount of time suction was applied, the number of times the client was suctioned on each shift, and any untoward effects of the suctioning. The client's reaction to the procedure and the understanding and acceptance of the family to the suctioning procedure should be addressed. Knowledge of possible complications and measures taken to prevent them should be reflected. Continual intermittent monitoring of vital signs should be noted, with explanations of any gross fluctuations.

Infection Control

The respiratory tract is susceptible to infection by pathogens in the hospital environment. Bronchopneumonia frequently is acquired in hospitals by susceptible persons, that is, those whose immunity response is compromised. Precautions, such as handwashing and cleaning and disinfection of equipment used consecutively for clients, are essential.

Technique Checklist

	YES	NO
Procedure explained to client and family with emphasis on desired results	_____	_____
Suctioning done		
Nasal _____		
Oral _____		
Frequency _____		
Results of suctioning noted on chart, including amount and appearance	_____	_____
Complications _____		
Desired results obtained	_____	_____

Overview

Definition

The process of removing material used to secure wound edges or body parts together

Rationale

Discontinue support that is no longer needed after surgical healing.

Remove substances that may act as foreign bodies in the tissue.

Promote continuation of the healing process.

Terminology

Continuous: Sutures formed by one continuous thread, alternating one lip of the wound to the other

Dehiscence: The spontaneous release of the sutures or suture line after healing has begun

Evisceration: The spontaneous protrusion of viscera through a surgical incision

Interrupted: Sutures formed by single stitches, inserted separately

Staples: Metal fasteners that penetrate the skin vertically to hold the incision closed

Assessment

Pertinent Anatomy and Physiology

1. See Appendix I: *skin.*
2. Wound healing can be of two types. Regeneration is the replacement of tissue with cells similar to those destroyed. When regeneration is not possible, as with some types of tissue, fibrous tissue formation occurs, with a scar as the result.
3. Wound healing occurs by *first* intention when the edges of the wound are brought together (as by sutures), and there is minimal tissue loss. Wound healing by *second* intention occurs when there is much tissue loss, and granular tissue must be generated to fill the gap. Wounds that are sutured enhance the healing process and prevent infection. Epithelialization of the wound, with the edges brought closely together by sutures, begins within 1 to 2 days.
4. The usual sequence of healing of a postoperative wound is inflammation with some redness, serous drainage, and the appearance of granulation tissue, which usually has covered the wound by the 7th to the 10th day.

Pathophysiological Concepts

1. The usual response of the body to any laceration is inflammation. Immediate vascular changes occur owing to the increased flow of blood to the area. The increased blood flow enables the body to bring leukocytes to the area to prevent infection. Exudate formation follows. The type of exudate depends on the type of wound, the location, and the degree of inflammatory response. The types of exudate are:

   Serous: A watery fluid comprised chiefly of serum from the blood and serous membranes (*e.g.,* a blister)

Purulent: A thicker, pus-filled drainage of various colors depending on the causative organism (e.g., an abscess)

Fibrinous: A clear, thick, sticky exudate that may cause objects to adhere to the wound (e.g., some burns)

Sanguineous: A red drainage that may be characterized as fresh bleeding when the color is bright red and as the release of previously lost blood when the color is dark (e.g., surgical wound drainage)

2. Factors that influence wound healing are age (healing takes longer in the elderly), nutrition (adequate nutrition is essential for proper wound healing), infection (infections slow the healing process and often cause an incision to heal by second intention), hormones (steriods are known to delay healing), circulatory efficiency (if the blood supply is compromised, the healing process is slowed), and the presence of foreign bodies (this includes sutures and staples, which can slow the healing process if left in too long).

3. Complications of poor incisional healing may be dehiscence and evisceration.

Assessment of the Client

1. Assess the progress of the healing process. Assess the presence of a foul odor or unusual discharge, either of which may indicate infection.

2. Assess the anxiety level of the client. If the client is very anxious, sensitivity may be heightened and the procedure may be more uncomfortable.

3. Assess the physical condition of the client. If the client is in a high-risk group (elderly, poorly nourished, or infected), assess the integrity of the suture line before removing the sutures. If there is any question about the ability of the incision to remain intact, contact the physician before removing the sutures. Alternate sutures may be removed. Then, after several days, the remaining sutures are removed. This gives a chance to assess the integrity of the suture line.

Plan

Nursing Objectives

Allay the client's fear and anxiety regarding wound rupture and pain as a result of the suture or staple removal.

Provide physical comfort.

Maintain asepsis.

Observe and promote the healing process.

Client Preparation

1. Explain to the client what will happen during suture removal. Emphasize that the wound has healed sufficiently so it no longer requires the support of sutures. Tell the client that some tickling and discomfort may occur, but the pain should be minimal. Inform the client that after the sutures are removed, some loss of incisional support may be felt, but this does not indicate weakness of the incision.

2. Place the client in a position of comfort without undue tension on the suture line. Suture removal may be accompanied by some nausea or dizziness; therefore, ask the client to recline during removal. Provide adequate lighting to see the sutures with ease.

Equipment Sterile suture removal set, including scissors, forceps, and hemostats, or a skin staple remover

Skin antiseptic (benzalkonium chloride [Zephiran] or alcohol)

Sterile cotton balls or gauze pads

Sterile gloves

Sterile dressings (if indicated)

Sterile strips of tape for adding support to the incision

Tape

Plastic bag

Implementation and Interventions

Procedural Aspects

ACTION

1. Determine the hospital policy concerning personnel who are allowed to remove sutures. Suture removal is a delegated medical function. A physician's order is required before sutures are removed.

2. Remove the dressing and cleanse the incision (see Technique No. 49, Dressings, Surgical). Cleanse from the center of the incision outward for an area of 5 cm (2 in). Use sterile forceps and a new cotton ball saturated with antiseptic for each stroke.

3. Grasp the knot of the first suture with a sterile hemostat or forceps and elevate it so that the portion below the knot is clearly visible.

4. Using sterile scissors, cut one side of the suture *below the knot*, close to the skin (Fig. 87-1). Avoid cutting the knot. Succeeding interrupted sutures are removed by repeating the cutting process for each suture. Succeeding continuous sutures are removed in the same manner, except that each portion to be cut is grasped by the suture itself since there is no knot for each stitch.

RATIONALE

Some hospitals allow only physicians or nurse specialists to remove sutures.

Remove as many pathogenic organisms as possible before suture removal.

Direct visualization aids in proper suture removal technique for thread sutures.

Cutting the suture near the skin prevents drawing the exposed contaminated portion of the suture through the tissues.

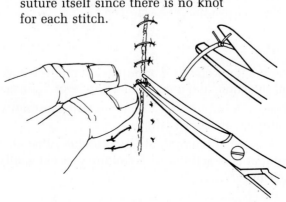

Figure 87.1

ACTION	*RATIONALE*
5. Remove each suture in a smooth, continuous motion. Remove every other suture from one end of the incision to the other. Check to see that tension on the wound does not cause dehiscence. If the integrity of the wound is satisfactory, remove the remaining sutures. Remove skin staples in one motion by placing the staple remover between the staple and the skin and gentle pulling the staple from the skin (Fig. 87-2). Remove every other staple to check for the integrity of the incision. If dehiscence begins, leave the remaining sutures intact and notify the physician.	A smooth, continuous motion decreases discomfort. If the wound begins to separate after removal of part of the supporting sutures, it will be more likely to separate with the removal of all of the sutures because tension on the suture line will be increased.

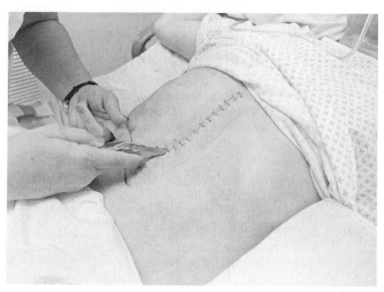

Figure 87.2

ACTION	*RATIONALE*
6. Cleanse the incision again with a disinfectant if drainage from the suture removal has occurred. Apply a sterile dressing if the physician orders it. Some physicians prefer to leave the incision open.	A small dressing may serve to minimize discomfort from clothing and bed linens rubbing over the incision.

Communicative Aspects

OBSERVATIONS

1. Observe the wound for approximation of the edges, signs of inflammation and infection, and amount and nature of drainage.

2. Observe the sutures for tissue reaction, continuity of suture line, and the possibility of embedded stitches.

3. During suture removal, observe carefully that all of the sutures are removed and that no small piece of a suture is accidentally cut and left in the incision.

CHARTING	DATE/TIME	OBSERVATIONS	SIGNATURE
	8/9 1330	Sutures removed by order of Dr. S. Abdominal incision cleaned, wound edges in close approximation. No drainage or redness. Tolerated well with no discomfort stated. Twelve sutures removed without difficulty. Sterile dressing applied as ordered. ———————————————	G. Ivers RN

Discharge Planning Aspects

CLIENT AND FAMILY EDUCATION

1. Instruct the client not to touch the wound until the healing is complete. Recommend cleansing and wound care after discharge according to the physician's wishes. Showering usually is advised.

2. Instruct the client and family to report any unusual changes in the incision. Explain that the incision should become less red and that only the scar line should remain in a few weeks.

3. Reinforce the physician's instructions regarding avoiding strain on the incision, restrictions on activities, and return visit to the physician's office or clinic.

Evaluation

Quality Assurance

Documentation should include the order from the physician regarding removal of the sutures. The reaction of the client to the procedure, the appearance of the suture line, and any problems should be reflected. The number of sutures or staples should be noted. Any drainage or signs of inflammation should be reflected in the client record. Discharge instructions regarding care of the incision should be on the chart.

Infection Control

1. The sutures project into the tissue of the client. This area is sterile and must be guarded from contamination. If the portion of the suture that has been on the outside of the body (and therefore considered contaminated) is pulled through the tissue, the tissue may be contaminated. Cut the sutures close to the skin on one side and pull them straight.

2. Suture removal is a sterile procedure. Thorough handwashing must be carried out. Sterile gloves and sterile equipment will help reduce the chance of introducing pathogenic organisms into the incision. Cleansing the wound with an antiseptic solution should precede suture removal.

3. Discard the dressings and the sutures or staples in a water-resistant bag so that drainage will not leak through and contaminate personnel.

Technique Checklist

	YES	NO
Procedure explained to client	_____	_____
Type of incisional closure		
Number of sutures _____		
Number of staples _____		
Removed with no problems	_____	_____
Appearance of wound noted on chart	_____	_____
Physician's instructions reinforced	_____	_____
Wound closed without complications	_____	_____

88   Teaching the Client and Family

Overview

Definition

A system of actions intended to produce learning by the client and family, any interpersonal influence aimed at changing the ways in which the client and family can and will behave

Rationale

Promote knowledge of health maintenance and prevention of disease.

Involve the client and family in nursing care during hospitalization.

Expand the client's information and knowledge about the condition necessitating hospitalization.

Assist the client and family in adjusting to stress during this time of illness or injury.

Prepare the client and family for discharge from the hospital.

Terminology

Learning: The discovery of meaning through the acquisition of new experiences and information

Learner objectives: Goals that identify the degree of competency that the client or family demonstrates by changes in behavior as a result of the teaching

Teaching: Activities by which the nurse helps the client and family to learn

Teaching plan: A plan developed by the nurse, with the assistance of the client and family, for use in implementing the basic concepts of teaching

Assessment

Assessment of the Client and Family

1. Assess the education level of the client and family. Assess their experiences, type of work environment, and familiarity with hospitals and health care.

2. Assess the degree of anxiety and stress being experienced by the client and family at this time in their lives. Anxiety can inhibit learning.

3. Assess the current knowledge levels of the client and family. Determine how much they know and how much they want to know in determining the best strategies to meet knowledge needs.

Planning Client and Family Teaching

Nursing Objectives

Assess the extent to which teaching should be incorporated in the provision of care to the client.

Incorporate the principles of the teaching–learning process in the teaching situation.

Identify the elements involved in assessing the client's and family's readiness for learning.

Develop a well-organized plan for client and family teaching based on individual needs.

Use appropriate teaching techniques or strategies.

Implement a teaching plan that is individualized, effective, and considerate of the client's needs and desires.

Evaluate the effects or results of the implementation of the teaching plan.

BASIC ASSUMPTIONS OF THE TEACHING–LEARNING PROCESS

The Client and Family As Learners

1. Knowledge is meaning, and because the person is an integrated whole, to be meaningful, knowledge must be viewed as integrated.

2. The process of learning is the process of becoming, through perceiving and behaving, based on one's field of perception.

3. Meaningful learning is more likely when clients and families select or help to select goals of real need or interest, or even more likely when they relate these goals to individual purposes.

4. When clients and families choose goals, they are more likely to assume the responsibility for the fulfillment of these goals.

5. Clients and families learn best when they are challenged within the range of their abilities and interests.

6. As more individual needs and purposes become the focus of learning, the greater is the depth of client and family involvement and commitment.

7. The most desirable form of learner discipline is self-discipline.

8. Freedom of choice in learning must be accompanied by the realization of responsibility for the behavior that ensues.

9. Learning experiences become most desirable and meaningful when they enable clients and families to fulfill present needs, interests, and goals. Learning experiences are not something apart from the learner but are an integral part of daily life.

10. The rate, depth, and intensity of learning vary according to individual abilities, drives, purposes, attitudes, and values, in relation to felt needs and that which is to be learned.

11. People respond better to learning experiences when there is a relevant relationship between the learning experiences and problems of daily life.

12. With dianostic help and a clear understanding of purposes, individual learners will select and organize learning experiences relevant to objectives.

13. The discovery of new knowledge and new meanings is more likely to occur when learners have the opportunity to identify and explore problems that interest them and for which no obvious solution is foreseeable at the time.

14. Transfer of knowledge into behavior occurs when clients and families are given the opportunity to act on that which they value; that is, knowledge that is meaningful to the client and family will transfer to behavior automatically.

15. The process of transferring knowledge and meaning into behavior is best achieved when clients and families have opportunities to related knowledge and meaning to unique situations, to unknown problems, and to areas of living.

16. Each person has an individual learning style, preferences for study, a specific rate of learning, and an individual degree of involvement in the learning process.

17. The physical condition of the client often affects learning capability. Decreased oxygen consumption and absorption interfere with the brain's ability to process and store information.

The Nurse As a Teacher

1. The nurse has access to many teaching techniques: art of questioning, lecture, small-group discussion, one-to-one relationships, and others.

2. The client and family, with the nurse, analyze learning errors, diagnose learner problems, and then seek methods to meet needs.

3. The nurse must know the client and family—their strengths, areas for improvement, needs, and goals.

4. Learning experiences should be planned by the client, family, and nurse together to provide satisfying experiences.

5. Planned learning experiences should promise a certain degree of achievement to the nurse, the client and the family.

6. When teaching techinques are varied and are directed toward the total development of the client and family, personal responsibility for effective learning is more likely to be realized.

7. People learn best through concrete, relevant, and predominantly first-hand experiences that elicit critical thinking, discovery, and total involvement.

8. The more intense the motivation of the client, family, and nurse, the greater is the possibility for the client's involvement, commitment, and responsibility for choice.

9. The nurse is responsible for applying knowledge about learners and learning to establish the best possible learning environment for the client and family.

Principles on Which Teaching Is Based

1. The teaching–learning process is a cooperative effort in which trust plays an important part.

2. Teaching what the learner already knows wastes time and lowers the learner's self-esteem.

3. A favorable environment facilitates learning.

   Anxiety reactions, such as denial, fear, or frustration, reduce the motivation to learn.

   Physical discomfort or a distracting environment impairs the learner's perceptions.

   An important criterion of readiness for learning is acceptance of the client's condition by the family and the client.

4. Reinforcement and repetition are necessary steps in learning.

5. Innovative ways of accomplishing goals must vary according to the needs of the learner.

   The process of trial and error is a way of learning.

   People interact differently, depending on age, culture, custom, education, environment, and language.

6. Starting at the client and family's level provides for continuity of learning and promotes teacher–learner dialogue, rather than merely a teacher's monologue.

7. Effective learning requires active participation.

8. Conceptualization, or the ability to form a mental image or idea of a situation, occurs in the learner's mind. It involves perception, ideas, emotions, facts, and symbols.

9. Accomplishment reinforces learning, and near-accomplishment motivates the learner.

Client Preparation

1. After the need for client and family teaching has been identified, evaluate their ability and readiness to learn. Prepare them for teaching by cooperatively establishing satisfactory learning objectives.

2. After careful study, decide in conjunction with the client and family the most appropriate teaching method for the particular learning–teaching situation.

Equipment   Depending on the information to be taught, teaching materials such as treatment equipment, teaching plan charts, brochures, and audiovisual aids may be brought into the teaching–learning situation.

Implementation and Interventions

Steps in Teaching
1. Demonstrate an interest in the needs of the client as an individual and in those of the family as a group.
2. Establish the extent of the client's and family's needs for learning, using observation, physician's requests, and direct communications with the client and family.
3. Plan the content, time span, and sequence (from simple to complex) of the learning experience.
4. Evaluate the client's and family's readiness for learning.
5. Enlist the aid of supporting or reinforcing persons in whom the client has faith and confidence.
6. Have well-defined objectives and a clear outline for the sessions, but avoid a stereotyped approach to individuals and groups.
7. Begin teaching at the client's and family's level, using terminology understandable to all and explaining those with which they are not familiar.
8. Teach concepts rather than procedures, and encourage the learners to express these concepts in their own ways.
9. Provide learning experiences in such a way that the client and family can have satisfying or nearly satisfying accomplishments.

Summary of Teaching Process
Assessment of need to learn

Assessment of readiness

Setting objectives

Teaching–learning situation

Evaluation of effectiveness

Evaluation

Quality Assurance   Each hospital should have a written plan for client education. This plan should be adaptable to the individual needs of each client and family. The methods used and information given to the client and family, as well as questions asked and interest shown, should be reflected in the chart. Behavior changes emanating from teaching should be noted.

Principles of Evaluating the Effectiveness of Techniques
1. Any evaluation of behavioral change or client and family progress is based on an on-going diagnosis of needs and ability to make choices.
2. Self-selected goals are the meaningful standards of behavioral change or progress.
3. Self-analyses by the client and family are the most valid forms of evaluation and the first prerequisites for behavior change. Evaluation is continuous; behavior is reinforced or modified, or new behavior is developed.
4. Nurse behavior is stimulated by a variety of inputs and is interdependent on the outcomes of instruction.
5. The nurse must determine how well the family and client are progressing in the process of learning.
6. The nurse, the client, and the family must have a joint understanding of what the achievement criteria are and must be able to secure evidence of progress toward those criteria.

89 Tracheostomy Care

Overview

Definition

Aspiration of secretions from an artificial opening in the neck by using a sterile catheter connected to a suction source; also cleansing of the inner cannula of the tracheostomy tube, the incisional area, and the anterior portion of the neck

Rationale

Facilitate adequate exchange of gases for maximal respiratory results.

Limit the introduction of pathogens into the tracheobronchial tree.

Terminology

Cannula: A tube for insertion or removal of secretions from the body

Hypoxia: Varying degrees of inadequacy of oxygen supply

Patent: Open, unobstructed

Tracheostomy: The surgical creation of a vertical slit in the anterior portion of the neck (usually below the first or second tracheal cartilage) and the introduction of a single- or double-lumen cannula airway to facilitate adequate exchange of gases (Fig. 89-1). The outer cannula is held in place by ties around the neck; the inner cannula is locked into the outer cannula.

Tracheostomy cuff: A rubber, balloon-type appliance located around the lower two thirds of the outer cannula of the tracheostomy tube. After inserting the obturator in place, the cuff can be inflated to prevent accidental removal, or air leaks, if positive-pressure respiratory devices are used.

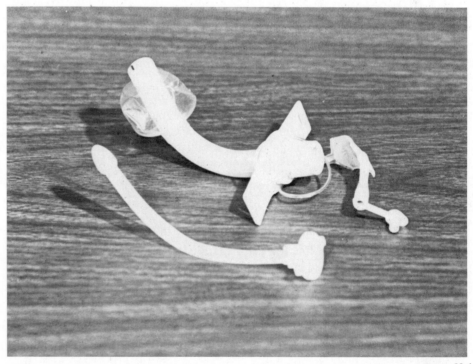

Figure 89.1

659

Assessment

Pertinent Anatomy and Physiology

1. See Appendix I: *lungs, trachea.*

2. The larynx, or voice box, serves as a passageway for air between the pharynx and the trachea. It lies in the midline of the neck. The larynx is a triangular box composed of nine cartilages that are joined together by ligaments and controlled by skeletal muscles. Three of the cartilages are paired. The remaining three are the cricoid, thyroid, and epiglottis. The epiglottis forms the fold that closes the larynx during the act of swallowing to prevent aspiration of food into the respiratory system. The thyroid cartilage is the largest. It is composed of two broad plates that meet and fuse in the midline of the throat. The ventral edges of these plates form the Adam's apple. The cricoid cartilage lies at the lower end of the larynx and is connected to the first cartilaginous ring of the trachea. The vocal cords and vocal ligaments are found in the upper anterior portion of the larynx. These are important to the production of sound.

Pathophysiological Concepts

Tracheostomy is a surgical procedure whereby an opening is made in the trachea to provide a free passageway for air. The incision is usually made into the tracheal cartilage below the level of the thyroid and cricoid cartilages. The thyroid gland lies in this area. Care must be taken not to injure the thyroid gland or the vocal cords. Clients with tracheostomy tubes are particularly susceptible to pulmonary infections because the air is not conditioned before it reaches the lungs.

Assessment of the Client

1. Assess the consciousness level of the client. Explain what will occur whether the client appears awake or not. If the client is alert, however, the suctioning process can be very frightening owing to the momentary inability to breathe. Explain during the procedure what is happening and coach the client about how to cooperate. Determine before beginning how much cooperation reasonably can be expected.

2. Assess the condition of the skin around the tracheostomy. Assess the patency of the tracheostomy tube, the amount of exudate, and the ability of the client to aerate the lungs successfully through the tube. Assess the sound of the client's breathing by means of auscultation and determine when to suction. Assess the need for cleaning the tracheostomy tube and changing the dressing.

3. Assess the understanding of the client and family of why the tracheostomy had to be performed, what the goals of the treatment are, and how long the tube will be necessary. Assess their acceptance of this alteration to body image and their concerns about current treatment. Determine educational deficits when deciding what and how to teach the client and family.

Plan

Nursing Objectives

Maintain a patent airway to facilitate the therapeutic exchange of gases.

Allay the fears and anxieties of the client and family concerning the altered breathing route and loss of speaking ability.

Prevent the transmission of pathogenic microorganisms.

Prevent encrustation around the tracheostomy area.

Provide adequate humidity.

Provide adequate aeration of the lungs and oxygenation of the blood.

Provide physical and emotional comfort for the client.

Client Preparation

1. Diversion of the respiratory flow by means of a tracheostomy also directly alters the client's ability to speak. Inability to speak or cry out adds to the emotional stress of the client. Obstruction of the airway may cause a client to panic. Observe the client closely at all times. Explain the suctioning procedure and any other care to enhance understanding and cooperation. Offer the explanations regardless of the apparent level of consciousness. The family, too, may exhibit increased anxiety over the inability of the client to communicate. Reassurance and clear explanations will help to allay this anxiety. Provide communication devices, such as writing materials or computerized communication tools, if the client is able to use such instruments.

2. Because of gravitational flow, secretions may collect in the tracheobronchial tree. Place the client in the side-lying position to facilitate drainage and aspiration of these secretions.

Equipment

Suction capability

Suction catheter, 10 F to 14 F and tubing

Sterile container with sterile water

Sterile gloves

Hydrogen peroxide

Cleaners (pipe cleaners or a soft brush)

Sterile dressings

Sterile scissors

Ties

Cool or warm mist apparatus (as prescribed by physician)

Implementation and Interventions

Procedural Aspects

ACTION

1. Wash hands carefully before and after tracheostomy care. Open the catheter package. Don sterile gloves and remove the catheter from the package.

2. Moisten the catheter tip in the basin of sterile water.

3. Insert the catheter through the tracheostomy tube with the suction off. Direct the catheter into the right or the left bronchus by positioning the client's head to the opposite side.

4. When the tube is inserted to the desired depth, cover the air escape valve on the tubing to create suction through the catheter. Withdraw the catheter slowly in a rotating motion (Fig. 89-2).

RATIONALE

Pathogenic organisms can grow and flourish in a warm, moist environment and are transmitted by direct contact.

Water will reduce the friction as the tube is inserted into the trachea.

The catheter will be guided by the anatomical structure of the bronchi. The suction is off during insertion to decrease trauma to the mucosal lining of the tracheobronchial tree.

Changes in pressure inside a tube will cause secretions to move from areas of greater pressure to areas of lower pressure. Rotating the catheter prevents excessive vacuum on one area, which may result in tissue damage.

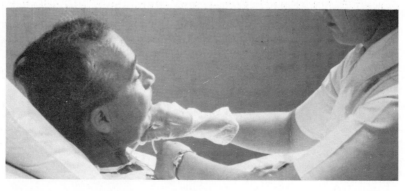

Figure 89.2

ACTION	*RATIONALE*
5. Do not suction continuously for more than 15 seconds. Stop and allow the client to breathe. Allow 3-minute rest periods between insertions of the suction catheter, if the safety of the client will not be compromised.	The client's airway is obstructed during suctioning, and hypoxia is intensified if the suction is maintained too long.
6. A tracheostomy cuff may be used to hold the tube in place. The soft balloon is inflated with air, which anchors it in place. The cuff must be deflated at regular intervals, such as once each shift, to prevent damage to the trachea. Low-pressure cuffs are available.	Continuous inflation of the cuff causes pressure on the walls of the trachea which may cause circulatory impairment and resulting tissue damage.
7. Position the client to facilitate adequate ventilation. Change the suction apparatus discarding the used catheter in a trash or waxed paper bag. Leave the suction equipment ready for immediate use in case emergency suctioning is necessary. Change or clean all equipment every 24 hours. If the equipment will be resterilized, place it in a waxed bag and label clearly with contents, date, and any special precautions to be taken. Tape the top shut and transport the bag to the cleaning area according to hospital protocol.	The client should be left feeling comfortable and secure. Changing the tubing frequently reduces the chance of microorganism growth and spread.
8. If a mist collar is ordered, ensure that it is positioned properly over the tracheostomy opening. Check frequently to prevent pooling of moisture in the collar itself. Keep the doors and windows closed in high-humidity environments.	Moist air keeps the delicate membranes of the respiratory tract from drying out and may help keep secretions from becoming thick and viscous.
9. Unless contraindicated, remove the inner cannula every 8 hours for cleaning. Wash the inner cannula with hydrogen peroxide on both the inside and outside using pipe cleaners or small, soft brushes to remove the secretions. Rinse thoroughly with sterile saline. Replace the obturator into the inner cannula and gently reinsert back into the outer cannula. Turn inner cannula to lock in place (Fig. 89-3).	The inner cannula becomes encrusted with mucus-containing proteins that may interfere with patency if allowed to accumulate. This exudate also provides a medium for the growth of bacteria. 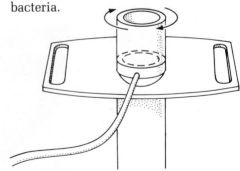

Figure 89.3

ACTION

10. Keep the area around the tracheostomy clean and dry. Wash and rinse the neck area and dry it thoroughly with a soft towel. Cleanse the area around the outer cannula with hydrogen peroxide to remove encrustations. Apply a bactericidal ointment and a sterile dressing to the skin around the outer cannula. With sterile scissors, cut a sterile 4 × 4 pad halfway to the center and place around the tube (Figs. 89-4, 89-5). If the material for the dressing will ravel, the pad may be unfolded into a rectangle (Fig. 89-6) and refolded so no loose edges are present to contaminate the tracheostomy opening (Figs. 89-7, 89-8). Tie the tracheostomy tube in place around the neck with the ties secure and comfortable.

RATIONALE

Keeping the area around the tracheostomy clean and dry will discourage pathogen growth and facilitate comfort. The sterile dressing will reduce skin irritation and absorb secretions. Ties are used to anchor the tube in place and to prevent accidental removal.

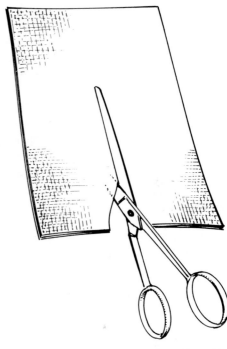

Figure 89.4

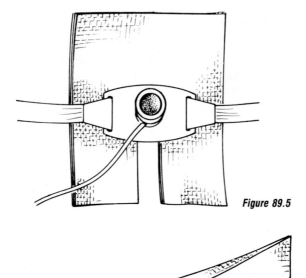

Figure 89.5

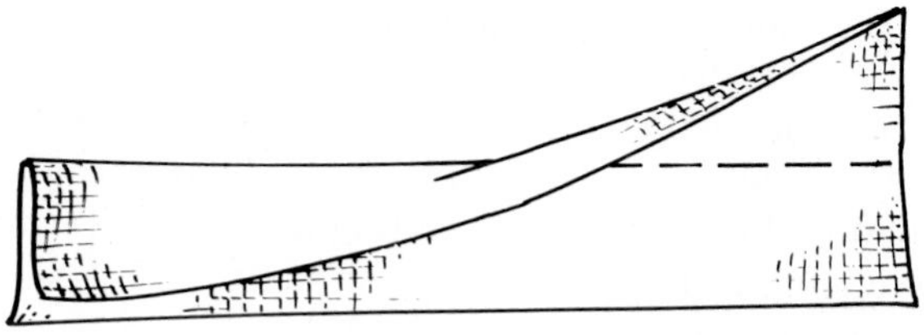

Figure 89.6

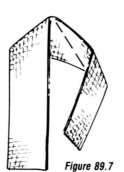

Figure 89.7

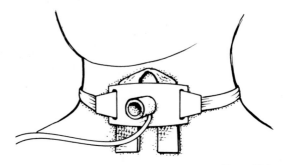

Figure 89.8

ACTION	*RATIONALE*

Special Modifications

Spontaneous extubation of the tracheostomy tube requires immediate attention. The outer cannula should be replaced under sterile conditions by a physician. Sterile forceps or any sterile dilating instrument may be used to hold open the tracheal opening to prevent suffocation until a new cannula can be inserted.

Accidental dislodgment of the tracheostomy tube may occur as a result of forceful coughing, confusion, or excessive movement.

Communicative Aspects

OBSERVATIONS

1. Observe the area around the tracheostomy site for edema and redness, which might indicate infection. Also note the presence of tissue breakdown.

2. Observe the amount, consistency, and color of the secretions suctioned from the tracheostomy.

3. Observe the client's reaction to the suctioning procedure. Note the approximate length of suctioning time. Observe the client's ability to cough up secretions and to turn as requested during suctioning.

CHARTING

DATE/TIME	OBSERVATIONS	SIGNATURE
5/23 1300	Tracheostomy suctioned for 15 seconds (2 ×) with good return of thick, viscous yellow secretions, approx. 12 ml from right bronchus and 4 ml from left bronchus. After 10-min rest period, the inner cannula was cleaned with hydrogen peroxide and reinserted. Clean tapes applied to outer cannula and the dressing changed. Bacteriostatic ointment applied to skin around tracheostomy as requested by Dr. J. Sterile dressing applied. Skin around incision is slightly red with no signs of tissue breakdown. Slightly apprehensive when cannula was removed; calmed considerably when reinserted. Reassured that the nurses are nearby and call signal placed near right hand. Dozing comfortably at this time. ————————————————————	G. Ivers RN

Discharge Planning Aspects

CLIENT AND FAMILY EDUCATION

1. A tracheostomy is frightening to the client and the family. Inability to speak adds to the fear of an unknown and uncontrolled situation. Provide the client with communication devices, such as tablets and pencils, digital communication boxes, or computerized communication boards. Assist the client and family in setting up a means of communication. Allay fear and embarrassment by anticipating this need and providing a method of speaking. Observe communication attempts and demonstrate or advise as needed.

2. Be sure that the client and family understand the purpose of the tracheostomy. They should also understand the basic anatomy and physiology of the altered respiratory method. Explain that the opening is much closer to the lungs than the nose or mouth, and that the air going into the lungs will not have the benefit of the warming, moisturizing, and cleansing effect of the nasal passage. For this reason, artificial warming and moisturizing apparatus may be necessary. In addition, whatever touches the tracheostomy tube should be sterile to prevent the entrance of pathogenic organisms into the tracheobronchial tree.

3. If the tracheostomy is permanent, the client and family should be taught care of the tube. Explain how to clean the inner cannula and how to change the dressing on the tube.

REFERRALS

If the tracheostomy is permanent, referral to a speech therapist for training in communication skills may be in order. In addition, the client and family should be referred to a hospital supply house where tracheostomy equipment may be purchased. Referral to a home health service may help in the transition from hospital to the home.

Evaluation

Quality Assurance

Documentation should include the appearance and the amount of the secretions, as well as indications of how the condition was progressing, evidenced by increasing or decreasing amounts of secretions throughout the hospitalization. Any ancillary devices, such as mist collars, should be noted, with references to their effectiveness. Cleaning and suctioning schedules should be noted. Notation of suctioning should be made as appropriate to indicate progress of condition. Teaching of the family and client should be recorded in the chart, with an appraisal of their understanding and acceptance of the client's altered condition. The chart should indicate that the nurse knew and understood the possible side-effects of tracheostomy care and took measures to ensure that client safety and well-being was maintained.

Infection Control

1. Tracheostomy care must be performed under sterile conditions. The proximity of the bronchial tissue makes the tracheostomy a perfect avenue for the entrance of pathogenic organisms into the lung tissue. All equipment coming in contact with the tracheostomy tube and site should be sterile. The client should be discouraged from touching the tracheostomy tube. If periodic plugging of the tube is allowed, it should be accomplished with a sterile obturator or sterile plug.

2. Strict handwashing should take place before and after tracheostomy care. Reusable equipment should be bagged and sent to the supply area for disinfection and cleaning.

3. If the client has a respiratory infection that is spread by the airborn route, a mask should be worn when suctioning or caring for the tracheostomy. Suctioning often causes coughing, which projects droplets into the atmosphere from the respiratory tract through the tracheostomy opening.

Technique Checklist

	YES	NO
Reason for tracheostomy explained to client and family	_____	_____
Suctioning procedure explained	_____	_____
Dressing change explained	_____	_____
Suctioned how often _____		
Return described in chart	_____	_____
Sterile technique maintained	_____	_____
Tracheostomy cleaned how often _____		
Inner cannula removed and cleaned	_____	_____
Outer cannula ties replaced as needed	_____	_____
Dressing changed q _____ hr		
Sterility maintained	_____	_____
Respiratory infection prevented	_____	_____
Mist collar present	_____	_____
Oxygen to tracheostomy _____ liters/hr		
Patency of tracheostomy maintained	_____	_____

	YES	NO
Tracheostomy removed before discharge	————	————
Client sent home with tracheostomy	————	————
Family and client understood how to care for tracheostomy	————	————
Follow-up care arranged	————	————

90

Traction, Nursing Care

Overview

Definition

A process of exerting a pulling force on portions of the body by means of pulleys and weights or both; support to a bone

Skin Traction: A weight that pulls on tape, sponge, rubber, or plastic materials attached to the skin; traction on the skin transmits traction to the musculoskeletal structures. Types of skin traction are the following:

Buck's extension: Traction applied to the lateral and medial aspects of an extremity with moleskin or adhesive. It may be unilateral (Fig. 90-1) or bilateral (Fig. 90-2).

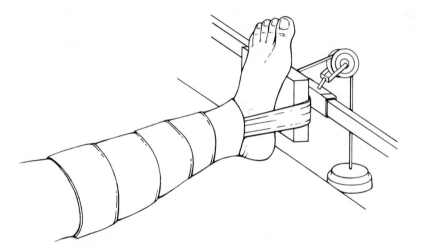

Figure 90.1

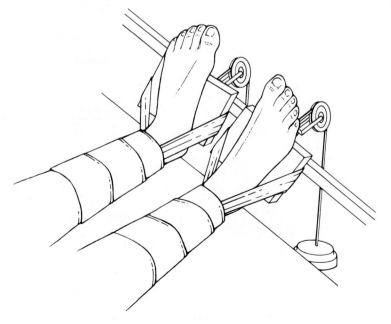

Figure 90.2

Russell's traction: Traction composed of Buck's extension on the foreleg, three pulleys at the foot, and a sling under the knee, which is attached to a rope and pulley above the knee (Fig. 90-3)

Cervical traction: Traction applied to the neck by use of a head halter and a series of pulleys and weights off of the head of the bed or over an elevated rod (Fig. 90-4)

Pelvic traction: Traction applied to the lumbosacral region by means of a pelvic belt (Fig. 90-5) or a pelvic sling (Fig. 90-6)

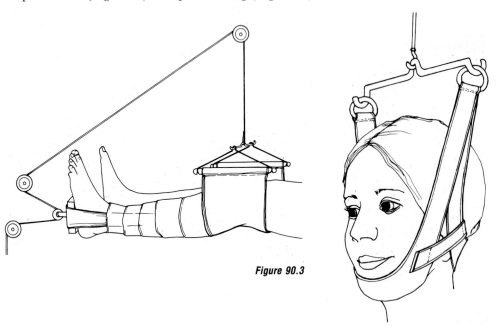

Figure 90.3

Figure 90.4

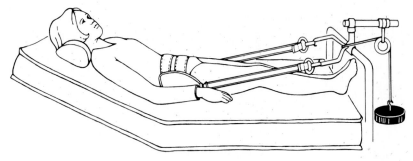

Figure 90.5

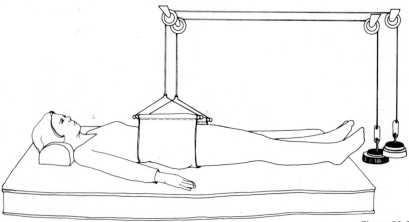

Figure 90.6

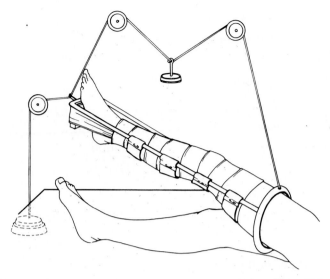

Figure 90.7

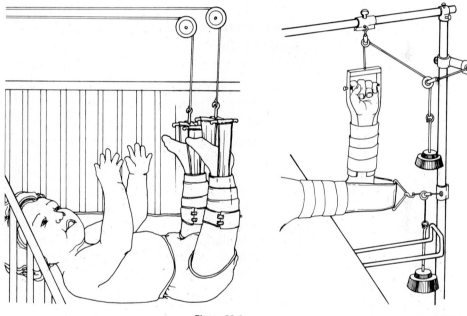

Figure 90.8   *Figure 90.9*

Thomas splint: A full-leg splint used in emergency transport situations or after amputation; keeps the leg fully extended and long bones in alignment. Pressure is on the ischium and perineal area, not on the knee (Fig. 90-7).

Bryant traction (pediatric): A method of vertical suspension skin traction, in which a child's pelvis is elevated from the bed. It is used to treat a fractured femur by reduction of the fracture, maintenance of normal alignment, and immobilization of legs. It is used mostly in small children (Fig. 90-8)

Side-arm traction: A method of traction similar to Buck's extension but placed on the arm (Fig. 90-9)

Skeletal traction: Immobilization by means of a pin surgically inserted through a bone

Rationale	Reduce and immobilize a fracture.
	Decrease or eliminate muscle spasm.
	Prevent fracture deformity or flexion contractures.
	Relieve pressure on nerve roots.
Terminology	***Contracture:*** Permanent shortening or tightening of a muscle from spasm or paralysis
	Reduction: Restoration to normal position

Assessment

Pertinent Anatomy and Physiology

See Appendix I: *bone repair, skeletal system, skin, vertebral column.*

Pathophysiological Concepts

1. Types of fractures are

   Simple or closed: The most common type of fracture, in which the bone is broken in one place without penetrating through the skin

   Compound or open: The bone may be broken in one or more places and a skin wound is present in the area of the fracture.

   Complete: The fracture extends all the way through the bone.

   Greenstick: The bone is not broken all the way through but is broken on one side; this is common in childhood when the bones are pliable.

   Comminuted: The bone is broken in more than two places or is splintered.

   Impacted: The bone pieces are driven into each other in a telescoping effect.

   Spontaneous or pathologic: A sudden fracture caused by simple pressure that would not normally cause a bone to break; common in persons with bone deficiencies or abnormalities, such as osteoporosis.

2. Healing of a fracture can be delayed by problems of union of the two or more sections of the broken bone. *Delayed union* is an abnormally long period required for the bones to heal. *Nonunion* refers to the situation in which satisfactory healing of the fracture never occurs. *Malunion* occurs when the segments of bone heal in an abnormal state, causing deformities. If the area around the fracture becomes infected, as may happen in compound fracture which is open to outside pathogens, healing may be delayed.

Assessment of the Client

1. Assess the condition of the client's limb, circulation, ability to move toes, swelling, and pain. Determine how much movement the client is allowed and can tolerate. Assess the skin before the traction is applied, if possible, to determine presence of breaks that might become infected.

2. Assess the client's experience with traction. Determine if this is the first broken bone ever experienced, and if the client has ever been in traction. Assess the anxiety levels of the client and family.

3. Assess the client's general physical condition. A debilitated state or presence of generalized infection may delay healing. Assess the client's nutritional state. Adequate nutrition is essential for proper healing.

Plan

Nursing Objectives

Maintain proper support to the musculoskeletal area until healing has occurred.

Prevent infection and complications of other body systems that may occur as a result of immobilization.

Maintain the client's mental and physical capabilities.

Teach the client exercises and other procedures that will assist in rapid and full recovery.

Client Preparation

1. Even when muscle tension is appropriate, as with the use of traction, it adds to the fatigue and pain of illness and injury. Back pain may be prevented by placing bed boards under the mattress. A regular schedule should be maintained for changing positions and exercising arms and legs to the extent possible.

2. Immobility fosters feelings of helplessness and dependence. Encourage the client to participate in care. A clear explanation of why the traction is being applied and the expected results may encourage the client to cooperate more actively.

3. Shaving the affected part and applying tincture of benzoin disinfects the skin and causes the traction strip to adhere better and more comfortably (see Technique No. 84, Shaving the Client).

Equipment

Adhesive, moleskin, or adhesive foam

Razor and tincture of benzoin

Specific traction equipment necessary to achieve the traction system prescribed by the physician

Sheepskin or eggcrate mattress

Bedboards

Pillows

Trochanter rolls (if indicated and allowed)

Sandbags (if indicated and allowed)

Implementation and Interventions

Procedural Aspects

ACTION	RATIONALE
1. Maintain the injured part in the position prescribed by the physician.	Traction must not be removed if the object is immobilization or reduction.
2. Ensure that the heel of the extremity in traction is free of pressure. Use a sheepskin or eggcrate mattress to relieve pressure on the hip. Check bandages frequently and rewrap as needed (if allowed) to correct constriction of circulation. Pressure areas under the traction may be discerned by gently rubbing the hand over skin surfaces, observing skin irritation and odor, and listening to the client's statements regarding pain and discomfort. If pressure is noted in a traction that is not to be removed, notify the physician.	Pressure on the skin constricts circulation and causes pressure areas, leading to the formation of pressure sores (decubiti).
3. Trochanter rolls or sandbags may be used to keep the limb in proper alignment. These items may cause pressure, however. Their position must be changed frequently, and the limb must be observed for signs of pressure or impaired circulation.	Props, such as sandbags, tend to localize the pressure and the patient must be observed carefully for signs of pressure sores. Pillows may be more beneficial for maintaining proper alignment.

ACTION	*RATIONALE*
4. Check the traction frequently to ensure that the weights are swinging freely, alignment is straight, pulleys are separated with ropes intact and free of knots, and the linens are not obstructing the pulley.	The line of traction should remain constant to achieve desired results.
5. When skeletal traction is used, inspect the area around the pin and clean it daily using sterile technique to clear the drainage that might occur. Watch for signs of infection including odor, redness, and profuse drainage, as well as changes in vital signs. Cover the area of pin insertion with a sterile dressing.	A serious complication resulting from skeletal traction is infection in or around the pin area. Microorganisms gain entrance through breaks in the skin and may infect the bone (osteomyelitis).
6. Encourage the client to do deep-breathing exercises regularly (q2hr). Offer soft, easily digestible food.	Adequate expansion of the respiratory system may help to prevent pneumonia and other respiratory complications. Constipation may be prevented by dietary modifications and adequate intake of fluids.
7. Provide suitable diversion.	Boredom frequently accompanies immobility.

Communicative Aspects

OBSERVATIONS

1. Monitor vital signs.
2. Check circulation to the part in traction every 2 hours.
3. Observe the condition of the skin.
4. Check the position and alignment of the limb or body part in traction.
5. Note the amount, odor, and appearance of drainage.
6. Observe for neuromuscular spasm or other pain.
7. Observe the client for respiratory and circulatory distress. Fat embolism may occur after fractures of long bones.

CHARTING

DATE/TIME	OBSERVATIONS	SIGNATURE
4/21	Application of bilateral Buck's extension traction, 7-lb weights to each leg.	
1700	Correct alignment at this time. States traction has not relieved back pain. ――	F. White RN
1715	Oral analgesic given. ―――――――――――――――――――――――――	F. White RN
1800	States backs feels better now. Some tingling in feet. No swelling or redness. Able to move toes well. Traction remains in alignment. ―――――――――	F. White RN

Discharge Planning Aspects

CLIENT AND FAMILY EDUCATION

1. Teach the appropriate exercises to maintain muscle tone and prevent muscle atrophy or circulatory and respiratory complications.
2. Teach the principles and purposes of traction to the client and family to ensure cooperation and therapeutic involvement in the treatment regimen.
3. Teach the client and family the observations that are essential to a successful outcome of the traction. They should know the signs of infection and pressure. Answer any questions candidly, and support the family and client.

REFERRALS

After prolonged immobilization of an extremity, the client may need assistance when beginning ambulation. Referral to a physical therapist may provide the guidance and assistance necessary for a successful and rapid return to full ambulation.

Evaluation

Quality Assurance

Documentation should include a description of the pain for which the traction is applied, observations about the site of application, and reaction of the client to traction application. The nurse should show in the chart that anticipated problems were checked and preventive measures were taken. The progress of the traction therapy should be noted in relation to relief of pain, condition of limbs and body parts, complications, and client reactions. Note the emotional outlook of the client. Boredom can predispose depression. Frequency of changing the traction wrappings should be noted, with observations each time about the condition of the part. Each hospital should have a policy regarding who may apply traction.

Infection Control

1. If the limb has any broken areas, sterile technique should be used in applying dressings. If the dressing is under the traction, periodic checking for signs of infection should be done.
2. Traction equipment that is used for consecutive clients must be cleaned between uses to prevent cross-contamination.
3. Careful handwashing should be done before and after handling or rewrapping the traction, or contact with the client.

Technique Checklist

	YES	NO
Procedure explained to client and family before traction was applied	_____	_____
Type of traction		
_____		
Amount of weight _____		
Right _____		
Left _____		
Frequency of reapplication of traction wrapping	_____	_____
Complications		
_____		
Desired results achieved	_____	_____
If traction will be used at home, client and family instructed on how to set up traction and principles involved	_____	_____

91 Turning Immobilized Clients on Frames

Overview

Definition

Changing the position of immobilized clients from the prone position to the supine and vice versa, with little or no active participation on the part of the client. A variety of devices are available for this purpose. Because the principles are basically similar, the frames that will be addressed are

Stryker wedge turning frame: A two-piece frame that allows turning of the client in a lateral rotating motion on a 360° axis. The frame is a wedge-shaped with the narrow edge of the wedge on the side to which the client is turned to prevent the possibility of falls; the Stryker wedge frame is adjustable to the height of the client

Foster frame: A two-piece frame that utilizes both sections locked together for the lateral turning process, and one piece to support the client between turning procedures; heavier and bulkier than the Stryker wedge

CircOLectric bed: A flat frame supported on a circular foundation, which allows vertical turning or progressive elevation of the angle of the body

Rationale

Secure a high degree of immobilization.

Maintain the desired body alignment while administering needed physical care.

Maintain a position of hyperextension at adjustable points and heights.

Maintain traction during the turning process, if desired.

Change points of greatest pressure on the body.

Terminology

Anterior frame: Frame on which the client rests when in the prone position

Posterior frame: Frame on which the client rests when in the supine position

Prone: Lying stomach down, with the face downward

Supine: Lying on the back, with the face upward

Assessment

Pertinent Anatomy and Physiology

See Appendix I: *skeletal system, vertebral column.*

Pathophysiological Concepts

The brain and spinal cord are enclosed within the protective, rigid structures of the skull and vertebral column. Although these structures protect the central nervous system (CNS) tissues, they also afford the potential for development of ischemic and traumatic nerve damage. This is because these structures cannot expand to accommodate the increase in volume that occurs when there is swelling within the nervous system, or the expanded volume that occurs when there is bleeding within these structures. The bony structures themselves also can cause injury to the nervous system. Fractures of the skull and vertebral column can compress sections of the nervous system, or they can splinter and cause penetrating injuries. After injury of the vertebral column, strict immobilization in correct alignment may be necessary until sufficient healing has occurred to ensure the integrity of the spinal cord and brain tissues.

Assessment of the Client

1. Assess the client's level of the consciousness. All actions should be explained to the client in advance of the turning maneuver.

2. Assess the client's level of mobility and sensation. Determine how much the client can do within the medical limitations imposed by the physical condition. Assess whether the client can assist in the turning and to what extent.

3. Assess the integrity of the turning apparatus. Assess the straps and safety devices to ensure the client's safety during the turning procedure.

4. Assess the condition of the client's skin before turning. If pressure areas are beginning, provide padding so that pressure is relieved. Assess the pain or discomfort as well as the presence of any neurologic symptoms (e.g., numbness, tingling, or impaired or renewed movement).

5. Assess the client's tolerance of the turning procedure. Assess tolerance of positions in determining time sequences for turning. Some clients cannot tolerate the prone position as long as the supine position. Some clients cannot tolerate the higher angles of elevation for very long periods. Assess the ability of the client to bear some weight on the legs. The CircOLectric bed usually is not recommended for clients who cannot bear weight on the legs because of spinal cord injuries.

Plan

Nursing Objectives

Allay the fear and anxieties of the client and family about the turning procedure.

Provide a safe and therapeutic environment.

Prevent complications of the turning process by attention to details and safety.

Prevent tissue breakdown from pressure.

Maintain correct alignment.

Observe the reaction of the client during turning.

Plan and adhere to a turning schedule compatible with client and family needs and medical necessity.

Record and report observations accurately.

Ensure that hydration and elimination needs are being met.

Provide some sources of diversional therapy.

Client Preparation

1. Thoroughly explain the procedure to the client before turning the first time. The client on a turning frame usually is unable to assist in self-care and is the victim of a some degree of helplessness. This feeling can cause additional fear as the turning procedure is approached. Emphasize the extra precautions taken to ensure safety and security during the turning procedure. Each time, reassure the client that measures have been taken to prevent falls and injury during turning.

2. Check all equipment before initiating turning to be sure that it is in proper working condition. If there is any question, have the equipment checked by the biomedical department or a knowledgeable person before attempting to turn the client. Place all equipment (*i.e.*, straps, pillows, linen) within easy reach before the turning procedure.

3. Explain to the client on the CircOLectric bed that dizziness is expected on initial elevation of the head and shoulders above the feet and legs.

Equipment	Stryker wedge frame (also Foster frame)
	Frames with canvas strips
	Pillows and foam pads
	Restraining straps
	Footboard and armrests
	Springs
	Linen and pads
	Security pins
	CircOLectric Bed
	Frames (basic and anterior)
	Foam mattress
	Special sheet
	Restraining straps
	Footboard and siderails
	Forehead and chin straps and hand straps (if needed)
	Pillows and foam pads

Implementation and Interventions

Procedural Aspects

ACTION	*RATIONALE*
Stryker Wedge Frame	
1. *To place the client on the frame:* Offer a thorough explanation of the purpose and method of using the turning frame if the client is conscious. Allow the client to see the frame before being placed on it. Put the posterior frame in place and lock into position. Place the client on the frame using the three-person carry, being careful to maintain proper body alignment. If the client is on a backboard, place the client and board onto the posterior frame. Apply the anterior frame and turn the client. Remove the posterior frame and the backboard. Reapply the posterior frame and turn the client back to the supine position.	The idea of being on a turning frame is frightening to the alert client. Adequate explanation can allay some of the anxiety and instill the confidence of the client in the nurses responsible for care and turning. The goal is to keep the vertebral column in straight alignment.

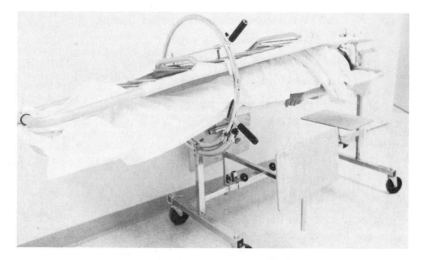

Figure 91.1

ACTION

2. *To turn the client from supine to prone position:* Lower the armboards before turning. Place pillows or sheepskin over the client's chest, lower legs, and anywhere else requested by the client to promote comfort. Open the turning circle and apply the anterior frame. Fasten the head end of the anterior frame on the securing bolt with a nut. Be sure the client is in proper alignment between the frames. Fasten the foot end of the frame with a nut. Have the client clasp hands around the posterior frame. If the client is unable to clasp the frame, place a safety strap at elbow level to maintain arm position. Close the turning circle until it locks automatically. Remove the bed-turning lock and turn the bed toward the client's right until it locks automatically (Fig. 91-2). Open the turning circle and remove the posterior frame. Relock the turning circle for safety.

RATIONALE

The Stryker wedge frame forms a pie-shaped wedge when both frames are in place (Fig. 91-1). The narrow edge is always on the client's right. This is the side to which the frame is always turned so that the chance of the client's falling is decreased. The frame will lock in place automatically when the bottom frame is horizontal. One nurse can turn the client on this frame using the turning circle.

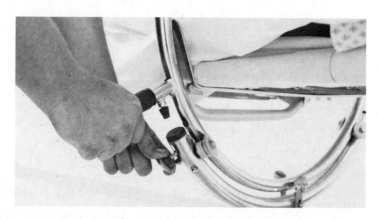

Figure 91.2

ACTION	**RATIONALE**
3. *To turn the client from prone to supine position:* Reverse the previous procedure. Place padding over back and lower legs unless contraindicated.	Padding should promote comfort without causing complications to physical condition.

Foster Frame

The Foster frame is used in a similar fashion to the Stryker wedge; however, two persons are required to turn it. Restraining straps encircle both frames while turning to protect the client (Fig. 91-3). Armrests should be replaced after turning to add support to the arms. When the client is supine on the posterior frame the armrests should be even with the frame (Fig. 91-4). When the client is in the prone position on the anterior frame, the rests should be at a comfortable level slightly below the frame (Fig. 91-5).	The Foster frame must be turned from head and foot simultaneously to ensure client safety. Armrests provide comfort and aid in maintenance of proper alignment.

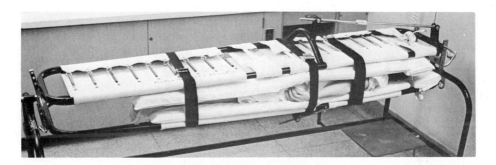

Figure 91.3

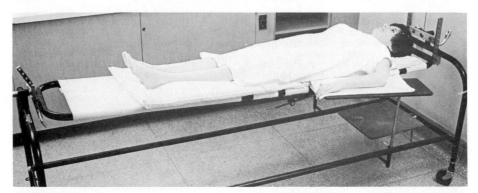

Figure 91.4

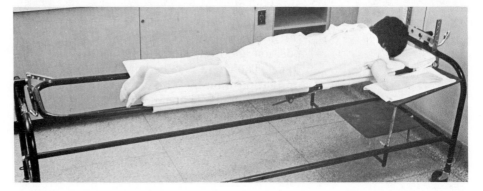

Figure 91.5

ACTION	RATIONALE
CircOLectric Bed	
1. *Placing the client on the CircO-Lectric bed:* Explain the reason for using the bed and the method of operation to the client and family. Show the client how the bed works. If the client is ambulatory, placement on the bed takes place from the standing position. Ask the client to step backward onto the footboard against the bed, which is in vertical position. Rotate the bed backward, adjusting the client's body in proper alignment. If the client is not ambulatory, explain the transfer technique and use of the bed to the client, if possible. Position the stretcher parallel to the CircOLectric bed. Transfer the client using the sheet or the three-person carry, keeping the client's body in correct alignment.	The goal is to keep the body in straight alignment. Minimize the client's anxiety by explanation and demonstration.
2. *Turning the client from the supine to the prone position:* Be familiar with the operation of the CircO-Lectric bed before trying to operate it in turning a client. Move the footboard and apply the anterior frame (Fig. 91-6). Attach the anterior frame to the head of the bed with the nut and bolt. Adjust the footboard on the anterior frame to fit against the client's feet. Attach the foot section of the anterior frame with the bolt and nut. The support bar of the anterior frame should support the client firmly but comfortably. Adjust the security collar knobs against the support bar. Place the headbands on the client's forehead and chin, if needed. Place the client's arms in slings for support. After double-checking all equipment, release the bed and turn the client slowly to the prone position. Lock the bed in position and remove the posterior frame. The client may be left in the upright position for a brief time, if there are no medical contraindications (Fig. 91-7).	The goal of the turning procedure is to keep the client's body in correct alignment while changing position for comfort and relief of pressure. The client should be turned slowly to prevent vertigo and loss of consciousness.

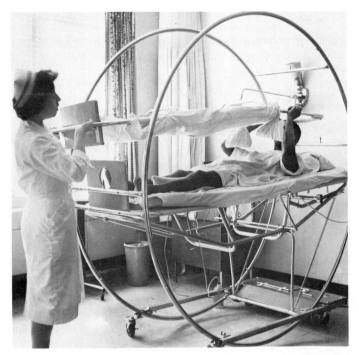

Figure 91.6

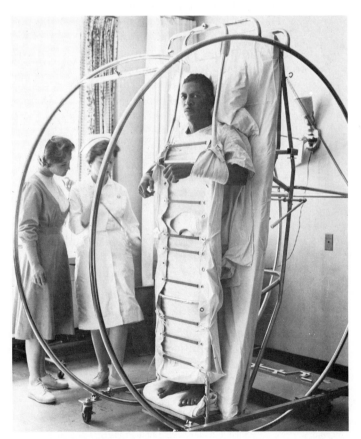

Figure 91.7

ACTION	RATIONALE
3. *To turn the client from the prone to the supine position:* Reverse the previous procedure. By manual adjustment, the bed may be placed in a sitting or semireclining position.	As the client is weaned from the bed, progressive positioning to the vertical position may build stamina and tolerance.

Special Modifications

ACTION	RATIONALE
1. To place and remove a bedpan, most turning frames have a removable section under the buttocks and perineal area. This section is removed and the surrounding area may be padded to prevent soiling. The bedpan is attached or held in place until the client is finished.	Proper elimination is difficult in an unnatural position; however, it is important to prevent constipation, a frequent side-effect of immobilization.
After removing the bedpan, cleanse and dry the client's perineal area and buttocks.	Cleansing and drying will help to prevent tissue breakdown.
2. Traction may be applied to clients on most turning frames. Fixed or skeletal traction may be applied. For fixed traction, the height of the frame determines the amount of traction. A table usually accompanies the bed to assist in determining how to achieve the prescribed goals of traction. Skeletal traction also may be applied. Care must be taken during turning to ensure that the ropes remain free and that traction is maintained.	Traction depends on a counterweight to achieve desired pull on the portion of the body for which is has been ordered. The benefit of the traction is lost if weights are allowed to rest on the floor.

Communicative Aspects

OBSERVATIONS

1. Observe and record the client's reaction during the turning. Observe the amount of understanding the client exhibits before turning and degree of compliance with any directions during turning.

2. Note the appearance of the skin in relation to the formation of pressure areas.

3. Note any treatments the client receives and reactions to them.

4. Observe the tubes or other devices (e.g., traction) during turning to ensure that they are not pulled or kinked. Secure any tubes before turning. The urinary drainage bag may be secured on the frame with the client, but take care that it does not rise above the level of the client's bladder during turning.

CHARTING

DATE/TIME	OBSERVATIONS	SIGNATURE
4/5 0900	Turned to the prone position on the Stryker wedge frame. Procedure explained before and during turning. Seemed apprehensive about turning, but tolerated procedure well. No reddened areas on posterior surface of body. Reading board adjusted. Reading at this time. ——————————	F. White RN
1100	Tolerated turning to supine position well; seemed less apprehensive. Bedpan requested; voided 300 ml. Requested bedpan be left in place so that she would not have to disturb nurses. Explanation given about need for support of buttocks area and willingness of nurses to replace bedpan at any time.	F. White RN
1200	Sleeping at this time. ——————————	F. White RN

Discharge Planning Aspects

CLIENT AND FAMILY EDUCATION

1. Instruct the client and family about the importance of frequent turning and good skin care. Explain how the turning will take place, and work with the client to determine how often to turn and how long the client will remain in each position.

2. Encourage the family to assist in diversional therapy for the client. Immobilization may cause time to pass very slowly. Spacing of visits from family and friends may help the time pass more quickly. Diversional activities such as television and reading may also occupy the client's time.

REFERRALS

If the client has a debilitating injury that may cause immobilization for a prolonged period, early referral to a physical therapy program may be made. Prepare the client for this action, and encourage full participation, emphasizing how it will help the client.

Evaluation

Quality Assurance

Document the time and manner of placing the client on the turning frame. Any explanations to the client or family regarding the turning device or procedure should be documented. Document each time the client is turned and any problems or complications associated with turning or prolonged bedrest. Some agencies may use a checklist or graphic display for documentation of turning times and position. Frequent notation of neurologic status should be made and charted. Any expressions of pain or complications should be addressed regarding assessment and outcomes. The status of transaction equipment should be noted each time the client is turned. If the goal of therapy is extended periods of elevation of the head or progress to the sitting position, the tolerance and progress of the client should be reflected in the chart. Each agency should have a mechanism for regular checking and maintenance of equipment (i.e., turning frames) to ensure that they are in proper working condition before a client is allowed to use them.

Infection Control

1. Handwashing should precede and follow turning of the client on the turning frame.

2. Equipment used for consecutive clients should be cleaned and disinfected before being used by other clients.

3. Equipment such as bedpans and urinals should be for the exclusive use of particular clients. Mark the client's toiletries and equipment and store them in an area where they will not be used for other clients.

4. Immobilization allows a favorable environment for the colonization of microorganisms. The client should be bathed daily while on the frame and should receive other routine care aimed at infection prevention, such as catheter care.

Technique Checklist

	YES	NO
Procedure for turning and need for placement on the turning frame explained to client and family	_____	_____
Proper body alignment maintained	_____	_____
Pressure areas prevented	_____	_____
Traction	_____	_____
Fixed _____		
Skeletal _____		
Family participated in diversion of client	_____	_____
Turning completed without complications	_____	_____
Frequency of turning _____		

Vaginal Examination

Overview

Definition

An internal examination of the vaginal area

Rationale

Examine internal structures of the female pelvis.

Ascertain possible pathologic or abnormal gynecologic conditions.

Obtain specimens for diagnostic purposes.

Remove a vaginal pack.

Evaluate the progress of labor.

Terminology

Lesion: Local change in tissue formation, an injury or wound

Leukorrhea: An abnormal white or yellowish mucous discharge from the cervical canal and vagina

Meconium: First feces of a newborn infant, greenish black and tarry in appearance. Intrauterine release of meconium may indicate fetal distress.

Assessment

Pertinent Anatomy and Physiology

See Appendix I: *genitalia (female), uterus, vagina, birthing process (labor).*

Pathophysiological Concepts

1. Three structures support the female abdominal viscera: the ilia, peritoneum, and the pelvic diaphragm. The pelvic diaphragm offers the main support; however, the inherent weakness of this structure is the opening through which passes the urethra, rectum, and the vagina. During pregnancy, the muscles of the pelvic diaphragm become stretched. After repeated pregnancies, the organs may slide out of the pelvis into the vagina. Three structures may protrude into the vaginal canal: the rectum (rectocele), uterus (uterine prolapse), and bladder (cystocele).

2. Cancer of the cervix is one of the most easily detected forms of cancer. The progress of cancer of the cervix begins with precursor cell changes, which form into atypical cells in the cervix. The next step is cancer in situ, which is a localized condition. The final step is invasive cancer of the cervix which spreads beyond the epithelial layer of the cervix. This condition can be readily diagnosed by a variety of laboratory tests, the most popular being the Papanicolaou (Pap) smear.

Assessment of the Client

1. Assess the condition of the client's external genitalia. Observe for lesions, rashes, inflammation, ulceration, discharge, swelling, or nodules.

2. Assess the physical mobility of the client. Determine if she is able to assume the lithotomy position.

3. Assess the previous experience of the client with vaginal examination. Assess the knowledge deficits to determine how much information is needed and how it can best be offered.

Plan

Nursing Objectives	Allay client fear and embarrassment.
	Reassure the client during the examination.
	Assist the examiner as needed.
	Record any unusual discharge or findings resulting from vaginal examination.
	Send specimens to the laboratory promptly.
	Record the effects of the examination and the information obtained.
	Note and record the progress of labor.

Client Preparation

1. The female client may face an impending vaginal examination with embarrassment. Explain the examination procedure and provide adequate draping. If this is the first time the client has had an vaginal examination, an in-depth explanation and reassurance may help her to feel more at ease.
2. Carry out the examination as quickly and efficiently as possible. Assemble all equipment ahead of time to avoid unnecessary delay.
3. A full bladder may displace the uterus and cause discomfort during the examination. Ask the client to void before the examination. Correct positioning will facilitate comfort further. Assist the client into the lithotomy position.
4. Determine the position and identify the presenting fetal part before beginning an obstetric vaginal examination. If there is a chance of placenta previa, do not undertake the examination.

Equipment

Vaginal examination tray containing vaginal specula (small, medium, and large), sponge forceps, tenaculum forceps, and sponges

Sterile gloves

Sterile lubricant

Gooseneck lamp or headlight

Specimen slides, containers, and fixative from the laboratory

Gauze packing (if needed)

Implementation and Interventions

Procedural Aspects

ACTION

1. The vaginal examination may be done by the physician with the assistance of the nurse or by the nurse who has had advanced clinical preparation and experience. Reassure the client during and after the examination. Interpret or explain findings in terms the client understands. It is usually desirable to have at least one other women present during the examination. This person may be the physician, the nurse, or an attendant.

RATIONALE

The client may feel more at ease with another woman present. There is also historical documentation of what occurs during the examination.

ACTION	**RATIONALE**
2. Cleanse the external genitalia if excessive drainage is present.	Organisms from the external genitalia may be transferred into the internal canal.
3. Lubricate the speculum by placing it in warm water or with a water-soluble lubricant, such as K–Y jelly.	Lubricants may impair the quality of the specimen and should be used only if requested by the examiner. Warm water not only lubricates the speculum but warms it to promote comfort and lessen reflex contraction of the muscles during insertion.
4. Provide a stool and lamp adjusted for maximum visualization. Place the client in the lithotomy position on the examining table with feet in stirrups, or in modified lithotomy position with the heels together when the examination is done in bed (Fig. 92-1). Drape with the sheet in triangular position, wrapping the corners around the client's ankles (Fig. 92-2). The examiner will don sterile gloves, lubricate the speculum (unless contraindicated), and gently insert it into the vagina (Fig. 92-3).	Visualization of the vagina and cervix requires a direct light source. Position to achieve the best view of internal structure but with the mobility and the comfort of the client in mind. Protect the client's modesty by adequate draping. The vagina is not sterile, and the vaginal examination usually is carried out under clean conditions. Most examiners wear sterile gloves, however.

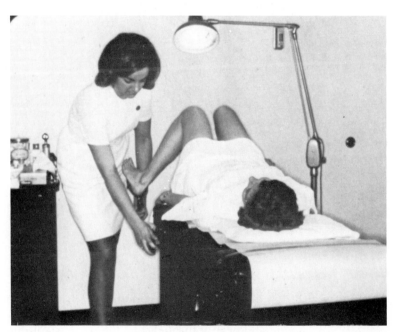

Figure 92.1

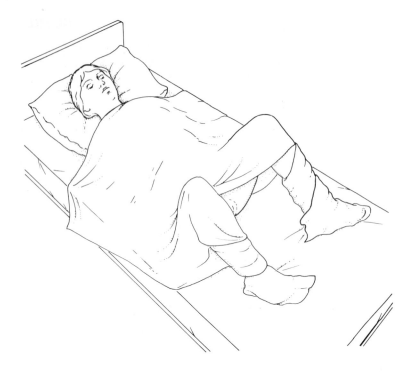

Figure 92.2

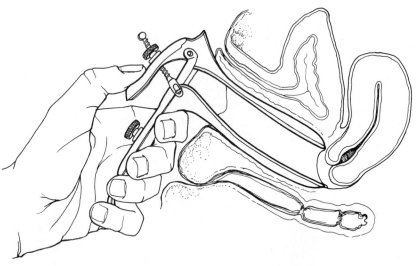

Figure 92.3

ACTION	*RATIONALE*
5. During the internal examination, encourage the client to breathe slowly and evenly through the mouth. If a smear is done, a slide and swab will be needed. A small layer of cells are scraped from around the cervix with a swab. The swab is rubbed across a glass slide, and fixative is sprayed on the smear. Transport this slide to the laboratory as soon as possible.	Mouth breathing promotes relaxation. Abdominal palpation aids in detecting cysts, tumors, or other abnormalities.

ACTION

    After removal of the speculum, the examiner usually will insert two fingers into the vagina and, with the other hand, palpate the lower abdomen.

6. On completion of the examination, cleanse the perineum of excess lubricant and any discharge. Assist the client to her room.

Special Modifications

Removal of Vaginal Packs

Remove vaginal packs under sterile conditions. With sterile gloves on, clean the labia with cotton balls and a disinfectant. Gently remove the vaginal pack. Apply a sanitary pad, if indicated.

Obstetric Examinations

1. Give the client a few seconds to relax at the end of a contraction. Cleanse the vulva with a disinfecting solution. Introduce the first and second fingers of a sterile, gloved hand into the introitus. Pause before advancing the fingers.

2. Locate the ischial spines as they indicate station 0 of the presenting part of the fetus.

3. Determine the extent of dilation and effacement by examination of the external os (see Technique No. 132, Labor and Delivery).

4. Limit vaginal examinations after the rupture of the membranes, to reduce the risk of infections.

5. Be alert for signs of complications and signs of fetal distress such as bleeding or the presence of meconium in the amniotic fluid.

RATIONALE

Leave the client dry and comfortable.

A vaginal pack usually is inserted in conjunction with a surgical procedure. To avoid contamination of the incision, the pack should be removed using sterile technique.

Contractions tire the client and cause muscular fatigue and anxiety. A short period to recover will enhance relaxation during the vaginal examination. Proper cleansing will decrease the chance of introducing pathogens into the birth canal.

Station 0 is a measurement guide, and the progress of the fetus below this level is referred to as station 1, 2, and so on.

A characteristic of normal labor is progressive dilation and thinning of the cervix. *Effacement* is the incorporation of the cervix into the lower uterine segment, during which thinning and softening occur.

The incidence of intrauterine infection and newborn infection are highest when prolonged rupture of membranes occurs.

In early labor, the mucus show is thin and pale pink. In the transitional phase, it is heavy and dark. At no time will this discharge clot, unless there is frank bleeding. Meconium-stained amniotic fluid indicates fetal distress and should be reported to the physician immediately.

Communicative Aspects

OBSERVATIONS

1. Observe the external genitalia for abnormalities or drainage. Note tenderness, rash, or redness.

2. Palpation of the vaginal canal will allow inspection for rectocele (along the posterior vaginal wall bulging forward), cystocele (anterior vaginal wall bulges downward), and uterine prolapse (bulging of the uterus into the vagina through the endocervical canal).

3. The cervix can be observed through the speculum. A purplish color may indicate pregnancy. Observe for lacerations, polyps or growths which may indicate cancerous tissue. As the speculum is withdrawn, observe the vagina for a greenish-yellow discharge which may indicate gonorrhea, inflammation of the vaginal wall (red spots which may indicate Trichimonas or white patches which may indicate monilia) or bleeding.

4. Observe the tolerance of the client during the examination. Watch for indicators of muscle contraction and nervousness, such as holding the breath and shaking knees.

5. Note the progress of cervical dilation and effacement in the obstetrical client, as well as the station of the presenting part.

CHARTING

DATE/TIME	OBSERVATIONS	SIGNATURE
7/27 0945	Vaginal exam by Dr. T. Cervical smear taken for pap exam and culture of client discharge sent to lab. No vaginal bleeding noted. Appeared to be slightly uncomfortable, instructed on relaxation techniques. ———	F. White RN
1020	Returned to room. Numerous questions raised about tests done. Seemed satisfied with answers to questions. ———	F. White RN

Discharge Planning Aspects

CLIENT AND FAMILY EDUCATION

1. Cervical cancer is the most common cancer of the reproductive system in women. The disease is always curable in its preinvasive state. Therefore, to discover the disease early every adult female should have a thorough gynecologic examination yearly.

2. Instruct the client not to douche before a gynecologic examination because such treatment will wash away cellular deposits used in diagnostic procedures.

3. Danger signals that every woman should report to her physician are spotting, irregular or excessive bleeding, any bleeding after menopause, persistent painful menstruation, leukorrhea, urinary disturbances, or pelvic discomfort.

4. Tell the client that in cleansing the external genitalia, particularly after elimination, women should begin at the urethral meatus and wipe backward toward the rectum. Otherwise, bacteria may be carried over the introitus and urethral meatus, which may predispose to vaginal and urinary tract infections.

5. The client and family should be kept informed about the progress of labor.

Evaluation

Quality Assurance

Documentation should include the name, title, or credentials of the examiner. Any specimens taken should be noted. The appearance of the external and internal vagina should be noted. Any abnormalities, including drainage, inflammation, or foul odor, should be noted. The instructions offered, degree of understanding, and the tolerance of the client should be noted.

Documentation of the vaginal examinations of the client in labor should reflect the progress of labor, any problems, and all information relayed to the family unit. Awareness of possible complications should be noted as well as precautions taken to prevent or reverse them. Sensitivity to when vaginal examinations are no longer indicated should be reflected.

Infection Control

1. The vaginal canal is not a sterile orifice, and the vaginal examination is carried out under clean conditions (with the exception of obstetric vaginal examinations). Care must be taken not to contaminate the lubricant once the gloved hand has been inserted into the vagina.

2. Cleanse the external genitalia with a disinfectant to prevent the introduction of pathogens into the vaginal canal. This is particularly important in the obstetric client. Pathogens must be prevented from entering the birth canal.

3. Thorough handwashing should be done before and after vaginal examination.

Technique Checklist

	YES	NO
Procedure explained to client	_____	_____
Client able to assume proper position for examination	_____	_____
Lithotomy _____		
Modified lithotomy _____		
Condition of external vagina observed	_____	_____
Inflammation _____		
Drainage _____		
Rash _____		
Lesions _____		
Condition of internal vagina observed	_____	_____
Lacerations _____		
Polyps _____		
Growths _____		
Irritation of the vaginal wall _____		
Progress of labor noted _____		
Smear or specimen taken	_____	_____
to laboratory at _____ (time)		

93   Vital Signs

Overview

Definition

Measurement of verifiable signs that reflect the physiologic state, which are governed by the body's vital organs (brain, heart, lungs), and are necessary to sustain life. Vital sign indicators are

Temperature: Oral, rectal, and axillary

Pulse: Radial, femoral, temporal, brachial, apical (auscultated), carotid, and pedal

Respiration: Visual or auscultated

Blood pressure: Auscultation, palpation (fingertips used instead of stethoscope; only systolic pressure can be determined accurately)

Rationale

Assess the client's condition on admission.

Determine the baseline values for future comparisons.

Detect as early as possible any deviation in the client's status.

Communicate with other members of the health team any observations relative to the client's well-being.

Terminology

Auscultation: Process of listening for sounds produced in a body cavity

Blood pressure: The force of blood exerted against the arterial wall; commonly measured in the antecubital fossa of the arm (brachial artery), and less frequently in the popliteal fossa of the leg (popliteal artery) and the wrist (radial artery)

Diastolic pressure: Lowest pressure exerted against the arterial wall, occurs during relaxation of the ventricles

Digital thermometer: A battery-operated device that contains a probe covered by disposable covers. Temperature readings may be determined in 2 to 60 seconds.

Palpation: Process of examining by application of the hands to external body surfaces

Pulse: The rhythmic throbbing caused by regular expansion (rise) and contraction (fall) of an artery as blood is forced into it by the contractions of the left ventricle of the heart

Respiration: The exchange of gases between an organism and its environment. The respiratory cycle includes inspiration (breathing in) and expiration (breathing out). Rate can be obtained by palpating, seeing, and listening.

Sphygmomanometer: Blood pressure cuff

Systolic pressure: Greatest pressure exerted against the arterial wall (during contraction of ventricles)

Temperature: Heat maintained by a living body, expressed in degrees; the balance between heat produced and heat lost

Assessment

Pertinent Anatomy and Physiology

1. See Appendix I: *blood vessels, heart.*

2. Heat is continuously lost and produced during life. Most of the heat loss occurs through the skin and is regulated by the amount of blood flowing through the cutaneous vessels and by the activity of the sweat glands. A delicate balance exists between heat loss and production. Heat is produced by the oxidation of foodstuffs in all cells. It is a by-product of the cellular production of energy. Heat production is influenced by muscular and by glandular activity. As body temperature rises, heat production also rises owing to the increase in metabolic rate. Temperature rises disturb metabolic patterns. Heat is lost by radiation into the air, conduction to another object, convection (the movement of air), and vaporization of liquids, especially through the skin. The hypothalamus is the center for body temperature regulation. The mouth, rectum, or axillae are used most often to determine body temperature because they most closely simulate the inside of the body. This is because of their abundant blood supply and the relation of the vascular system to heat regulation.

3. Blood pressure is the force exerted by the blood against the walls of the vessels. Arterial pressure is measured when the blood pressure is taken with a sphygmomanometer and stethoscope.

4. The medulla oblongata portion of the brain contains many of the vital centers that are essential to life. These include the cardiac center which speeds and slows the heart, the vasomotor center which constricts or dilates the blood vessels, and the respiratory center which changes the rate and depth of breathing.

Pathophysiological Concepts

1. The usual adult temperature range is 35.8° to 37.4° C (96.4° to 99.4° F), with the average being 37° C (98.6° F). Temperature regulation is diminished in the elderly; usually temperatures of older adults are subnormal. These persons are less active, the circulation is slower, and there is less power to compensate for fluctuations in external temperature. *Heat exhaustion* occurs when a person perspires so much that severe dehydration and sodium loss occur. *Heat stroke* develops when persons with decreased cutaneous blood supply have diminished sweating and finally circulatory failure. *Hypothermia* is subjecting the body to extremely cold external temperatures. *Fever* is an elevation of body temperature beyond the normal range. Causes may be viral or bacterial infection, drug reaction, brain lesion, or reaction to other body pathology. Fever-producing agents or pyrogens, act on the hypothalamus, stimulating heat production and conservation mechanisms. Vasoconstriction, decreased sweat gland activity, increased muscle tone, and shivering occur. Body temperature begins to climb.

2. Blood pressure is influenced by problems with cardiac output and peripheral resistance. Hypertension occurs when the arterial pressure is significantly above average for the person involved. Primary hypertension may be caused by obesity, heredity, or nervousness. Secondary hypertension is of unknown etiology but may accompany some other pathologic systemic condition. Arterial pressure is maintained by the elastic recoil of the arterial walls. When the walls become lined with atherosclerotic plaque, they lose their elasticity and the arterial pressure is compromised. This results in unusually high pressure during systole and low pressure during diastole.

3. Certain factors influence the regulation of breathing. Chemical factors depend on the presence and amount of carbon dioxide, which stimulates the chemoreceptors on the medulla and stimulates breathing. Physical factors include lung inflation, which stimulates nerve receptors and allows passive expiration to occur, and blood pressure changes, which cause breathing to become slower and shallower. Falling blood pressure, as in severe hemorrhage, causes the respiratory rate to increase. Irritation of the respiratory passages, such as in coughing, and an elevated body temperature, as in fever, cause an increase in the respiratory rate.

4. Pulse rate also is governed by the medulla. The rate is increased during conditions such as hemorrhage and shock. The elasticity of the vessels also affects the rate. During atherosclerosis, the plaque lining the vessels hardens and constricts the diameter. The amount of blood able to be pumped through the vessels is diminished. This causes conduction problems because the right ventricle has less space into which to push the blood and must exert more force to push the blood into the smaller vessels.

Assessment of the Client

1. Assess the familiarity of the client with vital sign procedures. If the client has never had blood pressure measured previously, explain that the cuff will feel very tight, but will not injure the arm and will be uncomfortable only momentarily. If rectal temperature is taken, be sure that the client understands what is happening, how long it will take, and what is expected of the client.

2. Assess the ability of the client to hold the thermometer in the mouth as well as safety factors involved. If the client is subject to seizure activity or is confused, the temperature should not be taken orally with a glass thermometer owing to the chance of breaking the thermometer in the mouth. If an electric thermometer is used, assess the ability of the client to comply with instructions. If *any* doubt exists about the safety of the client, axillary or rectal temperature should be taken. Oral temperature readings are done on all adult clients except those who are unconscious, confused, or subject to seizures, those receiving oxygen by nasal cannula, those who have nasogastric tube in place, those who have a pathologic condition of the nose, mouth, or throat, or those for whom the physician orders an alternative means.

Plan

Nursing Objectives

Recognize the interrelationships between vital signs, physiological activity, and pathophysiological change.

Recognize the periodic nature of physiological activity as a basis for evaluating measurement of vital signs.

Use the information offered by measurement of vital signs as a determinant of client progress, response to therapy, and nursing intervention.

Recognize and evaluate the response of the individual client to the environmental factors, internal and external, as indicated by the measurement of vital signs.

Initiate the measurement of vital signs above and beyond what is ordered if the client's condition warrants.

Communicate the measurement of vital signs to health team members in correct terminology and on correct records.

Recognize the changes in vital signs that require urgent medical or nursing intervention, and initiate action.

Client Preparation

1. Notify the client in advance if vital sign measurement will be taken during the night. Knowing the reason for being awakened may allow the client to accept these actions more positively.

2. The client should be at rest or normally active when vital signs are measured. Measurement should not occur immediately after the client has had a hot or cold drink, has been smoking, or has under gone unusual exertion. These activities can give false readings.

Equipment

Thermometer (glass or digital, oral or rectal)

Watch with a second hand

Sphygmomanometer

Stethoscope

Lubricant (if rectal temperature is being taken)

Alcohol sponge

Tissue

Implementation and Interventions

Procedural Aspects

ACTION

Temperature

1. Glass thermometer
Wipe soaking solution from the thermometer (Fig. 93-1). Hold it firmly between the thumb and forefingers and shake the mercury down to the base of the thermometer. Use a flicking motion of the wrist. Repeat until the mercury is below 35° C (94° F) (Fig. 93-2).

RATIONALE

Leaving the chemical solution on the thermometer may irritate the mucous membranes and skin. It can also have an objectionable taste and odor. The mercury rises in the glass tube according to a consistent ratio. It must be at the bottom of the thermometer before beginning to measure the temperature accurately.

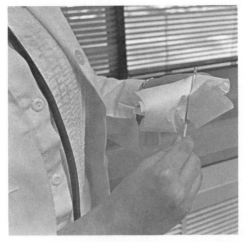

Figure 93.1

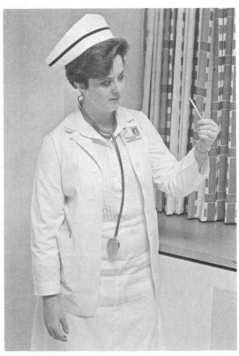

Figure 93.2

ACTION

Oral: Place the thermometer under the tongue and leave in place for 2 minutes. Remind the client to leave the lips closed around it (Figs. 93-3, 93-4). The normal oral temperature reading is 37.0° C (98.6° F).

RATIONALE

The lips should close around the thermometer rather than the teeth to prevent accidental biting and breaking the thermometer.

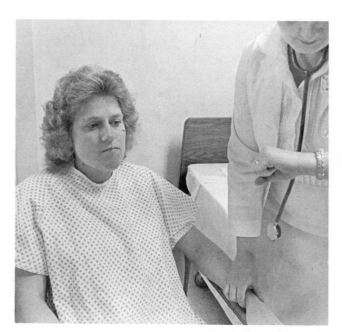

Figure 93.3

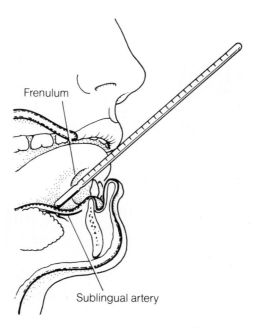

Frenulum

Sublingual artery

Figure 93.4

ACTION

Rectal: Wipe the thermometer and apply a lubricant (Fig. 93-5). Insert the thermometer gently into the rectum 2.5 cm to 3.5 cm (1 in–1½ in) in the adult (Fig. 93-6). Hold it in place for 3 to 5 min. (Fig. 93-7). The normal reading is 37.5° C (99.6° F). Cleanse the client's rectum after completion (Fig. 93-8).

RATIONALE

A lubricant will reduce the friction encountered as the thermometer is introduced into the rectum. The thermometer should be held in place to prevent accidental breakage or other trauma to the client's rectum.

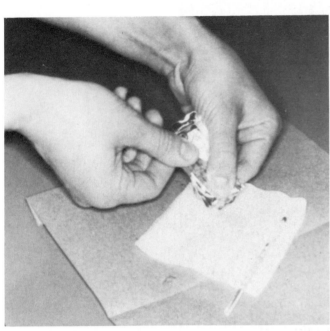

Figure 93.5

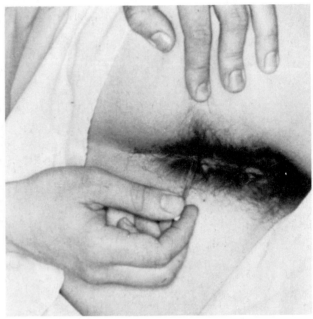

Figure 93.6

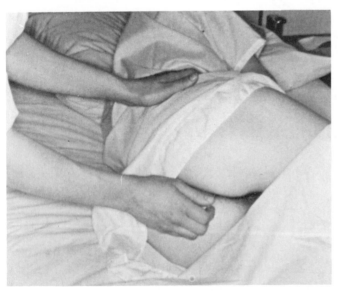

Figure 93.7

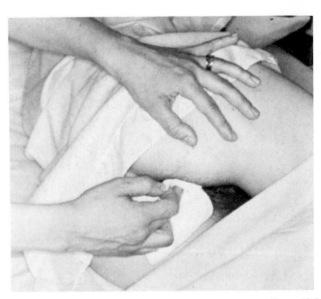

Figure 93.8

ACTION	RATIONALE
Axillary: Dry the client's axillary area. Hold the thermometer in place with the bulb against the client's axillary tissue for 7 to 10 min (Fig. 93-9). Fold the client's arm across the chest while the measurement is being taken.	Moisture in the axilla may cause incorrect temperature readings. The client's arm is folded across the chest to decrease air currents, which may cause an artificially low temperature reading.

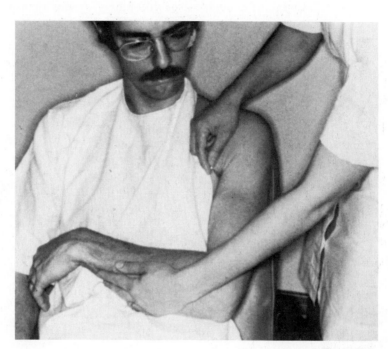

Figure 93.9

Reading the Thermometer

Wipe the thermometer with a rotating motion toward the bulb. Hold the thermometer at eye level and rotate it until the column of mercury comes into view. Read the value at the level of the mercury. If any fecal material remains on the rectal thermometer, it should be removed with warm water and mechanical drying.	Mercury expands when heated, according to the amount of heat applied. This allows the thermometer to record accurately the proper temperature consistently. The thermometer is wiped toward the bulb because this is going from the lesser contaminated area to the more contaminated area.

ACTION	RATIONALE
2. Digital thermometer Place the cover over the thermometer probe (Fig. 93-10). Place the covered probe into the area to be checked for temperature: the mouth, rectum, or axilla. Be sure that the appropriate circuit is engaged if the device uses different circuits for the various areas of measurement. Hold the probe in place during the entire measurement time (Fig. 93-11). When the device indicates that the measurement is complete, remove the probe and discard the cover in the trash (Fig. 93-12). Replace the probe to the appropriate place.	The probe cover is used to prevent cross-contamination and must be discarded after each use. Because the time needed for measurement is so short, it is a good safety precaution to hold the probe at all times when taking a temperature.

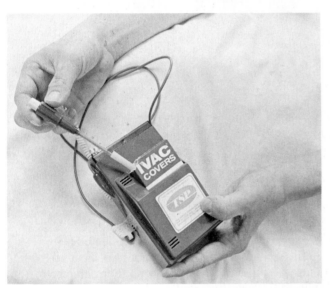

Figure 93.10

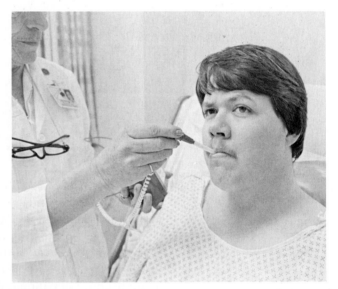

Figure 93.11

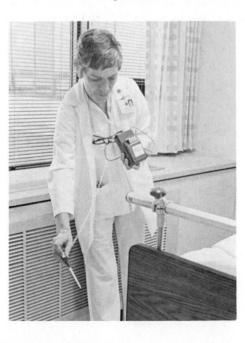

Figure 93.12

ACTION	**RATIONALE**

Pulse

1. Use the fingertips when taking the client's pulse, preferably the second and third (the middle and ring) fingers. Place them along the appropriate artery and gently press. Support the wrist on the bed or some firm surface.

The thumb and index fingers have pulses of their own which can be mistaken for that of the client; therefore, they should not be used to measure the pulse. Gentle pressure is necessary because too much pressure will obliterate the client's pulse, and too little will make it imperceptible.

2. Count the pulse for 30 to 60 seconds. If it is irregular, count it for at least 60 seconds. The normal ranges are 60 to 72 beats/min for men and 72 to 84 beats/min for women. Auscultate the apical pulse by placing the stethoscope over the apex of the heart and counting for 1 minute (Fig. 93-13).

Sufficient time must be allowed to detect irregularities in the pulse rate. The apical–radial measurement should be the same. If the apical rate is greater, however, it may indicate that insufficient force is being exerted on the blood leaving the heart for it to be felt in the peripheral pulse sites, or vascular disease may be interfering with the ability of the blood to reach the peripheral pulse points with sufficient strength. The radial pulse rate cannot be greater than the apical rate.

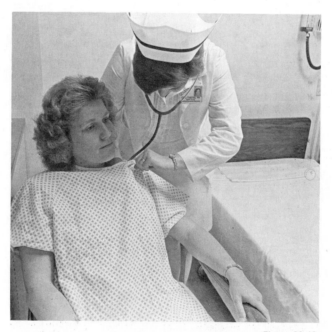

Figure 93.13

ACTION   **RATIONALE**

Measure the radial pulse on the inner aspect of the wrist (Figs. 93-14, 93-15). Locate the pedal pulse on top of the foot, over the instep (Figs. 93-16, 93-17). The femoral pulse is located in the groin area (Figs. 93-18, 93-19). The carotid pulse may be felt in the neck, about 2 in to 3 in below the mastoid process, under the mandible line (Figs. 93-20, 93-21). The apical–radial pulse is measured when two nurses take simultaneous pulse measurements, one taking the radial measurement and one taking the apical measurement. Various descriptions of the pulse are bounding, thready, weak, faint, and full.

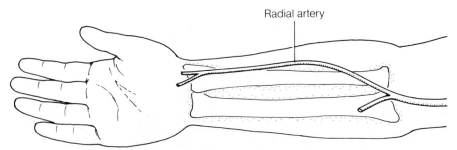

Radial artery

Figure 93.14

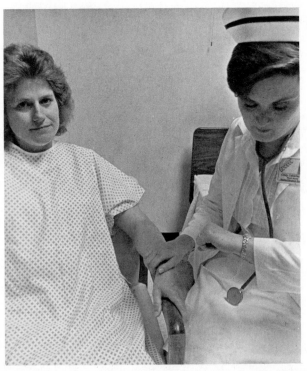

Figure 93.15

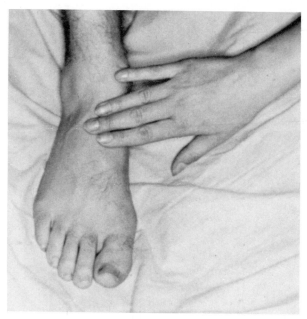

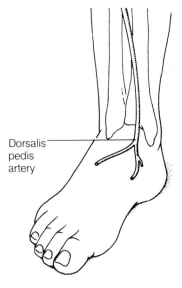

Dorsalis pedis artery

Figure 93.17

Figure 93.16

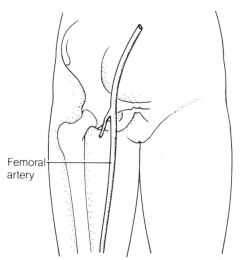

Femoral artery

Figure 93.18

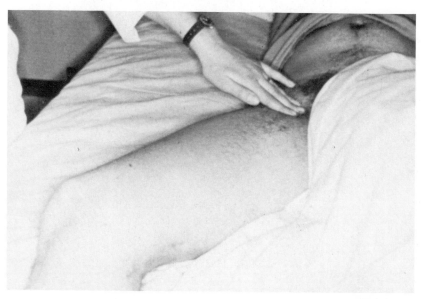

Figure 93.19

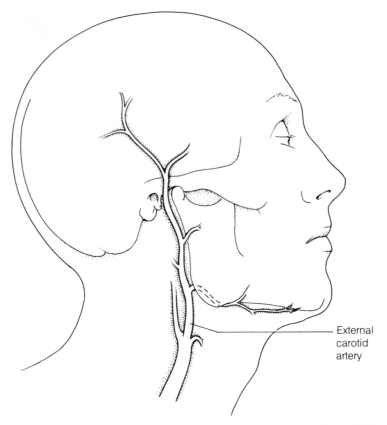

External
carotid
artery

Figure 93.20

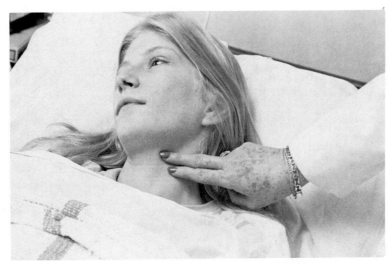

Figure 93.21

ACTION	RATIONALE

Respirations

1. Count the number of times the client takes a breath for 30 seconds. If abnormalities are present, count the respirations for a full minute. Note the respiratory rate by watching the rise and fall of the client's chest. The normal adult respiratory rate is considered to be 16/min to 20/min. Descriptions of the respirations include wheezing, labored, shallow, retracting, deep, irregular, unilateral, diaphragmatic, and Cheyne–Stokes.

A complete cycle of inspiration and expiration constitutes one respiration.

2. It may be helpful to count the respirations immediately after counting the pulse, with the fingertips still on the client's artery.

Awareness that the respiratory rate is being counted may cause the client to alter the normal rate.

Blood Pressure

1. Apply the sphygmomanometer cuff to the client's arm above the antecubital fossa (Fig. 93-22), or to the leg above the popliteal fossa (Fig. 93-23).

The examiner should be able to reach the antecubital area and see the pressure measurement gauge easily so that accurate measurement can be taken.

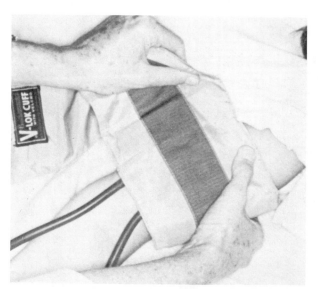

Figure 93.22

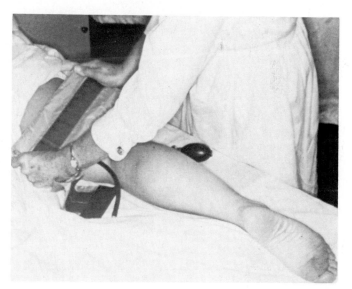

Figure 93.23

ACTION

2. Place the diaphragm of the stethoscope firmly over the artery so that sound can be transmitted without distortion. If in doubt about the location of the artery, palpate it with the fingertips and place the diaphragm directly over the area where pulse is felt (Fig. 93-24). On mercury manometers, read the level of the meniscus at eye level no more than 3 ft away (Fig. 93-25). The aneroid type has a dial indicator that measures the blood pressure (Fig. 93-26). Normal adult blood pressure is considered to be systolic, 110 to 130, and diastolic, 70 to 80, but this may vary greatly according to the client's age and condition.

RATIONALE

The edges of the diaphragm should all be flat against the skin to limit the amount of extraneous noise, but not so hard that the arterial pulse is modified or obliterated. A comparison of the blood pressure reading with what is normal for the client often is more important than the actual numerical reading at any one time.

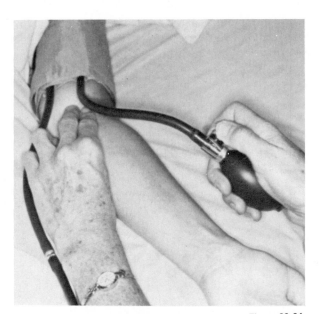

Figure 93.24

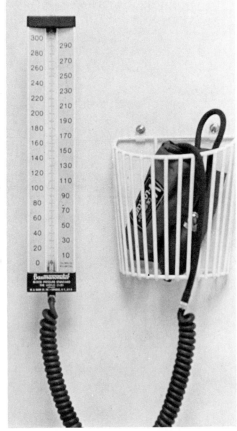

Figure 93.25

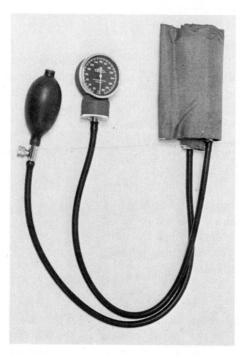

Figure 93.26

ACTION	RATIONALE
3. Inflate the cuff to a point about 20 to 30 mm Hg above the last systolic reading or until pulsation can be neither felt nor heard. Do not leave the cuff inflated any longer than necessary.	Pressure exerted by the inflated cuff prevents blood from flowing freely through the artery.
4. Determine the systolic pressure by slowly releasing the pressure valve. The point which the first pulse beat is heard is the systolic reading. Note the level of the mercury or the position of the arrow on the gauge.	Systolic pressure is the point at which blood in the artery is first able to force its way through against the pressure exerted by the inflated cuff.
5. Determine the diastolic pressure by noting the point at which the first muffled sound is hear (diastolic IV) and the point at which the sounds and the fluctuation of the gauge cease (diastolic V). Determine these pressures by the continuing slow and steady release of the pressure valve.	Diastolic pressure indicates the point at which blood flows freely in the artery and is equivalent to the amount of pressure normally exerted on the wall of the arteries when the heart is at rest.

ACTION	RATIONALE
6. The blood pressure also may be measured by the palpation method. Apply the cuff to the upper arm and locate the radial pulse. Inflate the cuff. The radial pulse will be obliterated at this point. As the cuff is slowly deflated, note the point at which the radial pulse is again palpable. The reading at which the first beat is felt is the systolic reading. It is generally 10 mm Hg below the systolic measurement by auscultation. Diastolic pressure is not measurable by the palpation method.	Occasionally the blood pressure is not audible through the stethoscope. This may happen in the critically ill client or one who is extremely obese.

Special Modifications

1. Take the temperature of children under 6 years of age by the axillary route. The rectal route is contraindicated if rectal abnormality is suspected or if the child has had recent rectal surgery. Initial temperatures of a newborn are take by the rectal route to ensure rectal patency as well as measuring body temperature. Never force the thermometer into the rectum. If it cannot be inserted easily, notify the physician. Thereafter, neonatal temperatures are usually taken by the axillary route (see Technique No. 119, Vital Signs in Children).	If the thermometer will not insert readily into the infant's rectum, the condition of imperforate anus may be indicated. This is an abnormal closure of the rectal canal that is very dangerous and must be corrected surgically. Forcing the thermometer may traumatize the tissue and cause severe complications.
2. Do not take a rectal temperature measurement on clients who have had rectal surgery recently. If the oral route is not possible, use the axillary route.	Insertion of the rectal thermometer after rectal surgery may cause trauma to the suture line and hemorrhage.

Communicative Aspects

OBSERVATIONS

1. Determine when to measure vital signs based on the client's condition and the physician's instructions. The following routine observation of vital signs is suggested: all new admissions; twice daily for all clients; every 4 hours or more often on all postoperative clients for 3 days; at least every 2 hours or more often on all critically ill clients and those with abnormal vital signs. Remeasure the vital signs of the newly admitted several hours after admission to ensure accuracy. Because of tension and anxiety of the situation, vital signs often are distorted on admission.

2. Pulse and respiration should be measured each time the temperature or blood pressure is taken to assist in a more comprehensive assessment of the client. The pulse usually increases 10 beats for each degree of temperature increase.

3. The rhythm, tension, and volume, as well as the rate, should be observed carefully when taking pulse and respiration to detect signs of irregularity.

4. The interval between systolic and diastolic pressures should be noted regularly. This measurement is called the *pulse pressure*. Because diastolic pressure remains relatively constant, the pulse pressure usually is considered to be a good indicator of stroke volume. In hypovolemic shock, the pulse pressure often is decreased. Report a steady decrease in pulse pressure to the physician or supervisor.

5. Steady or sudden decreases or increases in one or all vital signs should be reported at once. More frequent readings should then be taken for evaluation of client status until the measurements return to what is considered normal for this particular client.

CHARTING

1. Record vital signs on the unit worksheet, the client's record, and the bedside vital-sign sheet, if applicable.

2. Record observations of vital signs in the nurses' progress notes to assist in continued assessment of client condition.

DATE/TIME	OBSERVATIONS	SIGNATURE
5/5 0910	Pulse thready, rapid, and irregular. Rate 120. Stated, "My heart is pounding and feels as if it's going to explode." Respirations very short and shallow with rate of 28. B/P 190/120. Dr. D. notified. Attendant with client continuously.	F. White RN

Discharge Planning Aspects

CLIENT AND FAMILY EDUCATION

1. Instruct the client and family about the frequency of vital signs, especially if measurement will occur during the night. Explain the reasons for measurements and answer any questions.

2. Instruct the client concerning oral restriction before vital sign measurements (e.g., refraining from drinking hot or cold liquids, smoking).

3. Inform the client of any change in the schedule of measuring vital signs, such as more frequent checking after surgery, so that anxiety will be allayed. Relate the reason for the change and anticipated duration.

4. If the client will have unresolved problems after discharge, the family should be shown the technique for measuring vital signs. They should also be told where to purchase equipment and what type of equipment is the best buy.

Evaluation

Quality Assurance

Documentation should include a progressive record of the vital signs from admission to discharge. Any discrepencies should be addressed in the progress notes with regard to known causes and resolution. Policies should exist regarding routine procedures for measuring vital signs to ensure a certain standard of care. If the measurement is taken by a route other than the usual one, notation of the reason and any discrepancies should be made. Reactions of the client to the vital sign measurement should be noted.

Infection Control

1. Equipment that is used for consecutive clients must be cleaned carefully if it touches the client. When taking temperatures with glass thermometers, each client should have a thermometer for exclusive use. When the digital thermometer is used, take care that only the disposable probe cover touches the client. If the probe or any part of the device touches a client, clean it with the disinfectant recommended by the manufacturer.

2. The ear pieces of the stethoscope should be cleaned with an alcohol sponge after each use. This is especially important if the stethoscope is used by several personnel. The bell should be wiped with an alcohol sponge after it touches the client's arm or chest. No equipment should be used on consecutive clients without being disinfected.

3. Careful handwashing should occur between each client whose vital signs are taken. An explanation of why hands are washed after each client may help to instill confidence and may reassure the client that everything possible is being done to protect clientele from complications.

Technique Checklist

	YES	NO
Procedure explained to client	_____	_____
Temperature taken	_____	_____
How often _____		
Route _____		
Measurement device _____		
Abnormalities _____		
Reported to physician	_____	_____
Pulse taken	_____	_____
Route _____		
Abnormalities _____		
Reported to physician	_____	_____
Respirations noted	_____	_____
Abnormalities _____		
Blood pressure taken	_____	_____
Extremity _____		
Abnormalities _____		
Reported to physician	_____	_____
Vital signs recorded on the client's record	_____	_____
Family taught how to measure		
Temperature	_____	_____
Pulse	_____	_____
Respiration	_____	_____
Blood pressure	_____	_____

Wheelchair and Walker

Overview

Definition

Aids in client mobility. A wheelchair is a chair suspended between two large wheels in back and two smaller wheels in front. A walker is a support that accompanies the client during ambulation. It may have wheels or four legs that are lifted by the client with each step. The walker encircles the front of the client and has hand grips.

Rationale

Mobilize the client who is unable to walk or cannot walk unsupported.

Enhance the safety and security of the client while encouraging independence.

Assessment

Pertinent Anatomy and Physiology

See Appendix I: *skeletal muscles, skeletal system, skin.*

Pathophysiological Concepts

1. Abnormal stress on the bone results in structural problems. Muscle tone may be compromised owing to prolonged inactivity. With inactivity, muscles decrease in size and strength.

2. Changes in the joint result when the surrounding tissue is immobilized. When muscle movement decreases, the connective tissue in the joints, tendons, and ligaments becomes thickened and fibrotic. Chronic flexion or hyperextension of the joints can cause permanent contracture.

Assessment of the Client

1. Assess the client's degree of mobility, sense of balance, and desire to be ambulatory. If the client has been immobile or has had limited mobility, assess the client's potential for increasing extent of mobility.

2. Assess the client's physical condition in relation to sitting in the wheelchair or ambulating with a walker. If the client has physical limitations, assess the amount of assistance needed and ensure the client's safety by having an adequate number of personnel to assist.

3. Assess the client's skin, especially in areas around the bony prominences of the hips and buttocks. Look for pressure areas, abrasions, or rashes. Determine where padding may be needed.

Plan

Nursing Objectives

Maintain safety standards by locking the wheelchair, teaching proper body mechanics, and giving sufficient assistance during transfer from the bed or during ambulation.

Minimize client discomfort during transfer.

Make the client as comfortable as possible

Support dependent body parts adequately.

Prevent falls by teaching and encouraging proper technique.

Provide a safe environment in which to perfect mobilization skills.

Client Preparation

1. Tell the client how to assist with lifting and standing techniques. Assure the client that the nurses will assist as necessary and will be available to prevent falls or problems.

2. If the client is bathed before getting in the wheelchair or up to the walker, the bed can then be made while the client is up. This saves energy and exertion for the client.

3. Teach the client proper transfer techniques before attempting to ambulate or get up in the wheelchair for the first time. Have the chair prepared when the client is ready. Have the walker nearby and checked for safety before the client is ready to get up.

4. Assist the client in donning a robe and slippers. If the client will use a walker, properly fitting, nonskid shoes should be worn. A short robe is preferable so that the client's feet will be visible, and tripping over the robe will be prevented.

5. Most walkers are adjustable. Adjust the walker so that the hand bar is just below the client's waist.

Equipment

Wheelchair or walker   Sheet (if needed)
Pillows (if needed)   Slippers and robe

Implementation and Interventions

Procedural Aspects

ACTION

Wheelchair

1. Assist and support the client during transfer from the bed to the wheelchair. Lock the wheels of the chair according to manufacturer's instructions (Fig. 94-1). Move the foot and leg supports out of the way (Fig. 94-2). Hold the chair while the client is transported to it or sits in it without help. Place the bed in the lowest position.

RATIONALE

If the client is debilitated enough to need a wheelchair, assistance is probably needed to get into the wheelchair. Safety precautions should be taken to see that the client does not fall or get hurt during transfer. Even with the brakes locked, the chair should be secured to ensure that the client does not fall.

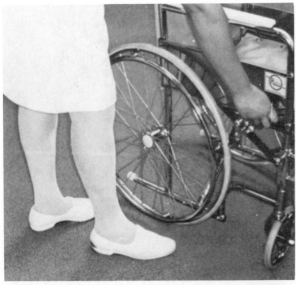

Figure 94.1

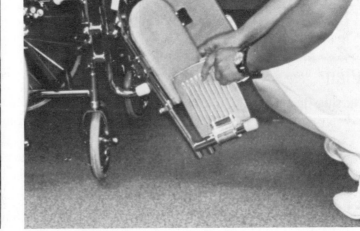

Figure 94.2

ACTION

2. *Pivot technique:* Position the chair next to and parallel to the bed. Assist the client into the sitting position on the side of the bed (Fig. 94-3). With one hand under each of the client axillae, two nurses assist the client into the standing position in front of the wheelchair (Figs. 94-4, 94-5). When upright and stable, the client slowly turns with a pivoting motion until in position to sit in the chair and slowly lowers into the chair still supported by the nurses (Fig. 94-6).

RATIONALE

This technique is used to minimize the distance that the client must move to get into the chair. The nurses provide support and leverage during the transfer. The client must be supported until safely and securely in the chair.

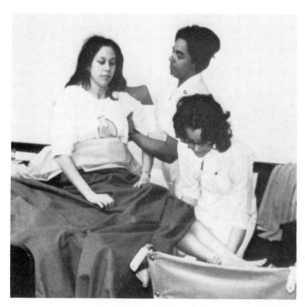

Figure 94.3

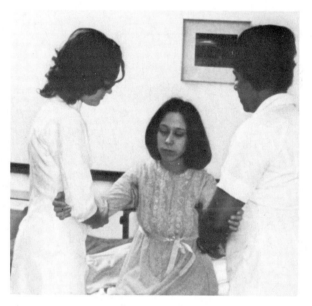

Figure 94.4

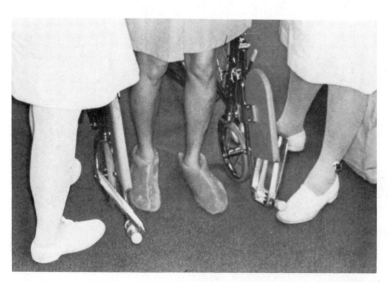

Figure 94.5

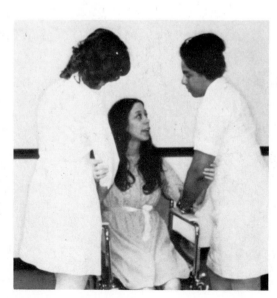

Figure 94.6

ACTION

3. *Lifting technique:* Position the chair parallel to the bed facing the foot of the bed. Raise the client into the sitting position in bed either manually or by raising the head of the bed. One person grasps the client under the axillae, one places hands under the hips, and one moves the legs. At a given signal, all simultaneously lift the client into the wheelchair.

4. To return to bed, the client may pivot or may be lifted using the three-man lift technique (see Technique No. 76, Position, Change of). To pivot, do the steps for getting the client out of bed in reverse order (Figs. 94-7 to 94-11).

RATIONALE

Minimize the distance the client must be moved by strategic positioning of the wheelchair. Support the client using proper body mechanics to prevent back strain.

The client may be tired after being up and may need additional support during pivoting.

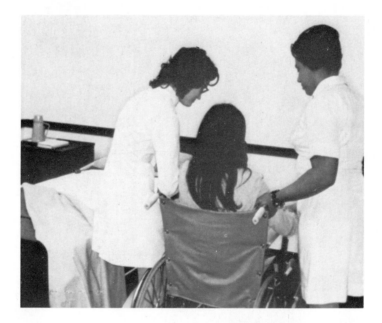

Figure 94.7

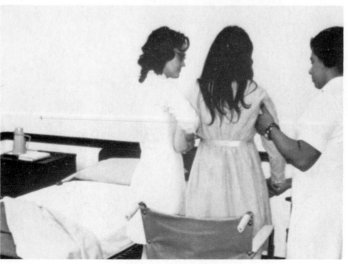

Figure 94.8

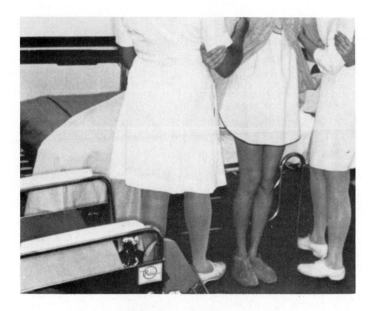

Figure 94.9

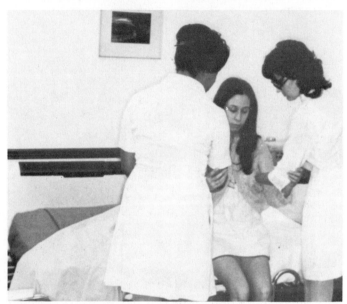

Figure 94.10

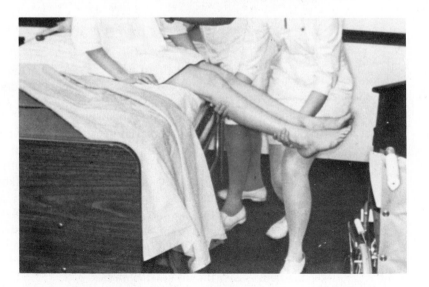

Figure 94.11

ACTION	RATIONALE
5. Place a safety belt or restraint around the client's waist while in the chair. If the client is unable to maintain proper posture while in the chair, a second belt may be secure around the chest area to prevent falling forward. Be certain that this second belt does not restrict breathing .	The client may be susceptible to falls owing to weakness or prolonged immobility. The safety belt(s) may provide security.
6. Place the client in proper alignment in the wheelchair with dependent parts supported. Elevate any limb with a cast on a pillow; do not allow it to dangle. Support the cast with a sling or restraining strap (Fig. 94-12).	A dangling cast places undue strain on the joint and casted limb. Elevated casts must be secured so that the limb does not fall.

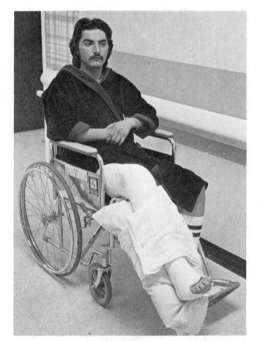

Figure 94.12

ACTION	RATIONALE
7. Place a sheet over the client's lap and knees.	A covering provides warmth and protects the client's modesty.

Walker

ACTION	RATIONALE
1. The walker is a device to assist in ambulation when the client requires more balance than can be provided with a cane but is able to ambulate without another person assisting. To approach the walker, place it at the client's bedside within reach. Assist the client into the sitting position on the side of the bed. Assist the client to stand, placing the bulk of the weight on	Some clients need the security and balance provided by the wide base of support offered when using a walker. If the walker is within reach, the client may be able to ambulate with little or no assistance. Be sure that the client is steady before allowing independent ambulation. The goal is to prevent falls.

ACTION

RATIONALE

the legs and the hands which hold the grips on the walker. Be sure that the walker is adjusted to fit the client.

2. To take a step with a walker, the client lifts or rolls the walker approximately 14 cm to 25 cm (6 in–10 in) away. Then, using the hand grips as a source of balance and support, the client takes a step into the center of the walker (Fig. 94-13).

The client's weight is supported by the legs while the walker is being moved, and by the walker while the legs are taking a step.

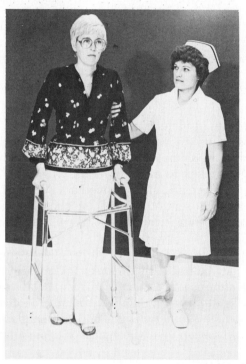

Figure 94.13

3. Assist the client the first time ambulation with a walker is attempted. Offer assistance until satisfied that the client understands the technique and is steady and safe.

Be certain the client can provide adequate balance and support to prevent falls.

Communicative Aspects

OBSERVATIONS

1. Check the client's general condition before ambulation or getting up in a wheelchair is attempted. Unusual fatigue, unstable vital signs, or recent administration of a narcotic, hypnotic, or sedative may be contraindications.

2. Check the client frequently for signs of fatigue or weakness that would indicate a need to return to bed.

3. Observe the client's alignment and position while up in the wheelchair. Use pillows to prop the client into proper position and support dependent parts. Do not allow the client to slip downward or to one side, resulting in unnatural curvature of the spine.

CHARTING

DATE/TIME	OBSERVATIONS	SIGNATURE
3/9 0700	Up in wheelchair for breakfast and remained up for 20 min. Hair braided while up. Slight discoloration of feet while up but no swelling noted. Tolerated much better today than yesterday. Balance better. ————————	B. Smith LVN

Discharge Planning Aspects

CLIENT AND FAMILY EDUCATION

1. Encourage independence to the extent possible for the client. Teach techniques, such as transfer and body mechanics, to facilitate self-care. Stress safety precautions, but allow the client as much flexibility as possible in determining self-care.

2. If the client will need a wheelchair or walker at home, teach the family proper techniques, safety measures, and body mechanics.

REFERRALS

If the client will require a walker or wheelchair after discharge assist the family in determining the benefits of renting or buying. Refer the family to hospital supply stores where they can get the best purchase for their particular needs.

Evaluation

Quality Assurance

Documentation should include an assessment of the client's ability and willingness to assist in techniques. The level of understanding of limitations and measures taken to overcome or compensate for these should be noted. Record the progress of the client as hospitalization progresses. Document safety precautions taken and teaching efforts aimed at client and family. Document any ambulation equipment sent home with the client or instructions to the family and client about obtaining wheelchairs or walkers outside the hospital.

Infection Control

Any equipment that is used for consecutive clients must be cleaned after each use. The chair may be padded with sheets or coverings; however, it should still be wiped clean after use by a client. Walkers usually are adjusted for one client. After the client is discharged, the walker should be cleaned and disinfected before being used for another client. Thorough handwashing should be done after assisting a client up in a wheelchair or to ambulate with a walker.

Technique Checklist

	YES	NO
Client understood procedure before beginning	———	
Client assisted to wheelchair		
Lifting technique ———		
Pivot technique ———		
Safety precautions used to prevent falls and strains	———	———
Family taught to assist client in and out of wheelchair	———	———
Walker adjusted to comfortable height for client	———	———
Client able to ambulate with walker safely before discharge	———	———
Client and family had proper equipment at discharge or knew where to obtain equipment	———	———

Unit 3

Techniques
for
Pediatric
Clients

95

Admission of the Pediatric Client

Overview

Definition

The incorporation of a series of activities that occur when a client enters the hospital

Rationale

Give basic, pertinent information to the parents and to the child, appropriate to the level of understanding.

Obtain valid information from the child and parents necessary to the provision of knowledgable care.

Make the child and family feel comfortable and secure in the hospital setting.

Terminology

Nursing history: Data obtained from the child and family on admission, which is used to establish a baseline of information about individual needs on which to base nursing diagnosis and interventions

Assessment

Pertinent Anatomy and Physiology

1. See Appendix I: *skin, skeletal system, vertebral column, ear (external), ear (internal), eye (external), eye (internal), teeth.*

2. Anatomy and physiology of the adult is generally applicable to the infant and child. Children must be assessed in relation to their own unique stage of growth and development, however. Many of the findings during physical examination of the child and their significance are very different from those of the adult client. (An in-depth discussion of normal growth and development is beyond the scope of this book. The reader is referred to Waechter EH, Phillips J, Holaday B: *Nursing Care of Children*, 10th ed., Philadelphia, JB Lippincott, 1985.)

3. The child in a strange environment has limited resources to call on for the reestablishment of equilibrium. Distrust is the usual emotional response to an unfamiliar and threatening setting, such as the hospital. The security of the presence and closeness of parents and familiar objects may allay some of the fear and anxiety surrounding admission to the hospital setting.

4. Play is one means used by children to cope with and adapt to new and stressful experiences. Play enables the child to act out aggression, fear, conflict, and anger regarding uncontrollable events.

Pathophysiological Concepts

Stress is a dynamic state within the body in response to a demand for adaptation. Whenever a child is hospitalized, stress is felt by the entire family. Stress takes many forms and affects many different levels of the body. Stress may cause changes in neural function, hormone release, and cardiorespiratory responses. Nausea, vomiting, and diarrhea may result from the stimulation of the nervous system by stress.

Assessment of the Client

1. Assess the activity level of the client. Determine if the activity currently being exhibited is usual, exaggerated, or depressed for this particular client.

2. Assess the behavior of the client in relation to whether it is indicative of discomfort or pain, fear, or restlessness. Assess the behavior in relation to the developmental stage of the client and expressed physical symptoms. Some children attempt to "cover up" or negate pain in hopes of returning to the security of their own home environment more quickly. Assessment of pain must include visual observation of symptoms and any attempts to mask those symptoms. Physical signs of pain include inflammation or abnormal posture, dependency of one part, or a pained facial expression when the child thinks that no one is watching. Use observational, as well as interviewer, skills in assessing the client.

3. Assess the physical signs of illness such as abnormalities of the skeletal system, the skin, the cardiorespiratory system, and any abnormality that indicates deviation from the normal patterns of growth and development.

4. Assess the child's usual patterns of nutrition and elimination at home. Determine words used by the child relating to eliminatory needs (i.e., what the child says when needing to urinate or move the bowels), whether the child is capable of self-care, and the child's usual bowel and bladder pattern. Determine what the child likes to eat, how often the child eats, any dietary restrictions and reasons for them, and the child's ability to eat without assistance.

5. Assess the anxiety level of the parents. Determine their understanding and acceptance of the need for hospitalization. Assess how much they know about the child's condition and prognosis. Determine if this is their first experience with hospitalization of a child. Assess their educational level and determine the type of teaching that will meet their needs best. Assess the home situation, the presence of other children, and who is caring or will care for them during the time the child is hospitalized. Ask whether both parents work, how this situation will be affected by having a child in the hospital, and the family's financial means.

6. Assess the allergy history of the child. Determine the presence of any past allergies to medications or other substances. Determine the presence of allergic manifestations in the family.

Plan

Nursing Objectives

Facilitate the adjustment of the child and parents to the hospital environment.

Observe, evaluate, and finally reevaluate the child's condition.

Institute primary diagnostic measures.

Maintain the individuality of the child and the family during the admitting procedure.

Institute the initial admission techniques such as measuring vital signs, securing specimens, and assessing needs.

Identify staff and hospital environment to the client and family to reduce stress and facilitate adaptation.

Client Preparation

1. Orient the client and family to the hospital environment. Explain the nurse call system, mealtimes, visiting hours for friends, any hospital regulations for who may visit, operation of the bed, lights, bathroom accessories, telephone, television, and any other environmental apparatus at the disposal of the client and family. Place the client in a bed appropriate for age and physical abilities. Be sure that the client and family understand how to call for assistance.

2. Some type of siderail or safety restraining rail or net should be placed on the beds of all infants and children.

3. Follow hospital regulations regarding who may stay with the client. Most hospitals encourage parents to remain with the client during hospitalization. Parents may help the child to adapt to a strange setting and may provide valuable information to the nurse regarding the client's condition and needs.

Equipment

Admission record

Portable scales

Admission pack

Hospital gown or client's own pajamas

Watch with a second hand

Stethoscope and sphygmomanometer

Otoscope

Ophthalmoscope

Tape measure

Specimen container

Implementation and Interventions

Procedural Aspects

ACTION

1. Greet the client and family courteously. If possible, introduce the child to other children in the immediate area and to the other personnel.

2. Take the nursing history as soon as possible after the client arrives on the unit. Most hospitals have an interview form to guide the initial assessment. Nursing histories usually contain the following general topics:

   Routines at home, including disciplinary methods

   Family relationships at home

   Emergency phone numbers

   Person who will remain in the hospital with the child

   Dietary habits of the client and family

   Peers, relatives, and friends

   School (if applicable)

   Favorite toys and games

   Activities, hobbies, and sports preferences

   Coping ability of the child in handling stress

   Previous experience with illness or hospitalization

   Hygienic practices of the child

   Sleeping patterns

   Elimination patterns

   Description of the child's physical and mental status

   Allergies and other medical problems

RATIONALE

Familiarizing the child and family with the unit may decrease anxiety and enhance feelings of self-worth and self-control.

Formulation of the care plan should begin on admission. The foundation of the plan of care should be a complete history and assessment of the client which will guide future planning and interventions.

ACTION

RATIONALE

3. Measure initial vital signs while the child is at rest. Measure the height and weight on admission. Blood pressure is generally taken on clients over age two. A complete assessment should be done according to hospital policy. This usually involves a complete systems review as well as ophthalmoscopic and otoscopic examinations (see Technique No. 17, Ophthalmoscopic Examination and Technique No. 18, Otoscopic Examination). Measure the frontal occipital circumference (FOC) of the child under age two. Measure the head at the point of greatest circumference (Fig. 95-1). If the child has abdominal problems, measure the abdominal girth at the level of the umbilicus.

Baseline measurements may be used during hospitalization to assess progress or complications. If the child is at rest and not crying or extremely active, the measurement will more accurately reflect the normal status of body systems.

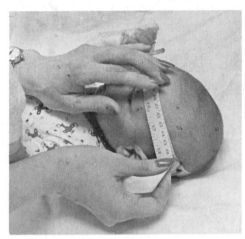

Figure 95.1

4. Obtain a urine specimen for urinalysis, if this is a hospital policy or a physician's order. If the child is toilet trained, ask the parents to assist in obtaining and saving the urine specimen. If the child is not toilet trained, place a disposable urine specimen collector over the external urinary meatus of the female client or the penis of the male (Fig. 95-2). Ask the parents to call as soon as the child urinates so that the collection bag can be removed.

The urine collection bag fits against the skin with an adhesive that holds it over the external opening of the urethra to catch the urine when it is discharged from the body. Because it is somewhat uncomfortable, the collection bag should be removed as soon as possible.

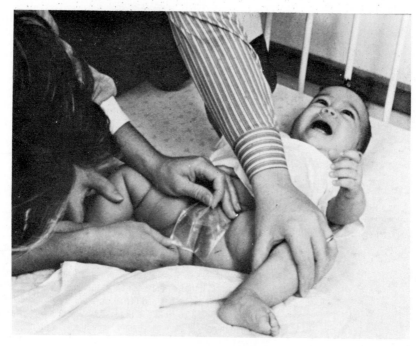

Figure 95.2

Communicative Aspects

OBSERVATIONS

1. Observe the parent–child interaction as a guide for evaluating the relationship.

2. Observe the reaction of the child and parents to the present hospitalization experience. Observe for knowledge deficits that may be amenable to teaching efforts.

3. Observe the comprehension level and cognitive achievements of the child when answering questions. Respond at a level appropriate to the child's age, level of understanding, and desire to know.

4. Observe the physical condition of the client. Observe the skin for any breaks, rashes, bruises, or dermatologic problems. Observe the body structure for abnormalities. Observe for tenderness over any areas, in addition to any stated or observed signs of pain.

5. Observe the emotional status of the client in relation to age and developmental stage, noting fear, anxiety, aggression, or maladaptive behavior. Observe for signs of stress and adaptive techniques in dealing with the stress.

CHARTING

1. Nursing history
2. Admission notes should include:

   Age and sex of child

   Time and manner of arrival

   Admitting information from parents or client

   Vital signs

   Physician visit and outcomes

   Observation and abnormal physical findings

   Allergies

   Medication taken at home

   Special dietary needs

   Any special information that would benefit the administration of safe, therapeutic care

3. Identify potential or present problems and note approaches toward their management on a written plan of care.

4. Written or graphic display of the following measurements:

Temperature

Pulse

Respirations

Blood pressure (for children over 2 years of age)

Weight and height

Frontal occipital circumference on children under age two

Abdominal girth for the child with known or suspected abdominal problems

DATE/TIME	OBSERVATIONS	SIGNATURE
2/5 0230	5-year-old girl admitted to room 565 by wheelchair; accompanied by mother. Scheduled for removal of tonsils and adenoids in the morning. Mother states that Dr. D. has fully explained the procedure and has no further questions. CBC and UA done. Mother states that the child is allergic to penicillin, no other allergies. She has had dental work done with no allergy to topical anesthetics. B/P 110/76, P 82, R 18, T 99.2° F rectally. Visual inspection shows small bruise, 1.25 cm in diameter, on left ankle with approximately 5 cm scraped area on side of left leg, states ''bicycle wreck skinned ankle.'' Takes daily vitamin at home, no other medications. Dietary intake the past several days has been soft foods, custards, ice cream, and lots of fluids (likes grape juice) because of sore throat. Weight 25.4 kg (56 lb), height 110 cm (44 in). No siblings. Mother will remain in room with client throughout hospitalization. Watching television. Does not seem apprehensive about surgery in the AM. ————————————————————————————————	B. Cole RN

Discharge Planning Aspects

CLIENT AND FAMILY EDUCATION

1. Explain to the parents that they will play an integral part in their child's hospitalization. Include them in goal setting and care planning. Encourage their input and solicit their advice in the care of their child. Make sure they understand that hospital personnel desire to have parents participate in the care of their child (Fig. 95-3).

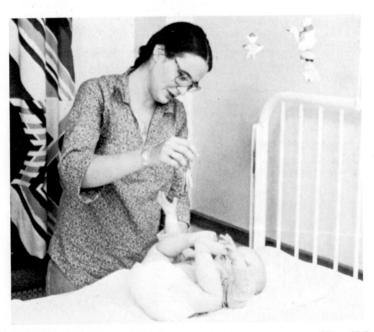

Figure 95.3

2. Explain that play is a natural part of a child's life and of the planned nursing care. Assure the family that attention will be given to this aspect of their child's life. Demonstrate appropriate play for the child's age and developmental task acquisition level. Explain the importance of eye contact and body contact to the family as they play with and observe the staff at play with the child.

Evaluation

Quality Assurance

The documentation should reflect attention to the child as a developing and interacting member of a family group. The nursing history should address any past health problems and their resolution. Allergies should be noted in a prominent place on the chart. Most hospitals have a written assessment form that should be completed during admission. Problems and abnormalities found on assessment should be reflected along with actions taken to report or correct these. Baseline vital signs, as well as height and weight measurements, should be noted. Any breaks or abnormalities in the skin should be noted. Evidence that the nurse took into account the history and present family situation should be reflected in the initiation of a written plan of care, which is begun on admission. Discharge planning goals should be initiated at this time.

Infection Control

1. Handwashing should be carried out before and after touching a client to prevent the spread of infection.
2. Equipment that is used for consecutive clients should be cleaned between uses to avoid cross-contamination. Toys that are available to children on a pediatric unit should be made of material that can be wiped clean with an antiseptic solution. All toys should be cleaned after use by a client.
3. If infectious processes are suspected or known, the client may be placed on some type of isolation restrictions (see Technique No. 66, Isolation Precautions).

Technique Checklist

	YES	NO
Age of client _____		
Client admitted by _____		
Client accompanied by _____		
Vital signs		
B/P _____		
Pulse _____		
Respirations _____		
Temperature _____		
Route _____		
Height _____		
Weight _____		
FOC _____		
Abdominal girth _____		
Previous hospitalizations	_____	_____
Allergies _____		
_____		
Physical assessment done	_____	_____
Care plan initiated	_____	_____

Orientation to bedside environment

    Nurse call system _____

    Telephone _____

    Televison _____

    Bed controls _____

    Siderails _____

    Heating/cooling devices _____

    Lighting _____

    Apparel _____

Orientation to hospital environment

    Visiting restrictions _____

    Meals _____

    Nursing staff _____

    Other children _____

    Playroom _____

    Physicians' rounds _____

    Public address system/paging system _____

    Cafeteria service _____

96

Bath of a Child Over 18 Months Old

Overview

Definition

The medium and method of cleansing the body of a child over 18 months of age. The type of bath is varied to meet the needs of each child, that is, a complete bath for an ill child, assistance in the self-bath for a convalescing or older child, and tub or shower bath for those children whose age and condition make either appropriate.

Rationale

Promote the comfort and cleanliness of the child.

Stimulate circulation systemically and locally.

Promote muscle tone by active or passive exercise or both.

Promote elimination from the skin.

Permit careful observation of the child.

Cleanse the skin of the child to remove microorganisms and debris to prevent infection and preserve the integrity of the skin.

Terminology

Complete bed bath: The entire body of the child is washed at the bedside by the nurse or parent

Foreskin: The fold of skin over the glans penis in the male

Partial bath: Only part of the client is bathed, usually at the sink or in the tub

Self-help bath: Bathing by the child without assistance

Assessment

Pertinent Anatomy and Physiology

See Appendix I: *skin.*

Pathophysiological Concepts

1. The skin acts as an exchange surface for body heat and as a vapor barrier to prevent water from leaving the body. Body fluids contain both water and chemical compounds. Electrolytes are compounds that dissociate in solution to form ions, which occurs during the breakdown of the salt ion, sodium chloride (NaCl) into the positively charged sodium ion (Na^+) and the negatively charged chloride ion (Cl^-). Body surface losses of sodium and water increase when there is excessive sweating (as in fever) or when large skin areas have been damaged (as in burns).

2. In adolescents, the sebaceous glands increase in activity as a result of higher hormone levels. The hair follicle openings enlarge to accommodate the greater amounts of sebum. Acne commonly occurs in adolescence. The hair follicle becomes obstructed, causing sebum to accumulate in the follicle. The sebaceous gland eventually is destroyed, releasing fatty acids into the surrounding tissues, causing inflammation. Cleanliness of the skin is important to prevent infection.

3. Moisture in contact with the skin for a prolonged period of time can cause irritation and predispose to the growth of bacteria.

Assessment of the Client

1. Assess the physical condition of the child in determining what type of bath is most suitable. Assess also the age, developmental level of the child, and degree of dexterity and self-control. Assess which bathing method will accomplish the purpose in the safest and most therapeutic way.

2. Assess the condition of the skin during the bath. Observe for signs of trauma, rashes, and abnormal markings or growths. Assess overall coloring.

3. Assess the emotional status of the child. Is the child withdrawn or frightened? Assess tenderness or dependency of a body part or a portion of the body to assess the presence of pain.

4. If the parent bathes the child, assess the parent–child relationship. Determine if the parent is at ease with the child, if the child is comfortable with the parent, if frequent eye contact is made, and the type of communication between the parent and child.

Plan

Nursing Objectives

Promote proper hygiene and comfort for the child.

Observe the child's skin.

Assess the child's range of motion, activity level, and behavior.

Assess the child's physical and emotional status.

Gain insight into the parent–child relationship.

Client Preparation

1. Explain to the child about the bath and encourage active participation to the extent that the child is able.

2. Ensure that the bathing room is warm and that drafts have been eliminated.

3. For a bed bath, remove all of the child's clothing and cover the child with a bath blanket.

4. If a tub bath is allowed, dress the child in a robe. Transport the child to the tub or shower in a manner appropriate to the physical condition. Remain with or near the child during the bath as dictated by the child's age, as well as safety and security needs. Gather all needed items before going to the bathing area so the child will not have to be left unattended.

Equipment

Linen for bed change

Bath blanket

Towel and wash cloth

Pajamas, gown, or hospital gown

Comb, toothbrush, and toothpaste

Orange stick for cleaning nails

Soap, lotion (if desired)

Bath basin for bed bath

Implementation and Interventions

Procedural Aspects

ACTION

RATIONALE

Bed Bath

1. Place the bath articles on the table top out of reach of the small child (Fig. 96-1). Invite and encourage parental participation in activities such as the bath.

Prevent delays caused from having to go after bath articles and promote safety by keeping the small articles out of the child's reach. Parent participation allows assessment and learning by demonstration and return demonstration.

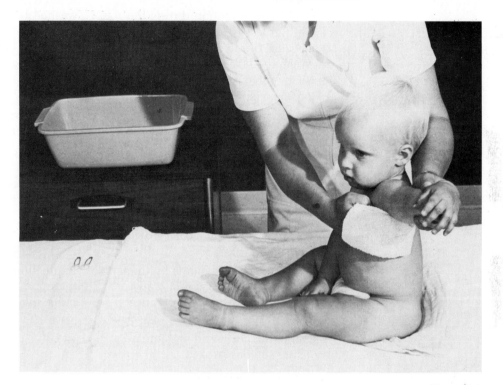

Figure 96.1

2. Fill the bath basin two thirds full of warm water, 43.3° C to 46° C (110° F–115° F). Change the water as necessary to maintain the proper temperature.

Warm temperature relaxes muscles and increases circulation by dilating the blood vessels without burning the child.

3. Perform oral care according to the age of the child (see Technique No. 107, Oral Hygiene for the Infant and Child).

Oral care as a part of the daily bath enhances feelings of comfort and cleanliness.

ACTION	RATIONALE
4. Remove the top linen from the bed and cover the child with a bath blanket.	A bath blanket covering the child during the bath will help to prevent chilling.
5. Fold the washcloth around the hand to prevent dangling against the child's skin. (Use the same technique as is described in Technique No. 28, Baths, Cleansing, in the adult section.)	The dangling washcloth is irritating and may cause water to splash or drip on the child or the linens. Folding the cloth keeps it warmer longer.
6. Bathe the child from top to bottom. Move all body parts through full range of motion during the bath unless contraindicated because of physical condition. Wash the face, with or without soap, depending on the condition of the skin.	The genital and rectal areas are considered contaminated and should be washed last. Moving through range of motion not only exercises the immobile child but allows the nurse to assess range-of-motion capabilities.
Use soap unless the child has a known allergy or unusually dry skin.	Soap decreases surface tension and allows more efficient cleaning.
Wash the child's neck and dry it thoroughly with particular attention given to creases and to the ears.	
Wash and dry the axillary regions and arms.	
Wash the child's hands by immersing them in the basin of water. Clean the nails with an orange stick, if needed.	Immersion aids in dissolving contaminants, removing debris, softens nails, and is refreshing to the child.
Bathe the chest and abdomen, using smooth strokes.	
Bathe and dry the back.	
Wash the legs and feet. The feet may be immersed in the basin of water, if possible.	
Wash and dry the external genitalia. Retract the foreskin of the uncircumcised male child to clean the glans by allowing water to drip over it from the washcloth. This area may be gently cleaned with a cotton swab. If the child is older, allow him to do this procedure for himself.	The glans is very sensitive and should not be roughly rubbed with a washcloth for cleaning; however, it is necessary to ensure that infection is prevented by cleansing the white accumulation of debris that forms under the foreskin.
Comb the child's hair, assist in donning pajamas or a gown, and make the bed.	The child should be returned to a clean environment after the bath.

ACTION	*RATIONALE*
Self-Help Bath	
1. Allow the child to do as much of the bath as possible. Assist only when asked or when the child tires or obviously needs assistance (Fig. 96-2).	Acquisition of self-care skills is a developmental task of the young child. Self-care builds ego and a sense of independence.

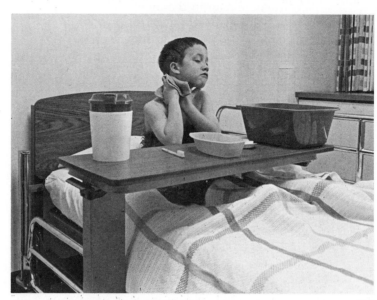

Figure 96.2

2. Remove the top covers and supply a bath blanket. Explain to the child that it may be used to keep warm during the bath. Assist in the removal of the pajamas or gown, if needed. The pajama bottoms or underwear may be left on until the end of the bath, if the child wishes. Place the bath articles within reach of the child.	Some children are extremely sensitive about modesty. Leaving on the pajama bottoms helps to protect the child's sense of modesty and self-image.
3. Assist the child as needed with oral care.	Oral care enhances feelings of well-being.
4. Observe the child's progress. Inspect the child's ears, neck and nails, and assist in care of the genitals as needed. Bathe and dry the child's back. Change the water as needed to keep it warm and comfortable.	Allow as much autonomy as possible, but not at the risk of sacrificing a thorough bath and adequate removal of dirt and debris, which may cause infection or discomfort.
5. Praise the child's efforts during the bath. Assist the child as needed into the gown or pajamas.	Praise and independence help build the concept of self.
6. Leave the child in a clean and comfortable environment. Be sure that toys and needed items are within reach and that siderails are raised to prevent falls.	Always ensure the safety of the client by keeping siderails raised.

Special Modifications

1. The older child may go to the bath tub or shower if physical condition permits. Keep the safety of the child in mind when deciding whether to remain in the room. If there is any danger of the child being accidently burned or drowned, remain in the room with the child. Stay nearby regardless of the child's age, in case assistance is needed.

Cleansing may be more complete when the child is allowed to go to the tub or shower. The safety of the child must be considered, however. Having the nurse nearby is reassuring.

2. The child with an IV may go to the tub or shower if the site is protected. Place a piece of plastic over the IV site and tape securely in place so that water will not penetrate to the site. Avoid prolonged soaking.

The plastic will protect the site from the water. If the area is allowed to soak for an extended time, however, the chance of contamination is greater.

Communicative Aspects

OBSERVATIONS

1. Observe the child during the bath to prevent falls. Do not turn away from the unrestrained child for even a second.
2. Observe the skin for abnormal conditions such as rash or chafing. Observe for abnormalities of the joints, limbs, and other body surfaces.
3. Observe the behavior of the child during the bath. Determine if the child is in pain. Observe for signs that the child is at the expected stage of growth and development. Note whether the child is able to converse with the nurse or parent in a manner expected for the age and condition.
4. Observe the physical condition of the child. Determine if the child is well nourished. Observe any symptoms relating to the condition for which the child is hospitalized.
5. Observe the hair and scalp during and after cleansing for signs of pediculosis, oiliness, scalp conditions, and cuts and abrasions of the scalp.

CHARTING

DATE/TIME	OBSERVATIONS	SIGNATURE
10/30 0930	Child bathed with mild soap. Good skin turgor. Slightly reddened papular rash on left scapula, diameter of area approximately 5 in. Playful during bath; washed own face, arms, and upper torso. Conversing with nurse, no anxiety about nor awareness of impending surgery voiced. ————————	B. Cole RN

Discharge Planning Aspects

CLIENT AND FAMILY EDUCATION

1. Instruct the child to test the water before getting into the tub or shower. This should be done before using the basin of water for a partial bath. This is a good habit to form to prevent accidental burns from getting into water that is too hot.
2. Teach the parents of young children the proper way to bathe a child, with emphasis on cleansing the contaminated areas last. Stress the necessity of cleansing from front to back when cleaning the genitals. If the male child is uncircumcised, the proper way to retract the foreskin and cleanse the glans penis should be taught. This may need to be discussed even with the older child if proper cleansing technique obviously has not been used in the past.

3. Teach the child the principles of good skin care. This is especially important to the prepubescent and pubescent client who already may be experiencing oily skin and acne-related problems.

4. Stress the importance of safety in bathing the child. Small children should *never* be left alone in the tub because they may drown or be burned by accidentally turning on the hot water. Older children should understand the hazards of standing or walking in the tub or shower without a nonskid material on the bottom to prevent falls. Water should always be tested before one gets into the tub or shower to prevent burns.

Evaluation

Quality Assurance

Documentation of the child's bath usually is not made every day unless something extraordinary occurs or is observed. The hospital policy should state the expected frequency of bathing and deviations from this should be addressed in the chart, however. Any observations during bathing should be noted on the chart.

Infection Control

1. Cleansing the accumulated microorganisms from the skin prevents colonization and proliferation into infection.

2. Label the client's equipment, such as the bath basin, so it will not be used for another client inadvertently.

3. Any equipment used for consecutive clients, such as the tub and shower, should be cleaned thoroughly after each use with an antiseptic cleaning solution to prevent cross-contamination.

4. Hands should be washed before and after assisting or bathing a child.

5. The skin is the natural protective barrier of the body. As long as the skin is intact, the chances of infection are minimized. Be careful not to scratch or otherwise traumatize the skin during bathing. Rings should be removed and long fingernails shortened.

Technique Checklist

	YES	NO
Explanation of procedure given before beginning	_____	_____
Hands washed before beginning	_____	_____
Type of bath		
Unassisted _____		
Assisted _____		
Complete _____		
By parent _____		
By nurse _____		
Chilling avoided	_____	_____
Condition of skin noted	_____	_____
Attendance while bathing	_____	_____
Teaching needs identified and addressed	_____	_____
Siderails raised after bath	_____	_____

97   Care of the Burned Child

Overview

Definition

The treatment regimen initiated when a child receives injury to the skin and mucous membranes from thermal, chemical, or electrical sources

Rationale

Reduce the amount of infection.

Prevent cross-contamination.

Enhance new tissue growth and regeneration.

Facilitate rehabilitation to realize maximal health potential.

Maintain a satisfactory psychological outlook.

Terminology

First-degree burn: Reddened skin area without blisters or areas of induration

Second-degree burn: Blistering and peeling of the skin, with some induration and pain on being touched

Third-degree burn: Skin has a leathery appearance with induration; no pain when lightly touched owing to nerve-end damage

Assessment

Pertinent Anatomy and Physiology

1. See Appendix I: *skin.*
2. The skin is about 1 mm thick at birth and increases to approximately twice that thickness at maturity. The ability of the infant and small child to self-moisturize the skin is limited. The skin of young children is more susceptible to superficial bacterial infection.

Pathophysiological Concepts

1. First-degree burns are superficial, with minimal tissue damage. The damaged epithelium peels off in small scalelike patches with no scarring.
2. Second-degree burns may be superficial or deeper, extending into the dermal layer. Superficial second-degree burns cause capillary damage with resulting edema. After 5 days a dried crust covers the wound to protect the regenerating tissue underneath. The crust separates in about 2 weeks with minimal scarring. Deeper second-degree burns heal more slowly, sometimes taking several months to heal completely. The skin is reddened and blisters may be present. Scarring is common and infection often complicates recovery, especially in children, whose skin is thinner than adults.
3. Third-degree burns involve the full thickness of the skin. The skin assumes a tough, leathery appearance. Blistering does not occur, although necrotic vesicles may appear. There is little pain because of anesthesia from destruction of the nerve endings. Skin grafting often is necessary to replace tissue. Systemic effects are usually devastating and involve every system in the body.
4. Systemic responses to burns include swelling in and around the wound as a result of increased capillary permeability and vasodilatation. If the edema is extensive, shock may result from loss of circulating fluid. Fluid loss also precipitates loss of protein and electrolytes.

Assessment of the Client

1. A thermal injury is assessed according to depth of the injury. First, second and third degree are generally used to describe the depth of the burn. First-degree burns involve the epidermal layer only, second-degree burns may involve superficial or deeper dermal depths, and third-degree burns involve full thickness of the skin.

2. Thermal injuries also are assessed according to the percentage of surface area burned. This is normally assessed by using age-related charts (Fig. 97-1). Because the young child has different body proportions than the adult, the "rule of nines" chart customarily used for adults does not reflect accurately the extent of the child's injuries.

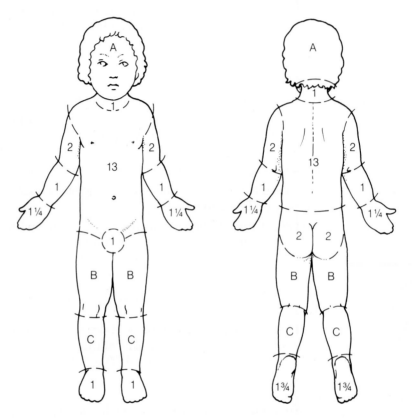

Relative percentages of areas affected by growth

Area	Age 0	1	5
A = ½ of head	9½	8½	6½
B = ½ of one thigh	2¾	3¼	4
C = ½ of one leg	2½	2½	2¾

A

Figure 97.1A

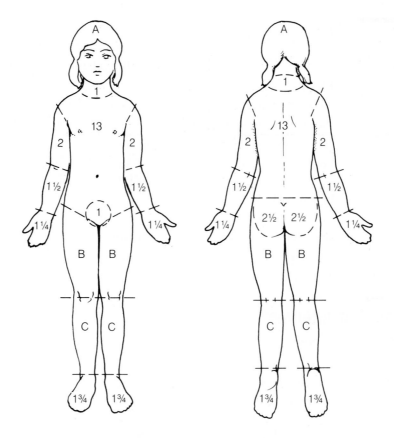

Relative percentages of areas affected by growth

Area	Age 10	Age 15	Adult
A = ½ of head	5½	4½	3½
B = ½ of one thigh	4½	4½	4¾
C = ½ of one leg	3	3¼	3½

B

Figure 97.1B

3. Assess the presence of secondary complications from the burns. Inhalation of heat or toxic fumes may cause serious complications for a child, whose airway may become obstructed from swelling.

4. Assess the type of burn. The burn may be chemical, thermal, or electrical. The preferred method of treatment usually depends on the type of burn to be treated.

5. Assess the health history of the child. Determine any allergies to antibiotics and other drugs. Determine the date of the last tetanus innoculation.

6. Assess the usual dietary habits of the child. Determine what foods the child likes and dislikes. During the recovery phase, adequate nutrition is of primary importance to tissue healing and regeneration. Burned children often suffer from anorexia. Nutrition may be enhanced if the child is offered foods that are desirable to individual taste.

Plan

Nursing Objectives

Provide immediate care to reduce the chance of complications.

Facilitate rehabilitative potential.

Assist the child and parents in coping with the problems of long-term therapy.

Provide psychological support and symptomatic relief.

Protect the client from cross-infection.

Provide fluid, nutrition, and exercise therapy to facilitate healing.

Equipment

Gowns and shoe covers

Intravenous equipment

Dressings and antimicrobial ointments

Graduated urine measurement device

Tracheostomy tray

Implementation and Interventions

Procedural Aspects

ACTION	*RATIONALE*
1. Determine the type of burn. In chemical burn, the priority is adequate cleansing of the exposed area to reduce the duration of exposure to the toxic chemical. Electrical burns may appear minimal and superficial. The full extent of the damage of electrical burns may not be known for several days. Postelectrical burn clients may be placed on a cardiac monitor for the first 48 hours after exposure. Identify the entry and exit points of the electrical current. Thermal burns require immediate attention to prevent shock and irreversible electrolyte imbalance.	The mechanism for tissue damage is contact of the skin with the toxic chemical. Once the chemical is removed, burning stops. Electrical burns may interfere with the electrical activity of the body, especially the brain and heart. Necrosis is possible at the entry and exit points of the electrical current. Thermal burns are a result of contact with a heat source. They may cause both internal and external damage.
2. Scrupulous handwashing must precede any care of burned clients. Wash hands well after care, also.	Mechanical removal of microorganisms by handwashing helps to prevent cross-contamination of clients.
3. Minor burns usually are treated on an outpatient basis. The wound is cleaned and all foreign matter is removed by scrubbing the area with cool water and a nonirritating soap. The wound is rinsed with sterile saline. An antiseptic cream may then be applied to the wound and the area covered by a sterile dressing.	Cool water relieves some of the discomfort and may help to reduce edema. Soap helps to remove microorganisms that may cause infection.

4. The major concern in the management of severe burn victims is airway maintenance. If there are signs of respiratory involvement, administer oxygen and assess blood gases. An endotracheal tube or nasotracheal tube may be inserted to ensure a patent airway. Keep a tracheostomy tray near the bed in case of emergency. Report any sign of respiratory difficulty to the physician at once.

Inhalation of flames may cause edema of the trachea and pulmonary system.

5. Ensure a patent intravenous route for replacement of lost fluids and electrolytes. Administer the fluids requested by the physician.

Water and sodium are lost through the exposed surface in burns. Plasma volume decreases and renal stability is compromised. The imbalance of electrolytes leads to acidosis, which must be corrected with fluid replacement therapy.

6. Reduce the chance of infection by using sterile technique when dressings are changed. Any object that touches the wound should be sterile. If the wound is open, sheets should be sterile. An antimicrobial cream may be applied during dressing change. Tetanus toxoid or booster also may be administered. The Centers for Disease Control recommend that care of the burned client involves efforts to prevent colonization and infection of the wound and precautions to prevent transmission to other clients.

The skin serves as the body's first line of defense against infective microorganisms. When the integrity of the skin is compromised, as it is in burns, infection is likely and care must be taken not to introduce microorganisms into the susceptible area.

7. Provide adequate nutrition to the burned child by whatever route is feasible. If the child is able to eat, offer small, high-calorie feedings at frequent intervals. Nasogastric feedings or total parenteral nutrition (TPN) may be necessary.

The metabolic requirements of burned children are significantly increased. Extra calories, the form of carbohydrates to spare the available protein, will offer the child necessary calories to meet metabolic needs. Calorie requirements may be doubled or tripled, and appetite may be suppressed.

ACTION	**RATIONALE**
8. Treatment of the wound will vary according to the location of the burn and the wishes of the physician. The wound may be cleaned and left exposed to the atmosphere. Strict isolation is usually necessary for this type of treatment. The wound may be covered with an adhesing water-soluble gauze that is covered with a large bandage. Sterile technique during dressing change is needed. Hydrotherapy may be used to soak off the bandages during dressing change, as well as to remove exudate. The wound may be débrided by trimming off loose or dead tissue. Débridement is done only by a physician, therapist, or nurse who has had advanced training in caring for burns. Prepare the child for débridement by administration of an analgesic about 30 minutes before the activity. After débridement, apply ointment to the wound surface with a sterile glove and apply the prescribed dressing. Skin grafting is also a method of treating burns.	The goals of treatment are regeneration of the skin and prevention of infection. Isolation should meet the needs of the situation.
9. Prevent chilling of the child. Heated environmental cribs or beds may be used. Heavy covers on the bed generally are too painful owing to their weight on the wound. If heaters in the room are used, they should be at least 5 ft away from the child. If heat cradles are used, the heat source must be situated away from the child's body and must be secured in such a way that it does not pose a threat to the safety of the child.	Burned skin is unable to regulate the temperature to prevent excessive heat loss. Maintaining the room temperature at an elevated level reduces evaporative loss.
10. Monitor the urine carefully for indications of the status of the child and possible complications. Urine volume should be done every hour. Specific gravity and pH levels should be measured regularly, such as every 8 hours, depending on the child's condition.	A primary goal of burn therapy is the prevention of shock. Infusion of fluids will be dependent on the urinary stability.

ACTION	*RATIONALE*
11. Prevent contractures by proper alignment of the body through positioning and splinting. Encourage the child to move as much as possible. Exercises may be prescribed during the healing phase.	Because of the pain involved, the natural movement of the child will be inhibited.
12. Allow the child to be involved in decisions about care. Burn rehabilitation is slow and tedious. Burns are painful and cause prolonged separation of the child from the family, therefore, their psychological impact is difficult for both the child and the family. Offer encouragement and reassurance. Show respect for the child's worth by allowing choices and supporting the child's decisions.	The psychological impact of burns may have long-lasting effect of the child. Show support, concern, and patience during the rehabilitative process.

Special Modifications

Skin grafts present a special challenge to the pediatric nurse. The grafted area must be immobilized to prevent trauma, bleeding or infection. Special splints or traction may be necessary to immobilize irregular surfaces. Grafts may be left open or covered. Sterile technique must be maintained to prevent infection of the graft area. The dressing on the donor site is undisturbed for about 2 weeks to prevent disruption of the regenerating epithelium.	Permanent grafts are tissues from healthy skin on the child's own body or skin from a compatible second person's body, such as an identical twin. Temporary grafts from other persons or animals may be used to reduce infection and evaporative loss. The object of the permanent graft is to grow and replace the destroyed tissue.

Communicative Aspects

OBSERVATIONS

1. Observe the child for adequate ventilation. If the child begins to show evidence of difficulty breathing, retractions, gasping for breath, or decreased breath sounds, notify the physician at once. Edema of the trachea and respiratory tract must be treated at once to prevent respiratory arrest. Observe the rate and depth of respirations.

2. Observe for adequate fluid and electrolyte balance. Vital constituents of the blood and lymph are lost from oozing through the burned tissue and must be replaced. Dehydration can occur quickly in a child and must be prevented. Overhydration is also a possibility, one that may result in pulmonary edema. Check hourly urine output and color. Note the specific gravity and pH every 8 hours. Note the child's sensorium, vital signs, and the condition of healthy skin as far as turgor to assess dehydration.

3. Observe the wound for signs of infection. Observe for redness around the edges of the wound and purulent drainage from the wound. Observe the progress of wound healing, the condition of the donor sites, movement of the nearby extremities, and the amount of pain that the child is experiencing. Observe the range of motion (ROM) of the child. Watch for drawing up of the ligaments, scar tissue, contracture formation, and the effectiveness of splinting and traction.

4. Observe the nutritional status of the child. Determine the amount eaten, ability to chew and swallow, and the frequency and consistency of bowel movements. If alternative methods of feeding are necessary, such as nasogastric or hyperalimentation fluid, observe to see that healing is taking place and the child is tolerating the feedings without problems (refer to the appropriate technique). Monitor the child's nutrition state by daily weighing and intake and output (I&O) measurement. Watch for vomiting, which may indicate ileus.

CHARTING

DATE/TIME	OBSERVATIONS	SIGNATURE
8/12 1130	Dressings to burned area of left thigh reapplied after whirlpool treatment of area. Silvadene ointment to area and sterile dressing. Areas of granular tissue increasing. No signs of redness or purulent drainage. ROM exercises to right leg with partial ROM to left lower leg and foot done by mother with nurse in attendance. Expressed readiness to learn how to change dressings in anticipation of going home on Tuesday. ———————————	P. Sanchez RN

Discharge Planning Aspects

CLIENT AND FAMILY EDUCATION

1. If the child is treated on an outpatient basis or is sent home with a dressing over the burn, dressing changes may be necessary. Reinforce the physician's directions regarding the frequency of dressing change. If the parents are to dress the burn, explain sterile technique. Show them how to soak the dressing in tepid water for several minutes before removal to reduce discomfort and trauma to the wound area during removal. Describe the signs of infection and ask them to notify their physician at once if infection should develop. Generally, the child may have to be hospitalized if the wound edges become reddened and purulent or if the child shows evidence of fever or cardiac arrhythmias. Show the parents how to measure the child's temperature and pulse. Allow the parents to return the demonstration of dressing change before discharge until they are comfortable with the procedure and perform it satisfactorily.

2. Offer emotional support to the family of the burned child. Often, they will fear for the child's life and will worry about disfigurement. Offer realistic encouragement and answer questions truthfully and as completely as possible. Involve the parents in the child's care to the extent to which they desire and can tolerate.

3. Explain the mechanism of skin grafting, if the child will receive grafts. Explain that temporary grafts are used only for a few days to aid in healing of the child's own skin. If a graft is taken from the child's body, explain about the appearance and care of the donor site and how the family and child can cooperate to enhance the chance of the graft succeeding.

REFERRALS

If the burn is treated on an outpatient basis, a referral to a home health provider may decrease the parents' anxiety about caring for the wound at home. For more extensive burns, the child may be referred to a hospital specializing in burn therapy. Physical therapy may help the child to regain ROM capabilities.

Evaluation

Quality Assurance

Documentation should include a description of the burned area upon admission. Emergency care should be noted along with preventive actions, such as administration of tetanus toxoid. The child's weight and vital signs should be measured to use as a baseline for evaluation of treatment. Attention to the possible development of complications should be noted on the chart. The I&O record should also reflect monitoring of hourly urine to detect renal complications. Any unusual findings should be noted and reported to the physician. The progress of tissue regeneration or graft acceptance or rejection should be noted. If the hydrotherapy is done in a different area, notes from that area should be available for the medical and nursing staff to guide actions and subsequent therapeutic directions. The notes should reflect attention to nutrition and prevention of infection. The nurse should show in the documentation that possible complications were understood and were avoided or reported to the proper person. All health teaching should be noted as well as an assessment of the physical and psychological status of the child. Referrals should be reflected, as well as method of follow-up, to ensure continuity of care.

Infection Control

1. The chief danger in the healing phase of burns is wound infection. Wound cultures should be done regularly, preferably two or three times a week. Dead tissue and exudate provide optimal conditions for the growth of pathogenic organisms. Sterile technique is maintained during care of the burn wound and the donor site.

2. Careful handwashing should be done before and after caring for the child with burns. Because most burns do become infected, the infecting organisms must not be transported to other clients. Isolation technique should meet the goals of preventing infection of the wound and preventing the spread of microorganisms.

3. Equipment used for the treatment of burns, such as whirlpool baths, must be cleaned and disinfected between uses. Equipment used for consecutive clients, such as transport carts, should be cleaned between uses and covered with a sterile sheet if any contact will be made with the burned area.

Technique Checklist

	YES	NO
Cause of burns _____		
Depth of burns _____		
Percentage of body surface involved _____		
Airway patent	_____	_____
Respiratory rate noted q_____hr		
Breath sounds noted q_____hr		
Dyspnea	_____	_____
Choking	_____	_____
Retracting	_____	_____
Nasotracheal tube inserted	_____	_____
Duration _____		
Endotracheal tube inserted	_____	_____
Duration _____		
Tracheostomy performed	_____	_____
Duration _____		

	YES	NO
Fluid and electrolyte balance maintained	_____	_____
Hourly urine noted on chart	_____	_____
Sensorium noted q _____ hr		
Vital signs noted q _____ hr		
IV infusion therapy	_____	_____
Duration _____		
Infection prevented	_____	_____
Cultures q _____ days		
Sterile technique used	_____	_____
Nutrition maintained by		
Oral feedings	_____	_____
Nasogastric feedings	_____	_____
Hyperalimentation fluid	_____	_____
Daily weight recorded	_____	_____
Wound condition noted		
Sterile dressings	_____	_____
Open air method of healing	_____	_____
Skin grafts	_____	_____
Permanent grafts	_____	_____
Temporary grafts _____ (no.)	_____	_____
Mobility maintained by ROM exercises	_____	_____
Splints used _____		
Traction used _____		
Physical therapy	_____	_____
Mobile on discharge	_____	_____
Parents understood		
How to change dressings	_____	_____
Sterile technique	_____	_____
How to do ROM exercises	_____	_____
How to prevent infection	_____	_____
Signs of infection	_____	_____
Complications to watch for	_____	_____
When to call for help	_____	_____

98　Cast Care for the Pediatric Client

Overview

Definition

Observation and nursing intervention that prevents or alleviates complications resulting from application of temporary external support to immobilize the bone and enhance healing

Rationale

Maintain the desired anatomical position of the appropriate part of the body.

Alleviate pain and swelling by preventing trauma to the periosteum and soft tissue.

Prevent or correct deformities and contractures.

Provide traction for reduction of a fracture.

Terminology

Blanching: Pressing the nailbed to ascertain circulatory impairment. If circulation is normal, the nail should whiten momentarily and quickly return to normal color.

Fracture: A break in the continuity of a bone; types of fractures are

Avulsion: Muscle damage with separation of small fragments of bone cortex at the site of attachment of a ligament or tendon (also called a ''chip'' fracture or sprain fracture)

Capillary: A fracture appearing on x-ray film as a fine, hairlike line; sometimes seen in fractures of the skull

Closed: A fracture in which there is no wound on the body surface that communicates with the break in the bone (also called a simple fracture)

Colles': A break in the lower end of the radius

Comminuted: A fracture in which two or more communicating breaks divide the bone into more than two fragments

Complete: A fracture involving the entire cross section of the bone

Compound: A fracture in which a wound communicates from the bone to the skin surface as the result of trauma to both soft tissues and bone (also called an open fracture)

Compression: A fracture resulting when one bony surface is forced against an adjacent surface

Depressed: A fracture in which a fragment of bone is forced beneath its normal contour line

Durverney's: A fracture of the ilium below the anterosuperior spine

Greenstick: An incomplete fracture of a long bone; only one side of the periosteum is affected (also called interperiosteal fracture)

Impacted: A fracture in which a portion of the fractured bone is driven into another portion

Monteggia's: A fracture in the proximal half of the shaft of the ulna with dislocation of the head of the radius

Oblique: A fracture occurring at a 45° angle to the bone shaft

Pathologic: A fracture occurring in diseased bone, with little or no trauma involved

Pott's: A fracture of the lower part of the fibula, with serious injury of the articulation of the lower tibia

Spiral: A fracture that twists around the bone shaft

Trophic: A fracture caused by a metabolic disturbance that weakens the bone

Full-leg cast: A cast extending from midthigh to toes

Hanging cast: A cast extending from the axilla to the fingers, usually with a bend in the elbow

Manual traction: Act of exerting pull by the hands distal to the injured site to achieve healing of the bone

Plaster of Paris: Quick-drying substance used in rolls as a casting material

Plastic cast (fiberglass cast): A cast made of a plasticlike material that performs the same function as the plaster cast but is lighter

Reduction of fracture: Restoration of the proper position of the fragments of a fractured bone. Types of reduction are

Closed: Reduction by external manipulation and application of a cast to maintain immobilization

Open: Reduction performed under direct visualization during surgery, with some sort of internal or external fixation

Short-leg cast: A cast extending from below the knee to the toes

Spica cast: A cast involving a great portion of the main trunk of the body, front and back, and possibly one or more extremities

Spreaders: An instrument used to spread or loosen a cast that is too tight

Stockinette: A soft cloth used under the cast, next to the skin, to protect delicate tissue and promote comfort

Assessment

Pertinent Anatomy and Physiology

See Appendix I: *bone repair, skin, skeletal system.*

Pathophysiological Concepts

1. During fracture repair, osteogenic cells move into the area within a relatively short period and fill the gap between the bone parts. If this does not occur, fibroblasts will enter the area and fill the gap with fibrous tissue. This tissue has no affinity for calcium, resulting in nonunion of the fracture ends.

2. There must be appropriate amounts of both organic and inorganic constituents to have functional bone tissue for support and protection. A dietary deficiency of calcium and phosphate interferes with normal calcification and results in a condition called rickets. This condition, found in infants and children, is usually the result of a deficiency of vitamin D.

Assessment of the Client

1. Assess the location and appearance of the fracture or the cast. Assess the amount and location of any pain. Assess the amount of physical limitation caused by the cast and its potential effect on the client. Assess any other physical problems that may or may not relate directly to the fracture but that may affect the hospitalization. Assess baseline vital signs.

2. Assess the developmental stage of the client. Determine the amount of mobility normally present and how the fracture will affect this. Determine the understanding level of the client in offering explanations for actions.

3. Assess the parent–child relationship. Determine the emotional status of the parent(s) and assess the amount of assistance that they can reasonably be expected to give in caring for the physical and emotional needs of the child. Determine also the amount of support they will need in coping with the hospitalization of their child.

4. Assess the home situation to which the child will be returning. Assess this situation in relation to the ability of the child in the cast to adapt to the environment. Note the presence of stairs, siblings, and any other environmental factors that will influence the child's ability to fit into the home environment in the altered state.

Plan

Nursing Objectives

Ensure that the activities of the child in a cast are as normal as possible.

Prevent excreta of the infant or young child from soiling the cast.

Maintain immobilization and desired anatomic position.

Provide adequate skin care.

Prevent pressure on nerves and pressure areas under the cast.

Prevent the child from damaging the cast or injuring the involved area.

Assist the family to feel and be competent in caring for the child after discharge.

Client Preparation

1. Be careful when removing the child's clothing on admission. Remove clothing from the unaffected extremity first, then from the affected extremity. Clothing removal should proceed in any manner that will disturb the injured part least. Handle the injured limb as little as possible.

2. A young child may be prepared for cast application by having a small cast put on one of the child's dolls. Some hospitals have sample casts made for clients to see before application.

3. Determine whether medication for pain is needed before cast application.

4. An explanation of what will happen during cast application should be made before beginning the procedure. This explanation should be given to the parents and to the child who is old enough to understand and benefit from such a discussion. Discussion of the need to remain still while the cast is drying should be offered. Explain that the cast will be warm at first because the casting material is dipped in warm water before being applied.

5. Bedboards may be placed under the mattress to support the weight and pressure of the cast.

6. Prepare the child for an extended period in bed by encouraging emptying of the bowels and bladder, if possible. Provide some type of diversionary material for the hours ahead.

Equipment

Cast application materials, which might include a container of warm water, stockinette and plaster in all sizes or plastic (fiberglass) casting material, and any other supplies requested or routinely used by the physician applying the cast

Implementation and Interventions

Procedural Aspects

ACTION

1. Assist the physician or practitioner who is applying the cast by holding the extremity in the desired alignment or by restraining the client as needed.

2. Keep the cast in correct alignment until drying is complete, which usually requires 24 hours. The cast should be turned frequently during this time, at least every 2 hours. Always handle the cast with the palms of the hands, not the fingers (Fig. 98-1). Do not apply bed covers over the casted limb until the cast is dry. The cast is dry when it no longer feels damp or slightly soft to the touch.

RATIONALE

The cast must be applied with the limb in normal alignment for proper healing to occur. The young child may need assistance in holding still during casting.

The goal of casting is to hold the extremity or bone immobile until healing is complete. The cast fits snugly when applied. Applying local pressure on the damp cast by handling it with the fingertips may cause abnormal pressure points. Exposing the cast to circulating air hastens drying.

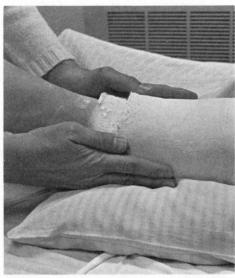

Figure 98.1

3. Check the toes or fingers every hour during the first 24 hours for early signs of circulatory impairment. These signs include numbness, tingling, unusual color, skin cool to touch, obvious edema, and continuous blanching of the nailbeds. If seepage of blood should occur through the cast material, encircle its exact perimeter and date it so that future seepage can be evaluated (Fig. 98-2). Call any new or additional drainage to the attention of the physician and note it in the chart. A warm spot on the cast may indicate infection. A window may be cut in the cast to

The cast tends to shrink slightly as it dries. This may cause inhibition of proper circulation and result in swelling of the affected area. Adequate documentation may provide a baseline against which future developments may be measured to determine the seriousness of swelling and drainage. Impairment of circulation can result in irreparable damage and even permanent loss of function.

ACTION

provide direct visualizaiton of the involved area. After the first 24 hours, the cast usually is checked every 4 hours or more often as indicated.

RATIONALE

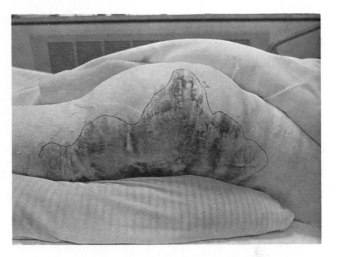

Figure 98.2

4. Poor venous return is common in an injured body part. After the cast is dry, the casted extremities should be elevated with all contours supported to prevent cracking. Ice may be ordered to reduce edema.

Cold applications constrict blood vessels, anesthetize nerve endings, and aid in blood coagulation.

5. Place protective, waterproof material on the casts of infants and children who cannot control urination or stools. Elevate the head of the bed slightly, if allowed. Line the edges of the cast with plastic or other waterproof material (Fig. 98-3).

Continuous contact with moisture breaks down the integrity of the cast. Elevating the head of the bed helps to prevent urine or stool from seeping under the cast.

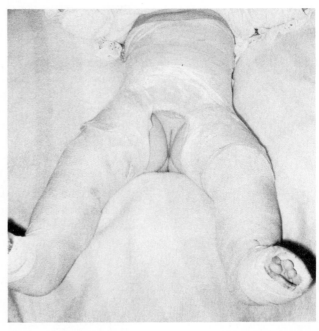

Figure 98.3

ACTION	*RATIONALE*
6. Line the rough edges of the cast with padding, if they have not been padded already, to prevent contact with moisture.	Padding promotes comfort and prevents trauma to the delicate skin.
7. Keep small toys and objects out of the reach of young children. Devices for scratching under the cast should not be used for infants and children no matter how much they itch. A musty odor coming from under the cast may indicate pus formation and infection	Foreign items pushed under the cast by the young child may result in pressure areas and skin irritation. Scratches under the cast can easily become infected because of the warm, dark, moist environment, which facilitates the growth of bacteria.
8. Two persons are needed to turn the child in the spica (body) cast. One should be on each side of the child's bed. Never use the support bar of the cast to turn the child.	Abnormal pressure on the suport bar may injure the child or complicate fracture healing. It also may compromise the integrity of the cast.
9. Proper body alignment and positioning are extremely important to the child in a cast. Change the child's position frequently. Pinching of skin and formation of pressure areas on bony prominences must be avoided.	Position change facilitates chest expansion and helps to prevent respiratory problems from stasis or pooling of secretions. Pinching or pressure on the skin areas may result in tissue breakdown. In proper alignment, no strain is placed on the joints, muscles, bones, or connective tissues. Strain may cause pain or structural problems.
10. Immobilize the infant or young child during cast removal. Support the involved limb on pillows following cast removal.	The casted limb may be sensitive or weakened owing to the forced immobility or restrictions of the cast.
11. Following cast removal, the skin may be flaky, and the muscles and joints sore and stiff. Wash these areas gently with a mild soap and warm water.	Careful removal of exudates and secretions may prevent trauma to the sensitive skin.

Communicative Aspects

OBSERVATIONS

1. Observe the child for signs and symptoms of pressure areas and skin breakdown. The main indicator is pain. It is usually continuous and intense at the site of the pressure. An older child will be able to show the nurse where the pressure is. The infant or younger child will be fussy and irritable. A sudden cessation of irritability after a period of several days may indicate that the pressure and skin breakdown have progressed to the point of numbing the nerve endings and loss of sensation. An odor generally characterizes skin breakdown; this may be a valid observation of cast problems.

2. Observe the skin around the edge of the cast for trauma. Observe the edges of the cast to see that they remain intact and do not break causing rough edges against the skin.

3. Check symptoms of nerve and circulatory impairments hourly until all symptoms are negative. Check the toes and fingers for the following signs:

   Color (blanching sign)

   Sensation (numbness and tingling)

   Edema

   Temperature

   Mobility

   Pain

   Skin irritation (around the cast edge)

4. Bleeding may occur is there is a wound. Observe for bleeding at frequent intervals. As previously noted, circumscribe the area on the cast to determine if bleeding or drainage is continuing.

5. Bony prominences, such as the heels, may develop pressure areas if allowed to remain on the bed. Check these areas frequently to determine if redness is present and to determine methods to alleviate any pressure.

6. Detection of a foul odor or a hot spot on the cast may indicate an infectious area beneath.

CHARTING

DATE/TIME	OBSERVATIONS	SIGNATURE
12/5 1345	Left leg elevated on pillows with knee supported. Toes show no swelling, movement without pain or difficulty, nails blanch well, and no pain or discomfort expressed. B/P 110/70, P 94, R 18, T 99.4°. ————————	P. Sanchez RN

Discharge Planning Aspects

CLIENT AND FAMILY EDUCATION

1. Involve the young child in the teaching plan and process. Encourage the parents to participate actively in the care of their child while in the hospital so that the transition from hospital to home will be less traumatic.

2. Instruct the child and family to observe for symptoms of nerve and circulatory impairment. Explain about the danger of the pressure areas, how to detect them, and when to call the physician.

3. Teach the child and family about the importance of isometric exercise to maintain muscle tone in the casted extremity. Simply tightening and relaxing the muscles will help maintain tone and prevent degeneration of the muscle tissue.

4. If the child will need aids after discharge, instruct the child and family about care of the sling, crutches, walker, or whatever aid is used. Demonstrate proper use of the aid and how to prevent accidents.

5. Explain to the child and family about the casting procedure and immediate care thereafter. Emphasize the importance of keeping the cast still for the first 24 hours while it is drying. Explain about safety factors, such as avoiding inserting anything under the cast and proper support when arising owing to the altered center of gravity.

REFERRALS

Give the family the name(s) of available orthopedic appliance suppliers in the event that they may need to replace such items as slings, crutch pads, or traction equipment after discharge. A home halth nurse referral might be in order if adjustment to the cast has been slow or if the home environment may pose hazards to recovery.

Evaluation

Quality Assurance

Documentation should include the child's initial reaction to the cast. Appearance and condition of the affected limb should be noted before and after application. The documentation should reflect that the nurse knew the signs of circulatory impairment and took precautions to avoid, recognize, or alleviate them. The child's progressive adaptation to the cast should be noted. The appearance of any side-effects should be documented, as well as the management and preventive efforts. Health teaching to the family and child should be noted. If demonstrations of care were offered and returned, assess the degree of understanding and anticipated compliance with medical restrictions after discharge.

Infection Control

1. Handwashing is essential before and after handling the child in a cast. Transmission of hospital-acquired infections must be avoided.

2. If a wound or incision is present under the cast, it is dressed using sterile technique before the cast is applied. The cast must be observed closely for signs of infection as healing progresses.

3. Scratching under the cast may cause tissue breakdown and result in infection. Pressure on surrounding parts also may result in tissue breakdown and eventual infection of otherwise healthy tissue.

Technique Checklist

	YES	NO
Cast application and restrictions		
Explained to child	_____	_____
Explained to parents	_____	_____
Extremity checked q_____ min		
For _____ hr		
Color _____		
Sensation _____		
Edema _____		
Temperature _____		
Mobility _____		
Pain _____		
Skin irritation _____		
Signs of bleeding on cast noted during hospitalization	_____	_____
Date _____		
Bleeding or drainage reported to physician	_____	_____
Date _____		
Cast dried without incident	_____	_____
Child mobile with cast	_____	_____
Discharge instructions on cast care at home	_____	_____

99   Endotracheal Intubation

(Note: Endotracheal intubation is a highly skilled procedure, which requires advanced training and experience. This technique is offered to provide insight into how the procedure is done so that adequate assistance may be given to the experienced intubator. This technique is *not* intended to be used as sole preparation for endotracheal intubation.)

Overview

Definition

Insertion of a hollow tube into the trachea to provide a patent airway; accomplished by means of a bladed instrument

Rationale

Provide adequate respiratory care.

Prevent aspiration.

Provide a means of mechanical ventilation or high concentrations of oxygen.

Facilitate suctioning of the bronchial tree.

Terminology

Hypoxia: Varying degrees of inadequacy of oxygen supply

Mucus: The liquid lining of the mucous membrane composed of secretions of the glands along with various inorganic salts, desquamated cells, and leukocytes

Patent: Open, unobstructed

Tracheostomy: The surgical creation of a vertical slit in the anterior portion of the neck (usually below the first and second tracheal cartilage) with the insertion of a cannula airway to facilitate adequate exchange of gases

Assessment

Pertinent Anatomy and Physiology

1. See Appendix I: *bronchial tree, lungs, trachea.*
2. Adequate oxygen must enter the lungs to aerate the blood. This oxygenated blood travels to the tissues, where it is exchanged for carbon dioxide; thus, metabolism is supported. If the amount of oxygen entering the lungs is insufficient to meet circulatory needs, acidosis results. Prolonged acidosis is incompatible with life.

Pathophysiological Concepts

1. The newborn usually is intubated immediately if the Apgar Score is less than 3. If the infant has traveled through a septic birth canal or one filled with meconium, intubation may be done to prevent the initial inspired breath from drawing the undesirable fluid into the lungs.
2. Excessive bronchial secretions often occur in diseases of children. These secretions cannot always be controlled or expelled by the child because of the narrowness of the tracheobronchial tree and the underdeveloped muscles of the thorax. If these secretions are allowed to build up and pool in the lungs, the fluid-filled air sacs cannot perform their function of gaseous exchange adequately. The blood does not receive enough oxygen to meet the needs of the body.

Assessment of the Client

1. Assess the respiratory adequacy of the infant to determine when endotracheal intubation may be necessary. Assess the infant or child to determine cyanosis, grunting respirations, nasal flaring, or other signs of respiratory distress. Blood determinations of PCO_2 and PO_2 levels will aid in assessment of the adequacy of respiratory effort.

2. Assess the child for history of respiratory problems, including asthma, bronchitis, and croup. Identify familial tendencies to respiratory difficulties.

3. Assess the presence of any loose teeth in the school-aged child. Tooth loss or damage is occasionally an unavoidable complication of endotracheal intubation. Knowledge about the presence of loose teeth may allow dislodged teeth to be recovered before they are aspirated.

Plan

Nursing Objectives

Establish a patent airway.

Provide adequate humidification of the respiratory system.

Prevent tracheal injury.

Avoid introduction of foreign particles into the respiratory system.

Maintain respiratory integrity by mechanical ventilation, if necessary.

Client Preparation

1. Ensure adequate ventilation until the endotracheal tube is inserted. This can be accomplished by mouth-to-mouth ventilation or by the use of a manual ventilatory assistance device (Figs. 99-1, 99-2).

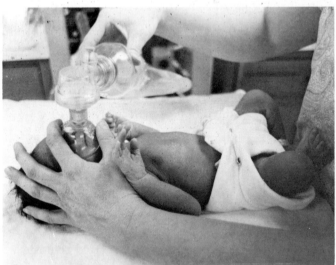
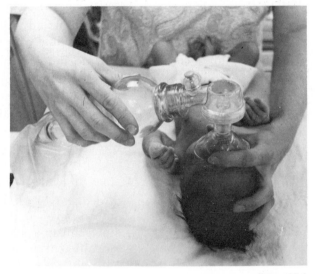

Figure 99.1   *Figure 99.2*

2. Explain what is happening to the parents if there is time. If they understand why the endotracheal tube is necessary and what will be accomplished by inserting it, they may be reassured and less anxious about the procedure.

3. Check the laryngoscope light before use to make sure it is in working order.

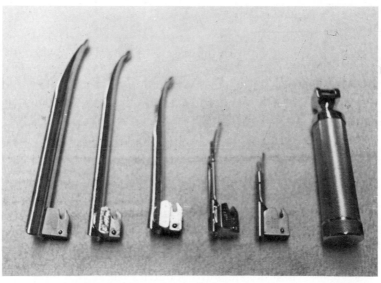

Figure 99.3

Equipment

Manual ventilatory assistance device
Oxygen source
Suction capacity
Suction tray (including sterile gloves, saline solution, and catheter)
Laryngoscope
Endotracheal tubes (varied sizes: 2.5, 3, 3.5, 4, 4.5) and stylets (Fig. 99-3)
Tapes and ties
Water-soluble lubricant

Implementation and Interventions

Procedural Aspects

ACTION	RATIONALE
1. Place the child on a flat surface. Tilt the head back but do not hyperextend. Elevate the shoulders with a rolled towel.	Hyperextension in the very young may cause collapse of the flexible airway and heighten asphyxia.
2. Determine what size of tube will fit comfortably and snugly into the child's trachea. Apply a lubricant to the endotracheal tube before insertion.	The endotracheal tube is a soft, malleable device that fits the contours of the child's airway. Although this soft texture facilitates comfort after insertion, it may make insertion more difficult. To provide the amount of strength and rigidity to insert the tube properly, a stylet may be inserted into the tube before the child is intubated. The stylet is made of a harder substance and can be bent to fit the insertion path. Once the endotracheal tube is in place, the stylet is removed. A lubricant helps decrease the resistance to insertion by reducing friction.

ACTION

RATIONALE

3. The experienced intubator will proceed with intubation in the following manner:

Hold the client's mouth open and tilt the head backward to provide a straight pathway for visualization and insertion. Introduce the laryngoscope blade along the right side of the mouth so that it pushes the tongue to the left. The epiglottis appears as a small flap of tissue. Lift gently to expose the vocal cords. Suction may be necessary at this time. The endotracheal tube is inserted into the larynx past the epiglottis about 1.5 cm beyond the vocal cords.

Damage to the trachea and vocal cords can cause permanent disability. It requires a great deal of practice and skill to intubate properly, and this technique should be undertaken only by qualified personnel.

4. After the intubation is complete, aspirate secretions from the tube and trachea. Suctioning should be done using sterile technique.

Suctioning of the endotracheal tube provides access to the tracheobronchial tree. Anything entering the lung area should be sterile to reduce the chance of infection.

5. Check the endotracheal tube for proper placement. Administer several quick breaths with a respiratory assistance device. Auscultate the lungs and stomach. If the "whooshing" sound of the air can be heard in the stomach, the tube is in the esophagus and must be removed and reinserted into the trachea. If the air can be heard upon auscultation of the lungs, the tube is probably placed properly. If air can be heard only on the right side, the tube may be inserted too far. Radiologic examination can verify the tube placement.

If the tube is placed in the esophagus, it will inflate the stomach, and the lungs will not benefit from aeration attempts. If the tube is inserted too far into the lungs, it may enter the right bronchus and aerate only the right lung.

6. Secure the tube by means of tape and ties around the back of the child's neck. Place a mark on the tube at the lip level so the tube can be checked for placement.

Coughing or movement of the child may cause the tube to become dislodged if it is not secured. A mark at lip level will allow the nurse to determine if the tube is slipping out.

7. The tube should be connected to a humidified oxygen source or to a mechanical ventilator.

The nose performs the task of warming and humidifying inspired air. When the inspired air bypasses the nose, it must be humidified to prevent drying out of lung tissue. A humidification device with sterile water can be attached to the oxygen source to provide inspired air of the proper oxygen concentration, temperature, and humidity.

Communicative Aspects

OBSERVATIONS

1. Observe to determine proper tube placement. Signs of esophageal intubation include abdominal distension, belching of air, absent or diminished breath sounds, and audible "whooshing" sound during manual ventilation when the stomach is auscultated.

2. Observe for possible complications of endotracheal intubation, such as lacerations of the mucous lining of the mouth and airway, tooth loss, hypoxemia, cardiac arrhythmia, aspiration, tracheal rupture, and tracheoesophageal fistula.

3. Observe the child's vital signs carefully after intubation. Observe for cardiac arrhythmias. It is vital to monitor the newborn's temperature because chilling increases oxygenation demands that have been compromised already.

4. Observe the amount, consistency, and color of the secretions suctioned from the child's respirtory tract. Note the position in which the best suctioning results are obtained. Observe the ability and willingness of the child to comply with the instructions during suctioning. Observe the child's reaction to the suctioning.

5. Observe the status of the tube to determine proper placement and to ensure that the tube is not being dislodged or slipping from its proper place. Signs of dislodgment include grunting or similar noises from the child, or speaking by the child. Auscultate the breath sounds. If the sounds can be heard in only one side of the chest, the tube probably has slipped into the bronchus.

6. Observe the extremities if restraints are used. Check frequently for adequate circulation and comfort.

7. Observe the blood gas evaluations to determine the adequacy of ventilation efforts.

8. Observe the child for signs of impending respiratory difficulty or tube blockage, which include restlessness, dyspnea, pallor, cyanosis, changes in vital signs, retractions, and noisy respirations.

CHARTING

DATE/TIME	OBSERVATIONS	SIGNATURE
4/9 0830	Endotracheal tube No. 3.5 F inserted by J.Ames, pediatric nurse practitioner with no complications. Audible breath sounds bilaterally. Connected to ventilator: Resp rate 60, 50% O_2, 20 cm pressure, 2–4 cm positive end-expiratory pressure (PEEP). Hands restrained. Child remains lethargic, color improved slightly. T 102.4° R, P 104, R 24 (with ventilator). Entire procedure explained to parents, who gave consent to procedure. Mother with child at this time. States that she understands what to watch for and will call the nurse if problems arise. Child remains in Pediatric ICU. ———————————	N. Jones RN

Discharge Planning Aspects

CLIENT AND FAMILY EDUCATION

1. The parents should be told why the procedure is to be done. They should understand why and how long the tube must remain in place. They should be told to report any signs of tube dislodgement (e.g., cyanosis, change in rate or quality of breathing, or physical appearance of tube).

2. Explain the need for restraints (i.e., the child might pull the tube out). Emphasize the importance of having someone remain in constant attendance. Inability to make a sound or cry out is very frightening to the child. Someone should maintain eye contact with the child in case of emergency. Older children can be taught to summon help with the call light. Writing materials or other communication tools should be available so the child can communicate with others.

Evaluation

Quality Assurance

Documentation should include signs and symptoms that precipitated the decision to intubate the child. The name and classification of the intubator also should be noted. Any problems with the intubation should be reflected, as well as outcome. The chart should show evidence that the nurse knew which parameters to monitor and acted accordingly. Teaching and reassurance of the parents should be reflected. Ventilatory assistance devices should be checked at regular intervals. These intervals usually will be determined by hospital policy. The chart should show evidence that monitoring of devices was done in accordance with hospital policy. Removal of the tube should be documented with an assessment of the child before and after tube removal.

Infection Control

1. Careful handwashing is essential before and after insertion, suctioning, or care of the endotracheal tube.
2. Secondary infection is a major concern when the air entering the lower airway (bronchi) bypasses the natural defense of the upper airway. All equipment coming in contact with the endotracheal tube therefore should be sterile.
3. If the child has a contagious respiratory infection, masks should be worn during intubation and subsequent care of the tube.
4. All reusable equipment should be sent for cleaning and disinfection. Equipment used consecutively for infants and children must be cleaned thoroughly between uses.
5. Intubation and suctioning of the tube should be done under sterile conditions.

Technique Checklist

	YES	NO
Procedure explained to parents	_____	_____
Procedure explained to child	_____	_____
Intubation done by _____		
Signs and symptoms that indicated the need for endotracheal intubation		
Apgar <3 _____		
Cyanosis _____		
Retracting _____		
Blood PO_2 and PCO_2 values _____		
Complications of intubation _____		
Humidification device _____		
Someone remained with child at all times	_____	_____
Adequate aeration accomplished	_____	_____
Endotracheal tube removed on _____		

100 Enema for the Pediatric Client

Overview

Definition

The process of introducing a stream of solution into the rectum or lower colon and draining it off by natural or artificial means

Rationale

Cleanse or remove accumulated solids or gases from the lower bowel.

Stimulate peristalsis in the bowel.

Cleanse the bowel in preparation for x-ray examination or surgery.

Terminology

Feces: Body wastes, including food residue, bacteria, epithelium, and mucus, discharged from the bowels by way of the anus

Flatus: Gas in the digestive tract

Peristalsis: Progressive contraction movement occurring involuntarily in the hollow body tubes (*i.e.,* alimentary canal). The contraction and relaxation of the musculature forces contents through the tube.

Assessment

Pertinent Anatomy and Physiology

1. See Appendix I: *anus, intestine (large), rectum.*
2. The rectum varies in length according to age of the child. Approximate length is: infant, 1 to 1½ in (2.5 cm–3.8 cm); toddler, 2 in (5 cm); preschool-aged child, 3 in (7.5 cm); school-aged child, 4 in (10 cm).
3. The infant or small child does not have the sensory control of the rectum and anus to retain the enema fluid; therefore, the enema usually is given over a bedpan or pad.

Pathophysiological Concepts

1. Diarrhea in infants is a fairly common symptom of a variety of conditions. It may be mild, with only a small amount of dehydration. If unchecked, however, normal alkaline secretions and fluids are lost, resulting in metabolic acidosis and dehydration. Inflammation and edema of the mucosal membranes results, which may develop into chronic diarrhea. Diarrhea often is associated with food allergy or contamination.
2. Hirschsprung's disease, or congenital aganglionic megacolon, is characterized by obstinate constipation resulting from partial or complete intestinal obstruction of mechanical origin. The condition is manifested after the congenital absence of parasympathetic ganglion cells within the wall of the colon and rectum results in an absence of peristalsis. This results in a narrowing of segments of the colon with reciprocal overfilling and dilatation of the segments above the affected area. Severe constipation with abnormal stools is common.

Assessment of the Client

1. Assess the child in relation to the reason for hospitalization. Assess past bowel habits and when the last bowel movement occurred. Determine whether the child is bowel trained and what words or phrases the child uses to signify the need to empty the bowels.

2. Assess the child's and parents' familiarity with the enema procedure. Determine the amount of teaching needed to meet the family's needs. Assess the age and understanding of the child when determining how much information to provide.

3. Assess the size and shape of the child's abdomen. Determine the usual form of the stool. When megacolon is present, the stool frequently will take the form of small pellets or small, ribbonlike bands.

Plan

Nursing Objectives

Enlist the child's cooperation, if possible.

Carry out the treatment as quickly and efficiently as possible to prevent trauma and discomfort.

Allay the anxiety of the parents by allowing them to stay with the child during the procedure, if desired, or by keeping them informed before and after the procedure.

Ensure a safe atmosphere by proper positioning, organizing and checking equipment before beginning, and adequate instruction to the child or restraint of the child as needed.

Observe and record carefully the child's reactions and results of the enema.

Client Preparation

1. Explain to the parents why the procedure is needed and what the expected outcomes are. Include the child in this explanation according to age and level of understanding. The child should know what is going to happen. The degree of detail of the explanation should be determined after discussion with the parents and determination of the anxiety and comprehension levels of the child.

2. Familiarize the child with the equipment. Explain the technique of mouth breathing, if the child can understand without becoming frightened. Explain that this type of breathing helps relax the muscles.

3. Position the child in the proper manner.

   Infant: Place a pillow lengthwise on the bed with the bedpan next to it (Fig. 100-1). Lay the infant on the pillow with the buttocks extended over the broad edge of the bedpan (Fig. 100-2). The assistance of the infant's parents may be enlisted to position or to divert the child's attention (Fig. 100-3).

   Older child: Because the descending colon is on the left side of the abdomen, gravity may be used to aid the flow of solution into the colon by positioning the child on the left side with knees flexed. Flexion of the knees produces abdominal relaxation, reducing discomfort and decreasing pressure. If the child is unable to retain the solution, however, give the enema with the child on the bedpan. Pad unsupported areas, such as the lower back, so that the child is comfortable.

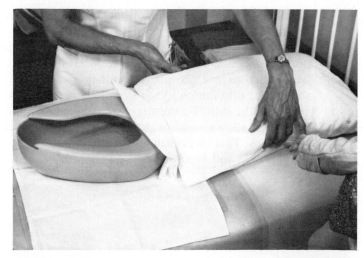

Figure 100.1

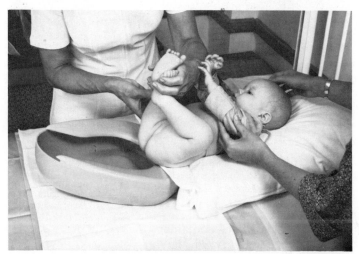

Figure 100.2

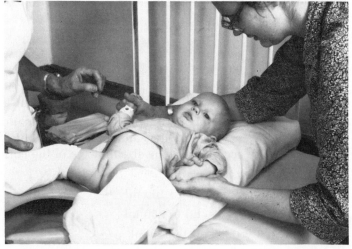

Figure 100.3

4. Ensure that the proper type of enema has been prepared according to the physician's prescribed treatment. Tap water enemas are not given to pediatric clients. It is essential to avoid giving a tap water enema to the child suffering from megacolon. The expanded surface of the colon, because of the accumulation of feces and gas, provides a larger-than-normal surface from which absorption into the child's system may occur. Water is hypotonic and causes a rapid fluid shift. Furthermore, the absence or decreased effectiveness of peristalsis allows additional time for the water to be absorbed into surrounding tissues. This can result in overhydration of the child, resulting in syncope, shock, and even death.

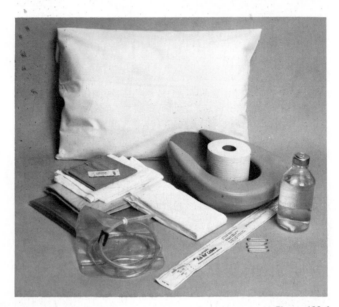

Figure 100.4

Equipment (Fig. 100-4)
Disposable enema container
Bath thermometer
Pediatric rectal tube
   Infant: #12 to #14 French
   Small child: #14 to #16 French
   School-aged child: #16 to #18 French
Bedpan and tissue (potty chair for toddlers)
Water-soluble lubricant
Linen: bath blanket, diaper for infants, hip pad, towel, pillow, and wash cloth
Solutions (as prescribed). Infants and preschool children usually are unable to retain as much solution as are older children; therefore, the amount given will vary according to the size and age of the child.

Suggested amounts
Birth to 3 mo: 30 ml to 100 ml
3 mo to 1 yr: 100 ml to 250 ml
1 yr to 6 yr: 200 ml to 500 ml
6 yr to 12 yr: 500 ml to 1000 ml

Types of solution
Soapsuds enema: 500 ml water, 2 dr soap
Saline enema: 500 ml water, 1 dr salt
Premixed, commercially prepared enemas: Administer according to directions on package.

Implementation and Interventions

Procedural Aspects

ACTION

1. Check the temperature of the solution with a bath thermometer. The proper temperature is 100° F (37.8° C)

2. Lubricate the lower 2 in to 3 in (5 cm–7.5 cm) of the rectal tube.

3. Expel air from the tubing before insertion into the rectum by allowing the solution to run down to the tip of the rectal tube.

4. Insert the rectal tube into the child's rectum slowly, to a depth of 2 in to 3 in (5 cm–7.5 cm) depending on the child's size (Fig. 100-5). Encourage mouth breathing during insertion.

RATIONALE

Heat is effective in stimulating the nerve plexus in the intestinal mucosa. The temperature of the solution, the length of the tubing, and the rate of flow all influence the temperature of the solution as it enters the bowel.

Friction and discomfort are reduced by lubrication of the intrusive surface.

Air introduced into the colon before the solution may overdistend the walls, stimulating peristalsis and discomfort.

Slow insertion of the tube minimizes spasms of the intestinal wall. Mouth breathing relaxes the anal sphincter and facilitates insertion.

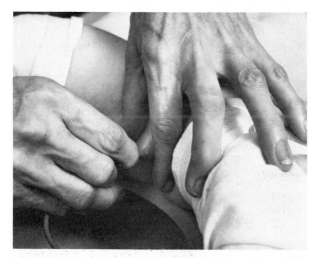

Figure 100.5

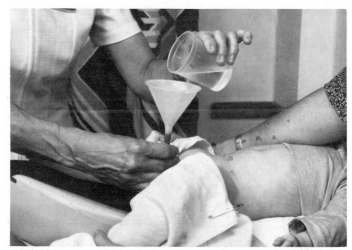

Figure 100.6

5. Elevate the enema container to a sufficient height to initiate flow of the solution. For an infant, the enema container is usually held no more than 3 in (7.5 cm) above the body level (Fig. 100-6). For older children, a height of 12 in (30 cm) or less usually is sufficient to instill the solution without causing cramping. The solution should not be elevated above a height of 18 in (45 cm). Mouth breathing may aid relaxation.

The higher the solution is held, the faster it flows into the rectum. Rapid insertion may cause cramping and discomfort. Relaxation of abdominal and rectal muscles helps relieve the discomfort.

ACTION	RATIONALE
6. Rotate the rectal tube gently during insertion.	Rotation prevents the tube from contacting the wall of the colon and stopping the flow of solution.
7. Clamp the tubing after all of the solution is in the colon.	Clamping prevents air from entering the colon, causing distension and discomfort.
8. The enema should be retained for 5 to 10 minutes. The young child usually is unable to hold the enema; retention may be assisted by manually holding the child's buttocks together for a short period while the solution dilutes bowel contents. The older child may be able to retain the enema, but a bedpan should be nearby in case of a sudden need to expel the enema. In the small baby, the buttocks may be taped together for the desired time with approximately 3 in (7.5 cm) of tape.	Retaining the enema offers an opportunity for the solution to dilute bowel contents so that they may be expelled more easily. Because young children cannot control the anal sphincter muscles, manual assistance is needed. Since older children may be embarrassed by accidental, premature expulsion of the enema, a bedpan should be handy.
9. For expulsion of the enema, place the child on a bedpan or commode, if condition permits. If the child is in bed, flexing the thighs upon the abdomen may facilitate expulsion of the enema. Depending upon the child's age and condition, someone should remain in attendance during enema expulsion.	Normal peristalsis should promote removal of the solution. Flexing the thighs on the abdomen may cause enough pressure to initiate removal of the bowel contents.
10. If after 1 hour the solution has not returned, place the child on the right side near the edge of the bed with the bedpan in a chair next to the bed. Remove the tubing from the enema container and place the attachment end in the bedpan. Reinsert the rectal end as before. Siphon the enema solution from the child's colon. Measure to be certain that all of the solution is returned. If the solution does not return, attach a funnel to the end of the tubing and fill the tubing with a small amount of the solution used for enema procedure. Reinsert the tubing into the rectum and allow a small amount of solution to run into the rectum. Then, quickly invert the funnel into the bedpan. Measure to be sure that all solution returns.	Fluid flows from an area of greater pressure to an area of lesser pressure. Holding the tubing lower than the bowel causes a pressure difference that should cause the solution to return spontaneously. It is essential to return all of the solution so that it will not be reabsorbed into the child's system.
11. Leave the child clean and in a comfortable position to rest.	The enema procedure is very tiring. Cleanliness promotes feelings of self-worth.

Communicative Aspects

OBSERVATIONS

1. Observe the color and consistency of the feces when the enema solution is expelled. Observe the amount of fluid returned. Note any unusual findings, such as blood, mucus, pus, or worms in the stool.

2. Observe the reaction of the child to the enema procedure. Watch for signs of pain, discomfort, cramping, or fatigue. Observe for signs that the child cannot tolerate any more enema solution and for signs that expulsion is imminent.

CHARTING

DATE/TIME	OBSERVATIONS	SIGNATURE
5/19 1000	170 ml saline solution instilled in rectum and retained for 6 min with coaching from mother. #14 Fr rectal tube inserted 2 in for instillation. Equipment and enema procedure explained before beginning. Some crying but after touching tubing and assured that his mother could stay with him, agreed to enema. Moderate amount of hard, dark brown stool returned with approximately 150 ml solution. No signs of bleeding. Abdomen soft and says he feels much better now. Praised for his cooperation. ————————	C. Day RN

Discharge Planning Aspects

CLIENT AND FAMILY EDUCATION

1. If the child will need enemas after discharge, teach the parents the correct technique and safety precautions. Explain basic anatomy, indications for enema, and expected results. Explain when to call the physician.

2. Teach the parents what constitutes normal elimination. Emphasize that "normal" does not necessarily mean daily bowel movements. Each person has an individual pattern. Because the child does not have a bowel movement for 24 hours is not an indication for an enema. Explain other rationale for determining when the child may be constipated, such as abdominal hardness or cramping, fussiness, poor appetite. Reliance on enemas or over-the-counter (OTC) laxatives for elimination is unnatural and dangerous. Explain the importance of adequate diet and fluids, exercise, and responding to the natural urge to empty the bowels in the promotion of normal elimination.

Evaluation

Quality Assurance

Documentation should include the type of enema, the amount of solution instilled, the amount of solution returned, and the results of the enema. The size of rectal tube and length of insertion should be noted. Any complications or unusual occurrences should be noted. The client's reaction to the procedure should be documented. Health teaching to the parents and when appropriate, to the child, should be noted on the chart.

Infection Control

1. Any procedure dealing with the eliminatory processes has the potential for cross-contamination of pathogenic microorganisms. Careful handwashing before and after the procedure are essential. The child should understand why it is important to wash the hands after bowel movements and to avoid transmitting rectal flora to the oral cavity.

2. When reusable equipment is stored in the bathroom or cabinet, it should be clearly marked to prevent the possibility of its being used for another client. Items such as bedpans should be for the exclusive use of one client until discharge. At that time, the equipment should be cleaned and terminally disinfected before being used for another client.

Technique Checklist

	YES	NO
Procedure explained to child	_____	_____
Procedure explained to parents	_____	_____
Reason for enema		
Surgical preparation _____		
Radiologic preparation _____		
Constipation _____		
Other _____		
Type of enema given _____		
Amount of solution given _____		
Amount of solution returned _____		
Child held the enema for _____ min		
Desired results obtained	_____	_____
Complications _____		
Complications reported to physician	_____	_____
Family teaching about judicious use of enemas and laxatives	_____	_____
Parents taught proper method of enema administration and indications for use of enemas.	_____	_____

101   Feeding Children

Overview

Definition   Feeding or assisting a child to eat

Rationale   Feed the child who is unable to eat alone.

Assist the child who can eat alone to some degree.

Provide adequate nutrition for the age, physical condition, and growth requirements of the child.

Terminology   *Ascites:* Accumulation of fluid in a body cavity

Urticaria: An inflammatory condition characterized by the eruption of wheals; hives

Assessment

Pertinent Anatomy and Physiology

1. See Appendix I: *esophagus, intestine (large), intestine (small), stomach.*

2. About the middle of the first year of life, the deciduous (primary) teeth begin to erupt. Calcification is complete during the the third year. The first teeth to erupt are usually the lower central incisors. The total number of primary teeth is 20. The permanent (secondary) teeth erupt beginning about 6 years of age. The permanent teeth develop under the primary teeth, the roots of which are slowly being absorbed. By the time the permanent teeth erupt, only the crowns of the deciduous teeth are left.

Pathophysiological Concepts

1. Colic involves paroxysmal abdominal cramping or pain. The child generally will cry loudly, often drawing the legs up to the abdomen. It is most common in very young infants, especially those under 3 months of age. Colic is believed to be caused by excessive fermentation and gas production in the intestines. It can be differentiated from more serious gastrointestinal (GI) problems by the fact that colic usually does not cause weight loss or inability to tolerate formula.

2. *Malnutrition* is a general term used to describe conditions associated with undernutrition as well as overnutrition. Childhood obesity is considered a form of malnutrition. Protein and calorie malnutrition are manifested in two conditions that are prevalent in the underdeveloped countries of the world, kwashiorkor and marasmus. Kwashiorkor, a protein deficiency, often develops in children between ages 1 and 4, when they are weaned at the birth of the next child. Classical symptoms are wasted extremities and a protruding abdomen resulting from ascites. Marasmus, a combination calorie and protein deficiency, can be a syndrome of physical and emotional deprivation. It is seen in extremely poor cultures as well as in failure-to-thrive children who lack emotional stimulation and interaction to eat a balanced diet. Marasmus involves gradual wasting and atrophy of body tissue, especially the subcutaneous fat.

3. Nutritional allergies are a common childhood problem. They are often the result of sensitivity to milk, eggs, wheat, vegetables, and fruit. The infant GI tract is immature and absorbs many proteins, which can stimulate an allergic response.

Assessment of the Client

1. Assess the past feeding patterns of the child. Elicit the mother's input in relation to what the child likes to eat. Determine the usual time and frequency of meals. Assess the usual dietary habits in relation to meeting the nutritional needs of the growing child. Determine if the diet included selections from the basic food groups.

2. Assess the state of the child's dentition. Determine the number of teeth, the presence of any loose teeth, and the condition of the teeth.

3. Assess the presence of food allergies. Note these allergies in a prominent place on the chart or care plan.

4. Assess the ability of the child to engage in self-feeding. Determine the ability of the child to hold an eating utensil and the degree of dexterity in handling food.

Plan

Nursing Objectives

Provide a pleasant atmosphere at mealtime.

Meet nutritional requirements.

Consider the child's food likes and dislikes.

Encourage the child to be independent by allowing self-feeding to the extent possible.

Allow the child the opportunity to enjoy meals.

Observe the child's state of hydration and nutrition.

Client Preparation

1. Allow the child the opportunity to void before mealtime.

2. Provide an opportunity for handwashing before eating. Assist as necessary.

3. Elevate the head of the bed unless contraindicated. If possible, allow the child to sit in a chair or in a high chair. *Do not leave the child unattended in a high chair.* Place in as near-normal position as can be tolerated by the child's condition.

Equipment

Overbed table

Bed tray

High chair (if appropriate)

Washcloth and towel

Implementation and Interventions

Procedural Aspects

ACTION	RATIONALE
1. Wash hands before beginning. If the child is young and soiling of the uniform is anticipated from spilled food, wear a gown.	Young children play and experiment with their food as a part of the growth and development process. Covering the uniform may save soiling.
2. Keep the eating utensils clean. If the child throws one on the floor, discard and get another or use the remaining utensils for the meal.	Bacteria tend to colonize on floors. Anything dropped on the floor is considered contaminated.

ACTION	RATIONALE
3. Identify the tray and the child by name and room number according to the dietary dispersal system of the hospital.	Different diets are appropriate for different ages and conditions. It is essential to give the right diet to the right client.
4. Assist the child as needed, but allow the child to enjoy as much independence as can be tolerated safely. Open any containers that the child cannot open. Cut the meat into bite-sized pieces, if needed. Offer the infant 8 months of age or older the opportunity to explore the food, if possible.	The opportunity for self-feeding and touching the food is consistent with the developmental need to explore and investigate as it relates to the handling of food at this age.
5. Be sure that the servings are small in proportion to the amount the child can eat. The food should be served attractively. Parents should be encouraged to participate in the feeding of their child (Fig. 101-1).	Desirable timing of meals and portion sizes can enhance the child's appetite and establish a pleasing association with the meal experience. Parental presence and encouragement also may promote adequate nourishment during hospitalization.

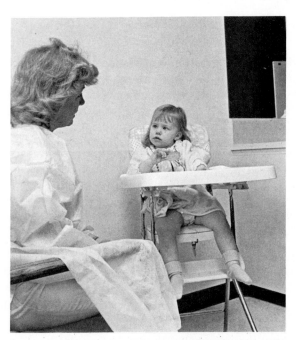

Figure 101.1

6. When the child finishes the meal, remove the tray and assist the child as needed with handwashing. Make sure that the child does not fall from the high chair while the restraining tray is removed.	Cleanliness is a habit that can be modeled or reinforced during hospitalization. The child can fall from the chair if not secured by hand while the tray is removed.

Communicative Aspects

OBSERVATIONS

1. Observe the child for likes and dislikes in relation to hospital food.
2. Observe any eating problems of the client such as difficulty with chewing and swallowing. Note the presence of loose teeth, which might impair the ability of the client to bite or chew certain types of food.
3. Note and record the child's progress in self-feeding.
4. Observe and record all aspects of the child's state of hydration and nutrition. This includes the amount of food eaten, the amount of fluids taken, the presence of vomiting or regurgitation with measurements (approximated if necessary), and the amount of urinary output.

CHARTING

Record fluid intake, if ordered, on the bedside record. In some institutions, a notation regarding the child's appetite is entered on the graphic record or the computerized graphic. Specific foods consumed by the child may be noted.

DATE/TIME	OBSERVATIONS	SIGNATURE
5/8 1130	Progressed to soft diet from full liquid. Ate all of the mashed potatoes and custard, none of the ground meat. Fed self with a spoon for half of meal; the remainder was fed to him by his mother. 70 ml milk taken from cup and retained without incident. Seemed to tolerate diet well. ————————	P. Sanchez RN

Discharge Planning Aspects

CLIENT AND FAMILY EDUCATION

1. Use the hospitalization experience as an opportunity to teach the parents how they can enhance the nourishment of their child. Offer these possible ways for parents to help their toddler and preschool child enjoy mealtime:

   Serve small portions. A child of this age is more likely to ask for a second serving of a small portion than to finish the first serving of a large portion.

   Serve food that is easy to handle, for example, apple slices, carrot sticks, toast slices, and crackers.

   Set an example at the table for the child to follow. If the parents demonstrate that they like the food and are relaxed and enjoying themselves, the child is also more likely to relax and enjoy the meal. If adults show a dislike for certain foods, the child usually will follow this example.

   Provide pleasant physical surroundings. If the child has a happy, cheerful atmosphere in which to eat, adequate food consumption is more likely.

   Be with the child at mealtime. Meals are a social experience. Having someone to share the meal is more conducive to a pleasant mealtime experience.

   Remind the parent that the goal of meals should not be eating everything on the plate. Childhood obesity is a growing problem. The child should eat until full, then should be encouraged to stop eating. Forcing the child to eat when full teaches poor eating habits and encourages stretching the stomach, which may predispose to weight problems.

2. The nutritional needs of children are extremely variable. The food needs of a school-aged child differ from the food needs of the preschool child mainly in quantity. The school-aged child can meet nutritional requirements with a diet that includes 3 to 4 cups of milk, three to four servings of bread and cereal, four servings of vegetables and fruits, and two servings of meat or other protein each day.

3. Nutritional requirements during teenage years are greatly increased. Inform parents of teenagers that because of rapid and extensive increase in height, weight, and mass, nutritional requirements of adolescents are increased. The peak requirement years are usually between the 10th and 12th years in girls and the 12th and 14th years in boys. Appetites soar, and food consumption increases greatly. Many of the social activities of teenagers are associated with the nutritional process. The adolescent boy and girl must be certain to get a sufficient amount of iron.

4. Teach the parents of the infant about identification of food allergies, a common childhood problem. Every effort should be made to determine the exact foods that are causing the allergic response. Following a schedule for a gradual introduction of new foods can help to indentify offending substances. Potentially allergy-causing foods should be offered in small quantities and should be well cooked since heat breaks down the proteins. If any local inflammation occurs, such as swelling of the lips or urticaria, the food should be avoided and should not be reintroduced for about 6 months. Reintroduction should be in small quantities.

REFERRALS

If the child will require special dietary considerations after discharge, a dietary consultant may visit with the parents to explain the diet and offer suggestions about meal preparation and dietary compliance.

Evaluation

Quality Assurance

Each institution should have some type of tray distribution system that ensures that the dietary trays arrive in the client's room at the desired temperature and appearance. There also must be a mechanism to ensure that each client receives the right tray. Documentation should include any problems with the diet. Generally, it is not necessary to document each meal except in regard to amount consumed. If the diagnosis is failure to thrive, however, documentation should include the ability of the child to take nourishment and the willingness of the mother to participate in this process. If the child has mobility impairment (e.g., a cast), alterations allowing the child to take nourishment should be documented and assessed. Any problems with feeding should be noted.

Infection Control

1. Handwashing should precede and follow meals for both the nurse and the child.

2. The alimentary canal is not sterile and contains acidic digestive juices that kill most of the bacteria consumed in food. The infantile digestive system is susceptible to gastric problems, however. Care should be taken to ensure that the child is not exposed to pathogenic organisms. Bottles, pacifiers, and eating utensils that have been tossed or dropped to the floor should be cleaned before being returned to the child.

Technique Checklist

	YES	NO
Proper feeding technique explained to parent(s)	_____	_____
Demonstration _____		
Return demonstration _____		
Child ate well during hospitalization	_____	_____
Gastric problems developed		
Regurgitation _____		
Vomiting _____		
Choking _____		
Inability to chew properly _____		
Inability to swallow _____		
Type of diet _____		
Diet instructions on discharge	_____	_____

102

Feeding Infants by Gastric Gavage and Nasojejunal Tube

Overview

Definition

Gastric gavage: Ingestion of food or medicine through a tube passed through the nares or mouth into the stomach

Nasojejunal tube feeding: The ingestion of food through a tube passed through the nares into the jejunum, bypassing the pylorus of the stomach; used to decrease complications such as gastric distension, aspiration, and regurgitation in infants who must rely on tube feedings for an extended period

Rationale

Provide nourishment for infants in whom sucking and swallowing reflexes are underdeveloped or lacking.

Provide nourishment for infants with respiratory problems or seizures who generally aspirate when fed with a nipple.

Decrease the possibility of complications in a child who must undergo long-term tube feedings.

Terminology

Aspirate: To withdraw fluid by negative pressure or suction

Emesis: The act of vomiting

   Nonprojectile vomiting: A nonexplosive, mild type of vomiting accompanied by contraction of the abdomen

   Projectile vomiting: An explosive type of vomiting with the material ejected with great force

Intubation: Insertion of a tube into any hollow organ for therapeutic or diagnostic purposes

Regurgitation: A backward, nonforceful flow of fluids and undigested food from the stomach to the oral cavity without contractions of the abdomen

Assessment

Pertinent Anatomy and Physiology

See Appendix I: *esophagus, intestine (large), intestine (small), stomach.*

Pathophysiological Concepts

Anomalies of the throat and esophagus, impaired swallowing capacity, severe debilitation, or respiratory distress in the infant may result in an inability of the child to consume adequate nourishment to meet the body's needs. Since metabolic processes continue at a high rate in the small child, nutrition must provide the energy required. If the food cannot be taken orally, it can be inserted directly into the stomach by means of a tube so that digestion and utilization of the food can begin. If the child may regurgitate or vomit the food, it may be inserted by means of a nasojejunum tube directly in the jejunum, where regurgitation is less likely.

Assessment of the Client

1. Assess the ability of the child to take food. Determine past dietary habits.

2. Assess the familiarity of the older child with hospital procedures, in particular with the nasogastric intubation procedure. Determine how much information to offer the child in relation to age and level of understanding as well as anxiety level.

3. Assess the length of the tube to be inserted. For nasal insertion, measure from the tip of the child's nose to the lobe of the ear, then to a point midway between the xiphoid process and the umbilicus (Fig. 102-1). For oral passage, measure the distance from the mouth to the lobe of the ear, then to a point midway between the xiphoid process and umbilicus (see Fig. 102-1).

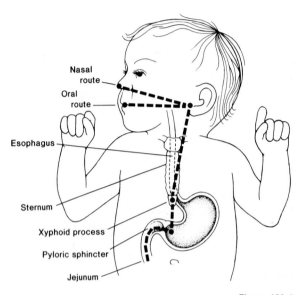

Nasal route
Oral route
Esophagus
Sternum
Xyphoid process
Pyloric sphincter
Jejunum

Figure 102.1

4. Assess the pulse rate, especially in small babies. Insertion of the tube may stimulate the vagal reflex and decrease the pulse rate. A baseline should be available for comparison.

Plan

Nursing Objectives

Adequately hydrate and nourish the infant or child.

Maintain comfort and safety throughout the procedure.

Inform the family about the purpose of and need for this procedure.

Maintain medical asepsis.

Observe signs and symptoms of tube displacement.

Observe and accurately record the effects and results of the procedure.

Observe for early signs of impending complications and take appropriate action.

Client Preparation

1. Offer to the child an explanation that is appropriate for age, anxiety level, and physical condition. Explain the procedure to the parents and enlist their assistance in explaining it to the child.

2. Apply restraints before beginning, if necessary, so that the child will not interfere with the tube insertion and will not dislodge the tube once it has been inserted. The use of restraints should be known and understood by the parents in advance of the gastric intubation. Commonly used restraints are the mummy restraint for infants and the elbow restraint for small children (see Technique No. 111, Restraints, Pediatric). Use the papoose board if a greater degree of immobilization is needed.

3. Elevate the child's head slightly before insertion. This lessens the possibility of aspiration as the tube is passed through the nasopharynx and also decreases the gag reflex.

4. For gavage feeding, position the child on the right side to facilitate the flow of fluid into the stomach and to prevent aspiration if the child regurgitates around the tube.

Equipment

GASTRIC INTUBATION

Gastric tube, 5 to 8 French for the infant; 10 to 14 French for the older child

Restraints, as needed

Disposable irrigation set

Water-soluble lubricant

Clamp

Tape (½ inch wide)

Stethoscope

Emesis basin

Gloves

GASTRIC GAVAGE

30-ml to 50-ml syringe

Sterile water and basin

Formula, as prescribed

NASOJEJUNAL TUBE FEEDING

30-ml syringe

Extension tubing

Venitubing

Adhesive tape (¼ inch wide)

Formula, as prescribed

Implementation and Interventions

Procedural Aspects

ACTION	*RATIONALE*
Gastric Intubation	
1. Wash hands thoroughly. Don sterile gloves and lubricate the tube for nasal passage by moistening the tip with sterile water or a water-soluble lubricant. If the tube is passed through the oral cavity, lubrication is not usually necessary. If the child's oral cavity is extremely dry, moisten the tip of the tube with sterile, water-soluble solution.	Lubrication facilitates tube insertion by decreasing friction and minimizing trauma to the delicate mucous membranes of the gastrointestinal (GI) tract. A water-soluble lubricant is used to decrease the complications arising from accidental insertion into the lungs or aspiration of the lubricant. Since the oral cavity is usually moist, oral passage of the tube does not usually require prior tube lubrication.
2. Once the tube has been introduced into the child's alimentary canal, advance it as the child swallows. Use a gentle rotating motion to facilitate insertion. If the child chokes or becomes cyanotic, remove the tube and reinsert it after the child's condition stabilizes.	The presence of a foreign substance in the esophagus or the mouth, whether a piece of food or the tube, initiates the secretion of saliva and mucus, which helps to lubricate the tube and facilitate insertion. Choking and cyanosis may indicate insertion into the pulmonary system.

ACTION

RATIONALE

3. Determine proper placement of the tube. Aspiration of stomach contents indicates that the tube is in the stomach. Place the bell of the stethoscope over the child's stomach and introduce a very small amount of air through the tube into the stomach (5 ml–10 ml of air is adequate). The sound of air entering the stomach should be definite.

Aspiration of stomach contents helps assure the nurse that the tube is in the stomach. Inserting air into the stomach may cause distension and discomfort due to the small capacity of the child's stomach.

4. If the tube is to remain in place, restrain the child's arms and secure the tube in place with tape (Fig. 102-2).

It is important that the tube not be accidentally dislodged.

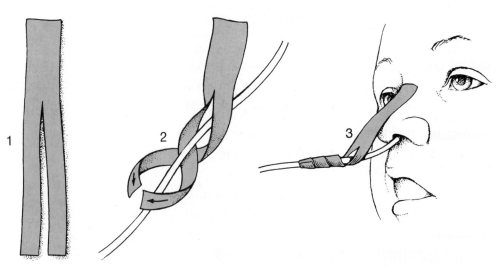

Figure 102.2

Gavage Feeding

1. Warm the formula to room temperature before administering it through the gavage tube.

Having the formula at room temperature facilitates digestion and decreases the chance of gastric spasms.

2. Attach the barrel of the syringe to the tube and check the placement of the tube by aspirating gastric contents. Clamp the tube to maintain the presence of this aspirated fluid in place until feeding begins.

Having the tube full of fluid prevents the instillation of unnecessary air into the child's stomach.

3. Pour the formula into the barrel of the syringe held 6 inches (15 cm) above the level of the child's body plane and allow it to flow slowly into the child's stomach by gravity. Do not exert pressure to instill the fluid. Be careful not to pull the tube because this will exert pressure on the mucous membranes of the child's nose and/or throat.

Pressure may stimulate and traumatize the gastric mucosa, causing aspiration and regurgitation.

ACTION	***RATIONALE***
4. Follow the formula with a small amount of sterile water, for newborns 5 ml–10 ml and for older children up to 30 ml.	Water serves to flush and clean the tube to prevent clogging.
5. If the tube is left in place, tape as described previously. Clamp the tube. If the tube is to be removed, pinch the catheter onto itself and withdraw quickly.	Taping prevents accidental removal. If the tube is removed quickly while it is pinched shut, leakage and aspiration may be prevented as the tube is withdrawn.
6. Position the child on the right side after feeding. If the child has difficulty turning, perform the feeding with the child on the right side.	Proper positioning decreases the chance of aspiration and hastens emptying of the stomach.

Nasojejunal Tube Feeding

1. Assist the physician as needed, during the insertion of the nasojejunal tube. The tube usually is passed into the nasotracheal tube, which is introduced using the same technique as in inserting the nasogastric tube. Once the nasojejunal tube is in the stomach, the larger tube is withdrawn over the smaller tube, which subsequently advances through the pylorus into the jejunum (Fig. 102-3). The physician usually requests an abdominal x-ray to ensure proper placement of the nasojejunal tube in the jejunum. A silicone tube with a weighted tip is also available. The tip flows through the GI system to the jejunum by peristalsis. Some control of the tube is possible by using a guide wire that comes with the tube.	The nasojejunal tube is very soft and pliable and lacks the rigidity to be inserted directly into the stomach without curling or kinking. The nasotracheal tube provides a structured pathway for tube insertion and is then removed to facilitate comfort. The tube is allowed to flow into the jejunum by normal peristaltic activity. For the weighted tube, the guide wire provides the structure to allow proper placement of the tube.

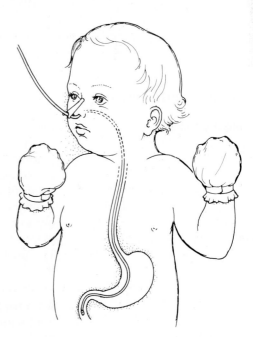

Figure 102.3

ACTION	RATIONALE
2. After the initial insertion of the tube, keep the infant or child on the right side with hips elevated for approximately 4 hours. After this time, the child may be turned to the abdomen or back.	Positioning the infant or child so that the tube is allowed to flow through the normal gastric passage by gravity and peristalsis facilitates proper placement of the tube.
3. An extension tubing is usually connected to the nasojejunal feeding tube. Small amounts of formula are given at frequent intervals. After each feeding, rinse the tube with distilled water. The contents of the tube should not be aspirated.	Because of the small lumen of the tube and the increased length to reach completely into the jejunum, the tube can be become blocked if it is not rinsed. Aspiration will cause collapse of the tube. Placement is verified by radiologic means.

Special Modifications

Gastrostomy Feedings

A gastrostomy is an artificial opening into the stomach by surgical incision for the placement of a feeding tube. The gastrostomy tube is used as a means to instill feedings directly into the stomach. The same principles apply as for tube feeding. Take care to keep the area around the gastrostomy clean and dry once healing has taken place. Avoid pulling the tube. Between feedings, place the child on the right side or in semi-Fowler's position. The tube is usually clamped between feedings.	Accidental pulling of the tube must be avoided because this may widen the incisional area, allowing gastric juices to escape. Because of its acidic nature, gastric juice is extremely irritating to the skin.

Communicative Aspects

OBSERVATIONS

1. Before gavage feeding, check proper placement of the tube. Aspirate the nasogastric tube. Carefully observe the return. If it is stomach contents, then the placement is verified. The stomach contents that are aspirated should be reinserted as a part of the count of the total milliliters for the feeding. The stomach contents contain the digestive enzymes that are valuable to proper nutrition and should not be discarded. If the aspirated solution is formula from the previous feeding, this may indicate that the child is being fed more than can be digested, and the amount of feedings may need to be reduced. The presence of undigested formula in the stomach may also indicate that the child is not able to digest this particular formula and that modifications in the type of formula may be necessary.

2. After feeding, observe the infant for regurgitation and vomiting. Observe how the infant tolerates the feeding, rate of respiration, and activity. Extreme fussiness or increased respiration may indicate distress from overfilling of the stomach.

3. Observe the infant during nasogastric intubation. Many infants experience bradycardia because of stimulation of the vagal reflex during insertion. Observe for cyanosis or choking, which might indicate that the tube has entered the bronchi or lung.

CHARTING

Gastric Gavage

DATE/TIME	OBSERVATIONS	SIGNATURE
9/10 0930	No. 8 French gastric tube inserted without difficulty. Restrained by mummy wrap. Mother understood what would happen and assisted with application of restraints, chose not to be present during insertion of tube. NG tube left in place per order of Dr. K. 50 ml formula followed by 5 ml sterile water. Tolerated feeding well. Left sleeping on right side. ————————————	R. Smith RN

Nasojejunal Feeding

DATE/TIME	OBSERVATIONS	SIGNATURE
6/14 1200	Nasojejunal tube remains in place to previously marked depth. No signs of movement of tube. 100 ml formula given by NJ tube. Tolerated well. Turned to right side after feeding. Mother in room, held baby during feeding. ———	R. Smith RN

Discharge Planning Aspects

CLIENT AND FAMILY EDUCATION

1. Explain the procedure for tube insertion and feeding to the parents and to the child who is old enough to understand. Be sure that they understand why the child cannot eat normally and have an understanding of approximately how long the tube feedings will be necessary.

2. Explain the restraint procedure before applying the restraints during tube insertion. Some children must be restrained after the tube is inserted so that they will not accidentally pull it out. The parents should understand why the restraints are necessary and how long they will remain in place.

3. If the child will require tube feedings at home, demonstrate to the parents how to insert the tube and to administer the feedings. Explain safety factors. Encourage the parents to hold the child during the feeding, if possible, to promote the infant–parent bond. A pacifier may be used during feeding to allow the infant to satisfy the sucking need.

Evaluation

Quality Assurance

Documentation should include symptoms that prompted the insertion of the tube in the first place. The presence of vomiting and/or regurgitation should be accompanied by a description of the return. Explanations given to the family should be documented, as well as an appraisal of their understanding and acceptance of the need for artificial feedings. The tolerance of the child to the insertion of the tube and any complications should be reflected. The amount, frequency and tolerance of each feeding should be recorded. Safety precautions should be noted. Hospital policy should dictate standards for lengths of time the tube is left in place.

Infection Control

1. The alimentary canal is not considered sterile. However, during intubation and feeding of infants, equipment and water to lubricate and flush the tube are sterile. The infant has an underdeveloped immune system and must be protected from cross-contamination.

2. Careful handwashing should be carried out before and after tube feedings.

Technique Checklist

	YES	NO
Procedure explained before beginning:		
To parents	_____	_____
To child	_____	_____

Type of tube inserted

Nasogastric _____

Nasojejunal _____

Gastrostomy in place _____

Size tube inserted _____

Complications during insertion

Choking and cyanosis _____

Vomiting _____

Other _____

	YES	NO
Tube left in place between feedings	_____	_____
Tube clamped between feedings	_____	_____
Formula fed at room temperature	_____	_____
Infant able to be held during feeding	_____	_____
Client positioned to facilitate absorption of feeding	_____	_____
Family encouraged to assist and participate in feedings	_____	_____
Child will have tube feedings at home	_____	_____
Parents shown how to do feedings	_____	_____
Return demonstration	_____	_____

103

Hyperalimentation
(Total Parenteral Nutrition)

Overview

Definition

A method of providing total and complete nutrition by the infusion of a hypertonic (30%) nutrient solution directly into a central vein, usually the superior vena cava, through a subclavian or a jugular vein. The mixture can be given in a peripheral vein; however, if the concentration of glucose is above 14%, irritation to the small veins is so great that the central vein method is desirable. The solution is a mixture of hypertonic solution of glucose with vitamins, water, electrolytes, a nitrogen source, and minerals.

Rationale

Sustain the life of a child when adequate nutrition is not possible for extended periods of time either by the oral or nasogastric intubation routes.

Terminology

Hypertonic: Having an osmotic pressure greater than that of the solution with which it is compared

Millipore filter: A filter interposed in the venous line to remove any particulate matter or microorganisms from the complex mixture of the hyperalimentation solution

Parenteral: Through a route other than the alimentary canal

Partial or supplemental alimentation: Parenteral nutrition supplements that can be given through the peripheral veins when central venous alimentation cannot be instituted.

Assessment

Pertinent Anatomy and Physiology

See Appendix I: *blood vessels.*

Pathophysiological Concepts

Hyperalimentation solution is a highly concentrated mixture, which can be very irritating to the surface of the veins. For this reason, hyperalimentation requires infusion into a vessel with sufficient diameter and blood flow to effect rapid dilution of the mixture immediately upon its entry into the bloodstream. The vessels usually selected are the superior vena cava and the intrathoracic subclavian veins.

Assessment of the Client

1. Assess the client's physical condition. Determine the history of the inability to ingest nutrients orally. Assess the condition of the oral cavity. Weight and skin turgor will also add insight into the client's nutritional status. Determine the head circumference and baseline vital signs. Assess color. Determine the presence of any urinary problems in the past.
2. Assess the allergy history of the client. Local anesthetic may be used for venous catheter insertion. Inquire about allergies to foods and drugs, particularly iodine.

Plan

Nursing Objectives

Prepare the hyperalimentation infusion setup under strict aseptic conditions.

Assist the physician with the insertion of the hyperalimentation catheter. (This is often done in the operating room.)

Successfully infuse the hyperalimentation solution at the rate ordered, using an infusion pump or other fluid control methods to prevent overinfusion.

Prevent contamination and reduce the possibility of infecting the client.

Record the total intake and output (I&O).

Observe for signs of complications from the hyperalimentation therapy.

Provide for the emotional well-being of the child and the parents.

Client Preparation

1. Offer a complete explanation to the client, if old enough to understand. The family should be given a detailed explanation of the rationale for and procedure of the infusion. Answer any questions simply and truthfully.

2. Properly restrain the young child or infant. If the external jugular is used, place the infant or small child in a mummy restraint with the head lowered over the side of the bed and held by the nurse's hands.

3. Clean the infusion site thoroughly with an antiseptic. A local anesthetic may be infiltrated into the infusion area.

Equipment

Hyperalimentation solution, as prescribed by the physician (Hyperalimentation solution is usually mixed in the pharmacy under a special laminar air flow hood to help ensure sterility of the infusion.)

Intravenous (IV) administration set with extension tubing

Hyperalimentation catheter, depending on size of child

Filter

Sterile cutdown tray

Local anesthetic

Antiseptic skin cleanser

Gauze pads or sponges

Hemostat for clamping tube if accidentally dislodged

Implementation and Interventions

Procedural Aspects

ACTION	RATIONALE
1. During tube insertion, hold the child's head in a dependent position turned to the side. Have the hyperalimentation solution ready by priming the IV tubing, ensuring that all of the air bubbles are removed. Label the solution with the time marked on the tape.	The child must be restrained to prevent accidental dislodgement of the tube or contamination during tube placement. All air must be removed from the tube to prevent air embolus. The head is held at a level lower than the body to distend the subclavian vein.
2. The physician will proceed with intubation of the vein by passing the catheter through the internal or external jugular, the facial, or the subclavian vein into the vena cava.	Tunneling the catheter to a site on the scalp gets the tubing out of the reach of the small child and reduces the need for elaborate restraints.

ACTION

The catheter may be tunneled under the skin of the head subcutaneously, exiting well up on the scalp, where it is secured with the tape.

3. Accompany the child to the x-ray department for confirmation of catheter placement. The patency of the infusion is usually maintained with an isotonic solution during this interim period.

4. Once the hyperalimentation solution has started infusing, assess the rate of infusion every 30 minutes to 1 hour to ensure that the rate prescribed by the physician is maintained. Place an infusion pump on the tubing to assist in monitoring of the rate (Fig. 103-1). If the amount of infusion is decreased for a period, *do not attempt to catch up* by infusion of the deficit amount over a shorter period.

RATIONALE

Proper positioning of the catheter must be ensured before infusion of the hyperalimentation solution is started.

Use of a pump will help ensure that the rate remains fairly stable. It will also prevent backflow into the tubing when the child's venous pressure is increased, such as during bouts of crying. If the rate is increased, there is a great risk of glucose overload. A rate of infusion that is too slow may produce hypoglycemia.

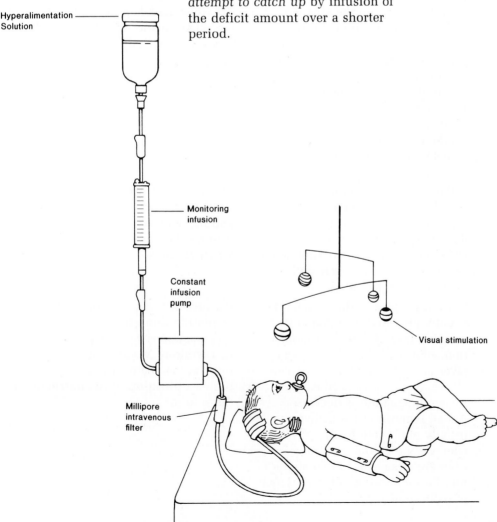

Hyperalimentation Solution

Monitoring infusion

Constant infusion pump

Visual stimulation

Millipore intravenous filter

Figure 103.1

ACTION	RATIONALE
5. Change the solution bottle and tubing with filter at least daily. All IV tubing connections should be secured with tape to prevent accidental disconnection. Chart the change of equipment and the time. Clamp the tubing with hemostats while the bottle is being changed. For the tubing change, place the child flat in bed or in the Trendelenburg position, and disconnect the tubing during *expiration*. If the catheter accidentally becomes dislodged, clamp immediately with a hemostat.	Hyperalimentation solution should not be allowed to hang at room temperature for longer than 24 hours because of the chance of growth of pathogenic microorganisms. Every precaution should be taken to prevent the occurrence of air embolism. If the child is exhaling when the tubing is disconnected, there is less chance for the air to be sucked in through the catheter.
6. Change the dressing on the catheter site according to the established hospital policy for hyperalimentation dressings. Use strict sterile technique during dressing change. Remove the dressing carefully to prevent accidental dislodging of the catheter. Clean the area surrounding the insertion site with a solution prescribed by the physician or hospital policy. An antibacterial ointment may be prescribed for application over the insertion site before reapplication of the dressing. Place a sterile dressing or synthetic skin dressing over the catheter area to prevent contamination.	The goal of frequent dressing change is to prevent contamination of the site by pathogenic organisms. Because of the concentrated nature and the constituency of the hyperalimentation solution, it is an excellent medium for the growth of microorganisms. Great care must be taken to keep the site and the infusion equipment free from pathogenic activity.
7. If the total parenteral nutrition solution runs out before the prescribed time, an interim infusion may used. The physician may order a concentrated solution such as 10% dextrose in water with sodium chloride added.	The 10% dextrose solution prevents a sudden drop in the serum glucose, and the sodium chloride helps prevent cerebral edema from infusion of a hypertonic solution.
8. Discontinuation of the infusion is usually preceded by a gradual weaning from the hyperalimentation solution. If insulin has been given with the solution, it is usually gradually decreased as the hyperalimentation is decreased. Actual removal of the catheter is usually performed by the physician. Cultures from the tubing and filter are often sent to the laboratory for monitoring of the presence of pathogenic organisms.	Because of the nature of the hyperalimentation fluid, the infant's system must compensate for its initiation and its cessation. Medications, such as insulin, may be necessary for the proper utilization of the nutrients in the solution.

ACTION	*RATIONALE*
Special Modifications	
Do not use the hyperalimentation catheter for infusion of other products, such as lipids or blood products. Medications are not usually given through the hyperalimentation catheter. If IV injection or infusion is needed, an additional peripheral IV infusion is usually instituted. Do not draw blood samples through the hyperalimentation catheter.	The hyperalimentation site must be preserved for the infusion of select substances because of its location so near the anterior chamber of the heart. Many medications are incompatible with hyperalimentation solution.

Communicative Aspects

OBSERVATIONS

1. Observe the infusion rate every 30 minutes to 1 hour. Determine the patency of the infusion, the reliability of the pump, and the timing of the infusion. Sudden cessation of the infusion could result in hypoglycemia. Observe for skin breakdown, since hyperalimentation does not provide fatty acids necessary to maintain fat pads in the bony prominences. Infiltration of the infusion into the tissues can cause sloughing of the tissue. Also observe the infusion site for signs and symptoms of infection.

2. Monitor the client's condition frequently (at least every 2 hours after stabilization on hyperalimentation solution). Note and record intake and output, the condition of the oral cavity, daily weight, condition of the site, and any signs of complications. Complications may involve the site (leaking, dislodgement of the catheter, bleeding), the infusion (loose connections, inpurities in the solution, allowing the solution to hang for over 24 hours), or the client (hyperglycemia, hypoglycemia, electrolyte imbalance, and fluid imbalance).

3. Closely monitor the blood glucose and acetone levels. Glucose levels are usually monitored at least every 8 hours. The potassium and sodium levels may also become deficient if no supplement is ordered or exaggerated if too much supplement is given. Serum electrolytes are usually monitored at least twice a week and more often if they are abnormal.

4. Weigh the child each day to ascertain the effect of the hyperalimentation infusion. Weigh the child at the same time each day on the same scale. Also make daily observation of head circumference.

5. Observe the child for prolonged bouts of vigorous crying because this will alter the venous pressure and may alter the infusion rate.

Charting

1. For catheter insertion, chart the date, time, place, location of catheter and type, amount, and rate of initial solution infusion. If the catheter placement was confirmed by radiologic means, note the condition of the infant or child during the radiologic procedure. Note any complications or difficulties with insertion.

2. For dressing change, note the time and date, the condition of the site, and application of any medication. Note the type of dressing applied and any complications.

3. For changing the filter, tubing, and infusion, note the time, whether or not a culture was sent to the laboratory (if so, its source or sources), patency of the infusion, and any problems.

4. Daily references should be made to weight and head circumference. Monitoring of intake and output should be done in a consistent manner, usually every 8 to 12 hours.

DATE/TIME	OBSERVATIONS	SIGNATURE
11/8 1130	Hyperalimentation solution continues to infuse at 50 cc/hr by infusion pump. Tubing and filter changed and new bottle of solution hung. Tubing (lower 6 inches) and milipore filter sent to lab for culture. Dressing dry. Elbow restraints continuous. Held by mother for 15 min. Sucking pacifier well. Mother seems to understand instructions about care of tubing when holding her daughter. No problems. Mother will return at 1330 to visit. No apnea, color pink. T 98.2° F, P 110, R 18. No crying. Sleeping now. ————	R. Smith RN

Discharge Planning Aspects

CLIENT AND FAMILY EDUCATION

1. Explain the need for the hyperalimentation infusions. Explain that these feedings will take the place of oral nutrition for a period of time so that the parents will not be alarmed that the child is not receiving any food by mouth. Answer any questions as simply and honestly as possible.

2. Inform the family about the need for restraints before these are applied. If the family understands how important it is for the catheter to remain in the exact location, they may be more accepting of the idea of restraints.

3. Explain about the danger of infection if the dressing or site is contaminated. Ask the family members to take care not to touch the site dressing, if possible. The child should also refrain from touching the tubing or site.

4. Explain to the family of the young infant that although the child's nutritional needs are being met by the infusion, the emotional needs associated with the nutritional process must also be met. Encourage the family to cuddle and rock the child at regular intervals while the child sucks on a pacifier. The rooting and sucking reflexes may be stimulated by stroking the child's cheek with a finger. These activities may allow the child to associate the sucking responses with a pleasurable activity even though the satisfaction of having a full stomach will be lacking.

Evaluation

Quality Assurance

Each facility should have a written policy about the administration of hyperalimentation solution to adults and children. The policy should address aspects such as the frequency of changing the tubing, site dressing, and infusion bottle. The method of dressing change should be addressed with recommendations about proper skin cleansers, disinfectants, antibiotic ointments and creams, and dressing material if these are not stipulated by the physician. Those persons who are considered qualified to change site dressings, tubing, and infusion bottles should be identified.

Documentation should include baseline measurements of weight and head circumference, as well as vital signs. Daily monitoring of weight and head circumference should be noted, as well as consistent monitoring of the intake and output. Methods of restraint should be noted and reassessed periodically. The rate of infusion and any complications should be reflected. The times, dates, and frequency of any procedures carried out regarding the hyperalimentation infusion should be noted in the nurse's progress notes. The physical condition of the child should be noted frequently along with assessment of possible complications. The nurse should show evidence by the charting that possible complications were understood and frequent observations for these complications were made. Any interventions to prevent or correct complications should be noted.

The teaching and acceptance of the family should be noted on the chart. The willingness of the parents to hold and cuddle the baby should be reflected. The persons who held and provided sensory stimulation of the baby, as well as a brief reference to the type of stimulation, should be noted. When the child begins to take oral nourishment again, the involvement of the parents in this process and a complete description of the process and assessment of the infant's tolerance should be reflected in the nurse's notes.

Infection Control

1. Strict sterile technique is necessary for changing dressings. Changing tubing for hyperalimentation infusions should also be done under sterile technique. The venipuncture site should be observed for signs and symptoms of infection. The hospital should have a detailed schedule for changing dressings and tubing, which should be followed. This schedule should reflect awareness of the latest Centers for Disease Control recommendations and the latest research on total parenteral nutrition.

2. Careful handwashing should be done before handling the infant who is receiving hyperalimentation.

3. The hyperalimentation solution provides optimal conditions for the growth and proliferation of microorganisms when it is at room temperature. Therefore, the bottle should not be allowed to hang for more than 24 hours. Even if it is not empty, it should be changed every 24 hours. The infusion should be prepared under strict sterile conditions, preferably under a laminar air flow hood. If any of the solution spills on the tubing, it should be cleaned off immediately to prevent bacterial growth. Prepared solutions should be kept refrigerated. If they are not used within 5 days, prepared hyperalimentation solutions should be discarded.

Technique Checklist

	YES	NO
Procedure explained to parents	_____	_____
Need for restraints explained to parents	_____	_____
Site of infusion catheter _____		
Date of placement _____		
Frequency of dressing change _____		
Sterile technique maintained	_____	_____
Leakage at site	_____	_____
Tubing changed _____		
Hemostat clamp nearby at all times	_____	_____
Child placed flat or in Trendelenburg's position	_____	_____
Tubing connections taped	_____	_____
Tubing remained patent	_____	_____
Tubing samples to laboratory for culture how often _____		
Hyperalimentation solution bottle changed every 24 hours	_____	_____
Rate of infusion _____		
Constant infusion pump in place	_____	_____
Solution mixed under sterile conditions	_____	_____

	YES	NO
Infant/child restrained	————	————
Consistent monitoring of:		
Vital signs	————	————
Weight	————	————
Head circumference	————	————
Blood glucose	————	————
Sodium levels	————	————
Postassium	————	————
Other _____		
_____		
Infant cuddled and rocked while sucking on pacifier at least 3 times a day for 15 minutes	————	————
Gradually weaned from hyperalimentation solution	————	————
Reintroduction to oral food	————	————

104 Interhospital Transport System for Critically Ill Infants

Overview

Definition

The system for transporting critically ill infants based on the expedient use of personnel, equipment, and vehicles coordinated to meet the specific requirements of the region served and the types of infants to be transported; communication and teamwork are the foundation of a successful transport system.

Rationale

The transport is initiated by a physician or practitioner requesting transfer of an infant to a specific destination, such as a neonatal intensive care unit. This request is influenced by past experience, training, local facilities, and overall ability to cope with the presenting problem.

The referring physician communicates the nature of the infant's problem and present condition to the physician controlling the transport system. This physician–controller relays the information to the destination area so that a plan of action may be prepared in anticipation of receiving the infant and necessary equipment may be obtained and prepared.

The timing of transport is important for the premature infant. Approximately one third of all neonatal deaths occur within the first 24 hours following birth. Early treatment of many conditions appears to alter the outcome favorably.

Assessment

Pertinent Anatomy and Physiology

See Technique No. 151, Neonatal Assessment, Initial and Continued.

Plan

Nursing Objectives

Coordinate personnel, equipment, and vehicles to transport the critically ill infant.

Have all available equipment in excellent working order.

Transport the infant in a safe and expeditious manner.

Meet the emotional needs of the parents.

Client Preparation

1. The physician–controller may serve as a consultant in the decisions to take such action as increasing the environmental oxygen, inserting an umbilical-vein catheter for fluid administration, assessment of the infant's blood glucose level, placement of the infant in a constant thermal environment, use of suction, and baseline measurements of such parameters as hemoglobin, hematocrit, and capillary blood gas levels.

2. The infant must be warmed and oxygenated before transfer. In addition to these measures, the referring facility usually prepares items such as a sample of the mother's blood, a copy of the mother's and infant's charts, and any other pertinent information for transport with the infant.

3. The parents must be kept informed of the reasons for and progress of the transfer. Some hospitals take a picture of the infant to give to the parents before transport and upon arrival at the receiving institution. A close relative usually accompanies the infant to the receiving agency to sign necessary legal documents to allow treatment.

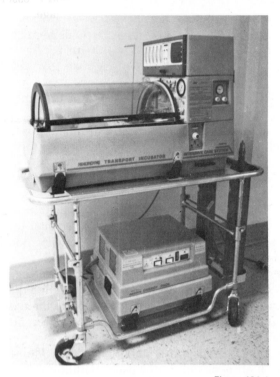

Figure 104.1

Equipment

Transport incubator or portable crib than can maintain the infant's temperature, allow easy visualization of and access to the infant, and provide for the controlled administration of oxygen (Fig. 104-1)

Battery-powered infusion pump

Masks, airways, and assisted ventilation bags or machines

Laryngoscope equipment with an assortment of endotracheal tubes

Intravenous infusion equipment, including umbilical-vessel catheters

Emergency medications

Implementation and Interventions

Procedural Aspects

ACTION	RATIONALE
Responsibilities of the Nurse Accompanying the Critically Ill Infant during Transportation	
1. Maintain the infant's position on the side with the neck extended.	This position facilitates breathing and lessens the pressure on the cardiovascular system. Hyperextension may cause collapse of the trachea.
2. Suction the infant as needed.	The accumulation of fluids in the infant's trachea may cause aspiration and choking.

ACTION	***RATIONALE***
3. Maintain the infant's color based on the clinical signs of cyanosis of the extremities, using the amount of oxygen ordered.	Administration of too much oxygen can cause blindness in the newborn. However, adequate oxygenation of the blood is essential to prevent brain damage.
4. Maintain the environmental temperature of the transport unit: minimal 90° to 95° F (32.2°–35° C); optimal, 95° to 97° F (35°–36.1° C).	The temperature-regulating mechanism of a premature infant is not sufficiently developed to provide internal regulation of temperature. This must be controlled environmentally.
5. Maintain the intravenous infusion at the specified rate.	It is essential not to overhydrate the critically ill neonate.

Communicative Aspects

OBSERVATIONS

Obtain vital signs before transport, en route, and upon reception at the receiving facility. Determine the following measurements:

Cardiac rate (taken apically for at least 1 minute, since the newborn may have an irregular heartbeat)

Respiratory rate (taken for at least 1 minute)

Degree of grunting or retracting

Muscle tone

Activity of the infant

Cyanosis and generalized color (plethora may indicate a hematocrit above 69%–70%)

Need for suctioning

Breath sounds

Evaluation

Quality Assurance

Documentation accompanying the neonate should include the labor and delivery record, the mother's prenatal record (if available) and hospital record, and the infant's record. A record of the activities during transport should be available, along with a complete list of techniques performed, medications administered, and vital sign measurements. In addition, the referring agency should be in voice communication with the receiving agency for a complete referral report. The transporting nurse should give a complete report of the transfer to the receiving nurse. The basic components of a successful transport are communication and teamwork.

Infection Control

1. The premature infant is particularly susceptible to infection. All equipment used should be sterile. The infant should be enclosed in a protective environment, if possible, to prevent cross-contamination.

2. Meticulous handwashing should be done by all persons who administer care to the neonate. Those who will transport the infant should wear gowns if they have been transporting other clients previous to the neonatal transfer.

Technique Checklist

	YES	NO
Parents understood the need for transfer	_____	_____
Infant transfer information recorded	_____	_____

Time of birth _____

Time of initial call to receiving agency _____

Time of actual transfer _____

Time of arrival at destination _____

Apgar scores

1 minute after birth _____

5 minutes after birth _____

| Vital signs monitored throughout transfer | _____ | _____ |

Treatments during transfer

_____

_____

_____

Medications during transfer

_____

_____

_____

| Transfer successfully completed | _____ | _____ |

Name of receiving agency _____

Name of receiving physician _____

Family member accompanying neonate _____

Relationship _____

105

Intravenous Infusion
for the Pediatric Client

Overview

Definition

The introduction of a substance directly into a vein of an infant or child

Rationale

Provide basic nutrition.

Provide a medium for medication administration.

Restore or maintain fluid and electrolyte balance.

Transfuse blood or blood derivatives for therapeutic purposes.

Terminology

Agglutination: Clumping of blood cells when incompatible blood types are mixed

Wingtip needle: A small needle used for unstable veins; also called butterfly needle because of the butterfly wing appearance of the upper portion of the appliance, which is used for guidance during insertion and for anchoring during infusion

Cutdown: Access to a vein by means of a surgical incision into the skin to locate and intubate a vein; the venous catheter is fed into the vein for a short distance and sutured in place. This is usually considered a medical function.

Derivatives of blood: Constituent parts of whole blood

Dripmeter: A chamber between the bottle or bag of infusate and the tubing with which to observe the rate of infusion

Edema: Accumulation of fluid in the tissues

Embolus: A foreign mass transported in the bloodstream

Hemolysis: The destruction of red blood cells

Infiltration: The deposit or diffusion into the tissue of substances not normally found there

Infusate: The solution to be infused

Ischemia: Interference with the blood flow to an area

Microdripmeter: A chamber between the bottle and the tubing that allows for accurate counting of drops; 60 drops = 1 ml of intravenous (IV) fluid

Phlebitis: Inflammation of a vein; in IV infusion, this is usually the result of injury to the vein by the introduction of the needle.

Plethora: Congestion causing distension of the blood vessels

Thrombus: A blood clot

Assessment

Pertinent Anatomy and Physiology

1. See Appendix I: *blood, blood vessels, skin.*
2. The site of IV infusion in the pediatric client depends on the size of the child and accessibility of the vein. In the older child, any accessible vein may be used. In the infant and small child, the superficial veins of the scalp, arms, legs, ankles, and feet are usually most accessible and most easily stabilized. Superficial veins in the scalp have no valves and can be infused in either direction.

Pathophysiological Concepts

1. See Technique No. 65, Intravenous (IV) Infusion Administration, in the Adult Unit.
2. Body water is located in the cells, in the spaces between the cells, and in the plasma and blood. Homeostasis is achieved by appropriate shifts of the fluids and electrolytes across the cell membrane and by the elimination of metabolic wastes and excess electrolytes. Failure to maintain homeostasis may be the result of some pathologic process in the body. Some of the disorders associated with water and electrolyte imbalance are pyloric stenosis, high fever, persistent or severe diarrhea and vomiting, and extensive burns. Intracellular fluid, which is contained within the body cells, accounts for nearly one half of the volume of body water in the infant. Extracellular water is located within the body spaces (interstitial fluid) or within the vascular system. Interstitial fluid decreases or increases in response to disease. In the infant, about 25% of the body weight is due to interstitial fluid. In the adult, only about 15% of the body weight is interstitial fluid. Infants and children become dehydrated much more easily than adults because of the increased metabolic rate and the increased proportional skin surface.

Assessment of the Client

1. Assess the infant's condition in relation to the present state of hydration. Determine how long the infant has been without fluid, the presence and duration of any vomiting or diarrhea, and the texture of the infant's skin. Assess baseline vital signs, with emphasis on weight and head circumference. Assess the condition of the fontanelles in an infant under 18 months of age.
2. Assess the presence of superficial veins. Determine the optimal site for insertion of the intravenous needle.
3. Determine the child's ability to cooperate during the procedure. Assess the extent of restraint required. Assess the client's level of understanding in determining how much explanation and information to offer. Assess the previous experience of the child and family with IV therapy.
4. Assess the parent–child relationship, as well as the parents' anxiety level. Determine whether or not to seek assistance from the parents when starting the IV infusion. If their presence will ease the child's anxiety and will not unduly upset the parents, their presence during the venipuncture may facilitate the procedure. Otherwise, they may participate in the explanation to the child and assist in preparing the child for the procedure.

Plan

Nursing Objectives

Adequately hydrate the pediatric client.

Reestablish fluid and electrolyte balance.

Meet the physical and emotional needs of the child and the family.

Prevent infection and complications.

Observe the client closely for adverse reactions.

Teach the parents safety precautions in handling their child with an IV.

Client Preparation

1. If the child is old enough, offer a thorough explanation of what will occur. Gear the explanation to the child's level of understanding and anxiety.

2. Explain to the parents why the child will have an IV infusion and what this will mean in regard to mobility and activity limitations. Explain about the use of restraints during the starting of the infusion, and prepare the parent if restraints will be necessary during the entire time the infusion is present.

3. Prepare all equipment before beginning the procedure so that delays will be avoided. It may be expeditious to remove the child to a well-lighted treatment area for initiation of the IV infusion so that venipuncture will be facilitated and the child's room will not be associated with painful or unpleasant activities. (Children usually consider their bed a place of safety.)

4. Calculate the rate of infusion to coincide with the prescribed rate. There are variances between the different delivery sets in the number of drops per milliliter delivered. Always check each time to be sure what the delivery rate is for the set being used. Two methods for calculating the flow rate of the IV infusion follow (see also Observations section of Technique No. 65):

   a. Microdrop or minidrop IV set yield approximately 60 drops/ml. The formula is as follows:

   Prescribed ml per hr = Flow rate in drops per min

   b. When not using microdrop or minidrop IV administration sets, the following formula may be used:

   $$\frac{\text{Drops per ml delivered by the IV set} \times \text{prescribed ml per hour}}{60}$$
   $$= \text{Rate of flow in drops per minute}$$

   For example: The administration set delivers 10 drops/ml; 24 ml/hr is the prescribed rate.

   $$\frac{10 \times 24}{60} = 4 \text{ drops/min rate of flow}$$

5. The rate of flow with an infusion pump should be set according to the directions that accompany the pump. This is the safest way to ensure an accurate rate of infusion; however, use of a pump does not excuse the nursing staff from checking on the infusion at least hourly to ensure that the infusion is progressing as ordered.

Equipment

IV solution, as ordered by the physician

IV tubing with a graduated measurement container for fluid located on line (such as the buret chamber on the pediatric Metriset)

IV tray with antiseptic solution, rubber band, razor blade, cotton balls, tape, 10-ml syringe with normal saline solution

IV stand

Scalp-vein needles, size #21, 22, 23, and 25, or a small gauge intracath, angiocath, or wingtip needle

Restraints

Infusion pump, for all children under the age of 12 years

Implementation and Interventions

Procedural Aspects

ACTION	*RATIONALE*
1. Check the bottle or bag of infusion solution to ensure the integrity of the container and the purity of the solution. If cracks or breaks are seen in the container, return it to the pharmacy. If the fluid is discolored or contains any small particles or sediment, return it. Check the expiration date on the bag or bottle to be sure it has not expired. Be sure that the solution is the one ordered for this particular child. Each IV solution should have some type of written documentation against which the nurse can verify the child's name, room number, and physician before hanging the solution. If any medication is added to the bottle, label the bottle with the name of the medication, the strength, the amount, the date and time it was added, and the name of the person who added it.	Proper identification prevents errors. Being sure that the right solution is administered to the right client is part of the nursing responsibility for the safety of the client. Proper documentation of the addition of medication may prevent duplication or omission.
2. Remove all air from the tubing by allowing the fluid to run through the tubing before clamping. Fill the graduated chamber to the desired level. Gently thump the tubing at the site of any remaining air bubbles, allow them to rise to the air space in the cylinder where they will not be infused into the child. Hang the solution on an IV stand at a level 24 to 30 inches above the venipuncture site.	Air can cause an air embolus. It should not be infused into the child. Gravity causes the fluid to drip, but the higher the level of the bag, the faster the fluid will drip. If an infusion pump is used, the height of the bag is not so critical, since the mechanical pump regulates to the rate of infusion.
3. Place the small child in a mummy restraint (see Technique No. 111, Restraints, Pediatric). The older child may be restrained on a papoose board or by another nurse. Shave the area around the intended venipuncture site. A large rubber band may be placed around the infant's head to distend the vein or a tourniquet may be used on the extremity of the older child.	The child must be immobilized during insertion of the needle to prevent unnecessary trauma and accidental contamination and/or dislodgement of the needle. Shaving the area helps reduce the risk of infection and facilitates visualization of the vein. Distension of the veins by pooling of blood aids in location and stabilization during venipuncture.

ACTION

4. Cleanse the area of intended veni-puncture thoroughly with an anti-septic solution.

5. Anchor the tubing from the IV bag or bottle to the treatment table or bed before making the venipuncture. Leave enough slack for easy maneuverability of the needle end of the tubing.

6. Insert the needle into the vein. Check the location within a blood vessel by one of several methods. Before venipuncture, the tubing on the scalp-vein needle may be attached to a 10-ml syringe filled with sterile saline solution. Once venipuncture is accomplished, one hand can anchor the needle in the vein while the other aspirates slightly on the syringe. A return of blood signifies that the needle is in the vein. Anchor the needle in place securely with tape (Fig. 105-1). Once the needle has been anchored in place, release the needle tubing from the syringe and fasten it to the IV tubing. If the tubing is already attached to the IV, the IV bag may be held at a level lower than the venipuncture site. If the needle is in the vein, a return of blood should be evident in the tubing. If this method is used, the bottle must be elevated and the fluid allowed to start infusing soon so that the blood will not clot in the needle. Once the infusion is instituted, apply a sterile dressing over the venipuncture site.

RATIONALE

Reduction of the number of micro-organisms in the area decreases the possibility of accidental contamination during venipuncture.

The weight of the freely swinging tubing is sufficient to pull the needle from the vein after venipuncture if it is not anchored.

The normal venous pressure is sufficient to push the blood out of the veins if there is no counterpressure. With the encouragement of gravitational pull or the negative pressure from aspirating the syringe, the blood will flow easily out of the vein, signifying location and patency. Application of a sterile dressing will help reduce the possibility of infection.

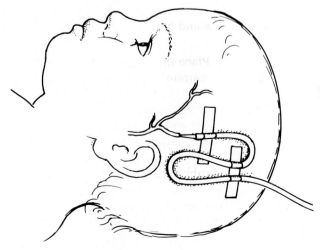

Figure 105.1

ACTION

RATIONALE

7. Set the rate of infusion at the level prescribed by the physician. For infants and children, a calibrated infusion pump is recommended as an added safety feature. Because of their small size, infants and small children cannot tolerate too much IV fluid too quickly. The rate should be adjusted while the infant is quiet. Check the rate every hour to ensure that the desired rate is being maintained.

Three major factors influencing the rate of flow are pressure, tubing size, and fluid viscosity. If the infant is crying, the vessels may be constricted, causing overinfusion later during a quiet period, when the vessels dilate. Too much fluid in a short time may cause fatal cardiac complications. An infusion pump will help ensure that the infusion runs at the proper rate.

8. Restrain the child in elbow restraints or on a pinned armboard to ensure that the needle does not become dislodged in the arm. An arm restraint may be applied and tied to the bed frame. Sandbags may be used to immobilize the infant's head. The infant's leg may be taped to a sandbag to provide immobilization (Fig. 105-2).

The goal of restraint is to limit movement of the child's extremities that causes tension on the vein and dislodges the needle. The restraints should be comfortable and should not produce undue pressure to any one area.

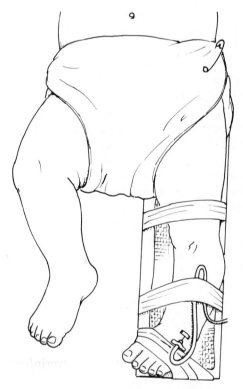

Figure 105.2

ACTION	RATIONALE
Special Modifications	
1. Wash hands thoroughly before and after handling blood and blood products. Transfusion of blood and blood derivatives to children involves the same precautions involved in transfusion of the adult. Infants and children are often given fractional amounts of the unit of blood or blood derivatives. Be sure that the proper amount for transfusion is stipulated in the physician's order. Check the child's type and cross-match the report with the label on the blood. There is usually an identification number, as well, which should be checked to ensure that the proper blood is given to the child. The needle for the infusion of blood must be of sufficient gauge to allow the blood to flow. This needle may be inserted by the physician by means of a cutdown. Frequent monitoring of the infusion is necessary to prevent the complications from infiltration of blood into the tissues.	Agglutination and hemolysis may occur from the transfusion of incompatible blood. A blood reaction may be life-threatening and must be avoided by careful scrutiny of the labels and identification information. Blood is thicker and more viscous than IV fluid and requires a larger lumen for transfusion. Because it does not drip uniformly, the rate cannot be accurately determined without the use of an infusion pump.
2. To discontinue the pediatric infusion, close the clamp on the IV tubing nearest the needle. Hold the needle firmly in place and gently loosen and remove the tape. With one hand, hold a cotton ball over the injection site and with the other, slowly withdraw the needle from the skin, keeping the hub of the needle flush with the skin. Do not drag the top of the needle against the posterior wall of the vein. Apply gentle pressure to the site until bleeding stops.	Tissue may be traumatized by improper needle removal. Any break in the skin is a potential entryway for bacteria and may lead to infection.

Communicative Aspects

OBSERVATIONS

1. Observe the infusion for proper rate. Overinfusion can be extremely dangerous for infants and small children. Underinfusion may compromise the treatment regimen.

2. Observe the site for signs of redness, tenderness, and pain, which might indicate inflammation. Observe for signs of infiltration, such as leaking or puffiness of the skin. Infiltration is often difficult to assess in infants, whose skin is normally puffy and firm. The larger proportional amount of subcutaneous fat and the larger amount of dressing and tape needed to secure the IV tubing in a small child obscure the presence of infiltration. Loosening the tape may allow visualization of the site. Check for the return of blood when the infusate is lowered. Observe dependent surfaces near the site, such as the palm of the hand or the occipital area to detect accumulation of fluid.

3. Observe the patency of the infusion hourly. Observe the IV to see that it is infusing according to the prescribed time frame. The microdrip chamber should contain fluid at all times. The clamp between the microdrip chamber and the infusion bottle should be clamped to prevent overinfusion. It is opened only to fill the microdrip chamber.

4. Observe the child's posture and reactions. If restraints are limiting the child's mobility, offer some time during which supervised mobility of the other extremities may occur to prevent discomfort. Observe the child for boredom and provide some type of diversion. Assist the parents to hold the infant, and observe their technique to ensure that the patency of the IV infusion set is not compromised (Fig. 105-3).

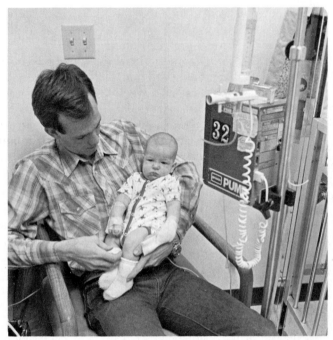

Figure 105.3

5. Observe the child receiving a blood transfusion very carefully for signs of a reaction or other transfusion complications. Baseline vital signs should be noted at the instigation of the transfusion for later comparisons in case of complications. Indications of complications include fever, hematuria, chills, nausea, vomiting, diarrhea, pain, dyspnea, shock, and allergic reaction. If reaction occurs, discontinue the blood transfusion at once. Notify the physician immediately. Keep the vein open with normal saline solution until the physician is notified and orders otherwise. Obtain a urine specimen and send it with the remainder of the blood to the laboratory immediately. All identifying tags, cards, and requisitions should accompany the blood.

CHARTING

Infusion Record: A cumulative record of the infusions given over a period of time should be present and should list the name of the solution, the size of the infusion bag (i.e., 250-ml bags for newborns and infants, 500-ml bags for children, and 1000-ml bags for adolescents), medications added, time of initiation and discontinuation, rate of infusion, site of infusion, and any problems.

Intake and Output Record: A complete record of intake and output (I&O) should be kept for all children and infants receiving IV fluids. The amount of intake will include oral intake as well as the infusions. Output will include emesis, urine, and drainage from any tubes (such as a nasogastric tube). If the infant is in diapers, the amount of urine should be measured according to hospital policy or physician stipulation, such as weighing the diapers, estimating the degree of wetness of the diapers, or counting the number of diaper changes. A suggested method is to weigh the diapers when dry and again when wet. The wet diaper weight gives the number of grams of urine which may be translated into output by using the following formula 1 gm of urine = 1 ml.

Nurses' Progress Notes: A notation about the status of the infusion should be made on each shift.

DATE/TIME	OBSERVATIONS	SIGNATURE
9/18 1130	IV infusing via infusion pump at 4 gtt/min. NPO at this time but sucking on a pacifier while being held by mother. Infusion site clear with no signs of leaking or bleeding.	P. Sanchez RN

Discharge Planning Aspects

CLIENT AND FAMILY EDUCATION

1. Explain to the family why the infant's hair must be shaved prior to initiation of the infusion. This is often very upsetting to parents. Assure them that the hair will grow back very soon. If restraints will be used during venipuncture and during infusion, explain this to the parents before they are applied. Be sure that they understand why the restraints are needed and how they will be applied. Show the parents how to hold their infant or small child with an IV infusion so that they will feel confident and the integrity of the infusion will be maintained. Tell the family the approximate length of time the IV line will be in place.

2. If the child is old enough, explain about the IV procedure and enlist the child's cooperation during venipuncture and infusion. Ask the child to notify the nurse if the infusion starts hurting or burning. Ask the child and family to notify the nurse if the infusion stops dripping or the infusion pump alarm sounds.

Evaluation

Quality Assurance

Documentation should include a description of the venipuncture process, including any problems encountered. Teaching of the parents and child should be documented. The rate of flow, type of infusate, additional medications, and additional measures to ensure safety (such as use of an infusion pump or microdrip chamber) should be noted in the chart. Accurate and ongoing assessment of the I&O should be reflected. Notation of frequent checking of the IV for infiltration, leaking, obstruction, and sterility should be made.

The hospital should have some type of policy addressing who may start pediatric infusions. If additional training of nurses is required for them to start infusions in children and/or infants, this should be stipulated in the policy. Also addressed in the IV policy is frequency of changing the IV site. A general policy on the assessment of the amount of output for the infant or small child in diapers should be stated. Every hospital should have a formal procedure for the administration of blood and blood products, which includes precautions to prevent transfusion of the wrong blood type or the wrong product.

Infection Control

1. Wash hands before and after handling blood and blood derivatives.
2. Engage in scrupulous handwashing preceding venipuncture, which is carried out under sterile conditions. Handwashing should also be done after venipuncture to prevent cross-contamination of other clients.
3. Take precautions to prevent accidental needle puncture of personnel. Be sure that the child is adequately restrained during needle insertion and removal. Dispose of needles in a designated container that is specially designed and handled to prevent accidents.

4. Prepare the skin by shaving the area if it is on the scalp and cleansing with an antiseptic. Hold the infant securely so that accidental contamination of the needle is prevented.

5. If the IV line must be in place for an extended period, adhere to the hospital policy for changing the tubing and site to prevent colonization of microorganism with resulting contamination of the vascular system. Tubing may be changed every 24 to 48 hours. Sites may be changed every 48 to 72 hours. Most hospitals recommend the infusate that hangs in the room for more than 24 hours be disposed of and new infusate be hung.

6. If the child is on isolation precautions that include blood, great care must be exercised during venipuncture to avoid accidental puncture of the nurses. Adequate restraint of the child is vital. Dispose of any equipment that contacts the child's blood in an unpenetrable sack that is taped shut. If any of the equipment is not disposable, wash and dry it in the client's room and place it in a sack, tape the sack shut, and label with the contents, the date, the client's name, and the type of isolation precautions required (see Technique No. 66, Isolation Precautions).

Technique Checklist

	YES	NO
Technique explained to child	_____	_____
Technique explained to parents	_____	_____
Baseline vital signs charted	_____	_____

B/P _____ P _____ R _____ T _____

Site of infusion _____

Type of needle used _____

   Size _____

Infusion rate precautions

Rate prescribed _____		
Infusion pump	_____	_____
Microdrip chamber	_____	_____
Filters	_____	_____
Hourly visual monitoring	_____	_____

   Other _____

Restraints necessary	_____	_____

Duration of infusions _____

Frequency of site changes _____

Frequency of tubing changes _____

Frequency of dressing changes _____

Blood or blood products transfused

   Type of infusion _____

   Amount _____

   Temperature at beginning of transfusion _____

   Temperature at end of transfusion _____

Complications _____

106

Medication Administration for Pediatric Clients

Overview

Definition

The process by which drugs are given to a pediatric client. Types include the following.

Oral administration: Drugs in liquid or solid state administered by mouth to infants or children. Tablets may be crushed and mixed with a small amount of liquid.

Topical administration: Administering drugs in the liquid (lotion, liniment, semi-solid (ointment, cream), or solid state (lozenges, suppositories) for absorption from the skin or mucous membranes

Inhalation administration: Administering drugs in a vapor or gaseous state for absorption from the respiratory tract (e.g., oxygen)

Parenteral administration: Administering drugs in a solution or suspension by injection; examples are the following:

Intradermal: The injection of a small amount of solution just below the surface of the skin

Subcutaneous (SC) or hypodermic (H): The injection of medication into the loose connective tissue under the skin when the oral route is not feasible or when slower action is desired than with the intramuscular route. Common sites include the upper arm and upper thigh.

Intramuscular (IM): The injection of medication into muscular tissue when a more rapid absorption is desired than is possible with SC injections or when the drug is irritating to subcutaneous tissue or injurious to a vein. The most common sites are the ventrogluteal muscle, the vastus lateralis muscle, the dorsogluteal muscle (in older children), and the deltoid muscle. IM injections are not given in the buttocks unless the child has walked for at least 1 year.

Intravenous (IV): The injection of a medication directly into a vein. With such rapid absorption, immediate systemic reactions are possible.

Rationale

Promote health and prevent disease.

Relieve symptoms of illness.

Aid in diagnosis.

Terminology

Aerosol: A pressurized dosage form containing the product and propellant capable of forcefully expelling that product through an opened valve

Diffusion: The movement of charged and uncharged particles along a concentration gradient

Edema: Accumulation of fluid in the tissues

Elixir: A sweetened, hydroalcoholic solution

Emulsion: The mixture of two liquids (usually water and an oil), one of which is disbursed in the form of droplets into the other

Enteric-coated tablet: A tablet coated with a composition of substances such as stearic acid, mastic, salol, cellulose, resins, or other substances that will not dissolve in the acid medium of the stomach, but will dissolve in the alkaline medium of the intestines

Lozenge: A flat disk of medication, containing sugar flavor and an adhesive substance, which is slowly dissolved in the mouth

Suppository: A solid dosage form for insertion into a body orifice

Vial: A glass bottle containing sterile medicine or solution, usually in multidose amounts, sealed with a rubber stopper

Assessment

Pertinent Anatomy and Physiology

1. See Appendix I: *blood vessels, skeletal muscles, skin, stomach.*

2. In an infant, the preferred sites for IM injection are the vastus lateralis muscle (Fig. 106-1) and the ventrogluteal muscle (Fig. 106-2).* The dorsogluteal muscle can be used in children after the child has walked for one year (Fig. 106-3). These muscles are free of important nerves and blood vessels, with the exception of the femoral artery on the medial aspect of the thigh. The vastus lateralis is the largest and best developed muscle in the infant. The dorsogluteal muscle is used for injections in the adult and older child, but is unsatisfactory as an injection site for the infant because it is small, poorly developed, and dangerously close to the sciatic nerve. Once the child begins walking, this muscle develops and is more satisfactory for IM injection. In the older child, the deltoid muscle may be used for injection (Fig. 106-4). Medication may be absorbed more quickly from this area than from the lower body. This muscle is avoided when selecting an injection site in infants and small children because of the small area available, the underdeveloped state of this muscle in small children, and the association of greater pain with injection in this area.

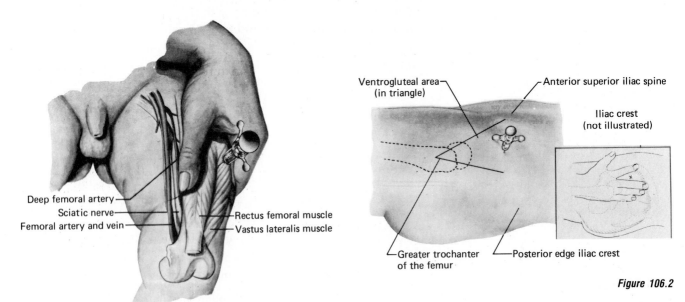

Deep femoral artery
Sciatic nerve
Femoral artery and vein
Rectus femoral muscle
Vastus lateralis muscle

Figure 106.1

Ventrogluteal area (in triangle)
Anterior superior iliac spine
Iliac crest (not illustrated)
Greater trochanter of the femur
Posterior edge iliac crest

Figure 106.2

* Figs. 106.1 to 106.4 are courtesy of Wyeth Laboratories.

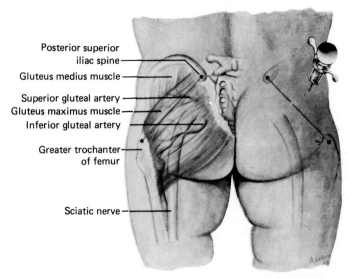

Posterior superior
iliac spine
Gluteus medius muscle
Superior gluteal artery
Gluteus maximus muscle
Inferior gluteal artery
Greater trochanter
of femur

Sciatic nerve

Figure 106.3

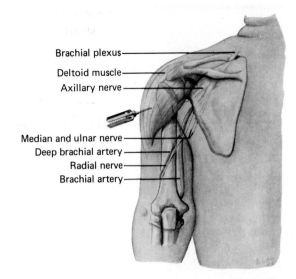

Brachial plexus
Deltoid muscle
Axillary nerve

Median and ulnar nerve
Deep brachial artery
Radial nerve
Brachial artery

Figure 106.4

3. Absorption of oral drugs occurs mainly in the small intestine. The intestinal folds greatly increase absorptive ability. Absorption occurs by active transport across the intestinal wall and by diffusion.

Pathophysiological Concepts

See Technique 67, Medications, Administration of, in the Adult Section.

Assessment of the Client

1. Assess the age and muscular development of the child in determining the site for intramuscular injection. Other factors to consider are the amount of medication to be injected and the desired rate of absorption. Assess the probable number of injections, the frequency of administration, preexisting physical conditions that might interfere with using the desired location, and the ability of the child to assume the position necessary to allow safe injection.

2. Assess the child's ability to swallow the pill or tablet. Determine whether or not to crush the tablet and the type of mixture that will most likely facilitate administration to the child. Assess the presence of vomiting and measures to decrease the chance of the child vomiting the medication once it has been administered.

3. Assess the parents' ability and willingness to assist with the medication administration procedure. Almost every parent has given their child some type of medication at one time or another. Assess the methods the parents have found effective and determine the appropriateness of using these methods in administering medication to the child in the hospital.

4. Assess the child's and parents' level of understanding of why the medication is needed, what its expected results are, and how the family unit can help the child by compliance with medication therapy.

5. Assess the child's allergy history. Determine the presence of any allergic responses in the past and the precipitating factors. Assess the presence of severe drug allergies in the parents.

Plan

Nursing Objectives

Allay the child's fear and anxiety by giving an explanation that is understandable and appropriate for age and level of interest.

Administer drugs according to the "Five Rights": right dose, right drug, right route, right time, and right client.

Know the safe dosage range of any medication administered, as well as its action and possible side-effects.

Observe, report, and record the desired therapeutic effects, the precautions taken, and any untoward reactions.

Answer truthfully the questions asked by the child and parents about the medication.

Establish a constructive relationship with the child.

Client Preparation

1. Offer an honest explanation to the child about the medications. The younger the child, the simpler and briefer the explanation should be. Explain what is to be done and what is expected of the child. Explain in terms the child understands and in a way appropriate to the child's level of comprehension.

2. If possible, disguise oral medications that are not palatable with small amounts of fruit juices, honey, jam, or some type of syrup. Most pills and tablets can be crushed and mixed with syrups and suspensions. Do not mix the medication with formula or foods from the basic food groups, which are important to adequate nutrition of the child.

3. Ensure the presence of equipment or personnel to provide adequate restraint of the child during medication administration.

Equipment

Medication

Medication card or sheet containing the child's name, identification number, name of the medication, dosage, route, and time of administration

Tray, if needed

Additional equipment for oral drugs

    Cup of water

    Syringe, dropper, or measurement spoon

    Syrup for mixing with drug

    Mortar and pestle for crushing drug

Additional equipment for inhalation drugs

    Inhaler

    Atomizer

Additional equipment for topical administration

    Gloves or applicator for lotions, liniments, and creams

    Gloves and lubricant for suppositories

Additional equipment for parenteral administration

    Syringe

    Needle

    Cotton ball and antiseptic cleanser

    Tourniquet (if IV is not present)

Calculating Dosage Formulas

1. Most medications come in prepackaged doses appropriate for administration to adults. Infants and children usually receive a portion of the dose. The determination of the dose to be given to the infant or child should be made as a fraction of the usual adult dose. The calculation of the pediatric dose is based on body weight or body surface area, as follows:

   a. Clark's rule (Calculation on the basis of weight): Divide the weight of the child by 150 and multiply by the usual adult dose:

   $$\frac{\text{Weight of child (in lb)} \times \text{adult dose}}{150} = \text{safe dosage for child}$$

   Example: To determine if the dosage ordered for a child who weighs 21 lb is within the safe dosage range, and knowing the usual adult dosage is 10 gr, the computation would be done as follows:

   $$\frac{21 \text{ lb} \times 10 \text{ gr}}{150} = \frac{210}{150} = 1\tfrac{2}{5} \text{ gr (safe dosage range for a child)}$$

   b. Calculation on the basis of body surface area: To calculate on the basis of body surface, a means of determining the body surface area (BSA) of the child must be used. Graphic numeric scales, called nomograms, are available for making this calculation. The formula is based on a 100% adult dose for a person weighing about 140 lb and having a BSA of about 1.7 square meters:

   $$\frac{\text{BSA of child in sq meters} \times \text{usual adult dose}}{1.7 \text{ sq meters}} = \text{safe dosage for child}$$

2. For some drugs, the manufacturer states the pediatric dosage.

3. For converting from one form of measurement to another, see the charts and formulas in Appendix III.

Safety Factors in Administration of Medications to Children

1. Use caution in obtaining drugs, calculating dosages, and measuring and administering medications to children. Check and double check. Be certain to properly indentify the child. Infants do not answer to their names; young children will often answer to any name; and older children will sometimes claim the identity of someone else as a game or jest, not realizing the danger of medication errors. Always check the medication sheet or card against the identification band of the child.

2. Never administer unfamiliar drugs without consulting a reliable reference.

3. Because of the danger of aspiration, never forcibly administer pills and tablets to a young child. The preferred and safest method is to crush the medicine and mix it in a solution. The danger of vomiting may be reduced by offering a sip of carbonated beverage on ice before and after taking the medication, if this is allowed in the child's diet.

4. Never leave drugs on the bedside table or within reach of the child.

5. Administer the medication slowly to prevent choking. Allow time for complete swallowing before continuing the administration.

6. Always double check the medication container, the card, and the physician's order for agreement.

Implementation and Interventions

Procedural Aspects

ACTION

RATIONALE

Preparation of Medications

1. Review drug literature carefully for any unfamiliar medication to ensure understanding of action and possible side-effects. If in doubt about any drug, consult the charge nurse, pharmacist, or physician until all doubts are resolved.

It is the responsibility of the professional nurse to be familiar with every drug administered.

2. Check the medication label three times: when the dose is removed from the cart, when the dose is poured or drawn from the container, and just before the container is returned to the shelf or discarded. Check the dosage calculation carefully. If there are any questions or doubts, verify computations with a co-worker or the physician.

Checking and rechecking help reduce the chance of medication errors.

3. Solid, stable dosage forms may be poured up to 1 hour before administration. Check any contraindications, such as the need to keep the medication refrigerated, before pouring.

Stable forms, such as tablets and capsules, will not decompose while standing.

4. When preparing a liquid oral preparation, shake the bottle or single-dose container well before opening, unless specifically contraindicated. Medication dosages can be most accurately regulated by drawing them into a graduated syringe to the exact level of the prescribed dose. A large-bore needle or the plain tip of the syringe can be used. Remove the needle before going into the client's room.

Particles held in suspension can be evenly dispersed throughout the medication by shaking the container. Exact dosages must be given to obtain maximum therapeutic effect. The needle must be removed before proceeding to the child's room to reduce the chance of accidental injury to the child or administration of the medication by the wrong route.

ACTION	***RATIONALE***
5. Parenteral medications are usually packaged in adult doses. After carefully calculating the proper dose, discard the excess medication from the syringe. If there is doubt about the accuracy of the dosage measurement, draw the proper amount into a small graduated syringe capable of measuring the dosages required. Because of the small amount of muscle mass in infants and small children, injections of more than 1 ml are usually not given. Medications for IV administration are often given by IV push high in the IV tubing. Be sure that these medications are compatible with the infusion, which will also act to dilute the medication.	It is imperative that the proper amount of medication be administered to the child. Administration of an adult dose to a child could be fatal. Diluting the IV medication may reduce irritation to the vein. However, if the intravenous medications are added to the bottle of infusion, they may lose their potency before reaching the child due to the slow infusion rate of pediatric IVs.
6. Do not administer drugs that have changed color, consistency, or odor. Do not give medications from an unlabeled container or one whose label is unreadable. In most states, only the pharmacist may legally fill and relabel medication bottles.	Changes in medications may indicate that they are no longer stable and cannot be depended upon to produce the desired therapeutic effects.
7. Exercise caution when mixing drugs. Do not give drugs if they change color or form a precipitate when mixed. Medications for IV infusion are usually given separately. All of the previous medication should be allowed to infuse and the tubing should be flushed with IV fluid before administration of another medication.	Some drugs react with each other when mixed and undergo chemical changes as evidenced by color change or formation of a percipitate. These altered medications may have detrimental effects on the child and must not be administered. Drugs that come in contact with drugs from previous doses may precipitate in the IV tubing.

Administration of Medications

1. Wash hands before administering medication to any client. Use a pleasant, positive approach. Assume that the child will take the medicine. Identify the child by comparing the written documentation for the medicine with the identification band on the child.	Prevent cross-contamination by diminishing the presence of microorganisms through handwashing. Take great care to administer the right medication to the right child.

ACTION

RATIONALE

2. Restrain the hands of the infant or young child to prevent accidental spilling of the oral medication (Fig. 106-5) or contamination of the needle during parenteral injection. Use reason and firmness with the older child who refuses medication. Use a positive approach and kindness. Allow the child to make some choices, if possible. For instance, say, "Here is your pill. Shall I pour your water or can you?"

The medication must be administered as ordered; however, the ego and self-confidence of the child should not be threatened. Allowing the child to participate in the decision-making process may enhance cooperation.

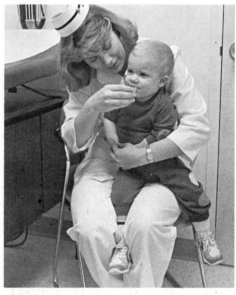

Figure 106.5

3. Oral medications may be diluted with water or sweet-tasting substances to disguise bad taste. Use only enough diluent to achieve the desired effect.

If too much diluent is used, the child may become full before the entire dose is consumed.

4. Infants may receive oral medication by dropper if the exact dosage can be ensured. Use only the dropper that comes with the medicine. If exact dosage is questionable, use a graduated syringe for administration. With the infant's head elevated, depress the infant's chin with the thumb to open the mouth and slowly drop the medication onto the middle of the tongue. Toddlers and young children may drink the medicine from a cup or individual container. Every effort should be made to make the medication as palatable as possible. Children over the age of 5 may be able to swallow a pill. Instruct the child to place the pill near the back of the tongue and drink the liquid, swallowing the pill with the liquid.

Since infants and small children receive minute amounts of some medications, it is essential to measure accurately. Drug manufacturers will only guarantee exact dosages if their dropper is used. Using a graduated syringe facilitates this procedure. The infant or child taking oral medications should always have the head on a higher plane than the rest of the body to prevent choking and aspiration.

ACTION

5. Identify the area for IM injection quickly. The length of the needle should be sufficient to place the medication deeply into the muscle tissue. If practical, the child may be allowed some input into the decision about where to place the medication.

6. Secure the child in such a way that movement that might dislodge or contaminate the needle is limited. For the infant, grasp the muscle mass of the thigh firmly and anchor it with one hand while injecting the medication with the other (Fig. 106-6).

RATIONALE

No one likes the pain that accompanies IM injection. Accomplish the injection as quickly as possible. The medication should be placed deeply into the tissue to facilitate absorption and to prevent irritation of outer tissues.

Anchoring the muscle of the thigh prevents the reflex jerk that occurs upon injection from dislodging the needle. Steady pressure allows the medication to be injected safely into the muscle without trauma to the surrounding tissue. Injection into a blood vessel may cause immediate absorption of the medication and untoward consequences.

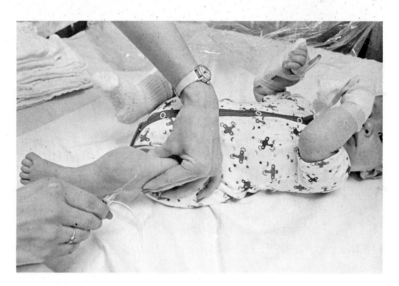

Figure 106.6

For the larger child, restrain the child's upper torso with the elbow and forearm while the hand holds the thigh (Fig. 106-7). Use the other hand to inject the medication. If the older child cannot be depended upon to hold still, assistance may be needed to ensure that the needle is not contaminated or dislodged. Insert the needle deeply into the muscle, aspirate to ensure that the needle is not in a small blood vessel, and inject the medication with a steady pressure. Withdraw the needle quickly and apply gentle pressure with a cotton ball until bleeding stops.

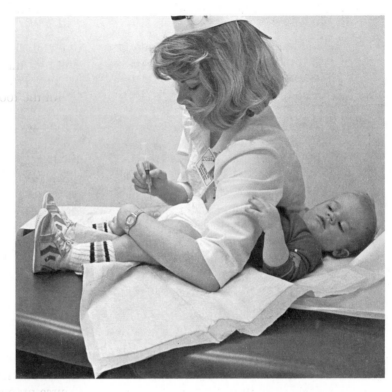

Figure 106.7

ACTION

7. Carry an extra needle and adhesive strip so that delays can be avoided. Replace the needle if it is contaminated. Apply an adhesive strip to the injection site. Praise the child and offer reassurance. It may be beneficial to hold the child for a few minutes after injection (Fig. 106-8).

RATIONALE

An extra needle may be placed on the syringe immediately in case the first needle is contaminated. Many children associate an adhesive strip with comfort. This small gesture also allows the nurse to acknowledge the child's bravery or cooperation and enhances feelings of self-worth. Re-establishment of a satisfactory relationship is beneficial after treatments that cause discomfort.

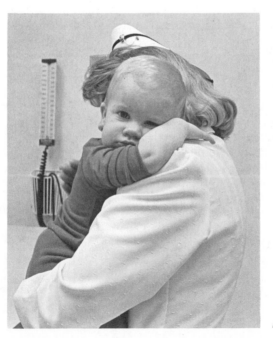

Figure 106.8

ACTION	*RATIONALE*
8. IV medication is usually added to the microdrip chamber of the IV tubing. Cleanse the injection port with an alcohol sponge and inject the medication into the chamber or hang an additional bag with a microdrip chamber. Placing the tubing in an infusion pump will help ensure that the medication is given at the desired rate.	IV medication is usually diluted and infused through a patent IV line. The injection port has been in contact with the room air and is considered contaminated until cleaned before injection.
9. Rectal medications may not be absorbed because of stool in the rectum. Use a finger cot or glove. Unwrap the suppository and insert it into the rectum beyond the anal sphincter. After the medication has been instilled, firmly squeeze the child's buttocks together for several minutes.	Pressure on the anal sphincter causes an urge to evacuate the bowel. Squeezing the child's buttocks together until this feeling passes helps ensure retention of the medication.
10. If the purpose of nose drops is to decrease stuffiness so that the child can nurse more easily, the nose drops are usually given 30 minutes before feeding time. Position the infant or child with a pillow under the shoulders, allowing the head to fall over the edge of the pillow. Place a hand on the child's forehead to stabilize it. Elevate the child's nares slightly with the thumb to facilitate insertion of the drops (Fig. 106-9). Allow the child to remain stationary for 1 minute after instillation.	Infants are nose breathers. Nasal stuffiness interferes with their ability to nurse properly. If the child remains in position for 1 minute, the medication has a better chance to come in contact with all of the nasal surface.

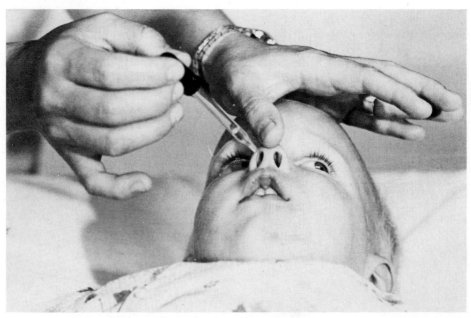

Figure 106.9

ACTION	RATIONALE
11. Ear drops should be warmed to room temperature. *Ear drops must not be hot.* Pull the auricle down and back gently and drop the desired number of drops into the ear (Fig. 106-10). For the child over 3 years of age, pull the auricle up and back gently and instill the drops. The child should be lying on the side opposite the ear into which the medication will be placed.	Hot substances will harm the delicate lining of the ear. Pulling the auricle down and back promotes the insertion and flow of the medication into the ear for the child under 3 years because the eustachian tube is short and straight. After age 3, the ear canal is curved like that of an adult.

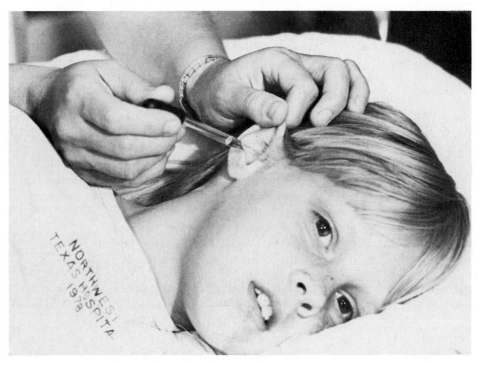

Figure 106.10

Special Modifications

1. If the child immediately vomits the medication, and its total presence in the emesis can be verified by sight, administration of the medication may be repeated. However, if the presence of the medication cannot be verified, it should not be given again without the physician's instructions.	Spontaneous vomiting of medicines, especially those with unpleasant taste, is not unusual. To ensure that the child is receiving the proper dose of medication, it must be ascertained that none of the first dose was absorbed before repeating the dose.
2. For other considerations affecting the administration of medications, refer to Technique 67, Medications, Administration of, in the adult section.	

Communicative Aspects

OBSERVATIONS

1. After the administration of any drug, observe the child's reactions. Observe for desired results, unexpected results, side-effects, and untoward reactions.
2. If the child vomits, observe the emesis for signs of the medication.
3. Observe the skin of the child who is receiving repeated injections for signs of tissue breakdown and inflammation. Encourage the child to move the limb and observe the degree of mobility and apparent discomfort associated with movement.

CHARTING

Medication Record.
A complete record of all medications received by the child during the hospitalization should be maintained. This should include the name of the drug, the amount, the route, and the person who gave the medication.

Nurses' Progress Notes.
Note any reaction to the medication, any problems associated with administration of the medication, and any omitted doses and the reason.

DATE/TIME	OBSERVATIONS	SIGNATURE
4/20 0830	IM injection in rt. ventral thigh. Alert and active. No problems and only slight crying after injection. Held for several minutes after injection. Playing at this time with mother in attendance. ———————————————————————	C. Day RN

Discharge Planning Aspects

CLIENT AND FAMILY EDUCATION

1. If the child will be sent home with medication, teach the parents and child, if appropriate, how to give the medications and what reactions to report to the physician. The parents should know the route of the medication and the technique for administration. They should know the times to administer the medication and should be cautioned about the importance of adhering to the prescribed schedule. Any expected side-effects, such as constipation or nausea, should be explained to the parents, along with suggestions for counteracting these problems.
2. If the client has an allergic reaction to a medication, tell the family the name of the drug (including the trade name and generic name). Caution them to alert health-care personnel about the allergy whenever they seek care in the future.
3. Caution the family about the judicious use of over-the-counter medications. The habitual use of laxatives and other home remedies may interfere with the action of prescribed drugs.

Evaluation

Quality Assurance

Documentation should include the complete record of all medications administered to the client during the hospitalization. The child's reactions to the medication should be documented in relation to relief of symptoms and progression of the condition for which the child was hospitalized. The documentation should reflect the names of the drugs, the amounts given, the routes, the names of the persons administering medications, any problems, and the resolution of any problems. Progress records should reflect that the nurse was aware of potential side-effects and took measures to identify and counteract these effects. Attention to the child's allergy history should be reflected.

Hospital continuing-education programs should address the problem of updating nurses' knowledge of the drugs used in health care. Pharmacology courses and courses in the latest methods of drug administration should be available. Pediatric drug administration is a specialty in its own right, and should be addressed by pharmacology courses.

Infection Control

1. Handwashing should be done after each client. In the administration of oral and topical medications, handwashing is important to prevent the spread of infection from one client to another. In the administration of parenteral medications, careful handwashing is important because the natural defensive barrier of the client—the skin—is broken. The potential for cross-contamination is increased. It is also important to remove as many pathogens as possible from the client's skin before administering parenteral medications.

2. Equipment that is used for consecutive clients, such as restraints, should be cleaned between uses.

Technique Checklist

	YES	NO
Explanation offered to child	_____	_____
Explanation offered to parents	_____	_____
Reason for medication	_____	_____
Name and dose of medication	_____	_____
Expected results of medication	_____	_____
Possible side-effects	_____	_____
Allergy history obtained on admission	_____	_____
All orders for medications were followed correctly	_____	_____
Dosage calculations checked		
Calculated by weight	_____	_____
Calculated by BSA	_____	_____
Complete written record of all medications received is on the chart	_____	_____
Unexpected reactions documented in nurses' progress notes	_____	_____
Follow-up actions documented	_____	_____
Complete instructions given before discharge in regard to take-home medications	_____	_____
Oral _____		
Written _____		
Allergies to medications experienced during hospitalization	_____	_____

107

Oral Hygiene for an Infant or Child

Overview

Definition

The process of cleaning and freshening the gums, mouth, and teeth (if present) of the infant or child

Rationale

Freshen the mouth and relieve it of offensive odors.
Remove food and debris on the surface of teeth that provide a reservoir for
microorganisms.
Keep the mouth, gums, and teeth in healthy condition.

Terminology

Malocclusion: Condition in which the upper and lower teeth do not fit together
when the mouth is closed

Plaque: The sticky layer of mucous material containing streptococcal bacteria that
forms on the teeth

Sordes: Accumulation of food particles, microorganisms, and dried mucous on
the teeth (also called materia alba)

Assessment

**Pertinent Anatomy
and Physiology**

See Appendix I: *mouth, teeth.*

**Pathophysiological
Concepts**

1. Healthy tissue and the presence of antibacterial enzymes in the saliva provide natural defense against oral infections. The oral cavity contains a balanced biological system of microorganisms, which serves the function of
beginning the digestive process. Antibiotic therapy can upset the normal flora
of the alimentary canal, including the mouth, causing greater susceptibility to
oral infection.

2. Dental caries (localized destruction of tooth tissue by bacterial action) is common in school-age children. Demineralization of the surface enamel occurs,
ultimately causing destruction of the dentin and pulp of the tooth. Caries are
actually caused by the acid produced by the bacteria that colonize on the
tooth surface. Untreated dental caries and malocclusion in childhood can
predispose the client to periodontal disease in adulthood. Dental caries, in
combination with fermentable carbohydrates, especially sucrose, cause destruction of the tooth structure. Children 4 to 8 years and 12 to 18 years old
are most susceptible.

3. As the teeth penetrate the gums during eruption, inflammation and sensitivity can occur. The child may become irritable. Delayed eruption of all
teeth may indicate a systemic or nutritional disturbance.

4. Periodontal disease usually occurs in adolescence, along with an increase in
dental caries. Drug-associated gingivitis of younger children can lead to
periodontal disease in adolescence. Facial growth during adolescent years
may add to the orthodontic problems of young people in this age-group.

Assessment of the Client

1. Assess the condition of the child's mouth. Determine the presence of caries and evidence of existing dental work. Inspect the gums for swelling, inflammation, and bleeding. Note whether or not the gums seem puffy, protrude down into the spaces between the teeth, or are discolored. Note foul odors, which may indicate the presence of infection in the mouth. Note the presence and location of loose, chipped, or broken teeth.

2. Assess the child's hygienic habits at home related to tooth care. Determine whether or not the child has ever visited a dentist. Determine the frequency of brushing and flossing and note the extent to which the child is able to perform or participate in these activities. Assess the child's and parents' knowledge of proper methods of caring for the teeth and mouth.

3. Assess factors that will alter the methods or increase the need for oral care, such as chemotherapy, antibiotic therapy, vomiting, nutritional deficiencies, immunologic deficiencies, and hereditary diseases.

Plan

Nursing Objectives

Carry out oral hygiene measures as often as necessary to maintain a healthy, fresh mouth.

Teach the child proper techniques for brushing and flossing the teeth.

Observe the teeth, gums, and mucous membranes carefully for early signs of infection and soreness.

Provide a role model for prioritizing oral care during daily activities.

Teach the child and family the role of proper nutrition in the formation of healthy teeth.

Client Preparation

1. Oral care is usually done with the daily bath. Assemble equipment and explain its use to the child who does not know about brushing and flossing.

2. Raise the child's head and shoulders for cleaning the teeth, unless medically contraindicated. If this is not possible, turn the child to the side and place the basin under the child's mouth to receive the water used to rinse the mouth.

3. The toothbrush for a child should be small enough to be effective in a small mouth. The preferred child's toothbrush has a short head and handle and soft natural bristles that are ½ inch long.

Equipment

Toothbrush and toothpaste

Curved basin

Dental floss

Towel

Cool water and cup

Lubricant for lips, if desired

Rinse for mouth (such as diluted hydrogen peroxide)

Bulb syringe (if needed)

Tongue blades (if needed)

Gloves (if needed)

Implementation and Interventions

Procedural Aspects

ACTION

1. Wash hands thoroughly before and after assisting the child with oral hygiene.

2. Brushing the teeth should be done for all children who have teeth. Even if the child has only a few teeth, these should be wiped gently with a soft towel during daily hygiene to establish the routine of consistent oral hygiene and to clean plaque from the teeth.

3. If the child can sit up, this is the position of choice for oral hygiene (Fig. 107-1). If not, turn the child to the side with a towel and basin under the side of the face (Fig. 107-2).

RATIONALE

Handwashing reduces the chance of cross-contamination. The oral cavity is the site of many normal bacteria, which may be pathogenic if introduced to susceptible persons.

Attention to oral hygiene establishes good habits and sets a good example for the child's parents.

Sitting or side-lying positions help prevent aspiration of liquids and choking by allowing the liquid to drain by gravitational flow.

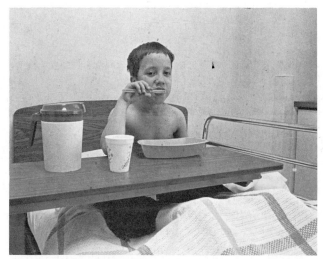

Figure 107.1

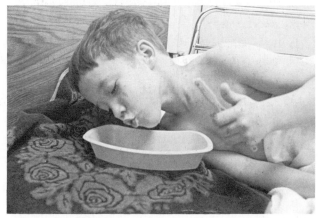

Figure 107.2

ACTION

RATIONALE

4. Rinse the toothbrush in cool water before applying the toothpaste. Assist the child or brush the child's teeth in the following manner: Place the brush flat against the teeth. The bristles of the brush should cover the teeth and extend slightly over the gumline. Turn the brush to a 45° angle and apply gentle pressure. Move the bristles gradually toward the biting surface of the teeth. Do one section of the mouth at a time. Turn the bristles toward the teeth with the sweeping stroke at least five times in each section of the mouth, on both the front and back of the teeth. Do not exert great pressure.

Brushing in the direction of tooth growth facilitates the removal of food particles and stimulates the gums. The child's oral mucosa is thin and easily damaged. Excessive force may cause bleeding.

5. Demonstrate and assist the child to floss the teeth. Place the child in the semi-Fowler's position. Wrap the dental floss around the middle finger of each hand and loop several times to stablize. Use the index finger to tighten the floss. Insert the floss between each of the child's teeth and move in a sawing manner along the sides of the teeth. To remove the floss, release it from the backmost finger and pull it through the teeth (see illustration in Technique No. 69, Oral Hygiene, in the adult section). Rinse the child's mouth with water after flossing.

Plaque continuously builds up on the teeth. If left in place, it can lead to gum and tooth disease. Flossing helps remove plaque. Rinsing will further wash the loosened plaque from the mouth.

6. Rinse the child's mouth with cool water and mouthwash, if the child desires. Rinse the toothbrush with cool water and hang it in a specified place to dry.

Rinsing the loosened food and toothpaste from the mouth leaves the child's mouth feeling fresh and clean. Warm or hot water may damage the bristles of the toothbrush.

Special Modifications

1. If the infant or child is febrile, be especially careful not to injure the gums. In addition, give special care to the lips, which tend to become dry, crusted, and cracked. Clean the lips and surrounding area gently and apply a lubricant.

Fever causes the delicate mucous membranes to be particularly susceptible to injury. Breaking the skin offers another entry point for infectious organisms.

2. For children on chemotherapy, special care must be taken. Use soft spongettes to clean the teeth and gums gently.

Chemotherapy renders the bucal membranes susceptible to ulceration. The gums bleed easily because of the decreased platelet count.

Communicative Aspects

OBSERVATIONS

1. Note the condition of the child's teeth and gums.
2. After teaching sessions, assess the effectiveness of the child's technique by observing the return demonstration.
3. Note signs of infection or irritation of the gums, mouth cavity, or tongue.
4. Note the condition of the lips and area around the child's mouth. Observe whether the lips are chapped, cracked, or crusted.

CHARTING

DATE/TIME	OBSERVATIONS	SIGNATURE
5/4 0830	Oral care given. Gums show no signs of redness or inflammation. Lips show some indication of cracking, lubricant applied and left with mother for reapplication as needed. Brushing technique demonstrated again. Return demonstration much better than yesterday. Continues to need assistance with flossing.	R. Smith RN

Discharge Planning Aspects

CLIENT AND FAMILY EDUCATION

1. Explain to the parents and the child the importance of regular daily brushing of the teeth. Parents should begin teaching about oral hygiene when the teeth erupt. Regular brushing after each meal should be started by age 3. Explain the importance of protecting the health of the primary teeth to contribute to the proper eruption and occlusion of the permanent teeth. Visits to the dentist should be instituted by age 3.
2. Demonstrate the technique for proper brushing of the teeth. Allow the child to return the demonstration with input and encouragement about proper technique. Be positive and encouraging so that the child will not become discouraged.
3. Many parents do not understand the proper technique for or the benefits to be derived from flossing the teeth. Demonstrate to the child and parents how to hold the dental floss. Explain that the benefits of flossing include removal of plaque that is missed by the toothbrush and massaging of the gums at the point of emergence of the tooth. Explain that the floss must be held tightly; however, discourage excessive force during flossing, which might cause bleeding of the gums.

Evaluation

Quality Assurance

Document the initial assessment of the child's dental condition. The status of detition and the presence of missing, broken, chipped, or loose teeth should be noted. This is particularly important if the child will undergo surgery. It is important for the anesthetist or anesthesiologist to be aware of any loose teeth before surgical intubation. The notes should reflect any complications of dental hygiene, including bleeding of the gums or pain. The ability of the child to participate in dental care should be noted. Dental history notations should include whether or not the child brushes regularly at home and if the child has seen or regularly sees a dentist. Teaching of the child and parents should be documented in the chart with an assessment of their degree of understanding.

Infection Control

1. Strains of the bacterium *Streptococcus mutans* most frequently cause tooth decay. The primary metabolic food of this group is sucrose. Carbohydrate in a typical diet is composed of 30% to 50% sucrose; therefore, the bacteria have ideal conditions for destruction of tooth enamel. Oral-hygiene measures help reduce the amount of bacteria in the mouth and prevent tooth decay and infections.

2. Cracked lips and bleeding gums provide an entry for pathogenic organisms into the body.

3. Meticulous handwashing before and after administering oral hygiene is necessary to prevent cross-contamination. Transmission of pathogenic micro-organisms can be greatly minimized by handwashing.

Technique Checklist

	YES	NO
Procedure explained to child before beginning	_____	_____
Proper technique demonstrated to child	_____	_____
Return demonstration of proper brushing technique	_____	_____
Flossing demonstrated		
To child	_____	_____
To parents	_____	_____
Return demonstration	_____	_____
Condition of teeth and gums noted	_____	_____
Loose teeth _____		
Swollen gums _____		
Bleeding gums _____		
Discoloration of gums _____		
Frequency of oral care _____		
Preventive-dentistry concepts explained to parents and child	_____	_____
Verbalized understanding of preventive dentistry	_____	_____

108 Oxygen Therapy for Children

Overview

Definition

Administration of oxygen, an element essential to life, in proper methods and quantities to ensure proper functioning of the heart, brain, and every cell in the body

Rationale

Oxygenate the child's arterial blood adequately and ensure adequate removal of carbon dioxide.

Enhance the quality of inspired air to decrease the amount of energy required for the infant or child to breathe.

Terminology

Anoxia: Oxygen deprivation, which if severe enough, may cause cell death in as short a time as 30 seconds

Retrolental fibroplasia: A condition in which an opaque fibrous membrane develops on the posterior surface of the lens of the eye, causing blindness

Ventilation: The movement of necessary gases from the atmosphere into the respiratory system

Assessment

Pertinent Anatomy and Physiology

1. See Appendix I: *bronchial tree, lungs, trachea.* See, also, Technique 82, Respiratory Care, in the Adult Section.

2. At birth, the respiratory tract is relatively small. After the first breath, the lungs grow rapidly. The volume of air inspired increases with the growth of the lungs. The chest has a rounded shape at birth, which gradually widens to achieve the oval shape, with flattened anterior and posterior surfaces, of adulthood. The infant relies almost entirely on diaphragmatic/abdominal breathing. The newborn's airway has little smooth muscle; however, by age 4 to 5 months, sufficient muscle is present to react to irritating stimuli. By age 1 year, the smooth muscle development of the airway is complete.

3. Because the muscles are immature and the skeletal structure is very pliant, the infant and small child must exert great energy to breathe. Their respirations are usually rapid and shallow. An infant's normal oxygen consumption per kilogram of body weight is almost double that of an adult. When oxygenation needs are intensified during stress periods, the infant tires quickly.

Pathophysiological Concepts	1. Prolonged exposure to high concentrations of oxygen can damage various body tissues, such as the retina of the premature infant and the lungs of infants and children.
	2. Asthma is one of the most common chronic conditions of children under the age of 17 years. This disease is characterized by bronchospasm in response to various stimuli. It is also causes edema of the mucosal surface of the bronchioles and increased production of mucus. Wheezing and dyspnea are a result of the airway obstruction. Bronchodilators and smooth-muscle relaxants are used to treat the condition. Preventive measures include avoidance of the triggering allergens.

Assessment of the Client	1. Assess the child's respiratory pattern. Determine rate, ease of inspiration and expiration, presence of cyanosis, and breath sounds. Premature infants usually have erratic breathing patterns; therefore, the respirations should be measured for a full minute to assess rate.
	2. Assess the child's past history of respiratory problems. Determine previous occurrences of pneumonia, asthma, bronchitis, croup, and other breathing difficulties.
	3. Assess the client's physical condition. Determine baseline vital signs for later comparisons.
	4. Assess the child's allergy history. Ask the parents if the child has allergies to any medications. Determine if the child has allergies that cause respiratory symptoms, such as hay fever.

Plan

Nursing Objectives	Provide the type and amount of respiratory assistance consistent with the child's needs and tolerance.
	Prevent oxygen toxicity caused by administration of too high a concentration of oxygen over too long a period of time.
	Decrease the parents' and child's anxiety level regarding the need for ventilatory assistance.

Client Preparation	1. Explain to the parents and to the child, if appropriate, why ventilatory assistance is needed and what form will be used. If ancillary equipment will be used, allow the child to see and touch the mask, cannula, or tent to overcome fear and anxiety.
	2. Allow the child to rest immediately prior to positive-pressure treatments. These treatments require effort on the part of the child and are tiring.

Equipment	Oxygen (O_2) source with regulator
	Cannula, catheter, mask, hood, tent, or ventilator
	Oxygen analyzer
	Distilled water
	Ice

Implementation and Interventions

Procedural Aspects

ACTION

1. Set the oxygen rate at the prescribed setting and monitor it carefully. Capillary oxygen determinations reflect the oxygen levels of the infant's blood (arterial for children). It will indicate if oxygen consumption is adequate to restore and maintain health. Oxygen can be administered by cannula or nasal catheter (50% O_2 delivered), masks (100% O_2 delivered), incubators (40%–100% O_2 delivered), and hoods (100% O_2 delivered). Tents deliver about 40% O_2. Ventilators deliver the concentration as preset on the controls. Fill the humidification source with distilled water. Be sure that water is present at all times. Never administer unhumidified oxygen.

2. Assess the oxygen concentration by using an oxygen analyzer at frequent intervals (such as q8h). Place the probe section in the oxygen enriched atmosphere (such as in the incubator or in the hood), and the oxygen concentration will register on the analyzer (Fig. 108-1).

RATIONALE

An inspired oxygen level of 30% to 100% is usually sufficient to relieve most oxygen deficits. Oxygen in the pediatric setting must be monitored carefully to prevent damage to immature systems and delicate tissues. An oxygen concentration of less than 40% is considered safe. Blood oxygen levels must be monitored regardless of the concentration being administered. Oxygen is humidified before delivery to prevent excessive drying of the respiratory tract. Infants usually receive oxygen in incubators or by hoods. Older children tolerate cannulas fairly well. Children do not tolerate masks or catheters well. Ventilators require the placement of an endotracheal tube or a tracheostomy tube.

The oxygen analyzer measures the oxygen concentration by contact with the sensitive probe. The concentration within the environment being measured registers on the dial of the analyzer.

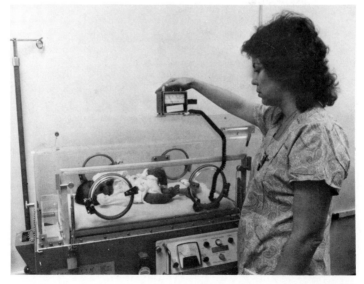

Figure 108.1

ACTION

3. The oxygen tent or canopy, such as the Croupette, is the common means of oxygen delivery to young children (Fig. 108-2). Allow the child to assist with setting up the tent. Touching the plastic and participating may decrease resistance to remaining in the tent. Tuck the edges of the tent under the mattress in such a manner that there is minimal escape of oxygen from around the edges of the tent. Plan nursing care so that the tent is not opened any more than is necessary. Monitor the temperature inside the tent. Mist may be ordered in conjunction with the oxygen therapy. Ice must be kept in the receptacle on the tent to ensure cool mist. Change the child's bedding and clothes as often as necessary to prevent chilling. Check any toys used by the child in the tent to ensure that they will not cause sparks.

RATIONALE

Children beyond infancy do not like equipment to be in contact with their faces. The tent provides a viable alternative. It is difficult, however, to maintain oxygen concentration unless the tent is kept closed as much as possible. Oxygen is heavier than air; therefore concentrations will be greatest at the bottom of the tent. Edges must be secured well to prevent dilution of the oxygen concentration within the tent. Mist will condense on the tent walls and dampen the linen and clothing inside the tent. Oxygen is an excellent supporter of combustion.

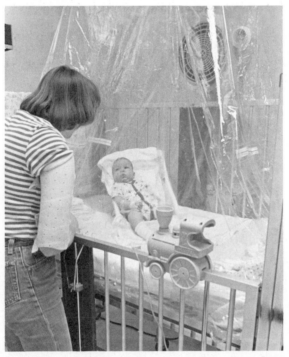

Figure 108.2

4. The oxygen hood is a clear plastic dome that fits over the infant's head with an opening at the neck area. Place the infant on the stomach or back with the head completely enclosed by the hood. The

Oxygen hoods can provide an oxygen-rich atmosphere at high concentrations. They are used primarily for infants who remain in a fairly stationary position.

ACTION

RATIONALE

neck opening should be large enough that it does not hinder the child's breathing or rub against the neck or shoulders (Fig. 108-3). Do not allow the oxygen to blow directly into the infant's face.

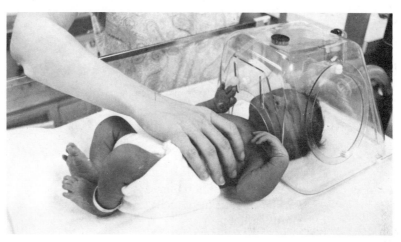

Figure 108.3

5. Incubators or self-contained environmental cribs may be used to maintain the infant's body temperature as well as to meet oxygen needs. Place the infant in the incubator in a position that facilitates breathing. Place IV tubing through access holes. Care for the child through the arm ports as much as possible (Figs. 108-4, 108-5).

Using the arm ports for care of the infant helps maintain consistency of the oxygen level. It also reduces the energy output of the infant who is already in a compromised position due to prematurity or illness.

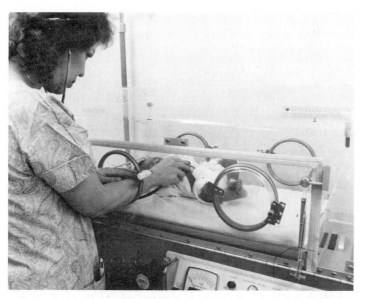

Figure 108.4

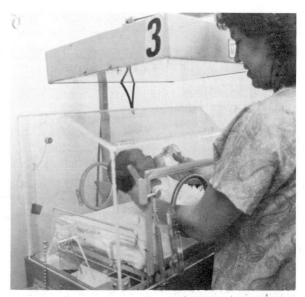

Figure 108.5

ACTION	*RATIONALE*
6. Mechanical ventilators are used only when skilled and experienced personnel are available to monitor them. Intermittent mandatory ventilation is often used in pediatrics. The infant breathes spontaneously, but the ventilator ensures that the rate of respiration does not fall below a specified number. If the rate falls below the preset amount, the machine is activated. If the infant breathes spontaneously at an adequate rate, the machine does not assist. Positive end expiratory pressure (PEEP) is used to keep the alveoli inflated in premature infants. Monitor the capillary blood gases frequently to determine the effectiveness of ventilation and to prevent complications.	Ventilatory assistance is used to keep the rate of respirations at a level capable of maintaining arterial oxygen levels to ensure adequate aeration of the infant's organs and tissues. PEEP is used when the alveoli are immature and tend to collapse. This system inflates the alveoli and leaves a residual amount of air pressure in them to prevent collapse, even during expiration.

Communicative Aspects

OBSERVATIONS

1. Observe the infant or child for signs of inadequate oxygenation, such as cyanosis, substernal respirations, rapid pulse, restlessness, and shallow, rapid respirations. Frequent monitoring of capillary blood gases will help determine the effectiveness of the oxygen-administration system.

2. Check the oxygen environment frequently to ensure that the desired concentration of oxygen is being delivered.

3. Observe the humidifying source to ensure that an adequate amount of water and/or ice is present.

CHARTING

DATE/TIME	OBSERVATIONS	SIGNATURE
5/7 0930	Oxygen by hood being delivered at 40%. Infant remains quiet under hood, skin pink, respirations 18 without retraction or any signs of distress. Out of the hood for 9 min. at 0900 to be fed by mother. Parents touching child and state they understand the need for the oxygen source.	C. Day RN

Discharge Planning Aspects

CLIENT AND FAMILY EDUCATION

1. Parents must be warned that oxygen supports combustion; therefore, smoking, friction toys, and anything that might cause a spark must be kept away from the oxygen area.

2. If the infant must be cared for inside an incubator, show the parents how to assist in the care, how the incubator works, and how to open and secure the arm ports. Encourage them to touch and cuddle their child as much as possible.

Evaluation

Quality Assurance

It is imperative that the child receive the amount of oxygen at the concentration and volume ordered. Frequent monitoring of the concentration levels for the duration of the treatment is essential. Documentation should reflect the frequency and results of oxygen analysis and blood gas monitoring. Signs and symptoms exhibited by the child previous to oxygen administration should be evaluated and progress noted after the oxygen was applied as part of the assessment of the effectiveness of the oxygen therapy. Documentation should reflect that the nurse understood the emotional aspects of separation from their child experienced by the parents and that attention was also given to the needs of the parents. A continuous record of the method and rate of oxygenation should be available throughout the duration of the oxygen therapy.

Each hospital should have a protocol for ensuring that oxygen concentrations are checked regularly (at least q8h in pediatrics). Protocol for the care of equipment should involve methods for ensuring that the humidification sources are not allowed to run dry and equipment is tested for effectiveness and safety regularly.

Infection Control

1. Handwashing is essential before and after caring for an infant. Infants in oxygenated atmospheres are usually weak and lack the natural immunity and physical strength to fight infection. Therefore, cross-infection must be avoided.

2. Equipment used consecutively for different children must be cleaned and disinfected between uses. This is particularly important for oxygen administration equipment, which is moist and offers an excellent medium for the proliferation of microorganisms. Regular cultures for oxygen-administration equipment should be done. Adequate disinfection measures must be a part of every hospital's respiratory services program.

3. If the child will require oxygen administration over an extended period of time, the equipment should be cleaned or changed at least once a week to prevent colonization of bacteria.

Technique Checklist

	YES	NO
Reason for oxygen administration explained to parents and child, if appropriate	____	____
Oxygen administered by		
Cannula	____	____
Catheter	____	____
Hood	____	____
Mask	____	____
Closed environment (incubator tent, Croupette)	____	____
Frequency of arterial/capillary blood gas studies _____		
Frequency of oxygen concentration analysis _____		
Duration of oxygen therapy _____		
Complications		
Cyanosis	____	____
Substernal breathing	____	____
Rapid pulse	____	____
Restlessness	____	____
Rapid respirations	____	____

Physical Examination of a Child, General Considerations

Overview

Definition

A systematic review of the body systems and structures of a child. (A description of the complete physical examination is beyond the scope of this text. The reader is referred to Bates B: A Guide to Physical Examination, 3rd ed. Philadelphia, JB Lippincott, 1983)

The four methods of examination are:

Inspection: Visual observation of a body part

Palpation: Examination of the body part by the use of touch

Auscultation: The process of listening for sounds produced within the body

Percussion: Assessment of the body by tapping with the fingers

Rationale

Observe, examine, and assess the client preliminary to determining nursing priorities in planning care.

Terminology

Asymmetry: Lack of correspondence in shape, size, and relative position of parts on opposite sides of the body

Ophthalmoscope: Instrument used for detailed examination of the eye

Otoscope: Instrument used to inspect the ears

Percussion hammer: Instrument shaped like a hammer with a head, often made of hard rubber or plastic, used for central nervous system reflex assessment

Speculum: Funnel-shaped instrument for widening the orifices and canals of the body for examination (e.g., nasal speculum)

Sphygomomanometer: Instrument used to measure blood pressure

Stethoscope: Instrument used to transmit sounds from the client's body to the examiner's ears

Assessment

Pertinent Anatomy and Physiology

1. See Appendix I: *skeletal system, skin, vertebral column.*
2. The newborn's skin is soft and smooth. Older infants who are fed yellow vegetables may develop a pale yellow–orange color, which is sometimes mistaken for jaundice. This condition, carotenemia, is usually limited to the palms of the hands, soles of the feet, and nasal folds. After 1 year of age, the normal child's skin is similar to that of the adult.
3. Skin characteristics may differ slightly in Asian or black children. Infants of dark-skinned parents are lightly pigmented at birth, except for the nailbeds and skin of the scrotum. The skin grows progressively darker until pigmentation peaks at about 6 to 8 weeks of age. Some dark-skinned children normally have bluish coloring of the lips and gums. Blacks may have brown

freckled pigmentation of the buccal mucosa. Pallor or paleness can be detected in the nail-beds, conjunctiva, oral mucosa, or tongue, which are normally reddish pink. Jaundice is best detected in the sclera or mucous membranes viewed in natural light. Carotenemia may be noted on the palms of the hands. A decrease or disappearance of normal pigmentation may be noted following diaper rash.

Pathophysiological Concepts

One of the objectives of the physical examination is to identify pathophysiologic conditions. Consult a textbook on pathophysiology for consideration of the wide variety of pathophysiologic conditions possible in infants and children.

Assessment of the Client

1. Assess the ability and willingness of the child to comply with instructions. Depending on the stage of growth and development, the child may be hesitant about following instructions, may be eager to follow instructions, or may intermittently combine both behaviors. Assess the anticipated behavior of the child to determine the approach to gaining compliance with the physical examination.

2. Assess the parent–child relationship. Note the amount of involvement of the parents in the examination. Note the amount of eye contact, whether the parents speak to the child, and their understanding of the findings of the examination.

3. Assess the reason for the hospitalization. Determine if the child's condition will affect the examination procedure. If the child is nauseated, weak, having diarrhea, or in pain, alterations in the usual examination procedure may need to be made.

Plan

Nursing Objectives

Facilitate the examination by having the necessary equipment in readiness and in proper working order.

Offer explanations to the parents and child, if appropriate, of what will happen during the procedure and why.

Protect the safety and modesty of the child.

Assist in the identification of normal and pathologic findings in the infant and child.

Client Preparation

1. Explain to the child in a matter-of-fact and calm manner what is going to be done, where the examination will take place, and who will be doing the procedure.

2. Ask the child to void before the examination. Anxiety about the procedure or palpation of the bladder musculature may cause involuntary emptying of the bladder during the examination, which might embarrass the child.

3. Take the child and parents to the treatment room or examination area. The procedure requires privacy and is best conducted in a well-lighted, quiet room. Allow the parents the flexibility of deciding whether or not to be present. Many parents become extremely anxious when seeking medical care for their children. Let the feelings of the parents and the needs of the child dictate which, if either, of the parents will be present during the examination.

4. Secure restraints, if needed, to use during the examination. It is generally considered better to gain the approval and compliance of the child with patience and understanding. If this is not possible, restraint may be necessary to prevent accidental injury to the child.

Equipment

Examining table
Sheet or towel for draping the client when indicated
Otoscope with speculum
Thermometer
Tongue blades
Stethoscope/sphygmomanometer
Percussion hammer
Ophthalmoscope
Tape measure
Rectal glove and lubricant

Implementation and Interventions

Procedural Aspects

ACTION

1. Place the child on the examining table (Fig. 109-1). Allow the child to remain dressed if possible. Stand near while the child is on the table to prevent falls. A screen may be used to protect the child's privacy. For the older child, drapes should be available during the examination.

RATIONALE

Staying clothed helps the child feel less threatened. The safety of the child must be considered at all times. Prepubescent females are modest and should be draped during auscultation of the chest and breast examination.

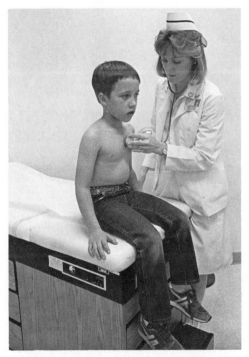

Figure 109.1

2. Gather all equipment before the examination and check it to see that it is in proper working order. All actions should be smooth, unhurried, and nonthreatening. Talk to the child during preparation. Ask simple questions that the

Every effort should be made to prevent delays and to do the examination in a smooth and efficient manner. Respect the child's autonomy and individualism by speaking and interacting directly with the child, not just the parent.

ACTION

RATIONALE

child can answer. Smile, make eye contact, and address the child by name.

3. During the examination, the child may be asked to assume different positions and to perform simple tasks of physical and mental dexterity. Take actual measurements rather than relying on parent's statements (Fig. 109-2, 109-3). Information about physical parameters, such as weight, height, temperature, head and chest circumference, and status of symptoms, should be available for comparison and/or consideration. Physical restraint may be necessary to prevent injury during certain procedures, such as the otoscopic examination.

Every effort should be made to facilitate the physical examination. Provision of baseline vital signs and physical parameters may aid in the physical assessment of the child.

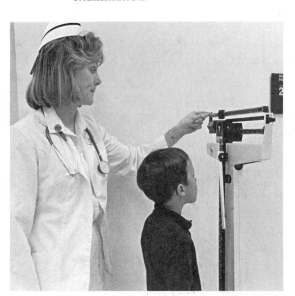

Figure 109.2

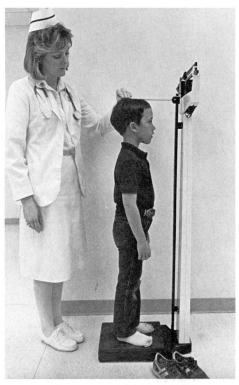

Figure 109.3

4. After the examination, return the child to the room. Clean off any lubricant and leave the child in a comfortable environment.

The physical examination can be very frightening. Leave the child in a safe and secure environment.

Special Modifications

For initial assessment of the newborn, see Technique 146, Neonatal Assessment, Initial, in the Neonatal Section.

Communicative Aspects

OBSERVATIONS

1. The actual examination usually proceeds from head to foot, including general review of body systems. The following observations may be made during examination.

   Head: look for bumps, cuts, and pediculosis; examine fontanelles and suture lines

   Eyes: Using an ophthalmoscope, check pupil size, reaction, and equality, and evidence of hemorrhage; externally, note turgor, puffiness, and excessive tearing or drainage

   Ears: Using an otoscope, examine for intact eardrum, lacerations, foreign objects, and excessive wax; note pain and tenderness

   Nose: Observe for drainage, blockage, and polyps; determine if the child is a nose- or mouth-breather.

   Mouth: Using a flashlight and tongue depressor, observe for rash or discoloration of throat, condition of teeth, gums, tongue, and tonsils; inspect the amount, color, and consistency of saliva and the condition of the hard and soft palates

   Face: Observe for paralysis, twitching, bilateral movement, and discoloration

   Neck: Observe for abnormalities of the thyroid gland and lymph nodes; test the swallowing reflex

   Skin: Observe the color, temperature and state of hydration, scars, birth marks, bruises, scratches, bites, swelling or lumps; note the texture of the skin and the presence of any rash and its extent

   Chest and lungs: Using a stethoscope, auscultate breath sounds, rales, wheezes, ronchi, and congestion; observe for asymmetry and retraction of the chest, scars, and rib abnormalities

   Heart: Using the stethoscope, auscultate heart sounds; determine cardiac margins by percussion; determine the presence of various pulses such as the carotid, radial, femoral, and pedal

   Abdomen: Ask the child to breathe through the mouth (flexing the child's knees may aid relaxation) and palpate the lower chest and inguinal areas (observe the inguinal area for masses or lymph node enlargment); palpate the liver, which should not be felt after 1 year of age (if the liver is felt, pathology may be present); observe the presence of peristalsis by auscultation of the bowel area

   Genitalia: Females—examine for vaginal or urethral discharge, clitoral enlargement, and masses in the labia major; *males*—observe for any urethral discharge, abnormalities of the penis and scrotum (check the presence and size of each testis), and the presence and condition of foreskin; using a glove and lubricant, check the anal region for rectal prolapse and abnormal masses

   Extremities: Observe for any lesions, abnormal masses, extra digits, or edema; observe the child walking to note any abnormal gait or asymmetry; examine each extremity for full range-of-motion capability; the percussion hammer may be used to check reflexes in the knee and ankle

   Back and spine: Note the alignment of the spine and the ability of the child to move freely, bend, sit, and stoop

   Nervous system: A developmental neurologic examination will elicit information about language, fine motor and gross motor development, and stage of socialization. The neurologic examination can offer evidence of muscular weakness, twitching, meningeal irritation, loss of muscle control, and febrile convulsions.

2. As each body structure is examined, observe for any abnormalities or deviations from that which is expected for a child of this age and diagnosis.

3. Note the emotional response of the child to the physical examination. Observe for crying, breath holding, or hyperventilation, which might alter the findings of the examination.

CHARTING

Most hospitals have a client assessment form, which allows the nurse to document physical findings easily and quickly by checking the appropriate responses and which has space for describing abnormalities and findings that require explanation. Document the child's response and any pertinent findings in the nurses' progress notes.

DATE/TIME	OBSERVATIONS	SIGNATURE
10/19 1420	Physical examination done by R. Tim PNP. Explanation given to mother and father this morning and both accepted it well. Exam done in treatment room with mother in attendance. Baby seemed at ease in mother's arms. No crying during exam. Petechiae noted on both legs. ———————	P. Sanchez RN

Discharge Planning Aspects

CLIENT AND FAMILY EDUCATION

1. Instruct the child's parents about the importance of periodic physical examinations.

2. Instruct the parents and the child, if old enough to understand, about the importance of reporting to the physician any new lesions, rashes, or abnormal signs and symptoms related to the physical condition.

REFERRALS

If conditions are discovered that will warrant therapy in the future, refer the parents to the proper health-care professional, such as a dentist, an orthodontist, a dermatolgist, or an orthopedist.

Evaluation

Quality Assurance

Documentation should include the explanation given to the parents and child before the examination, as well as the child's reaction to the examination. Any abnormal findings should be documented. The child's ability and willingness to comply with examination should be noted, as well as any occurrence that might alter the findings of the physical examination. The examiner's findings and interpretation of these findings provide a basis for future therapy and should be a permanent part of the chart.

Infection control

Equipment used for consecutive clients should be cleaned thoroughly between clients. Handwashing should precede and follow the physical examination. Any disposable equipment used during the examination should be disposed of in a paper or plastic container.

Technique Checklist

	YES	NO
Procedure explained to		
Parents	_____	_____
Child	_____	_____
Child complied with examiner's requests	_____	_____
Crying occurred during examination	_____	_____
Abnormalities noted during examination	_____	_____
Documentation of findings on chart	_____	_____

110 Postural Drainage and Breathing Exercises

Overview

Definition

Breathing exercises: Exercises used in conjunction with postural drainage to assist in the removal of pulmonary secretions. These exercises alone are helpful in the therapy used for respiratory diseases.

Postural drainage: Drainage of the bronchial airways by means of posture; uses gravity to enhance removal of secretions. Two types are:

Active: For the child who can actively assume various positions

Passive: For the weaker child, when position must be created by bed elevation or by holding the child in various positions.

Rationale

Clear secretions from the airway.

Mobilize the chest wall.

Reduce pain and discomfort associated with pulmonary distress.

Expel air and fluid from the pleural space.

Increase the input of oxygen and removal of carbon dioxide from blood flowing through pulmonary vessels.

Remove bronchial secretions.

Terminology

Alveoli: Minute air sacs in the lungs in which the gaseous exchange of oxygen and carbon dioxide takes place

Bronchodilators: Drugs that enlarge the passageways of the lungs

Chest physical therapy: Techniques of manual application of vibration and clapping over affected areas of the lungs. This helps dislodge retained mucus from the airways. Chest physical therapy is performed with the child in postural drainage positions. The usual sequence is positioning, clapping, vibrating, coughing, and removal of secretions.

Mucolytic medications: Drugs that liquefy secretions and facilitate expectoration

Assessment

Pertinent Anatomy and Physiology

1. See Appendix I: *bronchial tree, lungs.*
2. In the infant, the chest wall is thin with little musculature, and the rib cage is very soft and pliant. The respiratory rate of infants is more rapid than that of older children. Apneic episodes are normal in premature infants and, occasionally, in older children.

Pathophysiological Concepts

1. Dyspnea occurs if there is obstruction to the passage of air into the alveoli. This will be apparent by the extra effort required for respiration. In a baby, the soft tissues around the chest are drawn in with each respiration. The small muscles in the nose are also used. If the child has difficulty breathing out, the chest fills with air and changes shape as it becomes overinflated.

Children adjust their posture to ease their breathing.

2. Respiratory noises are due to a variety of causes. When the lower airway is obstructed, as in asthma and bronchiolitis, the child may hold the glottis closed to improve the expiratory movement, producing an expiratory grunt. Wheezing is also common. When the obstruction is in the upper airway, there is often a harsh inspiratory noise called stridor.

3. Cystic fibrosis is an inherited disease in which the secretions in the lungs are abnormally thick and viscous. Chest infections are common throughout the early years, resulting in lung damage. Postural drainage is frequently necessary.

Assessment of the Client

1. Assess the child's breathing pattern. Determine if the child has difficulty on inspiration or expiration. Assess the presence and amount of retraction. Determine if the respiratory rate is slower or faster than would be expected for the child's age and condition.

2. Assess the child's breath sounds. Auscultate the chest to determine the presence of wheezing, grunting, rales, or any other chest abnormality.

3. Assess the child's health history in relation to past respiratory problems. Determine if the child has frequent "colds," coughing, or congestion. Determine if the child has asthma, cystic fibrosis, or allergies that manifest in respiratory problems.

4. Assess the child's physical condition in relation to the ability to participate in breathing exercises and postural drainage positioning. If the child is very weak, the exercises may have to be scheduled more frequently and be of shorter duration. If the child has casts or physical deformities that preclude proper positioning, assess what alterations may be made to accomplish the desired purpose.

Plan

Nursing Objectives

Explain the procedure to the parents and child to allay fear and anxiety, which further compromise respiratory status.

Assess the child's respiratory status before and after the procedure.

Ensure the child's safety.

Place the child in the appropriate postural drainage position.

Allay the child's and parents' fear and anxiety.

Client Preparation

1. If the child is old enough to understand, explain how the various positions will help in clearing the fluid from the lungs. Demonstrate with a doll so that the child will understand the positioning involved. Be positive and forthright in answering any questions.

2. Before beginning the procedure, explain any physical percussion or vibrating that will take place. Allow the child to see the vibrator and hear it before being placed in an unusual position.

3. Offer a detailed explanation to the parents before beginning the procedure. Enlist their assistance in gaining the child's cooperation.

4. Remove any constricting clothing from the child before beginning. The child should be comfortable and capable of as much lung expansion as possible.

5. Generally, a radiologic examination of the chest is done to reveal the areas of greatest congestion where percussion should be focused.

Equipment

Vibrator

Emesis basin

Active postural drainage:

Covered pillow

Footstool, if needed

Passive postural drainage:

Bed elevator, if not built into bed

Implementation and Interventions

Procedural Aspects

ACTION

Postural Drainage

1. Position the child according to the portion of the lung that is involved. Position the infant or small child on a parent's or the nurse's lap (Fig. 110-1). The older child may be positioned on pillows or in a reclining chair. Encourage the child to cough up the secretions. Do not do postural drainage immediately before or for 1 hour after meals.

RATIONALE

Use gravity to assist in the evacuation of secretions from the lung. The area of congestion should be uppermost, above the area of entry of the bronchi into the lungs because this is the vehicle for expelling secretions from the lungs. The child should have time to rest before meals; however, postural drainage may allow the child to breathe more easily and thus improve appetite. If the procedure is done immediately after the meal, the child may vomit.

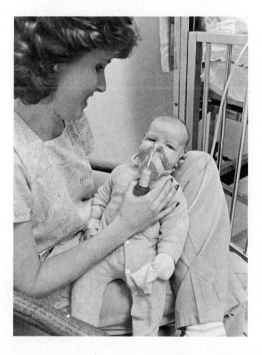

Figure 110.1

2. Use percussion by cupping the hand and striking the chest wall in the involved area. Vibration is done by placing a handheld vibrator on the chest. Have the child inhale deeply. During exhalation, vibrate the chest wall. Do this for approximately five exhalations in succession.

The objective is to loosen the secretions by the resonating thumping on the chest. The vibrations are meant to shake the secretions loose, allowing the child to expel them.

ACTION	**RATIONALE**
3. Active postural drainage occurs when the child assumes a position in which the affected area of the lung can be drained. This may involve the head being lower than the body. This can be accomplished by allowing the child to keep the body on the bed with the head over the side supported on a chair and pillow. It may also be accomplished by propping with pillows. The emesis basin should be conveniently located so that expectoration is facilitated. Encourage the child to cough vigorously for 2 to 3 minutes while being percussed or vibrated to assist in loosening the secretions.	Active postural drainage involves the child's active participation. The involved area of the lung should be encouraged to drain by gravity. Pillows and supervision will help eliminate the possibility of falls or injury. The emesis basin is used to contain the expectorated secretions.
4. Passive postural drainage occurs when the child is unable to participate actively in the exercises. It is accomplished by positioning. Place the child supine in the bed. Elevate the foot of the bed approximately 20 inches above the level of bed plane. Place the emesis basin nearby for the secretions. Leave the child in this position for approximately 15 minutes, with coughing during the last 2 to 3 minutes. Remain in attendance to encourage and observe the child (Fig. 110-2, 110-3).	For the weak and physically debilitated child, actively encouraging drainage of secretions from the lungs may be dangerously fatiguing. The lungs are encouraged to drain by gravity with some coughing after pooling of the secretions in the best area for evacuation (e.g., near the bronchi).

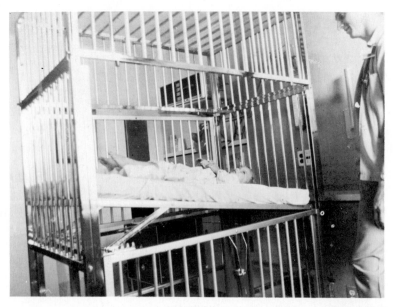

Figure 110.2

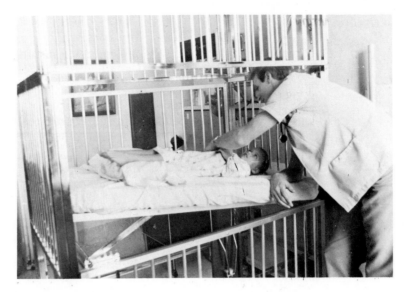

Figure 110.3

ACTION	**RATIONALE**
Breathing Exercises	
1. For exercising the diaphragm, place the fingers on the child's anterior lower ribs. During *inhalation*, ask the child to push the chest out forcefully against the light pressure of the nurse's fingers. During *exhalation*, ask the child to contract the abdominal muscles.	The diaphragm lines the lower thorax area. Expanding and contracting this muscle are means of strengthening it.
2. For exercising the apex of the lungs, apply light pressure just below the clavicle when the child *inhales*. When the child *exhales*, apply pressure to the sternum with the heel of the hand.	Counterpressure forces the child to bear down, thus strengthening the musculature used in breathing and aerating greater proportional areas of the lungs.
3. For exercising the posterior portions of the lungs, position the child on the side or abdomen. Place both hands over the lower portion of the child's thorax posteriorly. Apply pressure when the child *exhales*. Relax the pressure during *inhalation*.	Gravity is used as a counterpressure, along with the manual force of the hands.
4. For exercising the lateral lower rib area, encourage the child to *exhale* completely. Place both hands lightly on the lateral aspect of the child's lower ribs. Instruct the child to expand the ribs against the nurse's hands during *inhalation*. During *exhalation*, ask the child to tighten the abdomen and pull the ribs in while the nurse places pressure over the lower rib cage.	Tensing and relaxing of the muscles strengthens the muscles used in breathing. Complete exhalation encourages maximum expansion of the rib cage.

Communicative Aspects

OBSERVATIONS

1. Observe the child during the procedure to ensure that breathing is not compromised if the head is in a dependent position. Further, observe for fatigue and weakness. Observe for the successful evacuation of sputum and easing of breathing problems.

2. Observe the characteristics of the sputum returned after postural drainage. Determine if the viscosity has changed during the progress of drug and exercise therapy.

3. Observe the child for nausea. If the child vomits, observe for aspiration.

4. Observe vital signs throughout hospitalization. Determine baseline parameters upon admission. Observe the temperature because increases may indicate infection. Observe respiratory rate to determine if greater portions of the lung are being involved, requiring more rapid respiration and shallower breathing.

5. Observe the child's ability to comply with directions during active postural drainage. Note physical limitations that alter the possible positions.

CHARTING

DATE/TIME	OBSERVATIONS	SIGNATURE
12/9 1020	Passive postural drainage for 12 minutes with vigorous coughing for the last 2 minutes. Able to expel 10 cc thick, yellowish secretions. Very tired after coughing. Being held by mother at this time. T 99.2° F rectally, P 118, R 36. No vomiting. Color pale.	P. Sanchez RN

Discharge Planning Aspects

CLIENT AND FAMILY EDUCATION

1. If the child has chronic respiratory problems, it may be beneficial to teach the postural drainage methods and the breathing exercises to the parents before the child is discharged. Give detailed instructions regarding performance of these activities at home. Demonstrate and ask for a return demonstration to be sure that the parents understand the procedure and realize the importance of safety precautions. Assist in setting up a regular respiratory exercise program. Respiratory assistance devices may be available for use in the hospital and the home (Fig. 110-4). Teach the child and family how to use such devices.

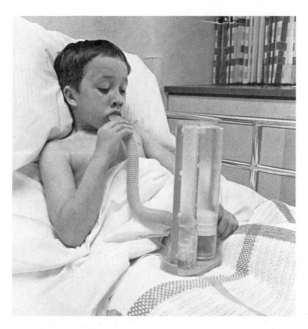

Figure 110.4

2. Encourage the child to engage in physical activities in accordance with the advice of the physician. Activities such as playing, swimming, and jumping usually tend to increase the efficiency of the ventilatory mechanisms.

3. Instruct the child to continue to cough as instructed after discharge. Explain the importance of coughing into a tissue to prevent the spread of droplets into the air.

REFERRALS

Inform the parents that hand vibrators and mechanical percussion devices are available at most hospital supply stores. Information, support, and some supplies may be available from the Cystic Fibrosis Foundation, 3091 Mayfield Road, Cleveland, OH 44118. The American Lung Association may also provide support and information.

Evaluation

Quality Assurance

Documentation should include the length of time of each procedure and the child's reaction to it. The various positions assumed by the child should be noted, as well as an assessment of the success of each. The vital signs should be monitored during the hospitalization. Significant discrepancies should be accounted for or reported. Any medications given should be recorded, along with an assessment of their effectiveness. The type and amount of secretions should be noted. Descriptions of the secretions should include comparisons with those produced during previous sessions. Use of mechanical devices or manual percussion should be noted. Any problems with breathing should be noted. Documentation during the hospitalization should include an assessment of the child's progress or lack of progress.

Infection Control

1. Equipment used for consecutive clients must be cleaned between uses to ensure that cross-contamination does not occur.

2. The child should be encouraged to cough into a tissue to prevent the spread of infection and contamination by droplet.

3. Because the child will most likely be in a weakened state, careful hand-washing should be done before breathing exercises or postural drainage to help eliminate the chance of cross-contamination. Handwashing also should follow the procedure.

Technique Checklist

	YES	NO
Procedure and technique explained		
To child	_____	_____
To parents	_____	_____
Postural drainage	_____	_____
Frequency _____		
Duration _____		
Positions _____		
_____		
Breathing exercises	_____	_____
Frequency _____		
Duration _____		
Target area(s) _____		
_____		
Respiratory status improved before discharge	_____	_____
Parents taught principles and techniques of postural drainage and breathing exercises	_____	_____
Family referred to support or informational agencies	_____	_____

Restraints, Pediatric

Overview

Definition

Limiting the physical movement of the child to facilitate examination and prevent injury

Rationale

Maintain the safety of the infant or child.

Allow healing or treatment in an uninterrupted manner.

Facilitate the physical examination and diagnostic measures.

Terminology

Slip knot: A knot used in restraints, most often to secure a tie to the bed frame; after one tie, the loose strap is brought as a loop through the second tie so it may be released easily in case of emergency (Fig. 111-1).

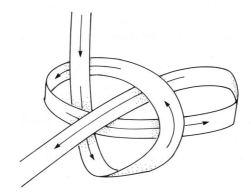

Figure 111.1

Assessment

Pertinent Anatomy and Physiology

1. See Appendix I: *skeletal muscles, skeletal system, vertebral column.*
2. Exercise has many positive effects on the cardiopulmonary system. The heart rate increases. Blood flow is redirected from nonexercising tissues to those areas of greater need, the heart and muscles. This redirection of blood increases the cardiac output and stimulates the heart muscle. Ventilation also increases, promoting removal of secretions from the bronchial area.
3. Metabolism includes all of the physical and chemical activity occurring in the body. The basal metabolic rate is the amount of energy used by the cells when the body is as much at rest as is possible during life. Exercise increases the metabolic rate according to the degree of exertion. The basal metabolic rate of infants is faster than that of adults.

Pathophysiological Concepts

Multisystem problems may result from prolonged inactivity and immobility. Respiratory activity is decreased, with resultant build-up or pooling of secretions. Circulation is slowed, and edema may result. Stasis of urine may result in the formation of stones or urinary infections. In addition, inability to move about freely is a source of irritation and frustration, even for the very young infant.

Assessment of the Client

1. Assess the child's activity level. Determine if the amount of activity will impair or interfere with the prescribed therapy.

2. Assess the child's level of understanding and potential ability and willingness to cooperate with therapy. If the child is too young to understand or remember those instructions necessary for the successful outcome of therapy, some type of restraint may be necessary.

3. Assess the parent's willingness and ability to assist with supervision. It may be possible to remove or alter the method of restraints when parents are present.

4. Assess the child's physical condition. Restraints may inhibit the child's activity to the point that they interfere with other aspects of the healing process, such as the ability to expel fluid build-up in the chest. Assess the needs of the child and determine priorities in managing health promotion and restoration.

5. Assess the best type of restraint to achieve desired results. The mummy restraint may be used for treatments to the head, such as eye examinations or insertion of a scalp-vein infusion. The elbow or wrist restraint may be used to discourage the baby from pulling out tubes, such as a scalp-vein needle or gastric tube. The ankle restraint may be used to prevent excessive movement of the leg in which an infusion is located. The bed net may be used for the child who is old enough to climb out of bed but too young to understand the danger of falling or the procedure for calling for assistance. The papoose board may be used for the infant or young child who is undergoing a cutdown, scalp-vein needle insertion, circumcision, or other procedures involving the ventral surface.

Plan

Nursing Objectives

Explain the purpose and expected therapeutic results of the restraints to the child and parents before they are applied.

Use restraints only when there is no alternative.

Check the restraints frequently and remove them at specified intervals to allow movement of the extremity.

Monitor the area below the restraint at regular intervals to ensure adequate circulation, especially of the hands and feet.

Prevent complications that might arise because of falls.

Apply the restraints so that they are comfortable and nonthreatening but still achieve the therapeutic goal of the restraint process.

Client Preparation

1. Thoroughly explain to the parents and to the child, if appropriate, why the restraints are necessary, approximately how long they will be used, and how the child can best comply with the restraint process to be comfortable and secure.

2. Place the child in a comfortable position. Be sure that the bed linens are clean and wrinkle-free to promote comfort. Place some diversional materials nearby if the child is restrained in bed.

Equipment

Mummy restraint
  Sheet or blanket
Elbow restraint
  12 Tongue depressors
  2 Elbow cuffs
  8 Safety pins
  Child's gown with long sleeves
Ankle/wrist restraints
  Strips of soft, tubular gauze or stockinette
Jacket restraint
Bed net restraint
  Bed net with ties
  Crib with head, foot, and siderails on the same level to permit the child to sit or stand up
Confined bed
Papoose board restraint
  Papoose board
  Towel or soft blanket

Implementation and Interventions

Procedural Aspects

ACTION	RATIONALE
Mummy Restraint	
1. Place a sheet or blanket flat on the bed. Place the infant supine on the top of the sheet. Place one of the arms close to the child's body and fold the sheet over arm and body under the opposite arm (Fig. 111-2). Tuck it under the infant's body (Fig. 111-3) Place the other arm close to the infant's body (Fig. 111-4) and fold the remaining side of the sheet over the entire body, tucking the excess under the child (Fig. 111-5). Grasp the long end of the sheet and gently but firmly pull it up over the child's feet and tuck it to one side and under the infant's body.	The goal of the restraint is to immobilize the infant's hands and feet so that these cannot be used to move the infant during treatment. Tucking the restraints under the infant will allow the child's own weight to provide the leverage to keep the restraints in place.

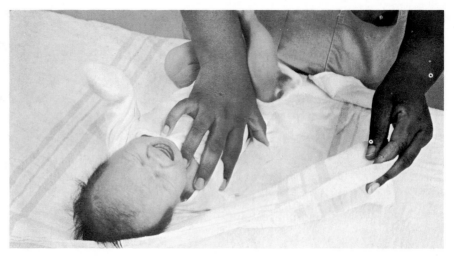

Figure 111.2

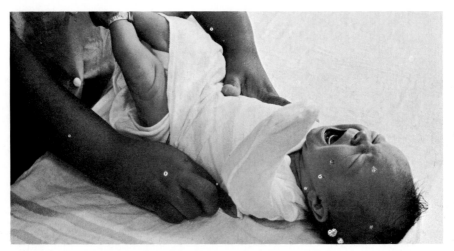

Figure 111.3

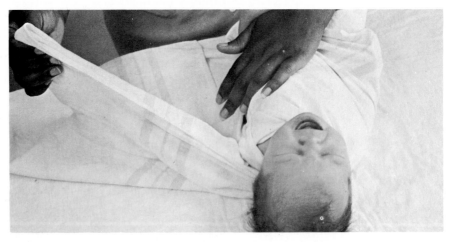

Figure 111.4

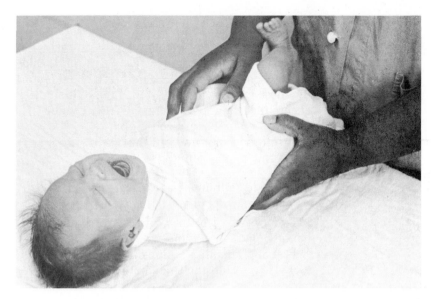

Figure 111.5

ACTION

2. Check the restraint at the child's neck to be sure that it is not too high, which might interfere with breathing. Also, check to see that the restraint is not so constricting across the chest that the child has respiratory difficulty.

Elbow Restraint

1. Insert tongue depressors into the slots in the cloth restraint.

2. Place the infant's elbow into the middle of the restraint and wrap the cloth around the child's arm. Secure with the self-adhesing fasteners or safety pins (Fig. 111-6).

RATIONALE

Restraints should immobilize the child without compromising respiratory status.

The tongue depressors hold the infant's arm straight, preventing the infant from reaching dressings, tubes, and wounds.

The bend of the elbow should be in the middle of the restraint so that the elbow cannot be flexed while the restraint is in place.

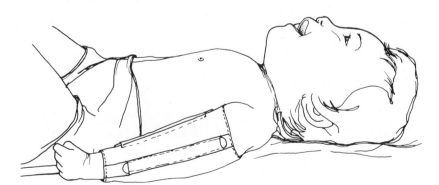

Figure 111.6

ACTION

3. Remove the restraint frequently and allow the infant to flex the elbow. Remain with the infant during these exercise periods and ensure that the intent of the restraint is not jeopardized (i.e., the child does not pull out the tube or reopen a wound).

Wrist/Ankle Restraint

1. Place a cylindrical piece of stockinette or gauze over the child's hand. Tape securely, but not so tight that circulation is impaired (Fig. 111-7). Fold the stockinette back over itself, pulling it over the child's hand (Fig. 111-8). Tie the long end of the stockinette to the bed frame in a slip knot (Fig. 111-9). Allow the child as much movement of the hand as possible while meeting the objectives for the restraint.

RATIONALE

Elbow restraints do not permit flexion of the elbow. This may become uncomfortable if periodic exercise, including elbow flexion, is not provided.

The child's hand and fingers are enclosed within the cylinder of stockinette or gauze so that the child cannot handle tubes and dressings. The child's range of motion can also be inhibited to prevent the child from placing the hands near areas such as IVs and dressings.

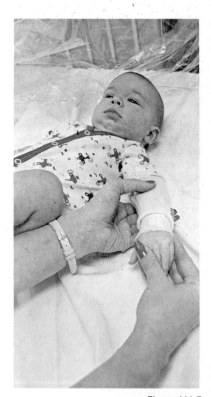

Figure 111.7

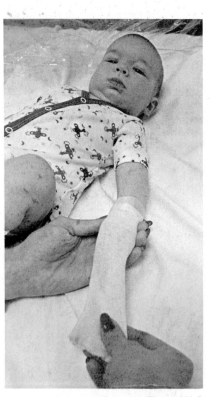

Figure 111.8

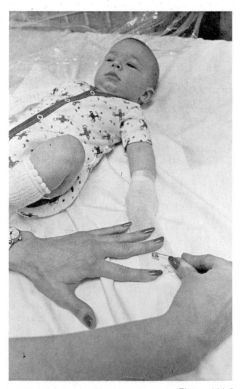

Figure 111.9

ACTION

RATIONALE

2. Apply the ankle restraint in the same way. Tie the ankle in such a way that as much motion as can safely be allowed is indeed allowed (Fig. 111-10).

The ankle restraint keeps the child from accidentally pulling out a tube or IV needle by rolling and tossing the hips and legs.

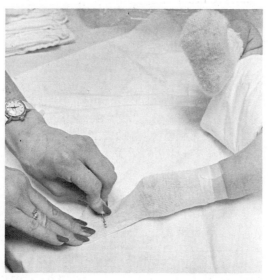

Figure 111.10

Bed Net

1. Apply the net snugly over the top of the crib. Secure the net to the mattress springs so that the side of the crib may be lowered by the parents or the nurse without removing the net (Fig. 111-11).

The function of the bed net is to prevent the child from climbing out of the bed and falling, while allowing freedom of movement in the crib area.

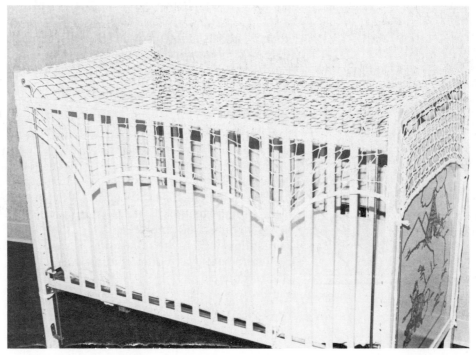

Figure 111.11

ACTION

RATIONALE

2. Tie the straps in a slip knot so that they may be removed quickly, if necessary.

The slip knot allows easy removal by anyone who can reach it. This is important in case of emergency.

Confined Bed

1. The confined bed provides limited mobility for the child without fear of the child falling from the bed. Both siderails must be secured in the "up" position after the child has been placed in the confined bed (Fig. 111-12).

The siderails prevent the child from climbing over the edge of the bed and falling.

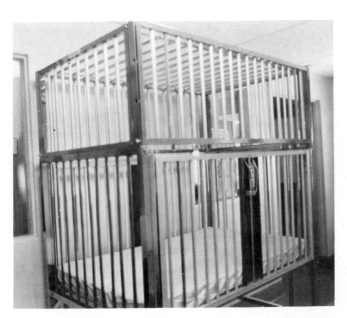

Figure 111.12

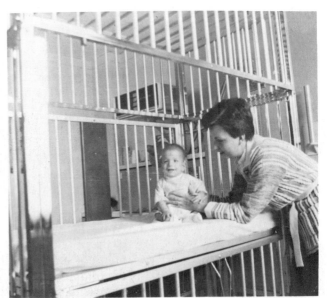

Figure 111.13

2. When a siderail is lowered, an adult must be present to ensure that the child does not fall (Fig. 111-13).

The height of the bed is such that the child cannot be left unattended when the siderails are down because of the possibility of falls.

Papoose Board

1. Place the board on the treatment table with the flaps of the board extended. Place a towel or soft blanket under the child for padding. Place the child on the board in the supine position. Carry out the restraining procedure in a calm, efficient manner. Talk soothingly to the child and offer continual reassurance.

The padding promotes comfort. The position of the child is important to ensure that discomfort is kept to a minimum. The child will probably be crying during the procedure because of being physically restrained. Removing the restraint as soon as possible will usually resolve the child's fears.

ACTION

2. Place the child's arms in the loops located at hip level. Bring the large center strap across the child's arms and abdomen and fasten securely. Fasten the large lower strap across the thighs and lower legs (Fig. 111-14). Be sure that the child's breathing is not impaired. Place the restraining strap across the child's head, if needed. The part of the body that will be treated may be made accessible by loosening one of the restraints or by using one of the arm-holes for the affected arm.

RATIONALE

The goal of using the papoose board is to immobilize the child so that treatments may be carried out without endangering the child's safety.

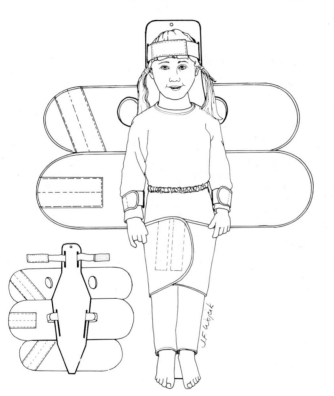

Figure 111.14

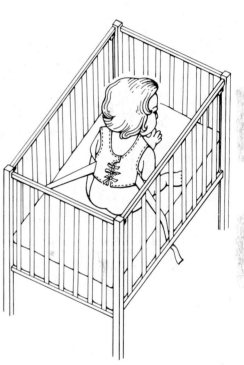

Figure 111.15

Jacket Restraint

1. Place the jacket on the child with the ties positioned in the back. Loosely secure the long straps to the bed frame out of the child's reach with a slip knot (Fig. 111-15).

2. Monitor the child frequently to ensure that the child does not become entangled in the restraint.

The ties and knots must be out of the child's reach to prevent accidental removal of the restraint.

Because of the length of the straps, it is important that the child not be tangled in the straps during normal play in bed.

Communicative Aspects

OBSERVATIONS

1. Observe the restraints frequently (q15–30min if the child is alone in the room). Restraints that are too tight will impair circulation. Observe for signs of impaired circulation, such as redness and swelling. Observe for signs of discomfort and release the restraints periodically to ensure good circulation and comfort.

2. Observe the child for signs of boredom and frustration. Place near the child safe diversional materials, such as toys, books, and magazines, according to the child's age.

3. Observe the patency of tubes and IV infusions which might be affected by the placement and positioning of restraints.

CHARTING

DATE/TIME	OBSERVATIONS	SIGNATURE
4/7 0700	Scalp vein IV started in R forehead. Wrist restraints to both wrists. Tied to frame of bed with 6 inches of slack allowed for movement. IV infusing well. Mother will return at 0930 to nurse infant.	P. Sanchez RN
0730	Wrist restraints checked for circulatory impairment. Hands are pink and fingers are flexible. Allowed to bend elbows for a few minutes with restraints untied. Retied. IV continues to infuse well.	P. Sanchez RN

Discharge Planning Aspects

CLIENT AND FAMILY EDUCATION

1. Instruct the family and the child, if appropriate, about the purpose and intended therapeutic outcome of the restraints. Tell them the expected duration of restraint. Explain carefully to the parent how and when they may remove the restraints if they will be in the room with the child. If this may pose a safety threat to the child, ask the parents not to remove the restraints unless a nurse is in the room.

2. Ask the parents and the child, if appropriate, to notify the nurse about any problems with the restraints. Describe for the family the signs that ankle and wrist restraints are too tight so that they may assist in assessment of the restraints.

3. Use this opportunity to explain and reiterate the importance of adequate restraints for infants and young children when riding in cars. Also explain the importance of restraining the infant in an infant seat or high chair or any place from which falls could occur.

Evaluation

Quality Assurance

Document the reason for the restraint. The notes should reflect the type of restraint, the extremeties involved, the safety precautions taken to prevent injury to the child, and the outcome of the restraining procedure. If the restraint is applied to enhance therapy, notation of the progress of the therapy should be made. Documentation should include evidence that the nurse knew the complications that may arise with restraint and took precautions to avoid them.

Infection Control

1. Restraints that are used for consecutive clients should be cleaned and disinfected between uses.

2. Handwashing should precede and follow restraining a child to prevent the possibility of cross-contamination.

3. Care should be taken when restraining a child near the area of skin breakdown because this is a possible entry point for pathogenic organisms. Clean restraints may be needed each time the dressing is changed if the restraints become contaminated by wound drainage.

Technique Checklist

	YES	NO
Procedure explained to		
Child	_____	_____
Parents	_____	_____
Type of Restraint used		
Mummy restraint	_____	_____
Elbow restraint	_____	_____
Right _____		
Left _____		
Bilateral _____		
Wrist restraint	_____	_____
Right _____		
Left _____		
Bilateral _____		
Ankle restraint	_____	_____
Right _____		
Left _____		
Bilateral _____		
Bed net	_____	_____
Confined bed	_____	_____
Papoose Board	_____	_____
Jacket restraint	_____	_____
Restraint checked q _____ hr		
Duration of restraints		
_____		
Therapeutic outcome of restraint realized	_____	_____

112   Resuscitation of Infants and Children

Overview

Definition

Restoring to life or conciousness infants and children who are apparently dead or whose respirations have ceased

Rationale

Maintain adequate circulation until definitive treatment is instituted.

Restore normal heart and lung functions after an unexpected failure of these organs.

Terminology

Abdominal thrust: Manual compression of the abdominal area used to dislodge a foreign body or food from the airway

Anoxia: Absence of oxygen

Cardiopulmonary resuscitation (CPR): The act of manually restoring the action of the heart and lungs

External cardiac massage: Compression of the heart in cardiopulmonary resuscitation

Hyperextension: In a resuscitation measure, an excessive extension of the neck

Positive pressure: Pressure greater than that of the atmosphere

Assessment

Pertinent Anatomy and Physiology

1. See Technique 36, Cardiopulmonary Resuscitation (CPR) in the Adult Section.
2. The carotid pulse of an infant is difficult to find because of the short, fat neck. During resuscitation, the pulse most easily palpable in infants is the brachial pulse, which may be felt midway between the shoulder and elbow on the inner aspect of the arm, or the femoral pulse, located in the groin area.

Pathophysiological Concepts

1. See Technique 36, Cardiopulmonary Resuscitation (CPR) in the Adult Section.
2. Most cardiopulmonary arrests in children are due to respiratory causes rather than cardiovascular problems. Cardiopulmonary arrest causes insufficient oxygen in the blood and a build-up of serum carbon dioxide. Anaerobic metabolism results, producing lactate. This causes a decreased pH in the blood and tissues. Increased vagal tone increases the possibility of bradycardia, asystole, and ventricular fibrillation. Symptoms include absent or poor chest movements, weak or absent pulses or heart sounds, marked bradycardia or tachycardia, cyanosis or pallor, and loss of consciousness.

Assessment of the Client

1. Assess the child's state of consciousness. Determine if the child is actually in a state of cardiopulmonary arrest.
2. Assess the child according to the ABC rule: **A**irway must be cleared of obstruction so that the child can breathe; **B**reathing must be assisted to prevent oxygen deprivation to the brain and vital organs; and **C**irculation must be maintained by external cardiac massage.

3. Assess the presence of wounds or injuries that might cause a modification in the usual method of administering cardiopulmonary resuscitation.

4. Each child should be assessed upon admission to a health-care facility in regard to normal sleeping patterns and any respiratory problems. A history of the occurrence of any cases of sudden infant death syndrome (crib death) within the family should be assessed.

Plan

Nursing Objectives

Maintain adequate ventilation and circulation of the infant or child.

Prepare for other emergency measures, such as intubation, tracheostomy, and administration of emergency medications.

Prevent anoxia and brain death.

Client Preparation

Cardiac arrest is usually sudden and unexpected. When arrest occurs, CPR must be initiated promptly. The best preparation is knowledge of the correct procedure.

Equipment

Pediatric airways

Self-inflating bag with pediatric mask

Intravenous (IV) infusion administration equipment

Emergency drugs in pediatric dosages

Implementation and Interventions

Procedural Aspects

ACTION	RATIONALE
1. Establish unresponsiveness by gently shaking the child's shoulder and shouting near the child's ear, "Are you OK?" Use the child's name or nickname to elicit a response. Call for help immediately.	It is dangerous to attempt to resuscitate someone who is not unconscious, but perhaps merely sleeping soundly or feigning unconsciousness.
2. Position the child on a hard, flat surface, such as a table or floor, in a supine position.	The horizontal position aids circulation.
3. Tip the head back—*DO NOT HYPEREXTEND.* Tilt the head back and lift the back of the neck or tilt the head back and lift the child's chin. Place an ear over the child's mouth to listen or feel for breathing. Look for the chest to rise and fall. Check the lip color. If the lips are pink, do not begin resuscitation. Cyanosis of the lips may indicate breathing difficulties;	Hyperextension in the infant and small child can collapse the trachea. The goal is to have a patent airway without interference from the tongue. A bluish tinge to the lips indicates that oxygen consumption is inadequate to oxygenate the blood.

ACTION

RATIONALE

however, this sign does not indicate the need for CPR. Check the inside of the child's mouth. If foreign material is present, clear it before beginning. If the airway is obstructed, use the abdominal thrust to remove the object (see Technique 23, Abdominal Thrust, in the Adult Section). If ventilation is not restored, begin resuscitation.

4. Assist breathing. For the infant, cover the mouth and nose with your mouth. For the older child, pinch the nose and cover the mouth with your mouth, as in adult resuscitation. Give 4 gentle, small breaths in rapid succession.

An airtight seal may be made over the infant's mouth and nose, since the infant's face is so small. Because the lung capacity of the infant and child is smaller than that of an adult, smaller breaths must be given to avoid overinflation of the lungs, which can result in gastric distension and vomiting. Rapid breaths allow the infant's lungs to remain partially inflated during the initial resuscitation attempt, a condition of positive end expiratory pressure.

5. Palpate the pulse. For the infant, use the brachial pulse. For older children, use the carotid pulse (Fig. 112-1). If no pulse is found, initiate compression of the heart.

The carotid pulse is difficult to locate in the infant because of the the short, fat neck.

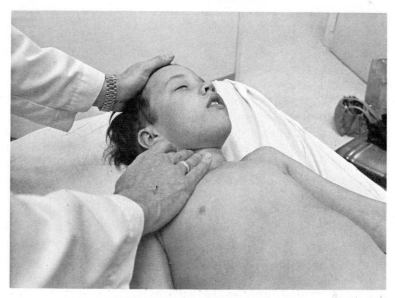

Figure 112.1

ACTION

6. Compress the heart at a rate of 5 compressions to 1 breath. For the infant, use 2 fingers in the mid-sternum area (Fig. 112-2). The rate is 100 compressions/minute. The mneumonic is "one, two, three...". The sternum should be compressed at a depth of ½ to 1 inch. For children, the heel of one adult hand is recommended for compression. A rate of 80 compressions/minute is desired. The mneumonic is "one and two and three and...". The area of compression is mid-sternum, and the depth of compression is 1 to 1½ inches.

RATIONALE

Infants and small children have a normally higher pulse rate than adults. The infant's mneumonic may be compared to that for the adult, which is "one–one thousand, two–one thousand, three–one thousand...". The depth of the compression should be only enough to compress the heart. Because of the pliancy of the infant chest and the smaller diameter, compression need not be as deep as in the adult. In addition, displacement by the liver in the child causes the ventricles to be located at midsternum level, slightly higher than in the adult.

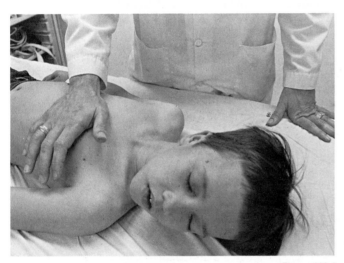

Figure 112.2

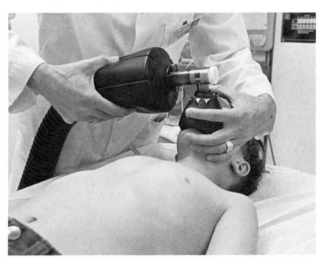

Figure 112.3

7. If an inflatable bag is used, adjust the mouthpiece to fit over the infant's or child's nose and mouth. It should form an airtight seal. Be sure that the right size is used or use mouth-to-mouth assisted ventilation to ensure adequate inflation of the lungs. An airway of appropriate size may be placed in the child's mouth (Fig. 112-3).

8. Periodically reassess the child to determine the effectiveness of CPR. Successful cardiac activity can be determined by the return of pulses, pupil movement, and possibly by spontaneous return of respirations. Reassess the need for continued CPR after 1 minute and then every 4 to 5 minutes during the duration of the resuscitation effort.

The inflatable bag provides a consistent source of air in a consistent amount. However, if the seal is not made, the air may escape from around the edges of the bag rather than being forced into the child's lungs. The airway is used to prevent the child's tongue from falling back into the throat and to provide a patent path for air to be forced into the lungs.

CPR should be stopped as soon as adequate circulation is ensured.

Communicative Aspects

OBSERVATIONS

1. Observe the child for reaction to the resuscitation efforts. Note signs of return to consciousness or adequate cardiac activity.

2. Observe any signs and symptoms that preceded the cardiopulmonary arrest. Carefully note the time of the arrest, the duration of resuscitation, and the time at which the child reacted, or was pronounced dead. Circulation must be restored within 4 minutes to prevent irreversible brain damage or death.

3. Keep a record of the following: when resuscitation began, when the physician arrived, when resuscitation ended, any drugs administered, techniques and equipment used, and the outcome of the procedure.

4. Observe for signs of airway obstruction, which would indicate use of the abdominal thrust procedure. Watch for signs of respiratory embarrassment, which might be caused by overextending the neck.

CHARTING

DATE/TIME	OBSERVATIONS	SIGNATURE
9/18 1300	Found in crib completely still, no noticeable respirations and no brachial pulse palpable. Lips blue, skin cool to touch. Resuscitation begun. "Code 99" called.	C. Day RN
1310	Dr. J. arrived. Spontaneous breathing returned. Brachial pulse 98 and weak. Respirations 18, very shallow.	C. Day RN
1320	IV started. Medications given intravenously as ordered. Pulse stronger, rate 110, resp. deeper and fast, rate 28. Beginning to move spontaneously.	C. Day RN
1325	Crying vigorously. Situation explained to parents, who are with infant now. Apnea monitor applied. IV continues to infuse. Pupils are equal and reactive to light. Blood to laboratory for tests.	C. Day RN

Discharge Planning Aspects

CLIENT AND FAMILY EDUCATION

1. Because time is a key factor during a cardiopulmonary arrest, teaching of the family is done after the emergency is resolved. The family should be notified of the arrest and kept informed of progress to the extent possible without further endangering the child.

2. Parents of infants who have suffered cardiac or respiratory arrest need a great deal of reassurance and education. Signs and symptoms of arrest should be carefully explained. An apnea monitor for the home, with instructions on how to use it, might alert the parents to problems after discharge from the hospital. However, inform the parents that as the child gets older, he or she may roll off of the monitor pad. Different types of monitors are available, with different types, styles, and sizes of apnea pads.

3. Teach the parents CPR techniques for the infant and child. Offer them booklets and material to enable them to teach the techniques to babysitters and friends who may care for the child. Be sure that they know the telephone number of the nearest emergency facility. Assist them to feel confident that they are prepared in case of an emergency after the child's discharge from the hospital.

REFERRALS

If the resuscitation efforts were unsuccessful, referral to a support group for grieving parents may be appropriate. Offer the suggestion for further reference. The parents will be dealing with their grief at this time, but later, the support of persons who have had the same experience may aid the parents' adjustment. There are many organizations that are studying sudden infant death syndrome (SIDS). If this is the suspected cause of the arrest, notification of one of these groups may aid in research of the cause and prevention of the phenomenon. This may be some comfort to the parents.

Evaluation

Quality Assurance

Document any factors that may have precipitated the cardiopulmonary arrest. The chart should reflect a progressive record of the arrest, those involved, the techniques and medications used, and the outcome. Follow-up care of the child and support of the parents should be reflected. Evidence of ongoing reassessment for signs of cardiopulmonary emergency should be reflected. Any education and referrals of the parents should be noted.

Each hospital should have a consistent method of certifying employees, at least yearly, in the latest techniques of CPR. The agency should also have a standard procedure for external cardiac massage and a protocol for obtaining skilled assistance in case of cardiopulmonary arrest. Nurses should know the location of emergency equipment and how to use it. If the agency has a special team to assist in CPR, the method for notifying and assisting the team should be known to every employee. Biomedical technicians should have a consistent means of ensuring that all emergency equipment is in proper working order.

Infection Control

Equipment that will be used for consecutive clients should be cleaned thoroughly between uses. This is particularly important for emergency equipment. There is no time to clean the equipment before use in an emergency situation. Because of tension and anxiety caused by the emergency, cleaning of equipment may be overlooked. It should be an assigned responsibility to make sure that all equipment is cleaned and ready for use as soon as possible after a cardiovascular emergency.

Technique Checklist

	YES	NO
Time CPR started _____		
Time CPR ended _____		
Outcome:		
Vital signs restored at _____		
Child pronounced dead at _____		
Abdominal thrust used	_____	_____
Number of times _____		
External cardiac massage	_____	_____
Assisted respiration		
Mouth-to-mouth _____		
Inflation device _____		
Airway used	_____	_____
Endotracheal intubation	_____	_____
Record of times, techniques, and medications on chart	_____	_____
Cardiac defibrillation ×_____		
Family notified at _____		
Family taught CPR techniques	_____	_____
Return demonstration of CPR	_____	_____
Apnea monitor sent home with family	_____	_____
Instructions in using monitor	_____	_____
Referral to support group	_____	_____
Name of group _____		

Subdural Tap and Ventricular Tap, Assisting With

Overview

Definition

Subdural tap is the introduction of a needle into the subdural space of the brain, between the arachnoid and the dura mater, for the removal of fluid.

Ventricular tap is the introduction of a needle into a ventricle of the brain to remove fluid.

Rationale

Obtain a specimen of cerebrospinal fluid (CSF).

Relieve intracranial pressure.

Allow the physician to make an accurate diagnosis.

Terminology

Subdural: Beneath the dura mater of the brain

Ventricle of the brain: One of the four small cavities in the brain

Assessment

Pertinent Anatomy and Physiology

1. See Appendix I: *brain*.
2. The head accounts for one third of the newborn's body weight. The bones of the skull are separated from one another by membranous tissue spaces called sutures. The points where the major sutures meet in the anterior and posterior portions of the skull are known as fontanelles (Fig. 113-1).

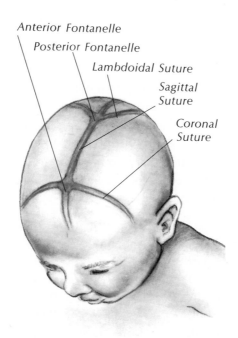

Anterior Fontanelle
Posterior Fontanelle
Lambdoidal Suture
Sagittal Suture
Coronal Suture

Figure 113.1

3. The cranial bones may overlap slightly in the newborn infant. This is the result of molding of the head as it passed through the birth canal. It usually disappears in a few days.

Pathophysiological Concepts

1. Increased intracranial pressure is found in infectious and neoplastic diseases of the central nervous system (CNS) and in conditions that obstruct the ventricular circulation. Intracranial pressure is reflected in the amount of tenseness and fullness seen and felt in the anterior fontanelle. Increased pressure is manifested by a bulging, full fontanelle. This is seen especially when the infant cries, coughs, or strains in any way. Dilated scalp veins are indicative of long-standing increased intracranial pressure.

2. Decreased intracranial pressure, reflected in a depressed fontanelle, is seen as a sign of dehydration in infants.

3. Hydrocephalus is an increase in the CSF volume within any part or all of the ventricular system of the brain. It is the result of overproduction of CSF or obstruction of the flow of CSF through the ventricular system. Communicating hydrocephalus occurs when there is obstruction to the flow within the subarachnoid space because of a condition such as congenital malformation, infection, or tumor. Noncommunicating hydrocephalus occurs when the CSF is not reabsorbed properly.

Assessment of the Client

1. Assess the size and shape of the infant's head. The sutures can be felt as slightly depressed ridges, and the fontanelles feel like soft cavities. The anterior fontanelle is best examined for tenseness and fullness while the baby is sitting quietly or being held in an upright position. The frontal occipital circumference should be measured around the infant's head, over the eyebrows and over the occipital area.

2. Assess the parents' familiarity with the procedure. Determine their level of anxiety and their ability and willingness to know about the procedure when deciding how much information to offer and when it can best be assimilated.

3. Assess any history of problems with blockage or poor reabsorption of CSF. Determine if the child has had the procedure done previously and the length of time elapsed between procedures.

4. Assess baseline vital signs for comparison after the procedure.

Plan

Nursing Objectives

Assist in the effective and efficient completion of the procedure.

Maintain surgical asepsis throughout the procedure.

Explain the procedure to the parents and to the child who is old enough to understand and is able to tolerate such an explanation.

Restrain the child, as necessary, to avoid injury caused by sudden movement.

Observe for signs and symptoms of impending complications, such as respiratory or cardiac abnormalities.

Client Preparation

1. If the client is an infant or small child, restraint may be accomplished by using a papoose board or mummy restraint (see Technique No. 111, Restraints, Pediatric).

2. If the child is older, explain the procedure and attempt to gain cooperation. Position the child's head at the edge of the treatment table for easy access. Physical restraint may be necessary to ensure immobility.

3. The area of needle insertion is shaved and prepared with an antibacterial agent.

Equipment

Tray containing needles, syringes, and receptacles

Antiseptic skin cleanser

Local anesthestic (for older children)

Razor and blades

Sterile gloves

Dry cotton balls

Suction capability or bulb syringe

Requisition for tests to be done

Implementation and Interventions

Procedural Aspects

ACTION	*RATIONALE*
1. Open the tray and gloves. Prepare the skin cleanser for application. Place the child in the dorsal recumbent position unless otherwise requested. The scalp area may be shaved at this time, or this may have been done previously.	Because of the proximity of the brain, strict aseptic technique is necessary. Cleansing of the skin reduces the number of bacteria normally found there, reducing the chance of infection.
2. The physician will insert the needle into the affected area and gently withdraw the fluid. The fluid is usually placed in a container for transport to the laboratory for analysis and testing as requested by the physician. Be sure that the containers are properly labeled with the child's name and hospital number, as well as identification of the type of fluid in the containers.	Analysis of the fluid may provide valuable diagnostic information. Proper identification will help prevent mistakes.
3. Some type of sealing solution may be applied to the skin to prevent leaking of CSF or a sterile dressing may be applied.	It is essential to prevent the leakage of CSF after the procedure because this is a potential entry point for infectious agents.

Communicative Aspects

OBSERVATIONS

1. Observe the tap site carefully and report any leakage from the puncture area.

2. Observe and record the child's tolerance and the procedure. Baseline vital signs should be taken before the procedure to compare with vital signs afterward. Monitor the child's vital signs for several hours after the procedure. Suggested monitoring schedule might be q15min for an hour, q1h for 4 hours, and then q2h for the next 12 hours. Observe the child for irritability, which may indicate pain.

3. Observe the amount and appearance of the fluid specimen.

CHARTING

DATE/TIME	OBSERVATIONS	SIGNATURE
3/10 0230	Subdural tap done in treatment room by Dr. J. Immobility ensured by using papoose board restraint. Initial crying but soon quieted. Puncture site shaved and cleaned with Betadine. Approx. 3 ml. clear fluid obtained. Specimen to lab. Child resting quietly in bed with parents in attendance. Procedure was explained to parents, who seemed to understand and voiced support of this measure as an attempt to diagnose their child's problems.	P. Sanchez RN

Discharge Planning Aspects

CLIENT AND FAMILY EDUCATION

1. Explain to the family and to the child, if appropriate, the reasons for the procedure being done and the expected outcomes. Explain the need for restraints during the procedure. Enlist the parent's assistance in gaining compliance from the older child.

2. Teach the parents how to measure the child's head circumference, if appropriate. Tell them how to determine if the baby's fontanelles are bulging and when to call their physician.

Evaluation

Quality Assurance

Documentation should include any teaching that was done prior to the procedure. Application of restraints should be documented, as well as the child's physical and emotional reaction to restraints. Document any problems occurring during the procedure. The amount and appearance of the fluid should be noted, as well as disposition of the specimen. Monitoring of the child's vital signs should be reflected on the progress notes or in a graphic section. Measures to prevent infection should be thoroughly noted.

Infection Control

1. Infection of the brain is an extremely dangerous complication of invasive procedures of the head and can result in death. It is essential to take every precaution to prevent the spread of infection by thoroughly cleaning and shaving the head, by application of an effective skin cleanser, and by strict adherence to sterile technique.

2. Equipment used in the procedure should be disposed in nonpenetrable containers or returned to the supply area for cleaning and disinfection. If infection is suspected, the equipment must be bagged and marked "contaminated" to prevent the possibility of spreading the infection to personnel.

Technique Checklist

	YES	NO
Technique explained to parents	_____	_____
Technique explained to child	_____	_____
Head area cleansed and shaved	_____	_____
Type of restraint used _____		
Disinfection of site done before insertion of needle	_____	_____
Amount of specimen _____		
Appearance of specimen _____		
Dressing applied	_____	_____
Skin adhesive applied	_____	_____
Vital signs before procedure		
T _____ P _____ R _____		
Vital signs after procedure		
T _____ P _____ R _____		
Frequency of monitoring _____		
Discharge instructions given	_____	_____

Overview

Definition

Aspiration of secretions from an artificial opening in the neck with a sterile catheter connected to suction; cleansing and dressing the incisional area; and changing the tube on a regular basis

Rationale

Facilitate adequate exchange of gases by enchancing respiratory effectiveness.

Limit the introduction of pathogens into the tracheobronchial tree.

Terminology

Hypoxia: Varying degrees of inadequacy of oxygen supply

Mucus: The liquid lining of the mucous membrane, composed of secretions of the glands, along with various inorganic salts, desquamated cells, and leukocytes

Patent: Open, unobstructed

Tracheopathy: Disease of the trachea

Tracheophony: A sound heard in auscultation over the trachea

Tracheostomy: The surgical creation of a vertical slit in the anterior portion of the neck (usually below the first and second tracheal cartilages), with the insertion of a cannula airway to facilitate adequate exchange of gases

Tracheostomy tube: A plastic or Silastic tube composed of two or three parts, the outer cannula, the obturator, and (for larger children) an inner cannula. Most pediatric tubes do not have inner cannulas or cuffs. The tube is inserted into the tracheostomy opening to provide a patent airway. Plastic and Silastic tubes soften at room temperature and more readily conform to the contours of the child's trachea. Their smooth surface also resists kinking and crust formation.

Tracheotomy: Incision of the trachea for exploration, removal of a foreign body, obtaining a biopsy specimen, or removing a local lesion

Assessment

Pertinent Anatomy and Physiology

1. See Appendix I: *lungs, trachea.* See also Technique No. 89, Tracheostomy Care, in the Adult Section.

2. The infant's neck is usually very short. In addition, the chin and cheeks tend to be puffy. For this reason, the neck may have to be supported to prevent the chin from occluding the tracheostomy opening. Hyperextension of the neck, however, may cause collapse of the trachea.

Pathophysiological Considerations

Excessive bronchial secretions often occur in diseases of children; these secretions cannot always be controlled by the child because of the narrowness of the tracheobronchial tree and the underdeveloped muscles of the thorax.

Assessment of the Client

1. Assess the child's age and development status. Determine the child's degree of understanding and anxiety when deciding how much detailed information to offer. Assess the child's previous experience with tracheostomy care.

2. Assess the parent's anxiety level. Determine their familiarity with the tracheostomy procedure and care. Assess their level of understanding and desire to know about the procedure and formulate educational objectives accordingly.

3. Assess the level of cooperation that can reasonably be expected of the child. Determine the need for restraints or assistance during tracheostomy procedure.

Plan

Nursing Objectives

Maintain a patent airway to facilitate gaseous exchange.

Keep the neck of the infant or young child extended to a degree sufficient to ensure that the tracheostomy tube is not obstructed.

Prevent the transmission of pathogenic microorganisms by using sterile technique.

Provide adequate warmth and humidification of the air entering the lungs by way of the tube.

Allay the child's and parent's fears and anxieties about the loss of speaking ability and altered breathing route.

Provide for physical and emotional comfort for the infant or child.

Prevent accidental dislodging of the tube.

Prevent encrustation around the tube and incisional site.

Client Preparation

1. Keep suction equipment in readiness at the child's bedside at all times. The obturator for plugging the child's tracheostomy tube should be kept in a sterile package taped to the head of the child's bed.

2. Depending on the age of the child, offer an explanation of the tracheostomy care. Explain about the inability to speak. If the condition is temporary, reassure the child that normal speech and breathing will return after the tube is removed. Try to help the child understand why and how long the tube must be in place. Since the tracheostomy is so frightening, a great deal of explanation and reassurance is necessary. If the child is old enough, provide communication tools such as a tablet and pencil or a computerized communication tool.

3. If the child is small and uncooperative, elbow restraints may be used to prevent accidental removal of the tube (see Technique 111, Restraints, Pediatric.)

4. Position the infant or small child with a rolled towel under the neck to keep the tracheostomy tube patent (Fig. 114-1). If the child can cooperate, turning to the side may facilitate drainage of secretions from the respiratory tract, preventing pooling of the secretions in the tracheobronchial tree.

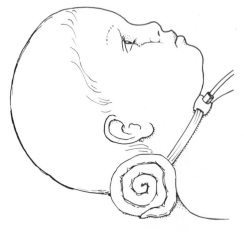

Figure 114.1

Equipment

Suction capability

Suction catheter: The size of the catheter is important for suctioning an infant or child. The diameter of the suction catheter should not be so large that it obstructs the tube for breathing during suctioning. Depending on the size of the tracheostomy tube, the following sizes of suction catheters should be used:

SIZE OF TRACHEOSTOMY TUBE	OUTER TUBE DIAMETER	SUCTION CATHETER SIZE
00	4.5 mm (#14 F)	#8 F
0	5.0 mm (#15 F)	#8 F
1	5.5 mm (#17 F)	#10 F
2	6.0 mm (#18 F)	#12 F
3	7.0 mm (#21 F)	#14 F
4	8.0 mm (#24 F)	#16–#18 F

Sterile gloves

Sterile container with sterile water

Sterile saline solution (0.9%)

Sterile syringe

Umbilical tape

Humidity apparatus, if prescribed

Sterile dressing (4 × 4)

Implementation and Interventions

Procedural Aspects

ACTION

RATIONALE

Suctioning

1. Wash hands before beginning suctioning. Open the catheter package. Don sterile gloves and remove the catheter from the package, maintaining sterility.

2. Moisten the tip of the suction catheter with sterile water.

3. Insert the catheter through the tracheostomy tube with the suction turned off. Direct the catheter into the right or the left bronchus by positioning the child's head to the opposite side (Figs. 114-2, 114-3).

Pathogenic organisms can grow and flourish in a warm, moist environment and may be transmitted by direct contact.

Water will reduce the friction as the tube is inserted into the trachea.

The catheter will be guided by the anatomical structure of the bronchi. The suction is turned off during insertion to decrease trauma to the mucosal lining of the tracheobronchial tree.

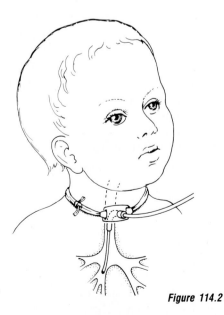

Figure 114.2

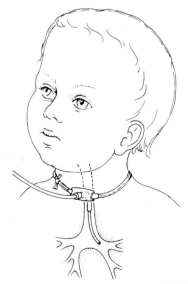

Figure 114.3

ACTION

RATIONALE

An assistant may hold the child's head in the desired position. The physician usually specifies the depth of insertion of the suction catheter. It is usually inserted deep enough to stimulate coughing and obtain secretions from the respiratory tract.

4. With the tube inserted to the desired depth, cover the air-escape valve on the tubing to create suction through the catheter. Withdraw the catheter slowly with a rotating motion.

Changes in pressure inside a tube will cause secretions to move from areas of greater pressure to areas of lower pressure. Rotating the catheter prevents excessive vacuum on one area, with resultant tissue damage.

5. Suction intermittently for no more than 15 seconds. Pause and allow the child to breathe at intervals. Allow the child to rest for 2 to 3 minutes before reinserting the suction catheter, unless the child is in respiratory distress.

The child's airway is obstructed during the suctioning process. Pausing will allow the child to breathe around the catheter. The child's respiratory status is already compromised; prolonged suctioning will intensify hypoxia.

6. If the secretions are very thick or the cannula tends to become encrusted, a small amount of sterile saline solution may be inserted into the tracheostomy tube and immediately suctioned back. The amount of saline solution (0.5 ml– 2.0 ml) depends on the child's size.

Sterile isotonic saline solution injected into the tube helps to loosen the crusts and secretions for easier aspiration.

7. Discard the used suction catheters in a waxed paper bag or plastic bag and label with contents, date, and any special precautions for handling. Send reusable catheters to the supply area for cleaning and disinfection.

Care must be taken not to cross-infect other clients or hospital personnel with careless handling of contaminated equipment.

Dressing Change

1. Remove the dressing and cleanse the area around the tracheostomy tube with hydrogen peroxide to remove encrustations. Replace the dressing by unfolding a 4 × 4 gauze. Fold it in half lengthwise and around the tube by turning each side under and downward (Figs. 114-4, 114-5).

Folding the gauze eliminates the need to cut the pad to fit around the tube, which may cause frayed edges that may be aspirated. The pad should fit around the tube to prevent trauma to tissues and to absorb secretions.

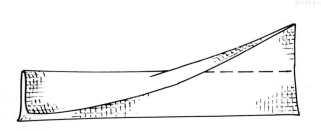
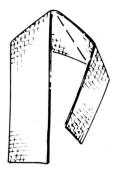

Figure 114.4

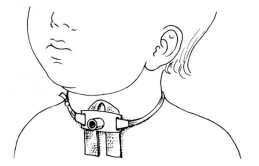

Figure 114.5

ACTION	**RATIONALE**

2. Replace the tracheostomy ties with clean umbilical tape if necessary. The tracheostomy tube should be held in place while the ties are off to ensure that the tube is not accidentally dislodged. After fastening the ties to each edge of the tube, tie them in the back with the child's neck flexed. Test for tension by placing one finger between the tape and the child's flexed neck. Flexion may cause coughing and should be done as quickly as possible.

Every precaution should be taken to prevent accidental removal of the tracheostomy tube. The ties are secured with the neck flexed because flexion decreases the circumference of the neck. Thus, when the neck is extended, the tube should be secure.

3. After dressing change, reapply moisturizing equipment. Check this equipment frequently for proper positioning and moisture build-up. Keep the doors and windows closed to maintain the high-humidity atmosphere.

Moist air keeps the delicate mucous membranes of the respiratory tract from drying out and prevents the secretions from becoming thick and viscous. The nasal passage usually serves this purpose.

Special Modifications

Accidental, spontaneous removal of the tracheostomy tube requires immediate attention. The cannula should be reinserted by a physician under sterile conditions. Sterile forceps or any sterile dilating instrument may be used to hold the tracheal incision open until a new cannula can be inserted to prevent suffocation.

Accidental dislodgment of the tracheostomy tube may occur as a result of forceful coughing or crying, excessive movement, or inadequate restraint of the child who pulls the tube out.

Communicative Aspects

OBSERVATIONS

1. Observe the area around the tracheostomy site for bleeding, crustation, edema, and redness. Note the condition of the tissue and any indication of chafing of the neck from the ties.

2. Observe the amount, consistency, and color of the secretions suctioned from the child's respiratory tract. Note the position in which the best suctioning results are obtained. Observe the ability and willingness of the child to comply with instructions during suctioning. Observe the child's reaction to the suctioning and dressing changes. Determine if the child is able to cough up the secretions.

3. Observe the extremities if restraints are used. Check frequently for adequate circulation and comfort.

4. Observe the child for signs of impending respiratory difficulty, which include restlessness, dyspnea, pallor, cyanosis, changes in vital signs, bleeding from the tracheostomy, retractions, and noisy respirations.

CHARTING

DATE/TIME	OBSERVATIONS	SIGNATURE
7/18 0430	Tracheostomy suctioned with child on left side. Elbow restraints in place. Large amount of thick, frothy secretions aspirated after 8 seconds of suctioning. Rested 3 min. Turned to the right side and suctioned for 5 seconds, very small return of viscous, white secretions returned. Mist collar continuous after suctioning. Remains lethargic with sporadic bouts of crying. Parents in room.	R. Smith RN

Discharge Planning Aspects

CLIENT AND FAMILY EDUCATION

1. Explain to the child and family why the tracheostomy must be done. Offer explanations of the anatomy and physiology consistent with their ability to understand and their desire to know. Explain that air is normally humidified, cleaned, and warmed as it passes through the nasal passage. Since this route is by-passed in tracheostomy, it is necessary to provide a means for adding moisture and warmth before the air enters the lungs.

2. Explain the need for restraints if the child might pull out the tracheostomy tube. If the child can be relied on not to pull out the tube, someone should be in attendance to see that the tube is not contaminated. Toys should be large enough so that the child cannot accidentally place one into the tracheostomy tube. Teach the family to observe the child so that toys or blankets are not allowed to occlude the tube. Clothing should not tie around the neck or cover the tube opening.

3. The child with a tracheostomy should not be left alone. Inability to make a sound can be very frightening. Someone should be in eye contact with the child in case of emergency. Older children can be taught to summon help with the call light or a bell. Writing materials or other communication tools should be available so that the child can communicate with others.

4. If the child will be discharged with a tracheostomy tube in place, be sure that the family understands how to care for the tube at home. Family members should have the opportunity to see a demonstration of caring for the tube and to return this demonstration until they can perform adequately. The parents should be involved in the child's care as soon as possible. Reinforce physician instructions on when to return for follow-up care. Tell the family where to get supplies for caring for the tracheostomy. The tracheostomy tube is usually changed weekly.

REFERRALS

If the child will have the tracheostomy tube for an extended period, referral to a speech therapist may be necessary. Refer the parents to a hospital supply store where they can obtain needed supplies. The supplies should be as similar as possible to those they used in the hospital to decrease the anxiety they will feel when caring for the tracheostomy at home. A home health nurse may provide support during the transition period.

Evaluation

Quality Assurance

Document the condition of the site and the appearance of the secretions at least every shift. Each time the dressing is changed, a notation of the appearance of the site should be made. If the child is restrained, evidence that the nurse monitored the restraints frequently should be present. Any ancillary devices, such as mist collar, humidifier, should be noted with reference to their effectiveness. Cleaning and suctioning schedules should be noted. Notation of suctioning should be made with a description of the results. Any teaching of the family and child should be noted on the chart, with an appraisal of their understanding and acceptance. The chart should indicate that the nurse knew and understood the possible complications of tracheostomy care and took measures to avoid them.

Infection Control

1. Scrupulous handwashing is essential before and after suctioning and dressing change. Reusable equipment should be bagged and sent to the supply area for disinfection and cleaning.
2. Secondary infection is a major concern because the air entering the lower airway bypasses the natural defenses of the upper airway. Every effort should be made to keep the area around the incision clean and free from pathogenic organisms. All equipment coming in contact with the tracheostomy should be sterile. Each procedure is carried out under sterile technique.
3. If the child has a contagious respiratory infection, masks should be worn for performing tracheostomy care. Suctioning causes coughing, which projects droplets into the air. The child should be in a room with no other clients.

Technique Checklist

	YES	NO
Reason for tracheostomy explained		
To parents	_____	_____
To child	_____	_____
Suctioning and dressing change explained		
To parents	_____	_____
To child	_____	_____
Frequency of suctioning _____		
Return described in chart	_____	_____
Sterile technique maintained	_____	_____
Frequency of dressing change _____		
Sterile technique maintained	_____	_____
Humidification device _____		
Patency of tracheostomy maintained	_____	_____
Complications _____		
Someone remained with child at all times	_____	_____
Tracheostomy removed before discharge	_____	_____

	YES	NO
Child sent home with tracheostomy	_____	_____
Parents understood care	_____	_____
Home health referral	_____	_____
Parents know where to get supplies	_____	_____
Speech therapy referral	_____	_____
Medical follow-up reinforced	_____	_____

Tuberculin Testing

Overview

Definition

Skin testing to determine the presence of the bacillus that causes tuberculosis. A positive result signifies that the child has been infected with the tubercule bacillus at one time or another. It does not prove there is active disease, nor does it define acuteness or chronicity. It provides a convenient screening method for skin tuberculin reactivity. The two most common types are:

Mantoux tuberculin test: Intradermal injection of purified protein derivative (PPD)

Tine tuberculin test: Puncture of the skin with a stainless steel disk containing four tines, 2 mm long, which are attached to a plastic handle. The tuberculin test solution is on the tines. The unit is covered and sterilized with ethylene oxide gas and the protected portion remains sterile until the plastic cap is removed. The unit is disposable which eliminates the need for special syringes, needles, and sterilization procedures. However, it is less reliable than the Mantoux test. (See Goroll AH, May LA, Mulley AG: Primary Care Medicine. Philadelphia, JB Lippincott, 1981)

Rationale

Aid in the diagnosis of past or present tuberculous infection.

Assist in differentiating tuberculosis from certain fungal infections, such as histoplasmosis.

Terminology

Antigens: A substance that stimulates an immune response in a sensitive individual

Induration: An area of hardened tissue

Intradermal: Within the substance of the skin

Papule: A circumscribed, solid elevated lesion of the skin, up to 5 mm in diameter

T lymphocytes: A type of immune cell which is responsible for forming the sensitized cells that provide cellular immunity

Wheal: A localized area of edema on the body surface; the dermal evidence of a skin test

Assessment

Pertinent Anatomy and Physiology

1. See Appendix I: *skin.*
2. *Cell-mediated hypersensitivity reactions* involve T lymphocytes that have been sensitized to locally deposited antigens. Cell-mediated immunity is also called delayed hypersensitivity, as compared with immediate hypersensitivity, which is caused by immunoglobulins. Two of the most common types of cell-mediated immunity are tuberculin tests and contact dermatitis. In the tuberculin test, a purified component of the tuberculosis bacillus is injected intradermally. In a previously sensitized person, there is redness and swelling at the site of injection as the sensitized T-type lymphocytes interact with

the tuberculin antigen. The reaction usually develops over a period of 48 to 72 hours. The tuberculin test merely indicates that an individual has been sensitized to the tuberculosis bacillus through previous exposure—it does not mean that the person has the disease.

Pathophysiological Concepts

Tuberculosis is an infectious disease caused by *Mycobacterium tuberculosis*. The mode of transmission is the airborne route. The nuclei remain suspended in the air and are circulated by air currents. They are so small that when inhaled, they travel directly to the alveoli. *Primary tuberculosis*, also known as childhood tuberculosis, begins with acute inflammatory response and progresses to a chronic granulomatous inflammation. *Secondary tuberculosis* results from reactivation of a previously healed primary lesion. Often the only evidence of primary tuberculosis is a positive skin test and the presence of calcified lesions on radiologic examination of the chest.

Assessment of the Client

1. Assess the history of the child in relation to exposure to known cases of tuberculosis. Tuberculin testing should be done with extreme caution in persons with active tuberculosis.

2. Assess the respiratory adequacy of the child. Determine if the child has any respiratory problems.

3. Assess the allergy history of the child. Tuberculin testing should be avoided if the child is known to be allergic to Tween 80, the stabilizer component in many tuberculin testing solutions.

4. Assess the child for possible supression of tuberculin reactivity, which may occur as a result of malnutrition, overwhelming tuberculous infection, administration of corticosteroids and immunosuppressive agents, and diseases associated with cellular immune deficiency. Certain viral infections and the use of live viral vaccines may suppress immunity for up to 4 weeks.

Plan

Nursing Objectives

Allay the fear and anxiety of the child and parents by offering a thorough explanation of the test and interpretation of results.

Administer the tuberculin test in the proper manner.

Read the test in 48 to 72 hours.

Provide follow-up as indicated by the results of the test.

Client Preparation

1. Secure the child in such a manner that the test may be properly administered. Restraint of the young child may be necessary. The older child may be sitting up with the left arm exposed.

2. Explain to the child and the parents what will occur during the test and why it is necessary for the child to remain still.

Equipment

Alcohol or acetone to cleanse the skin

Mantoux tuberculin test solution, tuberculin syringe, and intradermal needle with short bevel

Tine tuberculin unit consisting of a stainless steel disk with four tines or prongs, 2 mm long, attached to a plastic handle.

Implementation and Interventions

Procedural Aspects | *ACTION* | *RATIONALE*

Mantoux Tuberculin Testing

1. Cleanse the skin of the left forearm with acetone or alcohol and allow to dry. The area for testing is the flexor surface of the left forearm about 4 inches below the bend of the elbow. If this site is contra-indicated, use the right forearm.

    Extraneous substances on the skin may cause a reaction, thus skewing the test results.

2. With the needle bevel pointing upward, inject the testing solution into the most superficial layers of the skin (Fig. 115-1). A definite, white bleb will rise at the needle point. The bleb will be about 10 mm in diameter (Fig. 115-2).

    The bevel must be pointed upward so that the solution will be injected into the uppermost layers of the skin. Appearance of the bleb ensures proper placement of the solution.

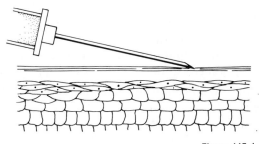

Figure 115.1

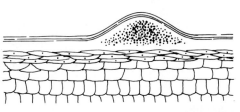

Figure 115.2

3. Interpret the test in 48 to 72 hours. Only *induration* is considered in reading the test. Palpate the induration using one index finger. Be sure the client's forearm is slightly flexed and in good light. Measure the induration transversely at the widest diameter.

    The width of the induration is indicative of the reaction. A negative reaction occurs when the induration is 00 mm to 4 mm in width. A doubtful reaction is 5 mm to 9 mm. A positive reaction occurs when the induration is 10 mm or more in width.

Tine Tuberculin Testing

1. Cleanse the upper forearm as in the Mantoux procedure. Expose the four tines by removing the protective cap while holding the plastic handle. Stretch the skin on the forearm tightly and apply the disk with the other hand. Exert enough pressure to puncture the skin with the tines. Hold approximately *1 second* before withdrawing. The four puncture sites and a circular depression of the skin from the base are visible.

    The tines of the testing unit are impregnated with the tuberculin testing solution. Sufficient time must be allowed for the solution to be deposited into the superficial layer of the skin. Visual evidence of proper puncture should be sought after removing the unit from the skin. Holding the skin tightly reduces the chance of scratching the skin.

ACTION	RATIONALE
2. Read the test in 48 to 72 hours in good light with the arm flexed. Induration is the only criterion for interpreting the test. Observe the diameter of the induration in reading the test.	The width of the induration indicates the extent of reaction. Less than 2 mm of induration is a negative reaction. 2 mm to 4 mm is a doubtful reaction. 5 mm or more is a positive reaction.

Special Precautions

1. Never reuse the tine test.	The chance of cross-contamination of infection would be very great by re-using the testing unit.
2. Avoid hairy areas and areas without adequate subcutaneous tissue, such as over a tendon or bone when doing tuberculin testing.	Excessive hair limits the successful reading of the test. The goal is to place the solution into the superficial layers of the skin. Satisfactory placement would be compromised if the skin was stretched tightly over a bone or tendon.

Communicative Aspects

OBSERVATIONS

1. In reading tuberculin tests, consider only the induration. Erythema is generally a good guide to induration because it usually occurs concomitantly. However, only the induration is indicative of the results of the test.

2. Observe for any untoward reactions to the tuberculin test, such as allergic response.

CHARTING

The date and time of the test should be recorded, as well as the interpretation.

DATE/TIME	OBSERVATIONS	SIGNATURE
3/10 1430	Mantoux tuberculin skin test on left inner forearm. States she has no allergies and has never had or been exposed to tuberculosis. Reason for test and date for reading results explained to child and parents. Emphasis placed on the fact that a positive test does *not* mean that the child has T.B. Parents have agreed to return the child for interpretation of test results on 3/12 or 3/13. Written instructions given.	C. Day RN
3/13 1600	Clinic Follow-up: seen in ambulatory clinic for interpretation of Mantoux skin test. No induration noted. Test interpreted as negative.	C. Hardin RN

Discharge Planning Aspects

CLIENT AND FAMILY EDUCATION

1. If the child is to be discharged before the time for reading the test, give the parents written instructions about when and where to return to have the tuberculin test read.

2. Instruct the child to avoid rubbing or scratching the injected site. No dressing is necessary; however, a long-sleeved blouse or shirt will protect the test area. Tell the family that usual bathing and hygiene measures are allowed.

3. Inform the parents and child that redness and swelling do not indicate that the child has tuberculosis. However, a positive test does indicate the need for further study. Emphasize the importance of follow-up of testing and treatment.

4. Stress the importance of follow-up for children tested for tuberculosis. Follow-up is of particular importance if the test is positive. Early institution of proper treatment can prevent many of the complications associated with tuberculosis.

Evaluation

Quality Assurance

Documentation of the placement of the skin test is very important. If this is not documented clearly, adequate interpretation of the test cannot be ensured. Instructions given to the client and family should be noted. Interpretation of the test should be reflected, along with follow-up plans and actions.

Hospitals should have a regular method of screening employees against contagious diseases such as tuberculosis. A consistent method of screening and follow-up is essential and may be carried out through such departments as Employee Health or Infection Control.

Infection Control

1. Tuberculosis is spread by droplet nuclei, which are suspended in the air and circulated by air currents. In cases of active tuberculosis, the method of prevention is careful handwashing and use of masks.

2. Scrupulous handwashing should precede and follow tuberculin skin testing.

3. Dispose of the needle or tine tuberculin unit after testing in such a way that the chance of accidental puncture is avoided.

Technique Checklist

	YES	NO
Procedure explained to parents and child	_____	_____

Type of test administered

    Mantoux test _____

    Tine test _____

    Date of administration _____

Site of test

    Left forearm _____

    Other _____

| Written instructions to parents about returning for interpretation | _____ | _____ |

Test interpretation

    Negative _____

    Doubtful _____

    Positive _____

    Date of interpretation _____

Type of follow-up care

    Chest x-ray _____

    Medication _____

    Other _____

Overview

Definition

Collection of part or all of a whole for the purpose of learning about the kind of quality of the whole; urine and stool specimens are samples used to aid in the diagnosis and treatment of diseases.

Rationale

Facilitate accurate and definitive laboratory analysis.

Assist in correct diagnosis and treatment.

Terminology

Clay-colored stool: Stool the color of clay (light gray or white) because of a lack or deficiency of bile in the intestinal tract. The bile pigment gives the characteristic brownish color to the stool.

Defecation: The elmination of wastes and undigested food, such as feces, from the rectum

Feces: Body wastes discharged from the intestine; also called stool, excreta or excrement

Incontinence: The inability to refrain from yielding to normal impulses, such as the urge to defecate or urinate

Retention: The condition existing when urine cannot be expelled from the bladder

Specific gravity of urine: The weight of a given volume of urine as compared with the weight of an equal volume of distilled water as measured by a urinometer. The specific gravity of urine varies, according the amount of dissolved solids in it, between 1.010 and 1.030.

Urea: A white, crystalline substance that is one of the chief nitrogenous constituents of urine. It is the chief end product of protein metabolism. The amount of urea in the urine increases with the quantity of protein in the diet.

Urology: The branch of medicine dealing with the urinary system in the female and the genitourinary system in the male

Assessment

Pertinent Anatomy and Physiology

1. See Appendix I: *anus, bladder, intestine (large), intestine (small), kidneys, rectum, ureters, urethra.*

2. The timing of specimen collection may have a bearing on the results of diagnostic tests. Early morning specimens are often desirable for urinalysis because the urine is more concentrated. This would not be valid, however, for the very young infant who still takes night feedings.

Pathophysiological Concepts

Diarrhea is the presence of loose, watery, sometimes explosive stools. Certain conditions cause water to be pulled into the bowel by the hyperosmotic nature of its contents. This occurs when there is failure to absorb osmotically active particles. Another cause of diarrhea is an increase in the secretory processes of the bowel. Most acute infectious diarrhea is of this type.

Assessment of the Client

1. Assess the age and understanding of the child in deciding how to get the best specimen while causing the least anxiety and discomfort to the child. Determine if the child is bowel and/or bladder trained. If the child is an adolescent, the reaction to this procedure may be embarrassment. Assess ways to relieve the child's anxiety. If the child is school-age, provide information about why the procedure is being done. Curiosity is a natural part of the school child's life. Assess the amount and type of information the child is seeking and the best time and way to provide it. For the young child and infant, assess ways in which to perform the procedure(s) quickly and efficiently with the least disruption.

2. Assess the parent's understanding and their willingness to assist in specimen collection.

3. Assess the presence of any bowel or urinary pathology. Determine if the child has any difficulties voiding or defecating. Assess the normal bowel and bladder patterns of the child. Determine the child's physical condition and the reason for hospitalization. Assess the impact of presenting symptoms on the normal bowel and bladder patterns.

Plan

Nursing Objectives

Gain the cooperation of the child by an adequate explanation appropriate to age and level of understanding.

Use the correct, labeled specimen container.

Obtain the specimen in the manner appropriate to producing the desired results.

Transfer specimens to the laboratory promptly.

Client Preparation

1. Explain to the parent and child the kind of specimen that is needed, the type of receptacle that will be used, and exactly what their part in the procedure will be.

2. Place the infant in Fowler's position for the collection of a urine specimen in order to take advantage of the gravitational pull to obtain the specimen.

3. Obtain equipment needed for specimen collection before approaching the infant. Plastic urine collection units are available for the small infant who cannot use a bedpan or commode (Fig. 116-1).

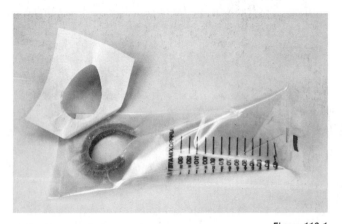

Figure 116.1

Equipment

URINE SPECIMEN

Bedpan, urinal, or commode container

Plastic urine collection container (for children who cannot use the bedpan, urinal, or commode).

STOOL SPECIMEN

Stool specimen container

Tongue blades

Diapers for infants

Bedpan and tissue for older children

Implementation and Interventions

Procedural Aspects

ACTION

RATIONALE

Urine Specimens

1. Urinalysis may be done on a minimum of 2 ml of urine. A minimum of 10 ml of urine is needed for specific gravity determination (see Technique No. 21, Specific Gravity of Urine, Measurement of).

Analysis of a part will yeild information about the quality and constituency of the whole.

2. Depending on the type of specimen needed, the older child may use one of several techniques to produce a urine specimen. Emptying the bladder into a urinal or container from which a small amount of urine is poured into a specimen container is satisfactory for urinalysis. It does not provide a sterile specimen. A midstream specimen may be obtained by allowing the child to void a small amount and then catching a small amount in a sterile container. A clean-catch specimen is obtained as a midstream specimen; however, the meatus must be cleaned first with sterile cotton balls and a soapy solution. The foreskin is retracted in the uncircumcised male until the specimen is obtained. The glans is cleaned with the cotton balls using a circular motion. The labia are separated in the female and remain separated until the specimen is obtained. The meatus and surrounding genitalia are cleaned with the cotton balls from front to back, using a clean cotton ball for each stroke.

The external portion of the urethra is considered contaminated. When the urine exits the body normally, it is no longer sterile. The type of test ordered will influence the type of specimen required. If a culture is ordered, the specimen should be as nearly sterile as possible. A carefully controlled clean-catch specimen is usually used for culture because of the trauma of catheterization on the young child.

ACTION

3. A urine specimen collection unit may be applied to the small child or infant who is not bladder trained. Cleanse the skin surface with cotton balls and disinfectant. Dry the skin thoroughly so that the adhesive will stick. Remove the protective paper and expose the adhesive surface on the bag (Fig. 116-2). Stretch the child's skin firmly and apply the bag with the receptacle portion downward. Apply adequate pressure to ensure adhesion. For the male infant, insert the penis through the bag opening (Fig. 116-3). For the female infant, place the bag opening over the upper portion of the external genitalia, completely enclosing the urinary meatus (Fig. 116-4). Replace the diaper loosely over the collection bag. Check the bag frequently. As soon as an adequate amount of urine is obtained, remove the bag.

RATIONALE

When the child voids, the urine will be trapped inside the urine bag. The adhesive prevents leakage of the urine out of the bag. The diaper should be loose so that it will not cause discomfort by compressing the urine bag against the skin.

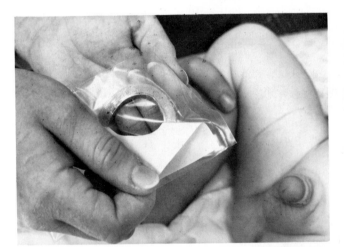

Figure 116.2

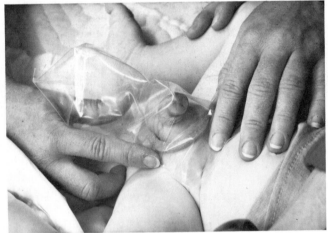

Figure 116.3

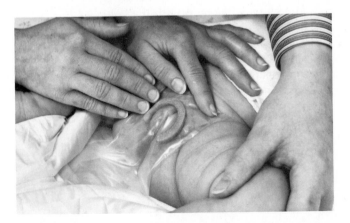

Figure 116.4

ACTION	**_RATIONALE_**
Stool Specimen	
1. If the child is older and capable of using a bedpan, offer the child the bedpan and an explanation that a specimen is needed. Allow the child as much privacy as possible. Use a tongue blade to obtain a small amount of feces from the bedpan. Wash hands carefully after handling the bedpan or stool specimen. If the child can go to the bathroom, place a commode container inside the commode and obtain the stool specimen from the container.	Maintain the child's self-esteem by attention to and respect for personal needs, such as privacy. The intestinal system contains a large amount of bacteria, which may be reduced by proper handwashing.
2. For the infant or very young child, remove the stool specimen from the diaper with a tongue blade and place it into the specimen container.	A small amount of fecal material is adequate for most examinations.
3. Label the specimen cup and transport it to the laboratory immediately. Do not place the specimen in the refridgerator. If the specimen is to be examined for parasites, it should be placed in an incubator.	Cold inhibits the action and growth of bacteria. Incubation promotes the growth of parasites so that they may be identified more easily and accurately.

Special Modifications

1. Catheterization of infants and children usually is avoided. If it is necessary, the procedure proceeds as with an adult catheterization (see Technique 39, Catheterization, Urethral in the Adult Section). However, it is necessary to use a light, gentle touch when cleaning the genitalia. Since most children will not willingly cooperate with this procedure, adequate restraint and assistance are important. For most infants, a size 8 to 10 French catheter is satisfactory. Special care must be taken when catheterizing young males to avoid injuring the delicate tissues in the urethral opening, which can result in sterility.	Catheterization is frightening and very uncomfortable to the young child. Adequate restraint can allow the procedure to proceed quickly and efficiently.

ACTION	*RATIONALE*
2. Suprapubic aspiration of bladder contents may be done by the physician. A 20- or 21-gauge needle is inserted into the bladder. This technique is usually done only when the infant has not voided for at least 1 hour and the bladder can be palpated above the level of the symphysis pubis. Thorough skin preparation is necessary.	Aspiration of bladder contents is done only when a sterile specimen is needed from a very young infant. Cleansing the skin will reduce the number of microorganisms and help prevent infection.
3. If the child is having watery diarrhea, a small piece of plastic across the inside of the child's diaper will catch the diarrhea before it soaks into the diaper.	Some diarrhea stools are so watery that they are absorbed into the diaper, making specimen collection extremely difficult.

Communicative Aspects

OBSERVATIONS

1. Observe the appearance of the urine and feces. Observe for unusual characteristics. Note the amount, odor, clarity, color, and cloudiness of the urine. Be alert to frequent voiding of small amounts of urine, buring upon urination, and a sense of urgency in the need to void. Note the color, odor, form, and consistency of the stool. Also, note if there is flatus associated with the bowel movements, abdominal cramping, distension, pain, or evidence of mucus or blood in the stool.

2. Observe the urine collection bag carefully. Remove the bag as soon as enough urine is obtained for a sample. If the urine is contaminated with feces, discard it and start the collection procedure again.

3. Observe the ability of the child to understand and comply with instructions for specimen collection. Protect the privacy of the child. Observe the level of understanding and amount of anxiety in assessing the adequacy of instructions.

CHARTING

DATE/TIME	OBSERVATIONS	SIGNATURE
6/5 1130	Urine specimen collection procedure explained to mother. Urine collection bag applied and diaper reapplied. Mother encouraged to feed baby at regular time. Shown how to hold baby so that urine bag is not uncomfortable. ——	D. Day RN
1205	Urine collection bag removed from baby. 25 ml urine obtained and sent to lab in labeled container. Urine yellow, clear. ——	C. Day RN

Discharge Planning Aspects

CLIENT AND FAMILY EDUCATION

1. Explain to the parents and child, if appropriate, why the specimen must be obtained and the procedure involved. Explain in terms that the child understands. Determine the words by which the child usually refers to the eliminative functions.

2. While inquiring about the child's normal bowel patterns, use this opportunity to emphasize the importance of a well-balanced diet and regular exercise for proper bowel habits. Caution the parents about the indiscriminate use of over-the-counter medicines and laxatives to stimulate "normal" bowel patterns. Emphasize that normal is whatever is normal for the individual, whether it is once-a-day evacuation, every-other-day, or more often.

Evaluation

Quality Assurance

Documentation should include the type of specimen required, description of the specimen, and notation about the procurement of the specimen. Instructions to the parents and child should be documented. Any precautions or actions taken to enhance the quality of the specimen should be reflected. The time the specimen was obtained and the time it was taken to the laboratory should be noted.

Each hospital should have a uniform protocol for the transportation of specimens throughout the hospital that ensures the quality of the specimen and protects against cross-contamination.

Infection Control

1. Careful handwashing should be done before and after collecting specimens. This is especially important in the collection of stool specimens because of the normal flora and bacteria that are present in the feces. Gloves may be worn while collecting feces to prevent contamination of the hands.

2. Transportation of the specimens should be done in such a manner that cross-contamination is prevented. The container should be closed securely and labeled. If the outside of the container is contaminated, the container should be enclosed in a sack or bag and clearly labeled before being sent to the laboratory. Persons transporting specimens should be taught the importance of handling the specimens carefully and avoiding contamination.

3. Equipment that is used for consecutive clients must be cleaned thoroughly between uses. This is particularly important for single-use equipment, such as a bedpan for the collection of specimens. Even if the equipment is used just one time, it must be returned to the supply area for disinfection or discarded if it is disposable.

Technique Checklist

	YES	NO
Procedure explained to parents	_____	_____
Procedure explained to child	_____	_____

Type of specimen _____

    Time obtained _____

    Time transported to laboratory _____

Complications _____

117 Vital Signs in Children

Overview

Definition

Measurement of verifiable signs that reflect the child's physiological state, which are governed by the body's vital organs (brain, heart, lungs), and which are necessary to sustain life. The vital signs are:

Blood pressure: Auscultation, palpation (fingertips used instead of stethoscope; only systolic pressure can be determined with any degree of accuracy)

Pulse: Radial, femoral, temporal, brachial, apical (auscultated), carotid, and pedal

Respiration: Visualized or auscultated

Temperature: Oral, rectal, and axillary

Rationale

Assess the child's condition.

Determine baseline values for future comparisons.

Detect any deviation in the child's status as early as possible.

Communicate any observations about the child's well-being to other members of the health-care team.

Terminology

Apnea: Absence of respiration

Arrhythmia: Any variation from normal rhythm

Blanch: A whitening of the skin under slight pressure

Bradycardia: An abnormally slow heartbeat

Crisis: Sudden decline of fever

Cyanosis: A bluish color of mucosa and skin due to the circulation of blood with reduced hemoglobin content

Extrasystole: An extra beat, usually at irregular intervals

Hyperpnea: Excessively rapid respiration

Hypertension: Abnormally high blood pressure

Hypotension: Abnormally low blood pressure

Lysis: Gradual decline of fever

Pulse: The rhythmic throbbing caused by regular expansion (rise) and contraction (fall) of an artery as the blood is forced into it by the contraction of the left ventricle of the heart

Respiration: The exchange of gases between an organism

Rhythm: The regularity of the heartbeats

Stertorous breathing: Noisy, snoring-type breathing

Tachycardia: An abnormally fast heartbeat

Temperature: Heat maintained by a living body expressed in degrees; the balance between heat produced and heat lost

Assessment

Pertinent Anatomy and Physiology

1. See Appendix I: *blood vessels, heart, lungs, skin.*

2. *Blood pressure* refers to the force of blood exerted against the wall of the artery (arterial pressure) in which it is contained. The *diastolic pressure* is the lowest pressure exerted against the arterial wall during relaxation of the ventricles. The *systolic pressure* is the greatest pressure exerted against the arterial wall during contraction of the ventricles. The *pulse pressure* is the difference between the systolic and diastolic pressures. This difference represents the volume output of the left ventricle. The level of systolic blood pressure climbs gradually throughout infancy and childhood. Normal systolic pressures are around 50 mg Hg at birth, 90 at age 1 year, 100 at age 6 years, and 120 in midadolescence. The muffled sound of the diastolic beat, detectable in adults, is often lacking in children. In early childhood, the heart sounds are often inaudible because of a narrow or deeply placed brachial artery.

3. The heart rate of infants and child is more sensitive to exercise, illness, and emotions than that of the adult. The average heart rate shows a gradual decrease as the infant grows. The average rate at birth is 140 beats/minute. At age 6 months, it may be 130, decreasing to 110 by age 2 years. The average heart rate for the school-age child is around 100 beats/minute.

4. The respiratory rate in infants and children has a greater range and is more responsive to illness, exercise, and emotion than in adults. The rate per minute ranges between 30 and 60 in the newborn, between 20 and 40 during early childhood, and between 15 and 25 during late childhood. In infancy and early childhood, diaphragmatic breathing is predominant.

5. Temperature regulation in infants and children is less well-controlled than in adults. The average rectal temperature is higher in infancy and early childhood, usually above 99.0° F (37.2° C) until the age of 3 years.

Pathophysiological Concepts

1. A state of anxiety in the young child may elevate the vital-sign readings. The pulse and blood pressure are both affected by this phenomenon.

2. The body temperature of infants may be normal or subnormal during massive infection. However, during early childhood, extremely high temperatures (103° to 105° F [39.5°–40.5° C]) may be present, even with minor infections. Infants do not tend to localize infections, as do adults.

Assessment of the Client

1. Assess the physical and emotional state of the child. Variations in blood pressure are brought about by exercise, crying, and emotional upset. Assess the condition for which the child is being hospitalized to determine any effect on vital signs.

2. Assess the size of the child and obtain the proper size cuff for blood pressure measurement. If the cuff is too large, a slight variation in the reading is possible; however, if the cuff is too small, an abnormally high reading is probable. The width of the cuff should be one-half to two-thirds the width of the upper arm or leg. The length should be sufficient to circle the extremity completely with at least a 20% overlap.

3. Assess the child's previous experience with vital-sign measurement. Determine if the child has ever had blood-pressure determination before. If not, anxiety may be eased by allowing the child to play with the equipment briefly before applying the cuff. Most children have had their temperatures taken. Assess the usual method of temperature measurement to determine how much information is needed. If the child is accustomed to oral temperature evaluation and will now have rectal measurement, an explanation of why and how the procedure will be done are in order. Allow the child to see that the stethoscope will not hurt before applying it to the child's body. Preschool children tend to view everything as alive and need reassurance that the equipment will not hurt them.

4. Consider the age level of the child when determining how to measure respiratory rate. The rate may vary greatly from moment to moment in premature and full-term newborns. Periods of rapid breathing may be interspersed with periods of apnea. Assess the length of time necessary to measure the true rate of repirations, which may be more than 1 minute if the rate is variable.

Plan

Nursing Objectives

Use the data from vital-sign measurement as a measurement of the child's progress in response to therapy and nursing interventions.

Understand the importance of using the proper size equipment in taking vital signs in children.

Recognize the interrelationships between the vital signs, physiologic activity, and pathophysiologic change.

Identify the changes in the vital signs that require urgent medical or nursing intervention.

Assess and evaluate the child's response to both internal and external factors as indicated by the measurments of vital signs.

Recognize the importance of keeping the child quiet and comfortable during the vital-signs measurement period.

Assess the periodic nature of physiologic activity as a basis for evaluating the measurement of the vital signs.

Communicate the measurements of vital signs to the health-team members in correct terminology and in accepted form.

Initiate nursing measures indicated by the change in the child's vital signs.

Client Preparation

The measurement of vital signs should be explained to the child according to age level and amount of anxiety. Explain that the procedure will not hurt and allow the child to handle equipment, if appropriate.

Equipment

Thermometer (mercury or electronic)

Stethoscope and sphygmomanometer

Watch with second hand

Tissue

Lubricant

Alcohol sponge

Implementation and Interventions

Procedural Aspects

ACTION

RATIONALE

Blood Pressure

1. Place the child in a comfortable, relaxed position. Using the correct size cuff, position the cuff approximately 1 inch above the antecubital fossa. Hold the lower arm straight, not hyperextended (Fig. 117-1). If the leg is used, place the cuff 1 inch above the popliteal fossa.

Anxiety can cause an increase in the blood pressure. The child should be relaxed, if possible. Hyperextension of the arm can obscure the sounds necessary for measurement of blood pressure.

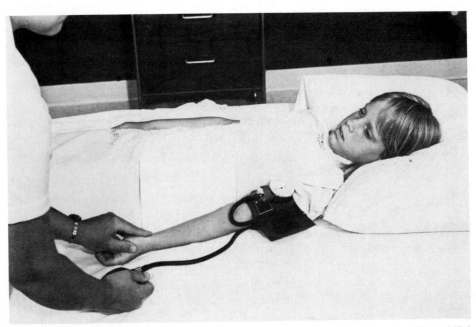

Figure 117.1

2. *Ausculatory method:* Apply the cuff ½ to 1 inch above the antecubital fossa with the arm supported in a slightly flexed and abducted position at the level of the child's heart. Palpate the brachial artery and inflate the cuff until the pulse is absent. Continue to inflate the cuff to approximately 20 mm Hg above the level where the pulse was last felt. Place the bell of the sphygmomanometer over the brachial artery. Keep the mercury-type manometer at eye level, no more than 3 ft away. Deflate the cuff slowly, about 5 mm Hg/second.

The sound of the pressure in the arteries is audible when amplified by using an instrument such as the stethoscope or other devices such as electronic or ultrasound amplifiers.

ACTION

RATIONALE

The systolic reading is the point at which the pulse becomes audible. The diastolic reading is the point at which the sound is muffled.

3. *Palpation method:* Apply the sphygmomanometer and palpate the brachial artery. Inflate the cuff to 150 mm Hg. Leave the fingers on the brachial pulse while deflating the cuff. Taking the reading when the pulse distal to the cuff becomes palpable.

The palpation method provides an indication of the approximate mean pressure between the systolic and diastolic pressures. It is useful in indicating an increasing or decreasing trend in blood pressure.

4. *Flush method:* Place the infant in a supine position with the cuff applied to the arm or leg just above the wrist or ankle. Apply pressure to the extremity from the fingers or toes toward the midline of the body by wrapping the extremity snugly with an elastic bandage. Inflate the manometer to approximately 120 mm Hg. Release the pressure bandage on the extremity. The extremity will be blanched. As the cuff is slowly deflated, take the pressure reading at the point when a sudden flushing of the extremity occurs, indicating return of blood to the foot or hand.

The flush blood pressure reflects the mean pressure between the systolic and diastolic.

Pulse

1. *Apical pulse:* Place the bell of the stethoscope between the infant's left nipple and sternum. Count the heart rate for a full 60 seconds. If significant abnormality is present, count the pulse for longer than a minute to ensure accurate measurement of the pulse rate.

The heart in the infant is located higher in the chest cavity than that of the adult. Auscultation at sternum level should provide clear sounds for measurement. Premature infants and some full-term infants have periods of apnea and periods of hyperpnea.

2. Measure the pulse of the older child at the radial, carotid, or temporal sites. Take the pulse for 30 seconds and multiply by 2. Use the second and third (middle and ring) fingers to palpate the child's pulse. Press *gently*. If there is any irregularity, measure the pulse for a full 60 seconds.

The thumb and forefinger have pulses of their own, which may be mistaken for that of the child if these fingers are used to measure the child's pulse. Too much pressure during palpation will obliterate the child's pulse and too little will make the pulse imperceptible.

ACTION	RATIONALE

Respiration

1. A complete cycle of inspiration and expiration constitutes one act of respiration. This cycle of the child's respirations is noted by the rise and fall of the child's chest and abdomen. For the infant, count the respirations for 1 full minute, noting chest and abdominal movement.

   The diaphragmatic breathing of the young infant make observation of the abdomen desirable for accurate respiratory rate determination.

2. For the older child, count the respirations for 30 seconds and multiply by 2. Visualize the rise and fall of the infant's chest. If abnormality is noted, count the respirations for 1 full minute.

   Older children move the thoracic cage, rather than the abdomen, during respiration unless pathology is present.

Temperature

1. Take the temperature last during vital-signs measurement.

   Temperature measurement may cause crying, which may elevate the pulse and blood pressure.

2. Wipe the soaking solution from the glass thermometer before placing it in the child's mouth. Shake the thermometer vigorously to ensure that the mercury is down to the 96° F level. Check to be sure that the proper type of thermometer is being used. The rectal glass mercurial thermometer has a more rounded bulb than the oral. If an electronic thermometer is used, place a protective sheath over the probe before placing the probe into the client's mouth or rectum. If rectal measurement is done, use the rectal probe.

   The soaking solution may be harmful to the delicate mucous membranes and the skin. The mercury expands when heated during temperature measurement. A constriction in the mercury line near the bulb of the thermometer prevents the mercury from receding to the lowest reading. Because the electronic device does not depend on mercury, shaking is unnecessary.

3. *Rectal* temperatures are recommended for any child who has had oral surgery, is receiving oxygen, or has a potential for convulsions. The initial temperature of a newborn is taken rectally. The average rectal reading is 99.6° F (37.5° C). To measure rectal temperature, lubricate the thermometer tip or probe with a water-soluble lubricant. Separate the child's buttocks and place the rounded tip of the thermometer gently into the child's rectum to a level of approximately 1 inch. Hold the mercury thermometer in place for 5 minutes. Hold the probe in place until the electronic thermometer signifies that

   Rectal readings offer an accurate measurement of the child's temperature. The initial temperature of a newborn is taken rectally to ensure patency of the rectum. Lubrication of the thermometer tip reduces friction and reduces discomfort.

ACTION

RATIONALE

the reading is complete. Keep one hand on the thermometer and the other on the child's legs so that sudden motion will not break or dislodge the thermometer (Fig. 117-2). After the rectal reading is taken, clean any excess lubricant off the child's buttocks.

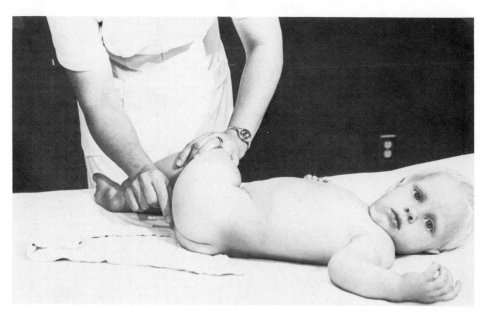

Figure 117.2

4. *Axillary* temperature is taken for most children under the age of 6 years. Dry the child's axilla. Hold the thermometer in the child's axilla for 7 to 10 minutes (Fig. 117-3). Hold the electronic probe in the axilla until the unit signals that the reading is complete.

The axillary route does not stimulate the reflex to empty the bowels. Since the axilla is not mucous membrane, it requires longer to obtain an accurate measurement. Children under the age of 6 years have difficulty holding the thermometer successfully under their tongues.

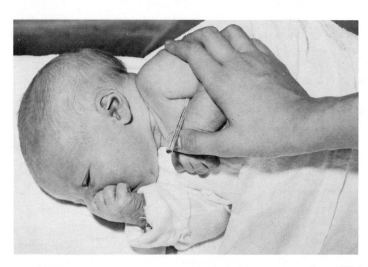

Figure 117.3

ACTION	*RATIONALE*
5. *Oral* temperature measurement is done on all children over the age of 6 years unless contraindicated. Place the thermometer under the child's tongue (Fig. 117-4). The child's lips must close around the thermometer. Leave the mercury thermometer in place for 2 to 3 minutes. Leave the electronic probe in place until the unit signals that the measurement is complete.	Oral measurement is usually the method to which most children are accustomed at home. The area under the tongue is particularly vascular and a good source of temperature measurement.

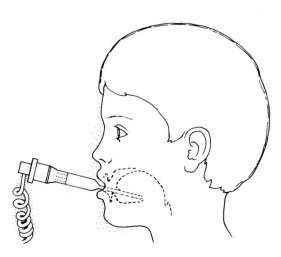

Figure 117.4

6. Read the mercury thermometer at eye level with the thermometer held horizontally.	The mercury in the thermometer expands when heated. The heat source is the body temperature as reflected by the vascular area in which the thermometer has been located.
7. Replace the glass thermometer in its proper place in soaking solution. Discard the sheath from the electronic probe in a waste receptacle.	The normal flora present in the rectum and in the mouth may proliferate and be cross-transmitted if not exposed to antibacterial solution.

Communicative Aspects

OBSERVATIONS

1. Measure the pulse and respiratory rates each time the temperature or blood pressure is taken to assist in the assessment of the child's total status.

2. Carefully observe the rhythm, tension, and volume, as well as the rate, when measuring pulse and respirations, to detect signs of irregularity or complications.

3. Never leave the child unattended during temperature measurement. Observe carefully to ensure the prevention of accidents.

4. Listen for abnormal respiratory sounds such as wheezing, expiratory grunts, fluid, or any sounds that might indicate that the child is having difficulty with adequate oxygen/carbon dioxide exchange. Observe the rise and fall of

the chest and/or abdomen. Determine if the child is using pectoral muscles, abdominal muscles, or other musculature in order to breathe. Observe the child's coloring. Determine if the lips are cyanotic and if the nailbeds are blanched. Observe for flaring of the nostrils, gasping, and anxiety, which might indicate that inadequate gaseous exchange is occurring.

CHARTING

1. Note the temperature, pulse, respirations, and blood pressure on the child's chart and any other unit worksheets or printouts where this information is compiled.

2. Record observations of vital signs in the nurses' notes, when appropriate, to complement nursing interventions and to provide ongoing assessment of the child's care.

3. Record the temperature and method used to measure it.

4. In measuring the pulse, record the following: rate, rhythm, strength, and activity of the child.

5. In measuring the respirations, note the following: quality of respirations, rate, and depth.

6. In taking the blood pressure reading, record the following: systolic reading, diastolic reading, pulse pressure (if applicable), location of cuff, method used (e.g., flushing), and activity of the child.

DATE/TIME	OBSERVATIONS	SIGNATURE
3/7 0800	Pulse appears rapid and thready. Rate 136. Resp. shallow and dyspneic. Rate 36. B/P 120/94. Crying and apprehensive. Dr. J. notified. Mother in attendance. Assured that nurse will remain with child until Dr. J. arrives. ——	P. Sanchez RN

Discharge Planning Aspects

CLIENT AND FAMILY EDUCATION

1. Explain to the parents the proper methods for taking vital signs at home. Explain temperature measurement. Caution the parents about the indiscriminate use of over-the-counter medications for temperature control. Severe complications have been found to occur with the treatment of fever in certain viral conditions. Some physicians feel that fever is the body's natural means of combating infection and should not be treated unless it is in the dangerously high range. Encourage the parents to contact their physician before giving their child any medication for fever.

2. Reassure the parents that the pulse, respirations, and blood pressure may vary greatly if the child is excited, apprehensive, or uncomfortable.

Evaluation

Quality Assurance

Documentation should include a progressive chart showing vital signs throughout hospitalization. This may be in graphic form or computerized chart form. It should be possible to trace the child's temperature, for instance, from admission to discharge. Deviations from the child's normal vital-signs readings should be noted, and explained, if possible, in the nurses' progress notes. Medication that might alter the vital signs should reflect the time administered, the vital signs before the medication was administered, and evidence that the vital signs were monitored after the medication was administered. The chart should reflect that the nurse knew and understood the significance of normal and abnormal vital-signs measurements and reported significant findings to the proper person.

Infection Control

1. Proper cleaning of equipment will retard the spread of infection. The earpieces and bell of the stethoscope should be cleaned with a distinfectant. Thermometers should be cleaned with a disinfectant between uses. If an electronic thermometer is used, the plastic sheaths used to cover the probe should be disposed of properly in a receptacle that is inaccessible to young clients. Equipment that is used for consecutive clients should be cleaned and disinfected between uses.

2. Thorough handwashing should precede and follow the taking of vital signs.

Technique Checklist

	YES	NO
Techiques explained to parents	_____	_____
Techniques explained to child	_____	_____
Blood pressure		
Arm measurement left _____ right _____		
Leg measurement left _____ right _____		
Pulse measured		
Apical	_____	_____
Radial	_____	_____
Brachial	_____	_____
Other _____		
Respirations measured		
Abnormalites _____		
Temperature measured		
Rectal _____		
Axillary _____		
Oral _____		
Mercurial thermometer _____		
Electronic thermometer _____		
Hands washed before and after procedure	_____	_____
Vital signs recorded on chart	_____	_____

Unit Four

Techniques for Obstetric Clients

118

Admission to the Labor Room

Overview

Definition

Activities that are performed during an expectant mother's entry into the hospital in preparation for the delivery of her baby

Rationale

Gather data regarding the pregnancy as a basis for planning.

Provide comprehensive assessment of the present status of the mother and fetus.

Provide individualized care for the mother and family.

Prepare the client and partner for the delivery process.

Monitor the progress of labor.

Prevent the spread of infection and cross-contamination.

Terminology

Acceleration: An increase in the fetal heart rate in response to uterine contractions

Amniocentesis: The introduction of a needle into the uterine cavity through the abdominal wall to withdraw a sample of amniotic fluid

Antepartal care: Refers to any health care given to the pregnant woman during the course of her pregnancy in preparation for a successful birth

Cesarean section: The removal of a fetus through an abdominal incision into the uterus

Crowning: A situation in which the head of the infant has progressed so far that its widest diameter is encircled by the vaginal opening; this is an indication that the infant will be delivered soon.

Deceleration: A decrease in the fetal heart rate in response to uterine contractions

Dorsal (supine) position: A position in which the client lies on the back with knees flexed and separated

External fetal monitor: A method used to provide a visual and audible record of the heart rate of an infant in the uterus by means of an electrical machine; used to keep a constant record of the fetal heart rate (FHR) during labor

False labor: Contractions, known as Braxton–Hicks contractions, that are actually an irregular tightening and relaxing of the uterine muscle with no accompanying dilatation or effacement of the cervix

Internal fetal monitoring: A method used to detect and display the FHR or the maternal contractions through an electrode placed into the scalp of the fetus while still in the uterus. Insertion is accomplished through an internal catheter inserted vaginally.

Lithotomy position: A position in which the client lies on the back with the knees separated and flexed on the abdomen or supported in stirrups

Perineum: The area between the vagina and the rectum in the female

Pregnancy-induced–hypertension (PIH): A condition unique to pregnant women in which the blood pressure becomes elevated and edema and albuminuria occur. This condition is among the leading causes of maternal and fetal deaths each year.

Stillborn: Any product of conception born dead that is 20 wks or more gestational age, 26 cm or more in length, more than 500 g in weight, or a combination of the latter two criteria regardless of gestational age. These parameters may vary from state to state.

Vulva: The external genitalia of the female, including the lower pubis to the perineum

Assessment

Pertinent Anatomy and Physiology

Pathophysiological Concepts

See Appendix I: *pregnancy*.

1. One of the signs of approaching labor is rupture of the amniotic sac. One danger associated with early rupture of the membranes is a prolapsed cord. In the case of a prolapsed cord, a portion of the umbilical cord is swept downward with the force of the released amniotic fluid. The cord may or may not emerge through the vagina. The descending infant may put pressure on the cord, thus cutting off fetal circulation. If this condition is not corrected, the infant may die from anoxia.

2. Another danger of premature rupture of membranes is infection. The enclosed membranes surrounding the fetus provide an impenetrable environment that protects the fetus from infection. When the sac ruptures, an avenue is provided for pathogenic organisms to infect the fetus. The longer the membranes are ruptured before birth, the greater the chance of infection.

Assessment of the Client

1. Assess the state of pregnancy. Determine if the client has had antepartal care. A complete medical and antepartal history is invaluable in assessing each client's needs and in anticipating complications. Some of the clients will have had no preparation at all; others may have attended various classes dealing with pregnancy and childbirth. If the birth is imminent, the minimal assessment should include vital signs, fetal heart tones, maternal allergies, blood type, status of membranes, previous pregnancies, physician or midwife contact, and whether the mother will keep the baby after it is born or release it for adoption. If time allows, a complete assessment will include the progress of the pregnancy and any complications. The presence of any type of infection, including venereal disease (particularly gonorrhea and herpes), should be noted. Assess the amount of weight gain and any edema. Determine if the client has been hypertensive or febrile. On the client's admission to the labor room, antepartal care in a broad sense refers to the physical, emotional, and social needs of the expectant mother and her family. The degree to which these needs have been met must be determined by the nurse in the assessment period.

2 Assess the client to determine whether labor has begun. If the client is in labor, determine the status of contractions. Assess when the contractions began and their frequency and duration. Assess any other indicators of the stage of labor, such as the discharge of pink mucus from the vagina or leaking or expulsion of the amniotic fluid.

3. Assess the status of the fetus by asking if there has been an increase or decrease in fetal activity since the onset of labor. (The entire admission procedure is an assessment process; further assessment activities will be covered in the Implementation and Interventions Section.)

4. Assess the psychosocial needs of the client and family. The psychosocial aspects of care are the extension of care beyond the physical–therapeutic realm of care. Assess the cultural background of the client and family. The nurse must have an understanding of cultural variations that influence attitudes and behavior. Recognize that all behavior is meaningful in understanding the specific needs of all ethnic groups. Assess the cultural norms relating to the father's role during the birthing process. Involve the father in making contributions that are consistent with his culturally accepted role. Consider the meaning of children in different cultures, and be nonjudgmental about parental behavior toward children. Assess the client's concept of the "mother role," which will also be based in part on the ethnic group and social class, as well as the culture of which she is a part and the socialization that has occurred in her life.

Plan

Nursing Objectives

Make the total labor process a meaningful learning experience.

Create an environment of trust and support.

Allay the fears and anxieties of the client and family by keeping them informed of the progress of labor and by offering information and reassurance.

Make an early assessment of the physical and emotional status of the client, encouraging her to express concerns and offering information to reduce anxiety.

Employ all appropriate methods to alleviate discomfort and fear.

Keep an accurate record of the observations of maternal and fetal status.

Obtain a complete obstetric history.

Client Preparation

1. Greet the client and her family in a kind and courteous manner (Fig. 118-1). Regardless of the urgency of the situation, it is imperative to present an image of competency and understanding. Admission to the labor suite will elicit a variety of responses from the client: relief that the waiting is nearly finished, fear of what lies ahead, excitement at the prospect of having a baby, and anxiety over her own helplessness in the situation. Her initial contact with the labor room personnel will have a profound and lasting effect.

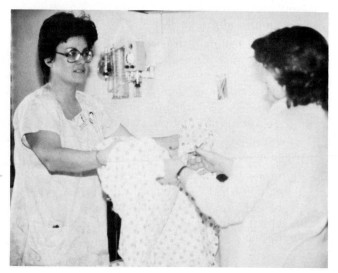

Figure 118.1

2. The family will look to the nurse to project an air of concern and expertise. Finding a person who knows what to do and who has consideration for their personal plans for the birthing process will greatly allay the anxiety of the family and will contribute to making the birthing process a pleasant and positive experience. Explain to the family members about such things as where to wait, where to get refreshments, and location of telephones and restrooms. Do this after the immediate needs of the client are met. Attention to the personal needs of the family will reinforce their part in the birthing process and may ease their anxiety.

Equipment

Labor record form and any forms required by the particular hospital

Medication and graphic record

Identification band for client and card for bed or door

Thermometer, sphygmomanometer, and stethoscope

Sterile gloves

Fetoscope or monitor

Clock (with second hand)

Prep kit (if a shave preparation is prescribed)

Enema setup, if prescribed

Bactericidal solution

Paper towels and soap

Sterile lubricant

Hospital gown

Implementation and Interventions

Procedural Aspects

ACTION	RATIONALE
1. Ascertain the status of the mother and the baby. Listen to the fetal heart tones (see Technique No. 125, Fetal Heart Tones). Measure the vital signs of the mother. Notify the physician or midwife of the client's admission.	Initially it is important to establish the state of health of the client and fetus to establish baseline measurements against which comparisons may be made during the birthing process.
2. Promote a feeling of trust by giving the appearance of competence and capability. Never appear rushed or anxious. Make eye contact with the client and spouse and provide feedback and information. Use "touch" in a soothing and appropriate manner.	During the admission process, it is the nurse who is perceived by the family as the expert who can handle the situation. They look to the nurse for information and security. The demeanor of the nurse must project confidence and competence.
3. Perform a vaginal examination (see Technique No. 127, Labor and Delivery, Nursing Care During) unless the client is bleeding or is in premature labor.	The vaginal examination provides a more precise indication of the progress of labor.

ACTION

4. Give the client's valuables to the family or secure them in the manner consistent with hospital policy. Secure clothing in a bag and label with the client's name and room number. Ask the client to remove any prosthetic devices, such as contact lenses or partial plates. These should be given to the family, placed with the client's belongings, or secured according to hospital policy. Document the dispersal of any personal items belonging to the client.

RATIONALE

The safety of the client's personal items should be ensured so that full attention can be given to the birth of the baby.

Communicative Aspects

OBSERVATIONS

1. Observe for signs of maternal distress:

   Sudden change in blood pressure

   Elevated temperature or pulse

   Continued sustained contraction with no relaxation phase

   Continuous extreme abdominal pain unrelated to contractions

   Extreme emotional distress

2. Observe for signs of fetal distress:

   Persistant fetal tachycardia

   Severe variable decelerations or late decelerations

   Passage of meconium (unless the infant is in the breech position)

   Prolapsed cord

   Bright red, frank bleeding

   Irregular fetal heart rate

   Fetal hyperactivity

3. Observe the status of the labor process by assessing the contractions, vital signs, and maternal responses.

4. Crowning is an indication that birth is imminent; take the client to the delivery room at once.

CHARTING

DATE/TIME	OBSERVATIONS	SIGNATURE
5/1 1330	Admitted to labor room No. 12, 24-year-old female, para i, grav ii, admitted in active labor with spontaneous rupture of membranes at 10 AM today. Dilated 6 cm, effacement 100%. B/P 128/82, P 78, R 14, T 99.2° F orally. Mrs. R, Certified Nurse Midwife, here. Rings given to husband. Contractions q3min., 45- to 60-sec duration. Husband in attendance; coaching wife with breathing technique. FHR 124 with acceleration to 130 during contractions. Client maintaining breathing posture and relaxation techniques without difficulty. Nurse in attendance. ————————————————————	D. Perez RN

Discharge Planning Aspects

CLIENT AND FAMILY EDUCATION

1. Teach or reinforce breathing techniques used during the different stages of labor. Explain when to breathe evenly and regularly (during the first stage of labor), more rapidly (during transition), and when to bear down (during the second stage of labor). Additional explanations and reassurance will be needed during the birthing process.

2. Use visual aids to explain the physiology of labor to the unprepared client or the prepared client who may need reiteration and clarification (Fig. 118-2). Give explanations consistent with the client's desire to know and ability to understand and assimilate the information.

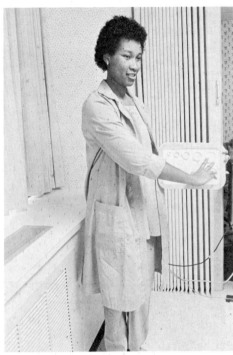

Figure 118.2

3. Assist the partner in coaching and helping the client through labor. Explain about assistance with breathing, rubbing the client's back, and physical reassurance of nearness and support.

Evaluation

Quality Assurance

Documentation of the admission process should include an assessment of the client and the status of the fetus. Baseline measurements should be recorded. The condition of the client should be noted along with evidence that suspected or possible complications were assessed and reported. Inclusion of the family in the admission process should be reflected. Disposition of personal articles should be documented along with names if they were given to family members. Procedures done during the admission process should be noted with results. The status of the membranes and degree of dilatation and effacement should be noted. If vaginal examination could not be performed, the reason should be noted. The duration and intensity of contractions should be noted.

Infection Control

1. Scrupulous handwashing must precede any care given to the client newly admitted into the labor and delivery suite.
2. If the membranes have ruptured, the chance for infection is intensified. All vaginal procedures are performed using sterile technique. After the membranes are ruptured, vaginal examinations are kept to a minimum. Care must be taken not to introduce microorganisms into the birth canal during the admitting process.

Technique Checklist

	YES	NO
Client accompanied by _____		
_____		
Status of pregnant client noted on chart	_____	_____
Membranes ruptured	_____	_____
Pink, mucous discharge	_____	_____
Contractions, frequency and duration _____		
Dilatation _____		
Effacement _____		
Vital signs		
T _____		
P _____		
R _____		
B/P _____		
Fetal heart tones _____		
Antepartum record available	_____	_____
Client had antepartal care	_____	_____
Prenatal classes	_____	_____
Lamaze classes	_____	_____
Other _____		
Other pregnancies _____		
Outcomes _____		
Dispersal of personal belongings documented in chart	_____	_____
Client reassured and comfortable	_____	_____

119   Amniocentesis

Overview

Definition

A procedure in which a needle is inserted through the abdominal and uterine walls into the amniotic fluid for the withdrawal of a fluid specimen

Rationale

Allow early prenatal detection, clinical diagnosis, and evaluation of genetic or acquired disorders and abnormalities.

Assess fetal maturity.

Relieve hydramnios.

Monitor isoimmune disease in clients.

Terminology

Amnion: Of the two fetal membranes, the innermost, which forms a sac and contains the fetus and amniotic fluid

Amniotic fluid: The liquid surrounding the fetus in the inner membrane

Assessment

Pertinent Anatomy and Physiology

1. See Appendix I: *pregnancy.*
2. The amniotic fluid is present from the second week of embryonic development. This fluid surrounds the embryo and then the fetus as it develops. The fluid, which is 98% water, is constantly replaced during the pregnancy. By the end of the pregnancy, the usual amount of amniotic fluid is 850 ml. The source of the fluid is unknown. It provides nutrients and protection for the developing baby. It protects the infant from injury by forming a cushion and by maintaining an equal pressure in fetal environment. Amniotic fluid also keeps the temperature stable and protects the fetal environment against bacterial invasion.

Pathophysiological Concepts

Hydramnios is the presence of an excessive amount of amniotic fluid. The normal amount of fluid is between 500 ml and 1000 ml. When the amount exceeds 3000 ml, hydramnios is considered significant. Hydramnios often is associated with fetal malformations and with maternal conditions such as diabetes and severe erythroblastosis. Amniocentesis as a treatment for hydramnios is controversial. Although the removal of 500 ml to 700 ml does provide temporary relief, it has been associated with premature labor.

Assessment of the Client

1. Assess the knowledge level of the client regarding what is involved and why the amniocentesis is being done. Determine if the client and family understand the procedure and its associated risks. Determine any questions that may arise, and answer them honestly or refer to the appropriate person.
2. Assess the ability of the client to lie in the supine position for the required period. Actual amniocentesis takes only about 5 minutes; however, with the preparation activities, the client may have to lie on her back for a long enough time to become uncomfortable from the weight of the fetus.

3. Assess fetal heart tones (FHT) before and immediately after the amniocentesis. If the amniotic fluid is an unusual color, more frequent monitoring of the FHT may be indicated. If blood is aspirated from the amniocentesis, it is imperative to check the FHT and to monitor them carefully by fetal heart monitor or by auscultation every 5 minutes for several hours or until fetal stability is indicated.

Plan

Nursing Objectives

Inform the client and family of the purpose of the examination and the procedure to be followed.

Provide emotional support before, during, and after the procedure.

Monitor the client's physical condition during the procedure to detect signs of complications.

Assist as needed during the procedure.

Client Preparation

1. Thoroughly explain the procedure to the client in terms that are understandable and meaningful to the client. Include the spouse and any other interested family members. Some states require written consent before amniocentesis is performed.

2. An ultrasound assessment of the fetus usually is done before amniocentesis to determine placental localization, fetal lie, and location of pockets of amniotic fluid.

3. Ask the client to empty her bladder before amniocentesis. A full bladder may displace the uterus somewhat and also increases the danger of penetration of the bladder.

4. Check the client's vital signs before amniocentesis; also measure the FHT before the procedure.

5. Assist the client into a comfortable position. It will be necessary that she be supine, but slight elevation of the head may be possible depending on the position of the fetus. Ask the client to change into a hospital gown to protect her clothing.

6. Supply a cool cloth for the client's head and keep an emesis basin nearby. Lying for extended periods in the supine position may cause postural hypotension owing to the pressure of the fetus on the abdominal vessels. It is not unusual for the client to feel faint, dizzy, clammy, and nauseated.

Equipment

Amniocentesis tray containing needles, syringes, sterile towels, and other equipment according to the particular hospital's procedure

Local anesthetic (as desired by physician)

Needles and syringes

Surgical preparation solution for skin cleansing

Sterile gloves

Sterile adhesive strip

Small brown bag or other light-excluding container if bilirubin is to be measured

Labels for tubes

For amniocentesis done for hydramnios, additional equipment:

Extra 20-ml syringes (about ten)

Sterile saline

Sterile basin

Measuring container

Implementation and Interventions

Procedural Aspects

ACTION	*RATIONALE*
1. Assist in determination of the position of the fetus. A conductive substance, such as mineral oil, is placed on the client's abdomen. Ultrasound radiography then is accomplished.	Ultrasound radiography will show the position of the fetus, the placenta, and the location of pools of amniotic fluid.
2. Cleanse and disinfect the client's abdomen by performing a surgical scrub with an antiseptic solution.	Because the needle is introduced directly into the protected fetal environment, care must be taken not to contaminate this environment with pathogenic microorganisms found on the skin.
3. The puncture site is injected with a local anesthetic. A needle then is introduced through the skin and into the pool of amniotic fluid. The desired amount is withdrawn (Fig. 119-1).	The local anesthetic reduces the discomfort during needle insertion. The needle can be inserted into the previously identified pool of fluid.

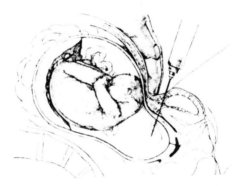

Figure 119.1

4. The specimens should be clearly labeled and sent to the laboratory for analysis. If the bilirubin level is to be determined, the specimens must not be exposed to light. Transport the specimens to the laboratory at once.	Labeling prevents errors in reporting of test results. Sunlight decomposes the bilirubin and alters the test results.
5. Check the FHT as soon as the procedure is completed. Allow the client to turn to her side to restore normal circulation before arising.	There is a small chance that the fetus could be injured during amniocentesis. Assessment of FHT will provide an indication of fetal status. Lying in the supine position places pressure on the abdominal vessels and may cause dizziness in the pregnant woman. This pressure is relieved by turning to the side.

Special Modifications

If blood was aspirated during amniocentesis, it should be sent to the laboratory at once for immediate analysis to determine if it is maternal or fetal blood. If it is fetal blood, continuous monitoring of the fetal status for the next 2 hours or until conditions are stable is recommended.

It is possible to puncture the fetal system during amniocentesis even though precautions have been taken to ensure the position of the fetus. Sudden movement by the fetus is always possible. The possibility of fetal distress must be eliminated before monitoring is discontinued.

Communicative Aspects

OBSERVATIONS

1. Monitor the vital signs of the mother and the FHT of the fetus before and after the procedure. Compare these with baseline measurements to assess deviations. The FHT are monitored until stable after the procedure, usually for a period of 1 hour. This may be done by electrical fetal monitoring or by auscultation every 15 minutes.

2. Observe for signs of premature or approaching labor as evidenced by vaginal mucus discharge, rupture of membranes, or contractions.

3. Watch closely for bleeding from the vagina. Observe for leaking of amniotic fluid.

CHARTING

DATE/TIME	OBSERVATIONS	SIGNATURE
9/10 0910	Amniocentesis performed by Dr. K. Complete explanation given to client and her husband. Both state that they understand and are anxious for the test. Fetal position determined by sonogram. 30 ml clear fluid withdrawn, labeled, and sent to the laboratory for examination. B/P 120/60, P 80, R 20, FHT 130. FHT monitored continuously for 1 hr by fetal monitor. No wide variations. No evidence of vaginal bleeding or leaking amniotic fluid. No contractions or discomfort. Was not nausated during procedure, although she did state that the pressure on her abdomen was very uncomfortable. Tolerated the procedure very well. Was turned to the right side after completion to remain for 15 min. ————————————————————	M. Brown RN
0925	Turning in bed without discomfort. FHT 136, B/P 114/58, P 76, R 16. No signs of complication from the procedure. ————————————————	M. Brown RN

Discharge Planning Aspects

CLIENT AND FAMILY EDUCATION

1. Make sure that the client and spouse understand why the amniocentesis is being performed and what the results will show. They should understand that if the test is being performed to determine the presence of a specific genetic defect, this defect may either be detected or eliminated. They are still as much at risk as the rest of the population for those birth defects that are not detectable by amniocentesis, however, such as cleft palate or mental retardation.

2. Explain to the client what will happen during the procedure and what she will feel. The feeling during removal of fluid has been described as a pulling sensation. Some cramping may occur for the several hours following amniocentesis. Explain that the preliminary examinations and radiographic studies are to ensure that the infant will be well away from the site of needle insertion. Reassure the client that every precaution will be taken to ensure the safety of her baby. There is a possibility of spontaneous abortion following amniocentesis, although the chances are very small.

3. If the client is stable and FHT remain stable, she may be discharged after the amniocentesis. She may experience slight cramping for the next 5 or 6 hours. It generally is considered appropriate for the woman to resume her normal activities. However, any bleeding, severe cramping, or leaking of amniotic fluid should be reported to her physician at once.

REFERRALS

It may be in the best interest of the client and her spouse to refer them for genetic counseling if abnormalities are discovered by the amniocentesis. Referral to family planning counselors also may be indicated.

Evaluation

Quality Assurance

Documentation should include a description of the preparations and any teaching that was done. An assessment of the client's understanding of the procedure should be noted. Amount of fluid withdrawn and its disposition should be reflected. The monitoring of the client and fetal vital signs after the procedure should be documented in the chart. Any measures to promote comfort should be noted with an assessment of their effectiveness. The nurse should show evidence that the possible complications following amniocentesis were understood and monitored. Measures to prevent or report complications should be noted. Any discharge instructions should be reflected in the chart.

Infection Control

1. Careful handwashing should precede any measures to prepare the client for amniocentesis. Thorough handwashing should be done after amniocentesis.

2. Amniocentesis is an invasive procedure providing access to the protective environment of the fetus. Penetration of this closed environment provides an avenue for invasion by pathogenic microorganisms. The skin harbors normal flora that may infect the infant if allowed to penetrate the fetal environment. A surgical skin preparation therefore should precede amniocentesis. The entire procedure is carried out using sterile technique. The bandage placed over the puncture site also should be sterile.

3. Equipment that will be used for subsequent clients should be returned for complete cleaning and sterilization before being reused. Disposable equipment should be disposed of in a manner that is consistent with hospital policy. Care to protect staff against needle stick is important and may be facilitated by proper labeling of recyclable equipment.

Technique Checklist

	YES	NO
Procedure explained to client and spouse	_____	_____
Reason for amniocentesis		
Genetic testing	_____	_____
Maturity testing	_____	_____
Hydramnios	_____	_____
Other _____		
Maternal vital signs checked		
Before procedure	_____	_____
After procedure	_____	_____
FHT checked		
Before procedure	_____	_____
After procedure	_____	_____
Frequency and duration _____		
Amount of fluid aspirated _____		

	YES	NO
Specimens labeled	_____	_____
Specimens to laboratory	_____	_____
How transported _____		
Complications _____		
Client discharged from hospital	_____	_____
Discharge instructions given	_____	_____
Client to remain in hospital	_____	_____
Interpretation of tests given	_____	_____

120   Amniotomy

Overview

Definition

Artificial rupture of the membranous sac surrounding the fetus and amniotic fluid

Rationale

Augment the labor process.

Terminology

Amnion: Inner membrane

Amniotic fluid: The approximately 800 ml to 1000 ml of fluid surrounding the fetus at term

Chorion: Outer membrane

Complete rupture of membranes: Penetration of both the chorion and amnion, with emptying of the amniotic fluid

Sepsis: The presence of pathogenic microorganisms or their toxins in the blood or other tissues

Assessment

Pertinent Anatomy and Physiology

1. See Appendix I: *labor and delivery.*
2. Amniotic fluid is the opaque fluid that surrounds the embryo from the second week of life until birth. The source of amniotic fluid is not known nor is the route of reabsorption understood. During pregnancy, the fetus swallows the fluid and excretes urine. The amniotic fluid is replaced continuously. The fluid is 98% water, with the remainder of the substance being electrolytes, glucose, proteins, lipids, enzymes, and hormones. As the pregnancy progresses, the fluid contains waste products from the fetus in increasing amounts. The amniotic fluid serves to cushion the fetus and to maintain temperature. It also facilitates fetal movement within the uterus. The fluid may act as a dilating force during labor as the fetus descends into the birth canal.
3. Labor usually begins within 12 hours after the membranes are ruptured.

Pathophysiological Concepts

Production of too much amniotic fluid is called *hydramnios.* Too little amniotic fluid is *oligohydramnios.* Both of these conditions often are associated with congenital abnormalities.

Assessment of the Client

1. Assess the client's stage of labor. The physician or midwife will make the decision about when to rupture the membranes based on the progress of the labor and the condition of the mother and baby.
2. Assess the fetal heart tones (FHT) before and after amniotomy. Assess the vital signs of the mother.
3. If the client is unsure about whether the membranes have ruptured, assess the acidity or alkalinity of fluid found in the vaginal tract by using Nitrazine tape. The tape may be placed into pooled secretions within the vaginal canal, which are apparent during examination with a speculum. If no fluid is present, a sterile cotten swab may be inserted into the cervical os and then

placed against a strip of Nitrazine tape. An alkaline reaction (tape will turn blue, blue green, or blue gray) indicates that the liquid is amniotic fluid. If the tape remains yellow, the secretions are probably urine or normal vaginal secretions that elicit an acidic reaction. The Nitrazine test is not useful in the presence of blood because blood is alkaline. Thus, a false-positive test result will occur.

Plan

Nursing Objectives

Ensure sterile techniques and prevention of infection.

Monitor the status of the fetus before and after amniotomy.

Allay the concerns of the client and family by explanations and reassurance.

Client Preparation

1. Explain to the client and family exactly what will happen during amniotomy and why it is done (Fig. 120-1). When the presenting part is already in place low in the pelvis and other conditions are right, amniotomy may be performed to hasten the onset of labor. Answer any questions honestly and in language that the client can understand. Explain that the client may have to remain in bed after the membranes are ruptured, although she may turn from side to side.

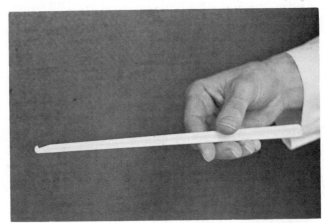

Figure 120.1

2. Measure the FHT immediately before the membranes are ruptured.
3. Have the client void before membrane rupture.
4. For the practitioner to rupture the membranes, the cervix must be accessible. Place the client in the lithotomy position and clean the vulva with an antiseptic solution. Provide an amniohook or sterile forceps.

Equipment

Antiseptic cleansing solution

Amniohook, sterile forceps, or whatever the practitioner prefers for breaking the amniotic sac

Sterile gloves

Lubricant

Fetoscope

Implementation and Interventions

Procedural Aspects

ACTION

1. Remain with the client and provide emotional support during amniotomy.

2. The membranes will be quite tense and are easily ruptured by nicking the sac with the forceps or hook. The procedure must be performed under sterile conditions and between contractions. Measure the FHT immediately after amniotomy to assess the status of the fetus and again after the first contraction after the amniotomy.

3. Give perineal care by drying the perineum with a sterile pad. Change the pad under the client. Determine if the client will be confined to bed after amniotomy.

4. Check the client's temperature every 2 hours after rupture of the membranes.

RATIONALE

Reassurance is need to calm the client and to gain her cooperation during the labor and delivery process.

The FHT is indicative of the status of the fetus. Complications resulting from amniotomy may be detectable by heart rate changes.

Leaving the client clean and dry increases her comfort. If the fetal head is well engaged and dilatation is less than 5 cm, the client may be allowed out of bed.

After the membranes are ruptured, the chance of infection is increased.

Communicative Aspects

OBSERVATIONS

1. Observe the color and odor of the amniotic fluid. Dark fluid may indicate meconium, which is not normal unless the presentation is breech. Blood in the amniotic fluid indicates the need for close observation. The obstetric care provider should be made aware of this occurrence so that fetal condition can be monitored closely and immediate emergency measures can be taken if indicated.

2. Observe for signs of prolapsed cord or any sign of fetal distress. Frequent monitoring of FHT is indicated. After contractions start, the FHT should be monitored every 15 to 30 minutes.

3. Observe for vaginal bleeding or fluid discharge after amniotomy. Such irregularities should be reported to the person responsible for the delivery.

4. Observe the progress of labor. Note frequency and duration of contractions.

CHARTING

Chart the time, appearance of fluid, and FHT before and after amniotomy.

DATE/TIME	OBSERVATIONS	SIGNATURE
6/21 1030	Amniotomy performed by Dr. K. Clear fluid returned. FHT 136 before amniotomy, FHT 140 after amniotomy. Tolerated the procedure well without discomfort. B/P 118/66, P 72, R 22, T 97.8° F. Amniotic fluid clear. Contractions have not started. Client to remain in bed. Explanations offered and client and husband seem very receptive. Turned to right side. ————	C. Parker RN

Discharge Planning Aspects

CLIENT AND FAMILY EDUCATION

1. Explain the need for the amniotomy. Be sure that the client and family understand why it is being done and what will happen. Emphasize that there is no danger to the baby and that the labor process may be hastened by this action. Answer any questions the family and client may have.

2. Tell the client and family about progress that is made after the amniotomy. This is encouraging to the mother.

Evaluation

Quality Assurance

Document the vital signs of the mother and the FHT rates before and after amniotomy. Any explanations should be documented and the receptivity of the client and family should be assessed. Document the appearance of the amniotic fluid and any unexpected findings. Any instructions given to the client should be noted. The progress of the labor should be reflected after amniotomy. The nurse should show evidence in the documentation that complications of amniotomy were understood and appropriate preventive or communicative measures were taken.

Infection Control

1. Handwashing is essential to prevent cross-contamination of the obstetric client and the fetus.

2. Amniotomy breaks the protective barrier that has been protecting the fetus from infection during the pregnancy. Any item or material that comes in contact with the fetal environment should be sterile. The entire procedure is carried out under sterile conditions.

3. The longer the membranes are ruptured, the greater the chance for infection. After rupture, the client usually is confined to bed.

4. Equipment used for amniotomy must be cleaned and disinfected after each use.

Technique Checklist

	YES	NO
Procedure explained to client and family	___	___
FHT measured		
Before amniotomy	___	___
After amniotomy	___	___
After first contraction following amniotomy	___	___
Frequency _____		
Client vital signs documented		
Before amniotomy	___	___
After amniotomy	___	___
Frequency _____		
Amniotomy successful	___	___
Appearance of fluid documented	___	___
Sterile techniques maintained	___	___
Labor started spontaneously	___	___
Labor already in progress before amniotomy performed	___	___

121 Antepartal Care

Overview

Definition

Health care teaching, monitoring, and procedures that occur from the time of conception to the onset of labor

Rationale

Provide adequate health care services and resources as well as thorough and consistent information regarding pregnancy and the birthing process.

Ensure and maintain the health of the expectant mother and infant.

Identify high-risk situations early and manage them successfully.

Reduce infant mortality. (The infant mortality rate has been reduced significantly when adequate antepartal care is made available and used.)

Terminology

Amenorrhea: Absence of menstruation

Amniocentesis: The introduction of a needle into the uterine cavity through the abdominal wall to withdraw a sample of amniotic fluid

Antenatal: Before birth; refers to fetal care

Antepartal: Before delivery; refers to maternal care

Auscultation: Listening to sounds produced within the body

Conception: The process of becoming pregnant, involving fertilization of the ovum and implantation into the uterine lining

Embryo: Early development of the unborn human from the 2nd week until the 7th and 8th weeks of gestation, when the skeleton begins to form

Family: A unit of individuals engaged in intimate interactions in daily living patterns

Fetus: The unborn human from the 7th week of gestation until birth

First trimester: The period between the last menstrual period until the 14th week of gestation, during which the fetus begins to develop. In the mother, physical and psychological changes are observable.

Gestation: The period of development of the fetus from conception through birth

Multigravida: A woman who has had two or more pregnancies

Nulligravida: A woman who has never been pregnant

Para: Delivery of a viable fetus or a woman who has produced a viable fetus

Primigravida: A woman who is pregnant for the first time

Quickening: The first fetal movements felt by the mother

Second trimester: The period from the 15th to the 28th week after the last menstrual period, during which the uterus extends to above the umbilicus and fetal movements are evident

Third trimester: The period from the end of the 28th week of gestation until delivery, during which fetal growth is rapid

Assessment

Pertinent Anatomy and Physiology

See Appendix I: *pregnancy.*

Pathophysiological Concepts

1. Pregnancy-induced hypertension (PIH), formerly called toxemia, is a common complication of pregnancy. It is characterized by hypertension, edema, and proteinuria usually occurring after the 24th week of gestation. The cause remains uncertain. The progressive forms of PIH range from mild pre-eclampsia to severe eclampsia; however, the order of presentation of symptoms does not necessarily follow this progressive pattern. Hypertension is considered a blood pressure above 140/90, or significant elevations in blood pressure parameters over those of baseline measurements (such as a 30 mm Hg rise in systolic or a 15 mm Hg rise in diastolic readings). Because edema is a common occurrence during pregnancy, significant findings include edema of the face and hands more than edema of the feet and legs. Weight gain of more than 1 lb/wk is also significant. Protein levels in the urine exceeding 500 mg/24 hr are also indicative of preeclampsia, although this usually is a late-occurring symptom. Convulsions and coma may occur. Resolution of the pregnancy generally improves the PIH condition, although it may recur within 24 hours following delivery. Prevention revolves around adequate antepartal care and awareness of symptoms.

2. Nausea and vomiting during pregnancy are common during the first trimester. These symptoms are called "morning sickness" because they occur most often in the morning. Persistent and prolonged bouts of vomiting are called pernicious vomiting (hyperemesis gravidarum), and may cause weight loss. If hospitalization is required, the condition is treated by parenteral infusion of fluids and nutrients and gradual reintroduction of solid foods. If the condition is treated quickly and effectively, there is usually no effect on the fetus.

3. *Placenta previa* is a condition resulting when the placenta grows partially or totally in the lower segment of the uterus instead of the upper portion. The placenta may totally or partially cover the cervical os. Vaginal bleeding without cramping or pain is a sign of placenta previa. Any woman who experiences painless bleeding during the third trimester usually is hospitalized and her blood typed and cross-matched for transfusion. Vaginal and rectal examinations are not performed when placenta previa is suspected unless immediate surgical capabilities are present for cesarean section. Postpartum hemorrhage is a possibility after delivery.

4. Premature separation of the placenta (abruptio placentae) occurs when part or all of the placenta detaches from the uterine wall before the delivery process. The resulting hemorrhage may be contained within the body or may escape to the outside. Bleeding from the vagina accompanied by abdominal pain is an indication of premature separation of the placenta. When the hemorrhage is concealed within the mother's body, the situation is very critical. Symptoms included abdominal pain and cramping accompanied by tenderness and rigidity of the uterus.

5. Isoimmune disease is a condition occurring when the fetus produces a red blood cell antigen that was inherited from the father and that is absent in the mother. The mother produces antibodies against this antigen, a situation that has the effect of "rejecting" the fetal tissue. The antibodies pass through the placental barrier and destroy fetal red blood cells. Isoimmune conditions may be due to ABO and other blood groups or to Rh incompatibility. Detection and treatment must begin very early in the pregnancy by screening of blood and, if indicated, of amniotic fluid. Anti-D immunoglobulin (RhoGam)

administered within the first 72 hours after delivery, prevents Rh sensitization in Rh-negative women. (It is of no benefit to Rh-negative women who are already sensitized, however.) Subsequent pregnancies must involve careful screening and surveillance.

Assessment of the Client

Care during the entire antepartal period involves continuous assessment and reassessment. Education and counseling should be based on physical, psychological, and social assessment of the client and her family.

Plan

Nursing Objectives

Promote the successful course of a normal pregnancy by providing essential services and information.

Teach parenting skills.

Arrange early detection and treatment of maternal diseases or conditions that may affect the course of the pregnancy.

Reassure and inform the client and family members to the extent indicated by their current level of knowledge and their degree of anxiety.

Identify abnormalities and other problems that may prevent the normal progress of a pregnancy.

Establish a therapeutic relationship with the client and her family.

Assist the client to provide a satisfactory environment for the growing fetus by attention to nutrition, exercise, habits, and general health.

Client Preparation

1. If the client will undergo physical examination of the pelvis, ask her to empty her bladder to promote relaxation and comfort during the examination.

2. Explain to the client what will happen during the visit. If it is a repeat of previous examinations, ask if there are any questions or concerns. If the examination will be something new or if it is the first examination, explain to the client what will be done and why. Many women have never undergone physical examination of such a personal nature. They may be frightened or intimidated. Kindness, understanding, and a matter-of-fact attitude will help to allay their embarrassment and anxiety.

Equipment

Equipment will vary according to the test, technique, or parameter to be measured.

For initial physical examination

Vaginal speculum

Sterile gloves for vaginal examination

Clean glove for rectal examination

Uterine swab

Sterile lubricant

Sponges

Applicator(s)

Vaginal pipette with aspirator

Slides

Spatula for Pap smear and fixative

Media for cultures

Cleansing solution

Implementation and Interventions

Procedural Aspects

ACTION

1. Recognize the common symptoms and signs of early pregnancy: amenorrhea, nausea and vomiting, urinary frequency, breast sensitivity, listlessness, fatigue, quickening, leukorrhea, abdominal enlargement, skin changes, and changes in the genitals.

2. Establish a general plan of antepartal care. Visits may be set up on a schedule such as once a month until the 8th month, then every 1 or 2 weeks depending on the needs and condition of the client.

3. The initial interview process includes gathering personal data, family history, health history, and emotional assessment. (Fig. 121-1).

RATIONALE

Adequate obstetrical care should be started as soon as possible. Many women present themselves to a clinic or hospital for treatment of symptoms without realizing that they are pregnant. Recognition of the signs and symptoms of pregnancy will provide an opportunity for early antepartal care.

Antepartal visits should be scheduled so that the pregnancy can be adequately monitored without disrupting the client's normal life-style.

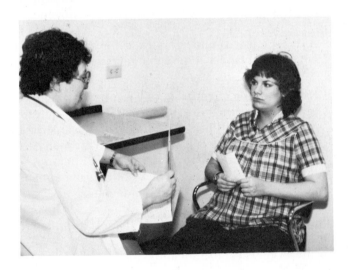

Figure 121.1

Personal data should include birthdate, occupation, education, number of children in the family, living habits, eating habits, and ethnic and cultural background.

Family history should include number of siblings, health status of family, serious illnesses, chronic diseases, hereditary diseases, familial deformities or mental illnesses, epilepsy, and multiple pregnancies.

Personal data allows the nurse to assess anticipated problems and to assist the client in meeting these problems realistically and with adequate information.

Because many birth problems and phenomena seem to reappear in families (e.g., twins), it is important to explore the family history to assess and prepare for unexpected events.

ACTION

    Health history should include childhood illnesses, operations, menstrual history, conditions relating to the body systems, obstetric history (including previous pregnancies, abortions, premature deliveries, outcomes, and problems), smoking, drug use, and current medications.

    Emotional status should include questions about feelings toward childbearing, past experience with pregnancy, plans for the infant (type of feeding, child care), future plans for self (return to school, return to job, stay at home), amount of assistance mother will have after leaving the hospital, and any anticipated problems.

4. Initial physical assessment will provide insight into current health status. Check the client's vital signs (Fig. 121-2). Measure height and weight (Fig. 121-3). Obtain a urine specimen by the clean-catch method (Fig. 121-4; see Technique No. 22, Urine Examinations, in the Adult Section) unless stipulated otherwise. A complete review of systems usually is done (see Technique No. 15, Physical Examination of the Adult). Assist the client to undress and drape for a complete examination (Fig. 121-5).

RATIONALE

Previous health problems may affect the pregnancy and will offer the nurse insight into health education deficits in developing the teaching plan.

Emotional status will affect the way in which the mother views her pregnancy and may indicate how much cooperation may reasonably be expected from her. Realistic goals may then be formulated with input from the client and the family.

Knowledge of current health status will provide a basis for teaching and formulation of goals throughout the pregnancy. Potential complications also can be identified and plans made for prevention or treatment.

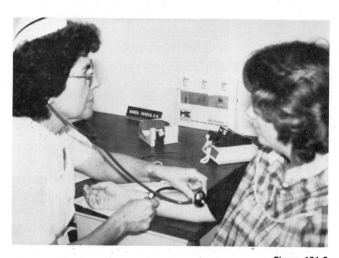

Figure 121.2

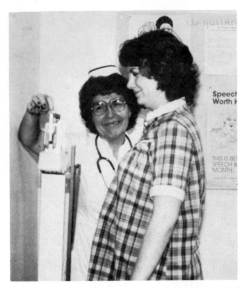

Figure 121.3

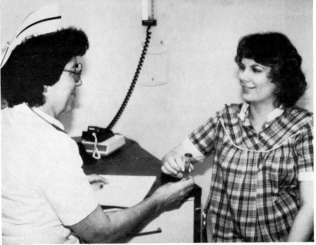

Figure 121.4

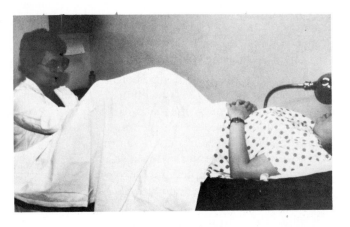

Figure 121.5

ACTION

Laboratory tests may include microscopic urinalysis, cervical smear for cancer, and cervical smear for gonorrhea. A blood specimen should be obtained for complete blood count, blood type, Rh factor, rubella antibodies, glucose level, and tests for sickle cell anemia and syphilis.

Place the client in the lithotomy position. The vaginal speculum may be warmed in a pan of warm water. Sterile lubricant may be applied to the speculum unless the client is to have a Pap smear. Instruct the client to breathe rapidly (pant), during any part of the examination which causes discomfort. The pelvic examination will reveal abnormalities of the vagina

RATIONALE

Assessment of the pelvis will indicate if the client requires evaluation for alternative birthing methods or if current pathology is present that may require attention. Shallow, rapid breathing relaxes the abdominal muscles and decreases discomfort during pelvic examination.

ACTION

(such as growths or weakness in the posterior or anterior walls), adequacy of the lower birth canal, and color and consistency of the cervix (see Technique No. 92, Vaginal Examination). Examine for height of fundus, outline of the fetus, and abnormalities of the external genitalia, anal sphincter, perineal body, and the urethral meatus.

5. Subsequent follow-up care generally includes the following nursing actions:

   Obtain data regarding vital signs, any symptoms, complications, or questions. Measure weight and ask about recent weight gains. Reinforce the overall plan for weight control. Perform a urinalysis using a specimen from the first morning voiding, which the client may be told to bring with her when she makes the appointment or from a clean-catch specimen. Check the urine for protein and glucose. Reassess the nutritional analysis and goals. Collect data about the family setting and discuss any concerns the client may have regarding the pregnancy. Review the profile of knowledge deficits, and assess the effectiveness of the teaching plan in meeting the identified needs of the client and her family. Involve the client and family in formation of goals.

6. Attention must be given to the psychosocial aspects of pregnancy. Assess the client's cultural background, which may have a profound effect on childbearing activities. When possible, include the father or significant family members in the planning and education sessions. Psychological outlook may change during the course of the pregnancy. The client's self-image may be greatly altered. Mood changes are also to be expected.

RATIONALE

Follow-up care is vital to successful antepartal care in providing monitoring of progress and clarification and reassessment of goals. It is important to establish a climate of acceptance and motivation during the initial visit. Establishing a relationship of confidence and concern may encourage the client to make and keep follow-up appointments.

Emotional support and acceptance during pregnancy is important to the client and her family. Understanding that variability in moods, tastes, and feelings is expected may relieve much of the tension and allay anxiety.

Communicative Aspects

OBSERVATIONS

1. Positive signs of pregnancy include laboratory tests showing the presence of human chorionic gonadatropin (HCG) in the urine and a fetal heartbeat, heard with a clinical stethoscope or electronically by means of fetal electro-cardiography.

2. Observe for signs of complications during the pregnancy. Be alert at each visit for unusual weight gains, blood pressure trends, edema, abnormal uterine enlargement, and distorted laboratory reports. Observe the client's emotional outlook and offer the opportunity to discuss questions and concerns.

3. Refer the client to any appropriate community agencies or classes that meet the criteria identified on the teaching plan. Community resources that might be used include prenatal classes, clinic services, Lamaze classes, and parenting classes.

CHARTING

A written plan of antepartal care should be developed in conjunction with the client and family. This plan should be shared with the family and altered to meet changing needs and expectations.

A written, ongoing record of antepartal care should be kept and made available when the client goes into labor.

Discharge Planning Aspects

CLIENT AND FAMILY EDUCATION

1. Inform the client about expected discomforts that may accompany pregnancy:

    Backache: Demonstrate the techniques for rest and relaxation; demonstrate desirable posture to minimize backache, which includes tilting the pelvis forward.

    Headaches: Discuss methods to lessen physical and emotional stress by identifying stressors and avoiding them when possible.

    Constipation: Encourage increased fluid intake, proper diet, and exercise.

    Leg cramps: Explain that these usually are caused by pressure on the nerves to the lower extremities; ensure that adequate calcium and phosphorus are consumed (milk is an excellent source of both). Loose-fitting clothing and frequent rest periods with the feet elevated are recommended.

    Nausea and vomiting: Causes may include anxiety, emotional stress, poor eating habits, altered hormone levels, and metabolic changes. Encourage eating small amounts of dry or bland foods during the day, delay breakfast if the nausea occurs in the morning, and rest before and after eating.

    Urinary frequency: Explain that this is usually due to the growth of the uterus resulting in pressure on the bladder. Encourage frequent emptying of the bladder, adequate fluid intake, withholding fluids near bedtime; relate the symptoms of bladder infection, which include burning and pain during urination and advise the client to report any such discomfort at once.

    Varicose veins: Supportive stockings may decrease the presence and severity of varicose veins.

    Swelling of the ankles and feet: Edema may be caused by sluggish venous return owing to pressure on the abdominal vessels. Advise the client to have her blood pressure checked; encourage elevation of the feet and ankles several times a day, as well as use of support hose and adequate fluid intake.

2. Inform the client about unexpected complications or problems that should be reported to the physician, midwife, or nurse practitioner at once: abdominal cramping, bleeding from the vagina with or without abdominal pain, leaking or sudden discharge of fluid from the vagina, continuous nausea and inability to keep food down, headaches, dizziness, vertigo, swelling of the hands and face, and rigidity or tightness in the abdomen.

3. Health counseling should involve the following topics:

Medications: No medications should be taken unless prescribed by the obstetric care provider. All medications, including aspirin and some of the more common self-treatment medications, can be dangerous, especially during the first trimester.

Alcohol and drugs: Excessive use of alcohol during pregnancy may result in premature delivery, fetal abnormalities, and other complications. Even occasional use of alcohol is controversial and should be discouraged. The use of any type of hallucinogenic drug, including marihuana, should be curtailed during pregnancy because the actual effect on the fetus is not fully understood. The drug-dependent mother-to-be presents a series of unique and complicated problems that will require patience and perseverance to address.

Smoking: Cigarette smoking during pregnancy has been clearly demonstrated to have a detrimental effect on the fetus, resulting in low birth weight and possibly fetal anoxia and mortality. Encourage women to stop smoking altogether or at least to cut down during pregnancy.

Clothing: Loose clothing is advised; constricting garments such as girdles, stretch pants, tight-waisted clothing, garters, and high heels should be avoided. Maternity clothing can be both comfortable and stylish. Maternity girdles may be indicated in some situations.

Exercise and physical activities: Simple exercises are encouraged because they improve circulation, enhance appetite, promote adequate bowel function, and encourage sleep. Walking is an excellent exercise. A physical exercise program patterned after the mother's prior activity regimen and present state of health is advisable.

Sexuality: Sexual desire may vary during the duration of the pregnancy. Desire may be heightened owing to release from fear of pregnancy or decreased because of fear of injuring the fetus or awkwardness from changing body size and coordination. Modifications of sexual activities during the various stages of pregnancy may be required owing to physical manifestations such as breast tenderness and increasing abdominal girth. Advise the couple that during normal pregnancy, there is no reason to prohibit sexual activity.

Personal care: Tub bathing is acceptable until the membranes rupture. Showering may be done throughout the pregnancy without problems; however, care should be taken to avoid falls from incoordination accompanying changing abdominal size. Efforts should be directed toward maintaining a positive self-concept, including exercise, breast support, nutrition, and cleanliness. Attention to dental problems is essential to prevent infections or dental caries.

4. The content of periodic instructional programs consistent with the period of gestation might include:

Developmental changes in the mother

Development of the embryo/fetus

Essential maternity care

Changes to note and report to the obstetric authority

Plans for hospitalization

Process of labor and what to expect

Postnatal period, plans and expectations

Care of the newborn

Breast care

Methods of feeding

Child growth and development

Evaluation

Quality Assurance

Each agency or hospital will have a particular form for recording the progress of the pregnancy. This form should provide evidence of ongoing assessment. Teaching should be noted, and client acceptance and understanding assessed. Tests and procedures should be noted and results portrayed graphically, when feasible, to obtain a comprehensive, progressive view of the pregnancy. Evidence should be available that complications were understood and either prevented or treated. The documentation should show evidence that the client was involved in goal-setting and reassessment. The outcome of treatments and the outcome of the pregnancy should be noted.

Infection Control

1. Handwashing between clients is essential to prevent cross-contamination.
2. All vaginal procedures performed on the pregnant client necessitate using sterile technique. Any instruments or equipment inserted into the vagina are to be sterile.
3. Equipment used for consecutive clients must be cleaned and disinfected between clients.

Technique Checklist

	YES	NO
Antepartal care explained		
To client	___	___
To family	___	___
Documentation of		
Physical examination	___	___
Health history	___	___
Psychosocial assessment	___	___
Initial assessment	___	___
Follow-up care	___	___
Frequency of visits _____		
Complications of pregnancy _____		
Documentation of observations during antepartal care	___	___
Documentation of education efforts	___	___

Breast Care

Overview

Definition

Care given to the supporting tissue, breast tissue, and nipples during pregnancy; care of the breasts after delivery of the non-nursing mother. (For care of the breasts after delivery of the nursing mother, see Technique No. 123, Breast-feeding.)

Rationale

Maintain proper support and cleanliness.

Prevent trauma and infection of the nipples and breasts.

Correct existing problems, such as inverted nipples.

Terminology

Everted: Turned outward

Inverted: Turned to the opposite of what would be normally expected

Assessment

Pertinent Anatomy and Physiology

1. See Appendix I: *breast.*
2. The breasts are covered with smooth skin, except for the pigmented areas surrounding the nipples called the areolae. The areolae become darker during pregnancy but gradually return to the lighter color after delivery. The nipples protrude from the breast tissue approximately 0.5 cm to 1 cm. The nipple is composed of erectile tissue that is permeated with openings of the milk ducts. During pregnancy the breasts also increase in size and thickness, becoming nodular and striated. The alveolar cells within the breast differentiate and become able to secrete milk. By the end of the second trimester, a small amount of the milk precursor, colostrum, is present in the breast ducts. By the end of the pregnancy, the ducts of the breast are filled with colostrum and ready to secrete milk. Hormonal changes taking place at delivery seem to initiate the secretion of milk, which begins in several days.

Pathophysiological Concepts

Mastitis (inflammation of the breast) occurs when pathogenic microorganisms invade the breast tissue through fissures in the nipple or trauma to the breast tissue. Stasis of milk or overdistension are not believed to cause infection; however, this pressure may be sufficient to traumatize the breasts, thereby allowing microorganisms to enter.

Assessment of the Client

1. Assess the condition of the breasts. Size has nothing to do with ability to breast-feed. Assess the nipples. Inverted nipples, those that recede into the breast tissue, require special attention for the client to breast-feed successfully. Assess the presence of fissures on the nipple.
2. Assess the client's dietary habits. If she does not eat a balanced diet, begin early to educate her about nutrition and successful breast-feeding.
3. Assess whether the client will breast-feed. If she will not, assess her knowledge of the importance of care of the breasts to maintain tone after delivery.

Plan

Nursing Objectives

Teach the client proper breast care.

Teach the client about expected changes in the breast tissue during pregnancy.

Prevent infection of the breast and nipple tissue.

Promote the satisfactory return of the non-nursing mother's breasts to the normal state after delivery.

Teach the technique and need for breast self-examination on a monthly basis for life.

Client Preparation

1. Special care of the breasts during pregnancy should begin with a thorough explanation of the anatomical and physiological changes occurring during pregnancy. Explain to the client the need for support and cleanliness.

2. If the mother chooses not to breast-feed her infant, she should be told to expect some discomfort for the first few days, which thereafter should be relieved and have no lasting effect on breast tissue. Explain that she may receive medication within the first few hours after delivery that will suppress lactation, or she may take oral medications for several weeks after delivery.

Equipment

Mild soap and warm water

Washcloths and towels

Well-fitted support bra

Implementation and Interventions

Procedural Aspects

ACTION	RATIONALE
Antepartal Care of the Client Who Will Breast-Feed	
1. Special care of the breasts and nipples during the antepartal period is essential in preparing to breast-feed the infant. Tell the client to do breast care daily by washing the nipples with warm water from the nipple outward. Tell her to rinse and dry the breasts. The hands should be washed before any type of breast care.	The breasts secrete colostrum early in the pregnancy. Unless this secretion is cleaned from the breasts regularly, infection may occur or the drying may result in crusts that irritate the breasts, causing cracking and a potential avenue for infection. Cross-transmission can be prevented by proper handwashing before doing breast care.
2. Advise the client to wear a good support bra during pregnancy.	The breasts become heavier and fuller during pregnancy. The hanging weight may cause strain or trauma, resulting in predisposition to mastitis.
3. Prepare the nipples for the sucking action of the infant by toughening them. This may be accomplished by rubbing them with a rough towel several times a day during the last trimester. Some practitioners advise clients to use a nipple cream.	The sucking action of the infant is traumatic to the sensitive tissue of the nipples until they become accustomed to this action. If they can be prepared before the baby is born, the transition to breast-feeding will be facilitated.

ACTION

RATIONALE

Antepartal and Postpartal Care of the Non-Nursing Client

1. Advise the client to wash her hands thoroughly before handling the breasts. Tell her to wash her breasts with warm water and soap on a washcloth, using circular motions from the nipple outward. Rinse and dry the breasts well but gently. This should be done throughout the pregnancy to prevent irritation of the breasts from colostrum secretion, which begins about the 28th week.

Pathogens on the skin and hands may cause infection in the breast tissue. A dry environment discourages bacterial growth. The presence of dried colostrum may cause cracking of the nipples or colonization of micro-organisms.

2. Non-nursing mothers may be given medications to suppress lactation. Once lactation begins, the breasts become engorged, or filled, with milk. If the milk is not removed by the sucking of the infant or by manual expression, the glands gradually will cease forming and secreting milk and lactation will be stopped. Engorgement is uncomfortable and may be painful, however. Advise the client to apply ice packs and a well-fitted, supporting bra. A mild analgesic may relieve some of the discomfort. The breasts should not be pumped for the purpose of relieving fullness in the non-nursing mother.

Palliative measures to decrease discomfort are usually successful. Heat may feel more soothing than ice packs. If the engorgement is relieved by expression of the milk either manually or by pump, the lactiferous glands will be stimulated to secrete more milk, and the problem will be compounded. A well-fitted bra is one that lifts the breasts upward and in the direction of the opposite shoulder. This serves not only to relieve discomfort, but also to encourage the breasts to return to normal muscle tone.

3. Advise the client to wear pads in the bra if the nipples leak. These pads should be changed as soon as they become soiled, however. Leaking should cease after a few weeks.

A warm, moist environment is conducive to bacterial growth.

4. Advise the client to perform breast self-examinations on a regular basis after the breasts return to normal.

The lactating breast contains nodules that make breast self-examination difficult during lactation and for several weeks thereafter.

ACTION

Special Modifications

The three types of nipples are normal (Fig. 122-1-A), flat (Fig. 122-1-B), and inverted (Fig. 122-1-C). Assist the client who wishes to breast-feed with correction of inverted nipple. Therapy to correct inversion should begin by the 5th month of pregnancy. Teach the client the following procedure: Place the thumbs close to the inverted nipple, press firmly into the breast tissue, and gradually push away from the areola (Fig. 122-2). Repeat this several times a day. Rolling the nipple very gently between the thumb and forefinger may also help to evert the nipple. Special breast shields are also available to place gentle pressure on the nipple.

RATIONALE

The infant must be able to grasp the nipple to nurse successfully. Any techniques applied to the breasts to remedy inverted nipples must be done gently, however, so that delicate breast tissue will not be traumatized.

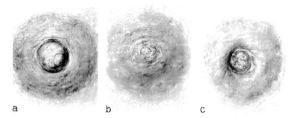

a   b   c

Figure 122.1

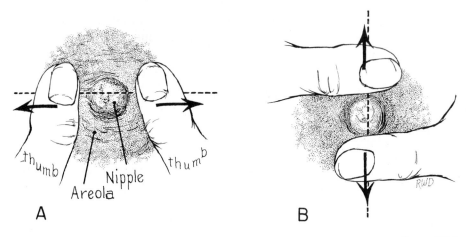

thumb   Nipple   thumb
Areola

A   B

Figure 122.2

Communicative Aspects

OBSERVATIONS

1. Observe the breasts periodically for integrity of the nipple. Cracks or fissures should be noted at once and treated by proper cleansing and prescribed medications. Determine if abnormalities of the nipple will require treatment for the client to successfully breast-feed.

2. Observe the client's bra to see that it is well supported by strong straps that both lift and support the breasts. Check to see that it is not too constricting around the chest area.

3. Observe for signs of infection such as redness or hardness of the breast.

4. Observe for secretion of colostrum.

CHARTING

DATE/TIME	OBSERVATIONS	SIGNATURE
9/12 1100	Supportive bra on at all times. Slight engorgement of both breasts with some discomfort. Ice packs to breasts while in bed. States some leaking of milk from breasts when she bottle-feeds the baby. Breasts are not reddened although they do feel firm. T 98.2° F, B/P 122/68, P 82, R 14. No cracking of nipples. States she hopes to go home tomorrow. ————————	C. Day RN

Discharge Planning Aspects

CLIENT AND FAMILY EDUCATION

1. Explain to all pregnant clients the need for a well-fitted supportive bra to protect breast tissue and promote comfort. Pads may be placed in the cup of the bra if leaking colostrum is a problem; however, stress the importance of removing these pads as soon as they become soiled to eliminate the chance of infection.

2. Advise the non-nursing mother that even with the lactation-suppressing medications, some milk will be present in the breasts. She should expect some secretion of milk from the breasts when she takes a warm shower, or perhaps when she is cuddling the infant. Secretion may also occur during sexual excitement. This secretion should not last more than a few weeks.

3. Explain palliative treatments to the non-nursing mother to relieve breast discomfort. Tell her that if the breasts become reddened and hard or feel hot to the touch, however, she should notify her obstetric care provider at once because infection may be present.

Evaluation

Quality Assurance

Documentation should include the teaching provided to the client and an assessment of her understanding and acceptance of advice offered. Any problems with the breasts should be noted along with referrals and outcomes. Techniques to correct any problems, such as inverted nipples, should be assessed for ability of client to perform the procedure and its effectiveness. Any medications for lactation suppression should be noted in the chart along with signs and symptoms relating to their effectiveness. Ongoing assessment of vital signs and comfort should be reflected. The nurse should show evidence that complications were understood and that the proper actions were taken to prevent or report them.

Infection Control

1. The breasts are susceptible to infection during the lactation process. Hands should be washed before breast care is done. The breasts should be washed from the nipple outward in an effort to decrease the amount of bacteria in the nipple area.

2. Bacteria thrive in a warm, moist environment. If the breasts leak, pads may be worn but pads and bras should be changed as often as necessary to prevent prolonged contact of the nipples with the moisture.

3. Cracks and fissures in the nipple area should be reported at once so that proper treatment can be started to prevent infection of the breast (mastitis) and possible abscess.

Technique Checklist

	YES	NO
Physiological changes of the breast during pregnancy explained to client	_____	_____
Proper technique for cleaning the breast explained	_____	_____
Pregnant client who will breast-feed advised of and checked for		
Condition of nipples	_____	_____
Normal _____		
Flat _____		
Inverted _____ Treatment _____		
Need for well-fitted support bra	_____	_____
Non-nursing mother advised of and checked for		
Need for well-fitting support bra	_____	_____
Engorgement of breasts	_____	_____
Application of ice (or heat) to prevent discomfort	_____	_____
Proper cleansing technique	_____	_____
Effectiveness of lactation-suppressing medication	_____	_____
Knowledge of breast self-examination technique	_____	_____

123 Breast-Feeding

Overview

Definition

Feeding the infant from the lactating breasts

Rationale

Provide the natural form of nourishment for the infant.

Facilitate involution of the uterus.

Foster a close mother-child relationshp.

Terminology

Lactation: Secretion of milk

Lactogenesis: The formation of milk within the breast

Assessment

Pertinent Anatomy and Physiology

1. See Appendix I: *breast.* (See also Technique No. 122, Breast Care.)
2. The thin, yellowish fluid filling the alveoli, ducts, and ampullae of the breasts is called *colostrum.* Colostrum is replaced by milk several days after birth. The nature of the milk changes through the first week from a watery substance to mature milk. Lactogenesis, or the formation of milk, is promoted by the infant's sucking and by emptying of the breasts. With complete emptying of the breasts, the milk flows more freely and copiously in subsequent feedings. The initial filling of the breast, known as the breast milk "coming in," may produce engorgement (fullness) and discomfort. After several days, congestion disappears. Fullness then is produced in response to the infant's needs and is relieved by the infant's feeding.

Pathophysiological Concepts

1. See Technique No. 122, Breast Care.
2. Breast infections may occur at any time during lactation but are most common during the first month. Symptoms include chills and fever accompanied by pain and redness in the breast, which feels hard to touch. Treatment must be started quickly to avoid abscess formation and progressive systemic effects. Antibiotic treatment generally is used to curtail the infection while ice packs and a supportive bra may relieve some of the discomfort. Authorities' opinions are divided about the advisability of continuing breast-feeding during mastitis. If breast-feeding is continued, the milk from the affected breast is manually or electronically expressed and discarded until the infection is under control. Breast-feeding usually can be restarted in 2 or 3 days.

Assessment of the Client

1. Assess the condition of the client's nipples to make sure that the infant is able to grasp the nipple and surrounding tissue in the mouth satisfactorily for successful sucking.
2. Assess the physical and emotional condition of the client because both of these may have a direct effect on lactation. Assess the motives for breast-feeding and reinforce the positive aspects of this method of feeding.
3. Assess the condition of the baby. A small or premature baby tends to tire easily and may become tired before receiving the desired or needed amount of milk.

4. Assess the client for engorgement of the breasts. Engorgement refers to excessive fullness of the breasts from buildup of milk, resulting in discomfort and possibly pain. The skin may appear shiny and the breasts feel hard to touch. Venous distention may be present, and the mother may relate that she feels a throbbing pain in her breasts.

Plan

Nursing Objectives

Assist the mother to see that the infant's nutritional needs are being met.

Assist the mother in becoming skillful and relaxed in nursing her infant.

Maintain the comfort of the mother and the safety of the infant during feeding.

Teach proper breast care.

Client Preparation

1. Make sure that the mother and infant are stable before the first feeding is offered. Vital signs should be within normal range. The infant's condition should be stabilized. Often the infant is put to breast immediately after birth if the birth was normal and there are no complications. Sometimes a small amount of sterile water is given by bottle before the initial feeding to assess the patency of the esophagus and the baby's ability to suck successfully.

2. Assist the mother into a comfortable position. Sitting erect usually is preferred. In the sitting position, the feet should be supported. A pillow may be used to support the infant (Fig. 123-1). If the mother remains in bed to nurse the infant, advise her to lie on her right side with the infant cradled in her right arm and allow the infant to nurse the right breast. When she wishes to nurse the infant at the left breast, she should turn to that side (Fig. 123-2).

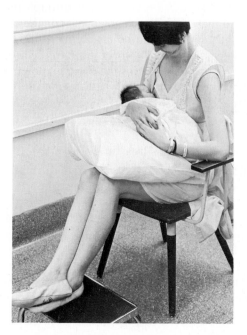

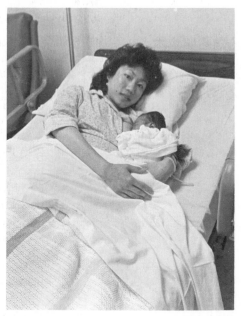

Figure 123.2

Figure 123.1

3. Offer encouragement and support of the nursing mother. If this is her first attempt at nursing her baby, it is especially important to have a positive attitude.

Equipment	Pillow
	Footstool
	Nursing bra and nursing pads
	Breast pump (if needed)

Implementation and Interventions

Procedural Aspects

	ACTION	**RATIONALE**
	1. With the mother in a comfortable position, assist her to position the infant. The infant's body may be supported with a pillow. The infant's mouth should be at the level of the breast so that the entire nipple and areola can be taken into the mouth. The infant's trunk should be lower than the head. Assist her with positioning so that the infant's abdomen is against the mother's abdomen.	The infant may be supported by the pillow but still should be cuddled in the mother's arms. The trunk is kept at a lower level than the head to prevent choking because gravity is used to facilitate swallowing of the milk by the baby.
	2. Assist the mother with the first feeding. Position the infant. If the nipple is flat or smooth because of fullness in the breast, tell the mother to gently compress the areola around the nipple with her thumb and forefinger or lightly massage around the nipple to make it stand up so the baby can grasp it. A brushing against the infant's cheek usually will stimulate the rooting reflex, which causes the infant to turn toward the stimulation with mouth open. As the infant nurses, observe for adequacy and proper positioning. Offer encouragement and reassurance if the infant does not suck well. Sometimes it is several weeks before the infant nurses satisfactorily.	To nurse, the infant must be able to grasp the nipple in the mouth. Stimulation usually will cause the nipple to project satisfactorily, enough for the infant to grasp. The sucking action of infants varies and may be unsatisfactory at first. The mother will require encouragement and reassurance to persevere in nursing attempts.
	3. Caution the mother that initial nursing efforts may cause some soreness of the nipples. The first breast-feeding times should be about 3 to 5 minutes at each breast. This will increase gradually to 15 to 20 minutes. Initially, the infant should be allowed to nurse at both breasts for each feeding; later the mother may choose to alternate breasts.	The soreness from initial nursing efforts will decrease as the nipples become toughened. If the infant is nursed at both breasts during each feeding for the first few feedings, nipple soreness may be reduced or prevented.

ACTION

RATIONALE

4. Observe subsequent feedings and be available to answer questions. Watch to see that the infant takes the nipple and surrounding tissue into the mouth. When the mother feels like sitting up to nurse, she may find that the infant can nurse more satisfactorily and she will be more comfortable.

The nursing mother needs continual reassurance and encouragement.

5. To remove the infant from the breast, advise the mother to depress the areola near one side of the infant's mouth. When the suction is broken, the nipple may be pulled out of the infant's grasp. If the nipple is pulled out without releasing the suction, trauma to the nipple and soreness may result.

Depression of the areola allows air to enter the infant's mouth, releasing the suction.

Special Modifications

1. If the breasts become engorged and the infant is unable to grasp the nipple, advise the mother to apply warm towels to the breast for 20 minutes before feeding time. Priming the breast with a breast pump may stimulate the milk flow. Encourage the mother to be patient and to keep trying.

Warmth may relax the tension enough to allow the infant to be able to grasp the nipple. Tension adds to the problem and should be prevented if possible.

2. If one or both nipples become cracked or sore, a nipple shield may prevent further trauma and ease the discomfort associated with nursing. Place the shield over the nipple and assist the infant to begin nursing. This may be done by advising the mother to express some milk manually into the nipple shield to stimulate the infant. If the infant is unable to nurse with the nipple shield, the affected breast may be pumped until the nipple is healed. The infant may require supplemental feedings during this time. If one breast is unaffected, the infant should be allowed to empty this breast; however, care must be taken not to make this nipple sore. Reassure the mother that the nipple will heal soon, and normal nursing may resume.

Cracked and fissured nipples may become infected if not allowed to heal. In addition, the infant's sucking may irritate the nipple further. The breast must be emptied; this can be done by pumping, which is less traumatic than the infant nursing.

Communicative Aspects

OBSERVATIONS

1. Observe the feedings to assess the breast-feeding technique. Watch to see that the baby has a firm grasp of the nipple, holding it well into the mouth to compress surrounding tissue and ducts. Note that the mother's breast tissue does not compress the infant's nose and inhibit breathing. Check the infant's technique to ensure that adequate nursing is occurring. Rapid sucking without swallowing may indicate that the infant is not grasping the nipple correctly.

2. Observe the mother's nipples for redness, cracking, and bleeding. Observe the breasts for engorgement, nodules, and tenderness. Note the breasts to see that they are being emptied adequately; that is, the breast should be soft after nursing, with no hardened areas or nodules. Observe the bra to see that it is adequate to support the breasts.

CHARTING

DATE/TIME	OBSERVATIONS	SIGNATURE
7/15 0830	Mother instructed on method for washing hands and nipples before nursing. Infant to breast for first breast-feeding attempt. Mother in chair with feet elevated. Positioning demonstrated. Infant nursed 3 min at each breast. Sucking reflex adequte. Mother stated she was comfortable and the feeding felt very natural to her. Praised for her efforts and encouraged. No discomfort noted. Breasts are firm but not distended. ————————————	M. Brown RN

Discharge Planning Aspects

CLIENT AND FAMILY EDUCATION

1. Nursing can be a very satisfying experience for both mother and baby. Not all babies nurse at the same rate. There is also great variation between babies regarding speed of learning to nurse. Some infants begin nursing successfully immediately after birth. Some must be coaxed and learn only after several weeks of patience and persistence. The infant who is slow to nurse may threaten the new mother's self-image. Emotions play a very important part in successful nursing. Offer continual reassurance and encouragement to the mother. A positive attitude is an important part of success, and the reassurance of the nurse that the baby's actions are normal may be the impetus she needs to persevere and nurse her infant successfully. Motivation plays a big part in successful nursing.

2. Tell the mother that the infant may suck intermittently with rest periods. Reassure the mother that the infant will nurse when hungry. The infant also will suck lightly after the milk feels as if it has stopped flowing. This seems to satisfy the infant's need to suck and should not be discouraged if the nipples are not sore. When possible, the infant will nurse most successfully when fed on demand, that is, when hungry.

3. Explain to the mother about manual expression of milk from the breasts. This is accomplished by grasping the breast tissue with the thumb on the upper portion of the breast and the forefinger on the lower portion (Fig. 123-3). The thumb and forefinger then gently but firmly compress the breast tissue. The thumb and forefinger are brought toward each other behind the areola, allowing the milk to flow out of the nipple (Fig. 123-4). The hand does not touch the nipple or the milk during this process. The milk may be expressed into a sterile cup or bottle. The milk should be expressed into a sterile plastic bag if it is to be frozen for later use. The hand may be positioned around the circumference of the breast to empty all sections. Manual (Fig. 123-5) or electrical (Fig. 123-6) breast pumps may be used. If the milk will be given to the baby, it should be covered and stored in a refrigerator or frozen until ready for use.

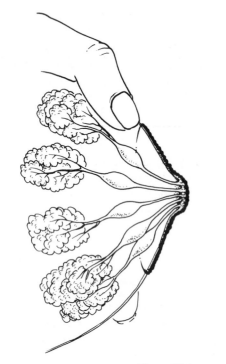

Figure 123.3

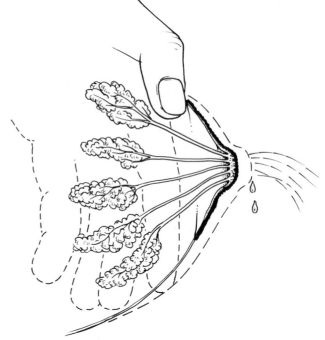

Figure 123.4

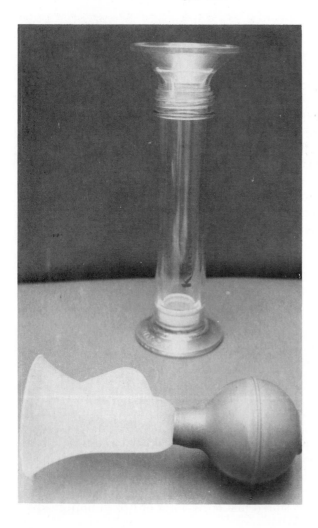

Figure 123.5

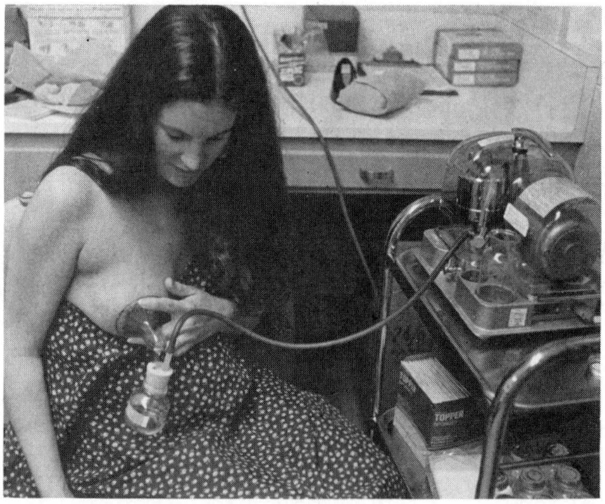

Figure 123.6

3. Teach the mother to recognize the baby's readiness for feeding. Behaviors such as swallowing, mouth activity, and sucking may indicate hunger.

4. Instruct the mother on adequate diet during lactation. Nutritional requirements are increased considerably above normal needs. An additional 500 calories per day generally are considered to be the minimum required to meet the needs of lactogenesis and to maintain the mother's energy level. An additional 20 g of protein and 400 g of calcium is recommended. Phosphorus, iron, and water-soluble vitamins also should be increased during lactation. Fluid intake is important to the production of an adequate milk supply. A fluid intake of about 3000 ml is needed. Foods that should be avoided are those that cause digestive problems during the nonlactating state. There is controversy about the effect of the foods eaten by the mother on the baby. The judicious action seems to be to advise the new mother that she may eat whatever she wishes. If it seems to cause digestive upset in the infant, she may wish to avoid that food during the remainder of the nursing period. All babies are different, and trial and error seems to be the best way to determine what the mother can and cannot eat.

5. Emphasize to the new parents that an occasional bottle of expressed milk or formula will not hurt the baby and will allow them to have some time to themselves. Stress the importance of physical and psychological care of self, and encourage the new mother to spend some time away from the baby occasionally.

6. Instruct the nursing mother to report to her obstetric care provider the presence of any nodules or masses in the breast which do not go away after nursing. Some nodules are due to pooling of milk, which constricts the duct and prevents its escape from the breast. Application of heat and massage of the area in the direction of the nipple usually will relieve the discomfort and allow the milk to drain from this area. If the nodule remains or becomes reddened or extremely tender, however, the obstetric care provider should be notified. Excessive breast tenderness or fever are also symptoms that should be reported.

Evaluation

Quality Assurance

Documentation should include instructions given to the mother and an assessment of her actions. The chart should reflect that the mother was taught the positions for nursing her infant, the principles involved, and possible complications. In addition, she should be taught about the importance of a support bra and methods to prevent infection in herself and her baby. The chart should contain some type of record of the breast-feeding routine established while in the hospital. This might include the time, as well as which breast was nursed and for how long. Discharge instructions should be noted. Advice about nutrition and exercise should be reflected.

Infection Control

1. Proper care of the nipples is extremely important in preventing transfer of microorganisms to the newborn. Because the immune system of newborns is immature, it is necessary to protect them against infection. A few simple actions will greatly reduce the chance of cross-contamination of the infant. Remind the mother to wash her hands before handling the infant, and especially before each feeding. The nipples should be washed with a fresh, clean cloth each day before the bath or shower.

2. Adequate handwashing is essential between clients and before handling any newborn baby.

3. Bras and nursing pads should be kept clean and dry. Advise the new mother to wear a clean bra each day. Nursing pads should be changed as soon as they become damp to prevent colonization of microorganisms in the warm, moist environment.

4. Manual expression of milk should be preceded by thorough handwashing. The container used to store the milk should be sterile. The mother's hands should not come in contact with the milk during expression. If a manual breast pump is used, it must have a receptacle that can be adequately cleaned to catch the milk. The milk should not flow into a rubber suction bulb because this cannot be cleaned to ensure sterility. The breast pump should be cleaned thoroughly between uses. Most can be cleaned in an electric dishwasher, although infant feeding equipment should be washed separately and should not be placed in the same load as other family dishes. The electric breast pump should be cleaned between clients. In addition, the portion that touches the client should be cleaned and sterilized between uses.

Technique Checklist

	YES	NO
Explanations to the client		
Lactogenesis	____	____
Breast-feeding the infant	____	____
Positioning	____	____
Times and duration	____	____
Breast support	____	____
Cleanliness	____	____
Client first fed infant _____ hr after birth		
Infant able to grasp nipple successfully	____	____
Breasts completely emptied	____	____
Infant gained weight	____	____
Engorgement of breasts	____	____
Sore or cracked nipples	____	____
Breast pump demonstrated	____	____
Nipple shield demonstrated	____	____
Discharge instructions documented	____	____

Cesarean Section, Preparation and Postoperative Care

Overview

Definition

A cesarean section is an operative procedure to deliver a fetus by an incision through the abdominal wall and the uterus. Types include:

Classic: The incision is made through the abdominal wall, peritoneum, and uterus from the umbilicus to the symphysis pubis

Low segment: The incision is made above the symphysis pubis into the lower part (the cervical end) of the uterus behind the bladder. The peritoneum is not incised.

Cesarean hysterectomy: Incision of the abdomen and uterus to remove the fetus and placenta followed by removal of the uterus

Postmortem cesarean: Incision of the abdominal wall and uterus and removal of the fetus after the death of the mother

Rationale

Enhance the chance of survival of the mother and infant when vaginal delivery or predisposing circumstances may threaten the lives of one or both.

Terminology

Dystocia: Difficult delivery, also prolonged labor because of size of the fetus, the pelvis of the mother, or inadequacy of the uterine contractions

Eclampsia: Severe complications of pregnancy characterized by high blood pressure, albuminuria, edema, convulsions, or coma, one of the forms of pregnancy-induced hypertension (PIH)

Hypoxia: Insufficient oxygen available to the tissues

Transabdominal: Through the abdomen

Assessment

Pertinent Anatomy and Physiology

1. Appendix I: *uterus.*

2. The peritoneum lines the abdominal cavity and covers the abdominal viscera. There is a difference between the peritoneum of the female and the male. The male peritoneum encloses the abdominal cavity completely. The female peritoneum is not a closed sac because the free ends of the fallopian tubes open directly into the peritoneal cavity. This means there is communication with the external environment through the uterus and vagina.

3. The female pelvis differs from that of the male in the smoothness of the bones, the larger capacity, and the flexibility of the coccyx. Four bones form the pelvis: the hipbones form the front and sides and the sacrum and coccyx form the back. If any of the diameters are too small, it may be impossible for the infant's skull to enter the true pelvis for a natural delivery.

Pathophysiological Concepts

1. Cephalopelvic disproportion (CPD) is the condition resulting when the infant's head is too large or the maternal pelvis is too small to allow passage through the birth canal. CPD is a common cause of dystocia. This is determined by such studies as a pelvimetry (which determines the size of the pelvis) and x-ray study.

2. Unusual presentation is also an indication for cesarean section. Breech refers to the buttocks (or lower limbs) being in the pelvis cavity ready to deliver first, rather than the head as in a normal cephalic delivery. Transverse lie is the condition of a fetus that has a shoulder as the presenting part. This is a serious complication and usually requires cesarean section.

3. Placenta previa is a condition resulting from the placenta growing partially or totally in the lower segment of the uterus instead of the upper portion. The placenta may cover the cervical os totally or partially. Normal vaginal delivery is impossible if the os is covered completely. Because of the chance of hemorrhage, these infants usually are delivered by cesarean section.

4. Premature separation of the placenta (abruptio placentae) occurs when part or all of the placenta detaches from the uterine wall before the delivery process. The resulting hemorrhage may be contained within the body or may escape to the outside.

Assessment of the Client

1. Assess the reason for the cesarean section. If the cause is cephalopelvic disproportion, the surgery should relieve the problem. If the reason is an obstetrical complication, such as placenta previa or premature separation of the placenta, however, postpartal complications also may occur. Watch these clients for hemorrhage. There is a good chance that clients with CPD will require repeat cesarean sections with subsequent pregnancies. If obstetrical complications do not arise in subsequent pregnancies, however, clients who have had previous cesarean sections may be able to deliver vaginally depending on the condition of the uterine scar.

2. Assess the client's understanding of the need for the cesarean section. Determine the client's emotional reaction. Many couples who have planned on using the natural childbirth method may be disappointed and feel "cheated" by this unexpected event. Guilt feelings are also common. Assess the anxiety level of the family and the need for further education and information.

3. Assess the client's general physical condition just as for any abdominal surgery. Determine the presence of any complicating factors, such as diabetes, allergies, or cardiac problems. Assess the vital signs and fetal heart tones (FHT) before surgery.

Plan

Nursing Objectives

Prepare the client mentally and physically for birth by an alternate method.

Maintain close contact with the family, assisting them through the birth process.

Provide preoperative care.

Assist in the evolution of a happy, family-centered birth experience to the extent desired by the couple and allowed by the medical limitations of the situation.

Assist the mother to a safe and expeditious recovery.

Make the birth experience positive by reinforcing the self-image of the parents and the family unit.

Client Preparation

1. The family may or may not know in advance that a cesarean section will be performed. Sometimes, after a trial labor, it becomes evident that the baby cannot be delivered safely or that complications make surgery the only safe alternative for the mother and the baby. Many times the cesarean section is

done on an emergency basis with little preparation. The abdomen and pubic area may be shaved and cleansed with a bactericidal solution. Regional or a general anesthetic may be used. A retention catheter is inserted (or may be inserted after anesthesia has begun), and an intravenous infusion is started.

2. If the surgery is planned in advance, the mother may check into the hospital the day before to have laboratory and other preparations completed. In this case, she may be given an enema to cleanse the lower bowel the night before the surgery. She may be fed a light diet and will probably be NPO (without oral food or fluids) for 12 hours before the surgery. A urinary retention catheter will be inserted to ensure that the bladder is empty. Blood typing and cross-matching may be done. An intravenous infusion will be started. Narcotics usually are withheld owing to their influence on the fetus. The anesthetic may be inhalation or regional. Inhalation anesthetic is not administered until all preparations are complete to reduce the amount of time the infant will be exposed. Other preparations will include teaching about what to expect during the surgery and recovery periods.

3. The father often is allowed to be with the client during cesarean section. This will depend on the wishes and emotional make-up of the father, the needs of the mother, the wishes of the physician, and hospital policy. If the father will attend the surgery, explain what will happen and how he can help his wife. Explain about the sterile field and inform him about what to touch and what not to touch to spare him embarrassment and reduce the chance of cross-infection.

4. Ensure that the client is properly identified before going to surgery. A matching identification of some type should be available for placing on the infant immediately after birth.

Equipment

Enema tray

Retention catheter setup

Surgical preparation tray include bactericidal solution and cleansing pad

Intravenous infusion tray and fluid

Gown

Fetoscope

Stethoscope and sphygmomanometer

Implementation and Interventions

Procedural Aspects

ACTION

1. Postoperatively, monitor the client's vital signs every 5 to 15 minutes until she has recovered fully from the anesthetic. If a spinal block was done, observe for return of function to the lower extremities. Observe vaginal flow, which should be red and free of clots. The uterus should be massaged for firmness. Gentleness must be exercised because of the nearness of the incision. The uterus must remain firm to prevent hemorrhage, however.

RATIONALE

The cesarean section client requires monitoring for both postoperative and postpartal complications. The placenta is removed from the uterine wall just as in vaginal birth. The exposed blood vessels may bleed if the uterus does not contract to close off the vessels. Firmness of the uterus signifies a state of contraction.

ACTION	*RATIONALE*
2. Maintain the intravenous infusion as requested by the physician. The client will probably receive liquids as soon as desired if nausea is absent. Solid foods usually are offered in 24 hours.	The bowels lie behind the uterus and are not manipulated during the cesarean birth. Therefore, there is usually little nausea or vomiting and the client is able to resume eating quickly.
3. Get the client out of bed when prescribed by the physician. The client usually gets up the same day as surgery. Assist her the first few times until she is stable.	Early ambulation hastens recovery and helps to prevent complications associated with immobility.
4. Change the dressing as prescribed. The dressing usually will be changed daily and as needed if it becomes soiled. The sutures should be cleaned with an antiseptic solution. Place the dressing in a paper bag and dispose of it in an appropriate container outside the room. Because the abdominal muscles have been stretched by the pregnancy and may provide little support, an abdominal binder may be ordered.	Frequent dressing changes and wound cleansing discourage the growth and colonization of pathogenic micro-organisms. An abdominal binder may provide support to the abdomen and prevent tension and strain on the suture line. The soiled dressing is not left in the room since the new mother may be particularly sensitive to odors and to the environment.
5. Administer pain medication as needed by the client. Be sure that she does not receive the baby unattended after she has had pain medication. If she is rooming in, the baby may be returned to the nursery. If the baby remains in the room, check the mother and infant frequently to ensure that accidents are prevented.	Most pain medications will make the mother drowsy. If she holds the baby or has the baby in bed with her, the infant could be dropped or smothered.

Special Modifications

Observe the fundus to see that it is contracted if the dressing is low enough. If the dressing is too high, release it for observing fundus contraction. Measure vital signs and watch the color and amount of vaginal flow. A weak thready pulse, increased vaginal flow, hypotension, and pallor are indications of hemorrhage.	Postpartum hemorrhage is a possible complication of cesarean section. The uterus may be less accessible. Fundus contraction must be maintained to prevent hemorrhage, however.

Communicative Aspects

OBSERVATIONS

1. Observe the client before cesarean section is performed for indications that labor has started. If labor has started, observe the FHT, fetal positioning, contractions (interval and duration), vital signs, and vaginal discharge. Observe for rupture of the membranes.

2. Observe the postoperative client for recovery from the anesthetic. Monitor vital signs. Observe the vaginal discharge. Observe the dressings for drainage. Maintain the patency of the catheter and the intravenous infusion.

3. Observe the incision during the healing period. Note signs of redness or pus formation that indicate infection.

4. Observe the breasts for engorgement and discomfort. Note the height of the fundus, if possible. Observe the lochia for amount and appearance.

CHARTING

DATE/TIME	OBSERVATIONS	SIGNATURE
9/23 0915	24-year-old client returned from OR after c-section. Delivered female infant, has seen baby. B/P 128/70, P 72, R 16, T 98.8° F. Lochia red, pad has been changed once since OR. Dressing dry. Foley patent and draining yellow, clear urine. IV infusing at keep-open rate. Able to move both legs and feet since spinal. Staying flat in bed at this time. No headache or pain stated. Husband is with her. To receive the baby in one hour for breast-feeding. ————	M. Brown RN

Discharge Planning Aspects

CLIENT AND FAMILY EDUCATION

1. Offer preoperative information to the extent desired by the client and family and allowed by the constraints of time. Be sure that the client understands why the cesarean section is being done and knows what to expect during the recuperation phase.

2. Whether the cesarean section was planned or is unexpected, the prospect of surgery usually carries a certain degree of apprehension and uncertainty. This may be compounded with feelings of guilt and frustration when the parents had planned on sharing a natural birth. The emotional climate may be very tense. Much understanding and reassurance are needed to ensure that the birthing experience is positive.

3. After surgery, explain the need for ambulation and resumption of normal activities. The catheter usually is removed on the first postoperative day. The client probably will have no difficulty voiding, although it may burn slightly for the first few days after the catheter is removed. Removal of the infusion should increase mobility. Ask the client to allow the nurses to assist her during early ambulation attempts. Once she is stable, she should be able to move about freely, however. Assure her that the stitches will not be affected by ambulation. She should stand up straight and look forward when ambulating.

4. Explain the need for pacing of activities to the mother who has had a cesarean section. This will be very important after discharge from the hospital as well. Explain that because of the excitement of having a baby and the new demands on her time, she may overestimate her capabilities. This results in overtiring and can lead to complications. She should allow frequent rest periods during the day. Offers for assistance should be accepted. Emphasize that when she cares for herself, she is also showing concern for her baby and the rest of her family.

5. Show the client how to use a pillow against her abdomen for splinting when she coughs. She may also use a pillow on her lap to hold her baby during feedings to relieve pressure and tension on the suture line.

6. Explain the normal pattern of postpartum recovery. The cesarean section client will have lochia and should be prepared for its gradual decrease and changing of color. The involution of the uterus should be explained. Breast-feeding is in no way contraindicated merely because of cesarean section. Care of the breasts should be explained (see Technique No. 122). Care of the infant should be explained and demonstrated. The need to avoid heavy lifting or overexertion should be emphasized.

REFERRALS

Referrals may include visits from a home health nurse if the client would bene-fit. Refer to diaper service or home-making services if the client will need assis-tance at home. Refer to parenting classes if the client does not have experience or feels the need for reinforcement in parenting skills. A referral to Planned Par-enthood may benefit those families wishing assistance with family planning.

Evaluation

Quality Assurance

Documentation should reflect a basis for the decision to perform a cesarean sec-tion by such means as radiology reports, symptomatology, or consultations. The information given to the parents should be reflected with an assessment of their understanding and acceptance of it. Preparations should be noted as well as results.

Postoperative documentation should reflect the progress of the recovery period. The appearance and care of the incision should be noted at least once each shift. The appearance of the lochia should be noted. Breast care should be reflected. Any teaching of the client and family should be documented. The vital signs should be monitored throughout the recovery period and may be displayed graphically on the chart. Evidence that the nurse was aware of the possible post-operative and postpartum complications should be in evidence, as well as any action taken to prevent or reverse them. Discharge instructions should be noted with an assessment of the degree of understanding and compliance expected. Any referrals should be noted.

Infection Control

1. Cesarean section is a major surgical procedure. Sterile technique is used when changing the dressings.

2. Careful handwashing should precede and follow any care given to the client. She should be told to keep her hands away from the incision until healing is complete. She should also be advised to wash her hands before handling her infant.

3. If the incision becomes infected, the mother will be placed on the appropri-ate isolation technique, such as wound and skin (see Technique No. 66, Iso-lation Precautions, in the Adult Section). The infant may be placed in the room with the mother or isolated from the other infants in the nursery to pre-vent the spread of infection among infants, whose immune systems are immature.

4. Any equipment used for subsequent clients should be cleaned thoroughly between clients and disinfected.

Technique Checklist

	YES	NO
Procedure explained to client	_____	_____
To father	_____	_____
To family	_____	_____
Elective cesarean section	_____	_____
Emergency cesarean section	_____	_____
Reason for cesarean section _____		
Vital signs and FHT noted on chart	_____	_____
Healthy baby delivered	_____	_____
Apgar 1 min _____		
Apgar 5 min _____		
Vital signs monitored		
Immediate postoperatively q _____ min		
During recuperation q _____ min		
Urinary catheter removed _____ (date)		
Voided without difficulty	_____	_____
Intravenous infusion removed _____ (date)		
Oral fluids without nausea	_____	_____
Solids without nausea	_____	_____
Dressing changes noted in chart at least every shift	_____	_____
Care of incision at home explained	_____	_____
Sutures or staples removed before leaving the hospital	_____	_____
Abdominal binder	_____	_____
Need for pacing of activities at home explained	_____	_____
Vaginal discharge explained	_____	_____
Referrals made _____		

125   Fetal Heart Tones

Overview

Definition

Periodic auscultation or monitoring of the heart beat of the fetus

Rationale

Evaluate the condition of the fetus and detect any fetal distress.

Diagnose a multiple pregnancy.

Ascertain fetal position

Terminology

Auscultation: The act of listening for sounds within the body

Funic souffle: A murmur or whizzing sound, caused by blood rushing through the umbilical cord, that is synchronous with the fetal heart rate

Uterine souffle: A murmur or rushing sound, caused by the blood rushing through the large vessels of the uterus, that is synchronous with the maternal heart rate

Villi: Tiny projections arising from the outermost layer of the fertilized ovum that penetrate into the uterine lining (called the decidua) and form the nutritive and eliminatory link between the developing embryo and the mother. Villi lay the groundwork for the placenta.

Assessment

Pertinent Anatomy and Physiology

1. See Appendix I: *uterus, labor and delivery.*
2. The normal heart rate of the fetus is 120 to 160 beats/ min. The heart beat usually can be heard around the 20th week with a fetoscope, and as early as the 5th week with ultrasound devices.
3. Fetal blood flows to the placenta through two umbilical arteries and returns to the fetus through the umbilical vein. On the maternal side, the blood enters the spaces between the villi. Exchange of nutrients and waste with the blood of the infant occurs through the capillary walls of the villi. Between 500 ml and 700 ml of maternal blood and 300 ml and 400 ml of fetal blood circulate through the placenta each minute. Although the maternal and fetal blood are in very close approximation over large surfaces for the exchange of nutrients and waste, they do not intermix.
4. Fetal heart measurements during labor must take into consideration the variations that occur in response to contractions. Sometimes there is no change at all during the contraction. Sometimes the fetal heart rate increases in response to the contraction; the is called *acceleration.* Sometimes the rate decreases in response to the uterine contractions; this is called *deceleration.*

Pathophysiological Concepts

1. Fetal tachycardia is considered a baseline rate over 160 beats/min or a rise of 10% over the previous baseline for at least a 10-minute period. One cause may be fetal hypoxia, which prompts an increase in the fetal heart rate in an attempt to make up for the decreased amount of oxygen available in the blood. Maternal fever or tachycardia may also cause fetal response. Immaturity of the fetal neurologic condition may cause irregularities in the fetal heart rate.

2. Fetal bradycardia is considered a baseline rate under 120 beats/min or a 10% drop from a previous baseline for at least a 10-minute period. The usual causes are fetal heart abnormalities and fetal distress. It may be relieved by changing the mother's position and by administration of oxygen to the mother. If not resolved, delivery must take place immediately.

Assessment of the Client

1. Assess the approximate position of the fetus when determining where to listen to the fetal heart rates. Assess by visualization and palpation of the maternal abdomen. Palpation of the abdomen to assess fetal position is accomplished by a procedure called Leopold's maneuvers (Fig. 125-1), which are summarized as follows:

   a. Palpate upper abdomen to determine contents of fundus.

   b. Locate fetal back in relation to right and left sides.

   c. Locate presenting part at inlet and check for engagement by evaluating mobility.

   d. Palpate just above the inguinal ligament on either side to determine the relationship of the presenting part to the pelvis.

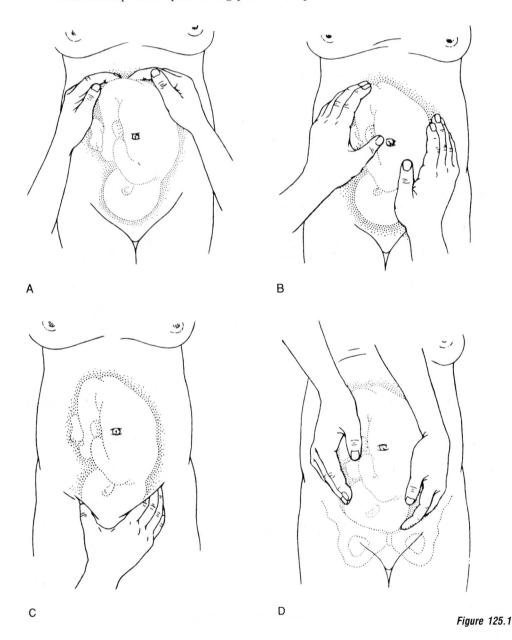

A   B

C   D

Figure 125.1

The sounds usually are heard through the thorax when the baby is in face presentation and through the back when the presentation is breech or vertex. In cephalic presentation, listen at the level of the umbilicus or slightly above.

2. Assess the level of understanding of the client and family regarding why the fetal heart rate must be ascertained and what is involved. Most clients who have had prenatal care will be accustomed to the procedure for auscultation of fetal heart rate. If electronic fetal monitoring will be done, be sure that the client and her family understand the reason for the procedure and know what will occur. They should be reassured that the procedure, although slightly uncomfortable to the client, is not harmful to the baby.

Plan

Nursing Objectives

Provide for the safety and welfare of the infant.

Measure and monitor the fetal heart rate throughout the labor and delivery process to provide continual assessment of fetal status.

Provide reassurance for the family.

Provide an accurate record of fetal cardiac status throughout labor.

Client Preparation

1. The client's abdomen should be exposed. Ask her to lower clothing to the hips for auscultation of the fetal heart tones.

2. Explain to the client about the need to press somewhat firmly against the abdomen with the fetoscope. Explain that it may be necessary to listen in several places to find the area where fetal heart tones (FHT) can be heard most clearly. Reassure her that moving the fetoscope around does not indicate that anything is wrong with her infant.

3. If the electronic monitor is applied, both parents should fully understand the methods used. If possible, during antepartal care, they should be prepared in a matter-of-fact way for the possibility of electronic fetal monitoring. Then, if electronic monitoring is needed, they will not be alarmed and completely unprepared. They should have an opportunity to see and examine the equipment. If internal monitoring is used, it is particularly important that they understand that the electrode is very small and will only be implanted into the infant's scalp to a depth of 1 mm. Explain to the mother any restrictions on her movement. Explain the procedure that will be used to introduce the internal monitor into the uterus. If external monitoring will be done, explain how the monitor will be attached to her abdomen. Have the client void before applying the monitor.

Equipment

Fetoscope, bell stethoscope, or ultrasound stethoscope

Electronic fetal monitor with transducer and belt (internal fetal monitoring requires a sterile tray containing the electrode, electrode guide tube, intrauterine pressure-monitoring catheter, leg plate, amniotomy equipment, and pads)

Transducer gel

Implementation and Interventions

Procedural Aspects

ACTION

1. Palpate the mother's abdomen to determine approximate position of the infant. Place the bell of the stethoscope on the abdomen and listen for a rapid, soft muffled sound. If the sound is not heard, move the bell around until the sound is audible. Move the bell from the umbilicus outward in a circular motion, stopping every 5 cm to 10 cm to listen for FHT. Reassure the mother that moving the bell is not indicative of a problem. When listening to the FHT, remove the hands from the fetoscope and apply pressure with the forehead to count the rate (Fig. 125-2).

RATIONALE

The fetal heart rate is best heard above the umbilicus in breech or vertex presentations. The mother's position also may affect the ability to hear FHT in various locations. The fetoscope is used because it works through the principle of conduction as well as hearing. The hands are removed from the fetoscope when listening to the fetal heart tones so they will not interfere with bone conduction.

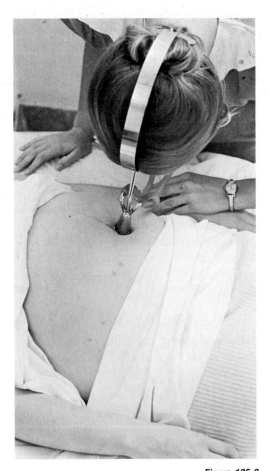

Figure 125.2

ACTION	RATIONALE
2. Determine the base fetal heart rate by counting the fetal heartbeat between contractions for at least two consecutive 15-second periods. The basal fetal heart rate also may be measured by counting for two consecutive 15-second periods, allowing a short rest period, then measuring for two additional 15-second periods.	The baseline rate assists in detecting early signs of fetal distress as labor progresses. It must be measured over a period of time and between contractions to get an accurate count, allowing for normal variability of 2 to 3 beats per minute.
3. If the fetal heart rate seems slow, it may be the uterine souffle that is being measured. Because the uterine souffle is synchronous with the maternal heart rate, the mother's pulse should be measured during FHT determination to differentiate the two rates.	The usual maternal heart rate is about 50 beats/min whereas the usual fetal heart rate is about 140 beats/min. If the fetal heart rate is low, it may be a sign of fetal distress.

Special Modifications

1. External electronic FHT monitoring takes place by amplifying the fetal heart beat through the use of a transducer. Apply the gel to the area where FHT can be heard most clearly. Place the transducer onto the gel and apply the elastic belt to hold the transducer in place. A second belt is applied to the lower abdomen to measure contractions.	The transducer both sends and receives ultrasound waves. The gel seals the transducer to the abdomen. The waves are deflected by movement of the fetal heart valves allowing for measurement of the fetal heart rate.
2. Internal fetal heart monitoring is accomplished by rupturing the fetal membranes and attaching an electrode to the infant's scalp. The electrode is placed by advancing the guide tube through the vagina until contact with the head is made. The electrode then is attached under the skin of the infant's scalp. This electrode is attached to the fetal monitor. A sterile, water-filled catheter is positioned inside the uterus to measure intrauterine pressure. Advanced experience and training are necessary to accomplish electronic fetal monitoring properly.	The fetal heart rate can be measured much more accurately by the internal route; however, the procedure is invasive and increases the risk of infection.

Communicative Aspects

OBSERVATIONS

1. Observe the fetal heart rate every hour during early labor. As the labor progresses, the FHT should be determined every 30 minutes. After 4-cm to 5-cm dilation, check the fetal heart rate every 15 minutes. When the contractions are very strong or when complications are suspected, the fetal heart rate is counted more frequently, every 5 to 10 minutes. Observe the FHT immediately after rupture of the membranes and for several contractions thereafter because prolapse of the cord is possible when the membranes rupture. During induction of labor and after regional anesthesia, the FHT should be closely observed. During the second stage of labor, determine the FHT after each pushing contraction.

2. Observe the basal fetal heart rate. This rate will be used to determine fluctuations as labor progresses. Normally, the basal fetal heart rate remains the same throughout labor. A rise or decrease of more than 10% indicates fetal distress.

3. Observe the client who is being monitored electronically to be sure that the belts remain in the proper position. Electronic monitors produce a graphic record of fetal and maternal measurements that should be observed. Reliance on mechanical means of determining fetal status should not replace the nurse's responsibility to observe carefully the clinical condition of the client, however. The client's vital signs should be measured regularly and contractions should be measured as an adjunct to electronic monitoring. FHT should be auscultated at intervals to ensure the proper functioning of the electronic equipment.

4. Observe the emotional status of the client and her family. The monitor must never replace the client as the focus of attention. When the monitor is checked, acknowledge the client as a person first. The monitor measurements should be interpreted in relation to their importance to the client and her baby.

CHARTING

Electronic fetal monitors produce a graphic record of the status of the fetal heart rate and intrauterine pressure (internal monitoring) or contraction (external monitoring). All of the monitoring record should be a permanent part of the chart.

The FHT should be charted when auscultated along with the location on the abdomen at which it was heard.

DATE/TIME	OBSERVATIONS	SIGNATURE
9/23 0910	FHT 142 beats/min heard in the lower right quadrant. Contractions q4min for 25 sec to 30 sec. Husband present and coaching during contractions.	M. Brown RN

Discharge Planning Aspects

CLIENT AND FAMILY EDUCATION

1. Explain to the client and spouse about the importance of monitoring the status of their baby during labor. Emphasize that the readings are taken frequently as a safeguard to ensure that the baby is safe and healthy during labor. Tell the parents that the measurements will be taken frequently during labor and will increase in frequency as the birth nears. Answer any questions that they may have. They must be reassured that the measurements are necessary and are for the benefit of the mother and baby.

2. If the electronic fetal monitoring is to be done, explain the procedure as completely as time and situation will allow. Tell the parents why this type of monitoring is necessary. Their agreement is necessary before the monitor is applied or the electrode is inserted. If the internal monitor is used, they should understand that the electrode will be placed directly into the infant's

scalp. They should be reassured that the depth of insertion is very superficial. The emphasis must remain on the mother and the infant, and not on the equipment and the procedure.

3. Allow the mother to listen to her infant's heartbeat throught the fetoscope, if time and situation allow. The father also may listen. This strengthens the family bond that has been developing throughout the pregnancy.

Evaluation

Quality Assurance

Documentation should include frequency of FHT measurements, the rate and rhythm, and any abnormalities. Graphic portrayal of the data may provide a comprehensive picture of the infant status during labor. The status of the labor process and the frequency and duration of contractions should be noted. Explanations to the parents should be reflected.

Each hospital will have protocols for the application of electronic fetal monitoring. These protocols should specify who may do the monitoring and what type of preparation is indicated to monitor the client successfully. Consult the hospital procedure manual to determine how much of the electronic monitoring graphic data is retained on the chart.

Infection Control

1. All equipment that is used for clients consecutively, such as fetoscope, bell stethoscope, and ultrasound stethoscope, should be cleaned and disinfected between uses. Each client should have one instrument for her exclusive use during the duration of her labor.

2. Application of the external fetal monitor should be accomplished using clean technique. All equipment touching the mother should be clean and disinfected.

3. Equipment used for internal fetal monitoring must be sterile. This is a sterile technique. One of the great hazards of this procedure is the risk of infection. The membranes are ruptured and direct contact with the fetus is made. Extreme care must be taken to protect the infant from cross-infection.

4. Careful handwashing should be carried out before and after touching any client in labor. Rings and jewelry should be kept to a minimum to reduce the chance of cross-infection.

Technique Checklist

	YES	NO
Technique explained to client and family	_____	_____
Type of monitoring		
Fetoscope _____		
Bell stethoscope _____		
Ultrasound stethoscope _____		
External fetal monitor _____		
Internal fetal monitor _____		
Baseline fetal heart rate determined	_____	_____
Documentation on chart of ongoing FHT monitoring	_____	_____
FHT variations		
Tachycardia _____ Bradycardia _____		
Reported to obstetric care provider	_____	_____

Overview

Definition

The assessment of uterine involution after birth

Rationale

Prevent or alleviate hemorrhage resulting from relaxation of the contracted state of the uterus after birth.

Check the progress of involution of the uterus.

Terminology

Atony: Lack of muscle tone; relaxation of the contractibility of the muscle tissue

Fingerbreadth: The width of any one of the examiner's fingers

Hemorrhage: Loss of blood at a rate above what would be expected (usually > 500 ml). In the postpartum period, saturating more than three pads in 15 minutes is considered excessive.

Involution: The retrogression of the female reproductive organs to the normal, nonpregnant state

Assessment

Pertinent Anatomy and Physiology

1. See Appendix I: *uterus.*
2. The uterus undergoes great change during the first week after the client's giving birth. Immediately after childbirth, the uterine muscle is firmly contracted to seal off the open vascular surfaces left on separation of the placenta. After the first 2 days, the size of the uterus decreases very rapidly. By the 10th day, it is usually at the level of the symphysis pubis. At the end of 6 weeks, the uterus usually has resumed its prepregnancy size and position. Involution usually progresses much faster in women who nurse than in those who do not because nursing stimulates uterine contractions.
3. Afterpains are caused by an alternating contraction and relaxation of the uterine muscle during the involution period. They are common in multiparas. These pains usually do not last more than 1 or 2 days and are relieved by analgesics.

Pathophysiological Concepts

1. Failure of the uterine muscle to contract properly may result in hemorrhage. Uterine *atony,* or impaired tone of the uterus, results when muscle fibers fail to contract and constrict vessels from the area of placental separation. If the labor has been especially prolonged, the muscle may lack the stamina to continue contracting, resulting in hemorrhage. Other causes of uterine atony may be precipitous labor, overdistension of the uterus (e.g., occurring in hydramnios, multiple pregnancy, or a very large fetus), or overmassage during the third stage of labor.
2. Retention of placental pieces or blood clots may interfere with the ability of the uterus to contract properly. If the placenta does not separate properly or completely, bleeding is probable. Afterpains that persist for longer than 48

hours or the appearance of severe afterpains in the primipara may indicate that fragments of the placenta or membranes have been retained in the uterus.

Assessment of the Client

1. Assess the client for expected discharge during the immediate postpartum period. Following birth, there should be a steady red discharge from the vagina. If the flow is interrupted, the client may have retained tissue or clots that are now blocking the cervix. Assess the amount of bleeding from the vagina and the color. Palpate the uterus. If the muscle feels boggy or soft, retention of blood may be suspected and massage of the fundus is indicated.

2. Assess the placenta as soon as it is expelled to see that it is intact. Retention of placenta fragments or portions will predispose to hemorrhage.

Plan

Nursing Objectives

Prevent the fundus from becoming boggy and soft.

Prevent shock and hemorrhage.

Evaluate the involutional process.

Help the client understand why frequent checking of the uterus is important.

Client Preparation

1. During prenatal instructions, the client should be told that frequent checking and periodic massaging of the uterus after birth will be necessary. Tell the client each time the fundus will be checked. Reassure her by telling her that it is normal to check the fundus frequently.

2. Allow the client to empty her bladder before checking the fundus. A full bladder may displace the fundus upward and to the side.

Equipment

Perineal pad

Implementation and Interventions

Procedural Aspects

ACTION	RATIONALE
1. Immediately after delivery, palpate the height of the fundus. Place one hand above the symphysis pubis. With the other hand, palpate the abdomen to locate the top of the uterus beginning above the umbilicus. The top of the uterus should feel firm and rounded (Fig. 126-1).	The contracted state of the uterine muscle makes it easily discernable beneath the softened tissue of the previously distended abdomen.

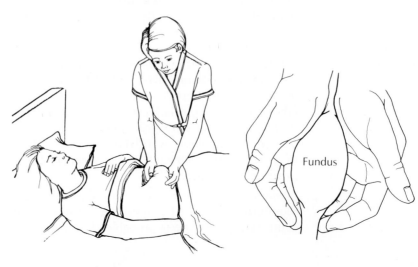

Fundus

Figure 126.1

ACTION	*RATIONALE*
2. Measure the height of the fundus, or top portion of the uterus, in relation to the umbilicus. Measure according to how many finger-breadths will fit above or below the umbilicus to the top of the fundus.	Immediately after birth, the height of the uterus will be at or slightly above the client's umbilicus. During the involutional period, the uterine height will recede beneath the umbilicus to the level of the symphysis pubis after about 10 days. Measuring in relation to the umbilicus provides a consistent method of recording and reporting the uterine height.
3. Gentle massage of the uterus to evacuate clots during the first hour after delivery should be done; however, do not massage vigorously unless the uterus is atonic. Replace the perineal pad if it is saturated.	Blood and clots may build up in the uterus if the cervix becomes blocked. Gentle massage usually relieves this blockage. Vigorous massage may fatigue the uterine muscle and cause relaxation, however. It is also uncomfortable for the client.

Special Modifications

If the uterus feels soft or boggy upon palpation, it is in a state of atony. It must contract to stop bleeding from the placental site. Massage by grasping the uterus with entire hand, holding the thumb toward the symphysis pubis and the fingers curved around the top of the fundus. Massage by grasping and releasing with firm pressure. Massage may also be done with both hands by placing one on top and one below the fundus. Proceed with a combined kneading and compressing motion of the fundus between the two hands. Stop as soon as the uterus contracts.	Massage will contract the uterine muscle and assist in evacuation of retained clots and blood. Overmassage will tire the muscle and further contribute to atony.

Communicative Aspects

OBSERVATIONS

1. The first 2 hours after delivery often are considered the most critical and hazardous of the entire pregnancy. For this reason, careful observation is essential. Observe the size, height, and consistency of the uterus. Palpate the fundus every 10 to 15 minutes for the first hour after delivery. The uterus should be firm and rounded at or near the area of the mother's umbilicus. Monitor the mother's vital signs every 15 minutes. An increase in pulse rate and decrease in volume may indicate hemorrhage. Observe for early signs of shock, which may include restlessness and anxiety. Observe the vaginal discharge (lochia).

2. If the uterus has remained contracted during the first hour, the client is less likely to have hemorrhagic complications. The height of the fundus and amount and consistency of the lochia should be observed frequently during the first 24 hours after delivery, however. Observations should be made at least every 4 hours.

3. Observe the involution of the uterus during the postpartum period by measuring the height of the uterus daily. The common method of reporting the height of the uterus is in fingerbreadths above or below the umbilicus (Fig. 126-2):

1/U: Uterus 1 fingerbreadth above the umbilicus

U/U: Uterus level with umbilicus

U/1: Uterus 1 fingerbreadth below the umbilicus

U/4: Uterus 4 fingerbreadths below the umbilicus

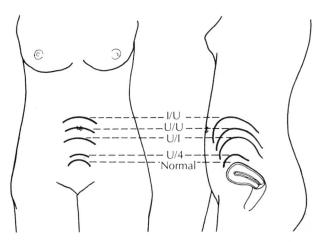

Figure 126.2

CHARTING

DATE/TIME	OBSERVATIONS	SIGNATURE
9/14 1100	Fundus U/1. Firm and midline. Lochia moderate, red, with no clots. Voiding without difficulty, 320 ml clear urine.	C. Parker RN

Discharge Planning Aspects

CLIENT AND FAMILY EDUCATION

1. Explain to the client and her family why the uterus must be observed closely during the first hour after birth. Also explain that the fundus will be checked frequently during the postpartum hospitalization period. Show the mother how to check her own fundus. Explain the involution process and tell her how the uterus should feel. Explain that if the uterus feels soft or boggy, the uterine muscle has relaxed, and advise her to call for assistance immediately. Tell her how to massage the uterus.

2. Explain about the involution process that will occur. Tell the mother that her uterus will return to its prepregnancy state in about 6 weeks. If she has had previous pregnancies, explain that she may experience afterpains. Present these in relation to their part in returning the uterus to its normal state. Advise her to take the analgesic prescribed by her obstetric care provider to relieve the discomfort accompanying afterpains.

Evaluation

Quality Assurance

Documentation should reflect that frequent and careful assessment and observation was provided for the first hour after delivery. Massage for evacuation of drainage or vigorous massage for uterine atony should be documented with a description of the effectiveness of the procedure. Periodic assessment of the height of the fundus throughout the hospital stay should be documented. An explanation of the reasons for checking the fundus and possible complications after discharge should be reflected.

Infection Control

Careful handwashing should precede and follow care of any client. Because of the presence of open vessel endings in the uterus, it is especially important not to cross-contaminate the newly delivered obstetric client. Instruct the client in the importance of handwashing before perineal care.

Technique Checklist

	YES	NO
Technique explained to the client	___	___
Fundus checked q15min during first hour postpartum	___	___
Fundus checked q ___ during remainder of postpartum stay		
Afterpains experienced	___	___

Complications

Uterine atony ___

Hemorrhage ___

Cramping ___

Excessive afterpains ___

127 Labor and Delivery, Nursing Care During

Overview

Definition

Care given to the family during the preparations for and birth of their baby

Rationale

Provide a warm and caring environment that will contribute to safe delivery of the infant.

Provide an integrated support system to care for expected and unexpected needs of the family.

Contribute to a family-centered birth within the parameters of safety and consideration for the health and welfare of the mother and baby.

Terminology

Dilation of the cervix: Enlargement of the cervical os from a few centimeters in size to 10 cm, which is fully dilated

Effacement: Shortening of the cervical canal from 1 cm or 2 cm in length to a paper-thin length in preparation for birth of the baby

Episiotomy: Surgical enlargement of the external birth canal by incision into the perineum to prevent tearing when the infant is born

Fetus: A child *in utero* from approximately 8 weeks gestation to birth

Infant: A child under 1 year of age

Assessment

Pertinent Anatomy and Physiology

1. See Appendix I: *labor and delivery.*
2. Uterine contractions are a rhythmic, progressive muscular activity of the body of the uterus that results in shortening and thickening of the upper uterine segment and dilation and thinning of the lower segment. The height of the contraction is called the *acme.* The *increment* is an increase in intensity of the contraction; the *decrement* is the release and decrease in intensity. The duration of the contraction is the time from the beginning of the contraction to the end. In active labor, it usually ranges from 45 to 60 seconds. The interval is the time from the end of one contraction until the beginning of the next one. The time between contractions is the time between the beginning of one contraction and the beginning of the next contraction.
3. The first stage of labor is considered the time from the beginning of cervical dilation and effacement until the cervix is fully dilated. Although the time may vary greatly between clients and between multiparas and primiparas, the usual duration of the first stage of labor is 8 to 10 hours. The second stage of labor is from full dilation to the birth of the baby. The usual duration is 2 hours; however, this time may be shorter for a multipara. The third stage involves separation and delivery of the placenta.

Pathophysiological Concepts	See Technique No. 121, Antepartal Care.
Assessment of the Client	1. Assess the client for actual labor. Braxton–Hicks contractions (intermittent, somewhat painful contractions that do not cause dilation of the cervix) often cease after several hours.
	2. Assess for rupture of membranes (see Technique No. 120, Amniotomy). Determine the presence of vaginal discharge ("show" or bleeding). Assess the maternal vital signs. Determine the stage and phase of labor by a vaginal or rectal examination. If the client is having vaginal bleeding or cramping, do *not* perform a vaginal examination.
	3. Assess the status of the client on admission (see Technique No. 118, Admission to the Labor Room).
	4. Assess the knowledge level of the client. Determine if she has attended prenatal classes or has had previous pregnancies. Assess the client and her spouse in relation to their knowledge of breathing and comfort techniques during labor.

Plan

Nursing Objectives	Prepare and assist the client to have a safe and positive labor and delivery process.
	Include the family to the extent desired and possible in the birth of the baby.
	Provide safe, efficient care in such a manner that the individuality of the client and her family is recognized and the uniqueness of their baby is fostered.
	Develop a relationship of trust and confidence with the client and family.
	Provide information and education in the amount and manner best suited to the needs and desires of the family.
	Monitor the condition of the fetus and the mother throughout the labor process.
	Assist in a safe and successful delivery.
Client Preparation	If the mother has attended prenatal classes, she will be better prepared for the labor and delivery process. If she has not, it will be necessary to offer a brief description of what to expect and how she can best help herself and her baby during the birthing process.
Equipment	Prenatal records
	Hospital record forms for the labor and delivery process
	Client identification tags (one attached to the client and one for the baby)
	Clothing container and identification tags
	Thermometer, sphygmomanometer, stethoscope, and fetoscope
	Sterile gloves for vaginal examinations, clean gloves for rectal examinations
	Hospital gown, hip pads, and washcloths
	Clock (with second hand)
	Amniohook
	Skin preparation tray containing cleansing solutions and pads
	Lubricant
	Enema setup

Implementation and Interventions

Procedural Aspects

ACTION	*RATIONALE*
First Stage of Labor	
1. Interact with the client in a caring and concerned manner. Labor and delivery are highly emotional times. The sensitivities of the client and her spouse may be heightened because of their anxiety and anticipation. Always acknowledge the client and her family when entering the room. Show concern for their feelings and needs. Treat them as individuals and recognize that their concerns, no matter how trivial they may seem, are very important to them and deserve whatever time and attention is required for resolution.	Because the birthing process is fairly consistent for most people, there may be a tendency to treat the uncomplicated birth as routine. Remember that the birth is indeed very special to the couple and that they want and deserve to be treated as a unique family.
2. Check the client during the labor process for progress of cervical dilation and effacement. Vaginal examinations also will assist in identifying the presenting part. The examination includes determination of the station and palpation of the sagittal suture. The posterior and anterior fontanelles may also be identified (Fig. 127-1, *A*, *B*, and *C*). Limit these examinations.	The amount of dilation provides an excellent indication of how soon the baby will arrive. Frequent vaginal examinations increase the chances of cross-contamination, however. Vaginal examinations are extremely dangerous in the client who has placenta previa or abruptio placentae.
3. Make periodic assessments of the contractions including their frequency, duration, and quality. To time the contractions, place a hand on the skin of the client's abdomen over the fundus. Press the fingertips lightly into the skin. When the muscle begins to get firm, start timing. Note whether the uterus becomes slightly firm, moderately firm, or very firm. The tightness will reach a peak and begin to relax. When the uterus is completely relaxed, note the time, but keep a hand on the client's abdomen. When the next contraction begins, note the time again. The duration of the contraction is the time from the beginning to the end of the contraction. The time between contractions is the time between the start of one contraction and the start of the next one.	The character and frequency of the contractions will change as the labor progresses.

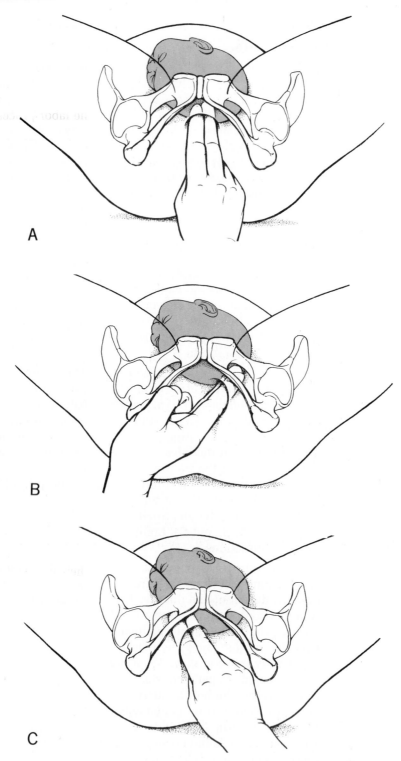

A

B

C

Figure 127.1

ACTION	**RATIONALE**
4. Monitor the client's vital signs throughout the labor process.	Vital signs provide an indicator of the physical status of the mother.
5. Observe the fetal heart tones (FHT) using a fetoscope at least every hour during early labor; every 30 minutes after labor gets under way; and every 15 minutes after dilation reaches 4 cm to 5 cm. An electronic fetal monitor may be used (see Technique No. 125, Fetal Heart Tones).	Fetal heart tones provide a means to monitor the status of the infant during the labor process.
6. The client may receive an enema. Skin preparation may include cleansing with a germicidal soap and possibly shaving all or part of the perineal area. The pubic area may be shaved.	The client strains during the delivery process. If the bowel is not evacuated, involuntary defecation may occur during the delivery. Hair can harbor pathogenic microorganisms; shaving therefore helps to reduce the chance of contamination.
7. Observe for the rupture of the membranes. Note the time of the rupture, the appearance and odor of the amniotic fluid. If the membranes do not rupture spontaneously, the physician may perform an amniotomy (see Technique No. 120, Amniotomy).	The membranes assist in dilating the cervix during early labor.
8. Assist the mother with positioning to promote comfort. Most clients are mobile and active until the cervix is dilated to about 5 cm. If the membranes are not ruptured, the client may be up and about. As labor progresses, the client may remain in bed. Proper positioning will help to relieve some of the discomfort and pressure on the abdominal vessels. Position the client on her side with the uppermost arm and leg propped on pillows (Fig. 127-2).	Positioning to relieve the pressure on the abdominal organs and vessels may enhance the mother's comfort greatly. After the membranes are ruptured, there is a greater chance of infection. The client usually remains in bed thereafter until the baby is born.

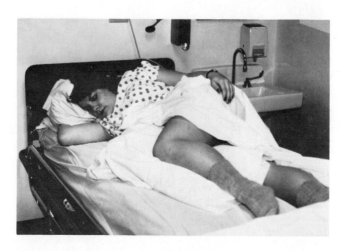

Figure 127.2

ACTION	*RATIONALE*
9. Observe the client's vaginal discharge. The pink, scanty "show" is usually absent during the period of 2-cm to 5-cm dilation. When the cervix has dilated to about 6 cm, there will be a dark, red, mucuos discharge. Change the pads beneath the client's hips as often as necessary to keep her clean and fresh. Explain that the vaginal discharge is expected and indicates that the birth is getting closer.	The vaginal discharge is sloughing of the lining of the uterus as the organ prepares for expulsion of the baby.
10. Assist the client to empty her bladder. Watch for the outline of the bladder above the symphysis pubis when the cervix is dilated to 6 cm to 10 cm. The bladder should be emptied every 2 hours during labor.	The bladder must be emptied. A full bladder retards the progress of labor and increases feelings of discomfort.
11. Encourage the client's spouse or a family member to provide comfort measures. A backrub, wet washcloth, and change of position may enhance comfort greatly (Fig. 127-3). Provide these if the client has no family member with her. Several medications are available for the client to provide relaxation during labor. These will be prescribed by the obstetric care provider, depending on the status of the client and the fetus.	Participation in the labor process may strengthen the family bond and allow the spouse to feel that he is part of the birthing process. Attention to small matters of comfort provide distraction and support for the laboring client.

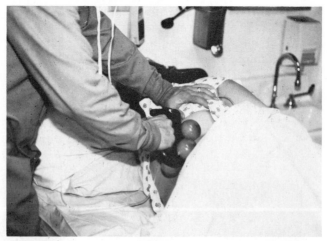

Figure 127.3

Second Stage of Labor

1. Cervical dilation will be complete upon vaginal examination. The perinuem may be bulging. The contractions are more frequent and cause greater discomfort. The client may show signs of frustration, fear, loss of control, total preoccupation with contractions, irritability, and signs of exhaustion. She may also experience nausea, profuse perspiration, a need to defecate, pallor, and headache. The client may have difficulty following instructions and may be vague in communicating. Reassurance and reinforcement of instructions is essential at this time.

   The head or presenting part will descend during this stage of labor. Total preoccupation with self and the labor process is expected.

2. Encourage the client about effective pushing and breathing techniques (Fig. 127-4). With each contraction, instruct the client to take a deep, cleansing breath, then take a short breath in and out. Instruct her to take another deep breath, hold it, and then push for 10 seconds. This process should be repeated until the contraction ends.

   Pushing with the contractions helps the uterine muscle to guide the infant into and through the birth canal.

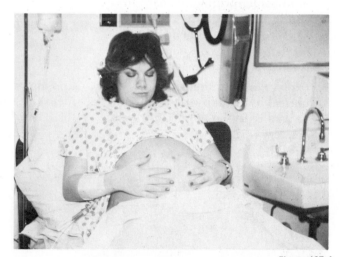

Figure 127.4

3. Place the client in semi-Fowler's position, with legs abducted, hands grasping the legs behind the knees, chin on the chest. If the upper part of the body is elevated about 30°, the client can bear down more effectively. Drape the client.

   Proper positioning, using the principles of direct pressure and gravity, can facilitate the birthing process.

ACTION

RATIONALE

4. Involve the father in the labor process as much as possible. He may coach about breathing techniques. He should be reminded that any unwillingness or inability to follow his suggestions or irritability on the part of the mother is due to her preoccupation with the labor and should not be taken personally. If the father can be prepared for such reactions before the labor, he will be better able to help and understand the mother's needs as the labor progresses.

Feelings of frustration and anxiety are common during labor. The father may feel helpless to assist the mother and fearful of her ability to withstand the rigors of the birthing process. He should be reassured and made to feel that he has an important role in the birth.

5. Take the client to the delivery room early enough to prepare her for the birth but not so early that she will have to labor for a long time on the delivery table. The proper time usually is determined by the duration of the other phases of labor, previous labor experiences, and the pattern of the labor. For the multipara, transport to the labor room usually occurs after dilation of the cervix. For the primipara, it is usually when the head of the infant is visible at the introitus (crowning). Remain in close contact with the client in the delivery room by touch and speaking softly. Offer continual reassurance and encouragement.

The delivery room offers the advantage of a sterile atmosphere and the latest equipment for the safety of the mother and the infant. It lacks the comfort and intimacy of the labor room, however.

6. Explain to the father, if he is present at the delivery, about how he can assist the mother during the delivery (Fig. 127-5).

It is important to the formation and identification of the family unit that the father be involved in the birth.

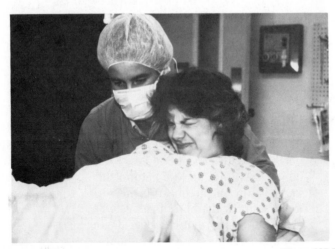

Figure 127.5

ACTION

7. Provide immediate attention to the infant. Position the infant to one side and ascertain that the airway is patent. Use a suction bulb to clear mucus from the infant's mouth and nose. Dry the infant and record the Apgar score (see Technique No. 146, Neonatal Assessment, Initial). Cover the infant and allow the parents to see and hold their baby. Identify the infant according to hospital and state requirements (Figs. 127-6, 127-7). If the father is not present in the delivery room, notify him as soon as possible of the sex and status of his baby and the condition of the mother.

RATIONALE

Attention to the needs of the baby is important. The infant must be aerated and warmed during the first moments outside of the warmth and security of the womb. Make every effort to maintain the identity of the family unit by including the father as much as possible. The bond between the mother and infant appears to be strengthened by early contact between them.

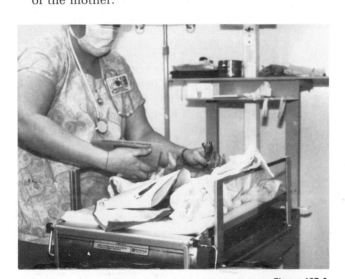

Figure 127.6

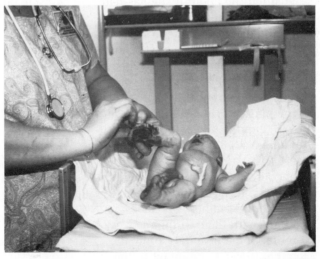

Figure 127.7

ACTION	*RATIONALE*
Third Stage of Labor	
1. Prepare a sample of the cord blood for analysis by the laboratory. Send the specimen to the laboratory as soon as possible.	Fetal problems may be detected early if the cord blood is analyzed. In addition, if there is an Rh incompatibility, the mother must receive RhoGam within the first 72 hours after birth to decrease sensitization.
2. Assist the mother in the expulsion of the placenta by telling her when to bear down. If she is unable to do so because of anesthesia, apply gentle pressure on the fundus. Be sure that the fundus is firm and contracted before applying any manual pressure. Oxytocic drugs may be used after the placenta has separated.	Pressure assists the uterus in expelling the placenta, which should be separated completely from the uterine wall. Oxytocic drugs stimulate the uterus to contract and help to prevent hemorrhage.
3. Examine the placenta carefully to ascertain if any fragments may have been retained in the uterus.	Retained placental fragments or blood clots can cause hemorrhage
4. Assist the obstetric care provider in examining the client's perineum by supplying new sterile gloves and sterile water to rinse the perineum. If an episiotomy was performed it will be sutured at this time.	The vagina, cervix, and perineum are examined closely for hematomas, placental fragments, and lacerations.
5. If the mother will not be breast-feeding her infant, administer an antilactogenic hormone as prescribed.	Antilactogenic hormones discourage the production of milk and decrease the discomfort of the breasts during the postpartum period.
6. Assist the mother to the transport cart. She should be clean and warm. Apply a sterile perineal pad to absorb the vaginal discharge. Position the client if she has had anesthetic and is unable to position herself. Continue to observe the client during the next hour for return of function if she has had anesthetic. Observe carefully for continued contraction of the uterine muscle (see Technique No. 126, Fundus, Checking, and Technique No. 132, Postpartum Recovery Care). Continue to support and encourage interaction between the parents. If the infant is stable, the mother and father may keep the infant with them in the recovery room. Some hospitals allow the father to carry the infant to the nursery.	The first hour after delivery has been called the most hazardous of the entire pregnancy. The threat of hemorrhage from relaxation of the uterine muscle demands continual observation of the fundus. This particular period following the birth is also an important time to establish the identity of the family as an entity that now includes a new member.

ACTION

Special Modifications

1. The location of the actual birth will vary with the wishes of the family and the facilities of the hospital. If the client is having a family-centered birth, she may have labored in the birthing room, where her baby also will be delivered (Fig. 127-8). Many hospitals have homelike suites that allow family members to be together during the birth. Nursing intervention is minimal unless there are complications.

RATIONALE

Family-centered births in a birthing room allows the benefits of a home birth along with the safety features of a hospital delivery.

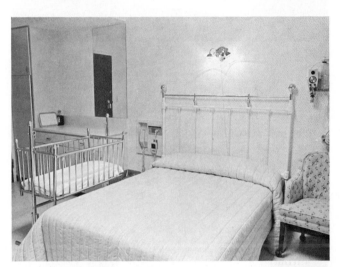

Figure 127.8

2. The birthing chair may be used for the actual birth of the baby. It allows a natural sitting position for delivery of the infant. The chair will tilt backward after delivery for the comfort of the mother and to facilitate the completion of the labor process (Fig. 127-9 to 127-11).

The birthing chair allows the natural force of gravity to facilitate the birth of the infant. It also promotes the natural position for birth.

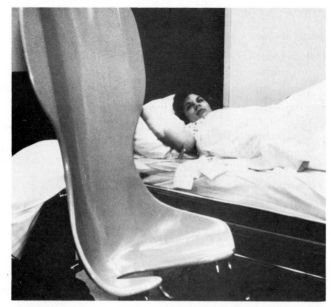

Figure 127.9

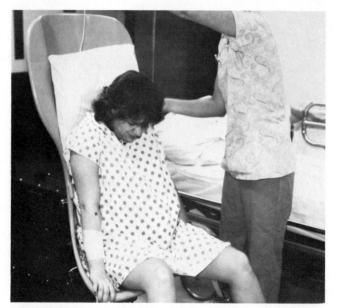

Figure 127.10

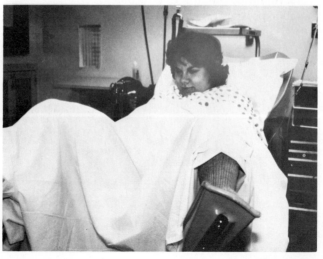

Figure 127.11

Communicative Aspects

OBSERVATIONS

1. Observe the client and family during the labor and delivery period for signs of anxiety, fear and apprehension. Offer reassurance and support during the process.

2. Observe the client for amount of anxiety and discomfort experienced during labor. The amount of discomfort will depend on a number of factors, including general emotional makeup, coping mechanisms, cultural expectations of the birthing process, instructions and preparations for the birth, and physical conditions. The amount of discomfort is not necessarily proportional to the force of contractions or the duration of the labor. The amount of discomfort varies widely from person to person and should be addressed in relation to the individual in labor. Generalizations and comparisons in regard to pain tolerance should be avoided. Pain medication should be administered in accordance with the wishes of the client and obstetric care provider.

3. Observe for deviations from the normal birthing process. Immediately identify potential problems such as unusual abdominal shape, unusual presenting part, arrest of dilation, or arrest of descent of presenting part. Meconium-stained amniotic fluid may indicate fetal distress, although this is expected when the presentation is breech. Presentation of the fetus' foot or the presence of the umbilical cord on the perineum are indications of complications. Communicate to the obstetric care provider any bright red bleeding that does not clot. Fetal distress is indicated when the fetal heart rate is below 120 or above 160 beats/min. Changes in FHT should be closely monitored and reported.

4. Check the blood pressure every 4 hours if it is in the normal range for this client. If it is higher or lower than it has been during the pregnancy, monitor blood pressure every hour or even more frequently. Report elevations above 140 (systolic) and 90 (diastolic) to the physician or care provider. Examine the client for swelling of the hands, feet, and face. A urine test for albumin may also help to determine if the client is suffering from pregnancy-induced hypertension (PIH).

5. Temperature, pulse, and respirations should be checked every 4 hours until after the membranes rupture. They should then be checked every hour. Elevated temperature may indicate that the client is not receiving enough fluids. An intravenous infusion may alleviate this problem. Note the time of the rupture of the membranes because premature rupture may predispose to infection.

6. Observe the contractions for frequency, duration, and effectiveness. Determine if the client is experiencing cervical dilation by vaginal or rectal examination. Contractions should be assessed every hour during early labor and every 15 minutes during the active phase of labor.

7. Observe the amount and type of vaginal discharge. Record the time of the observations and the color and odor of the discharge. When the membranes rupture, observe the time, in addition to the color, amount, and odor of the fluid.

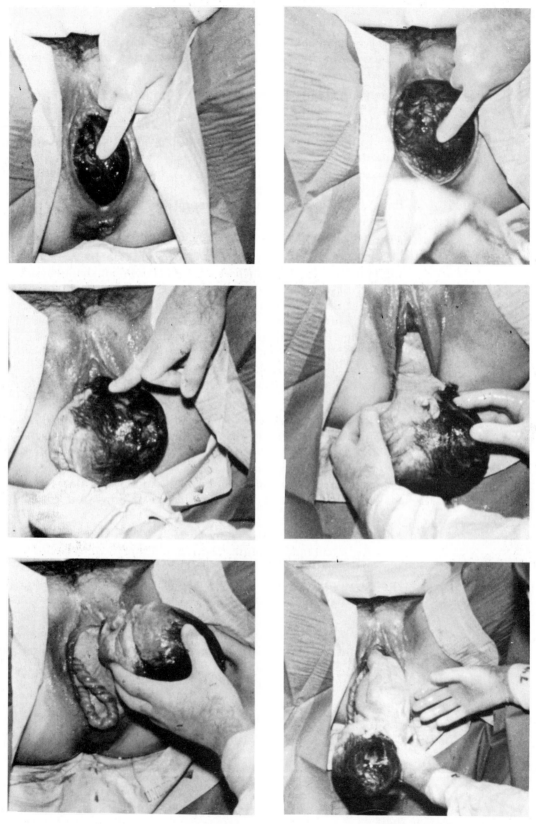

Figure 127.12 (continued opposite)

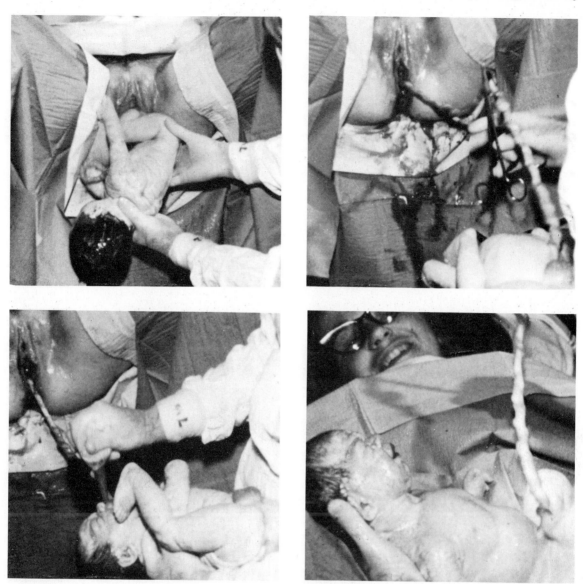

Figure 127.12

8. Observe the mother for impending birth. It is a fine art to get the client to the labor room at the right time. If crowning has occurred or the client feels the need to push, she should be in the delivery room. Once the multipara is fully dilated, birth usually takes place very shortly thereafter. In primiparas it usually takes longer to expel the baby. Other signs of impending birth are more frequent contractions of longer duration, increase in bloody show, rupture of the membranes, increasing restlessness, nausea, bulging perineum, pressure and pain the lower back and rectal area, and an uncontrollable urge to bear down.

9. Observe for the expected progress of the labor. Internal rotation will occur within the birth canal. In vertex presentation there is crowning, delivery of the head, external rotation, then delivery of the shoulders, anterior then posterior, with the entire body following (Fig. 127-12).

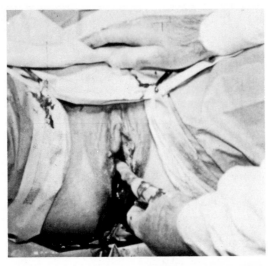

Figure 127.13

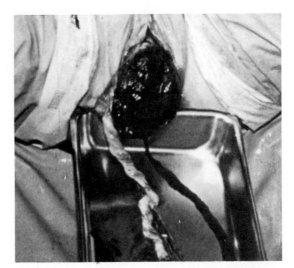

Figure 127.14

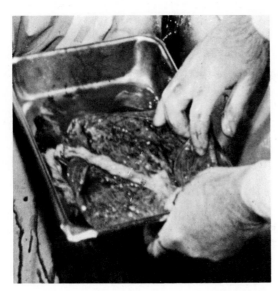

Figure 127.15

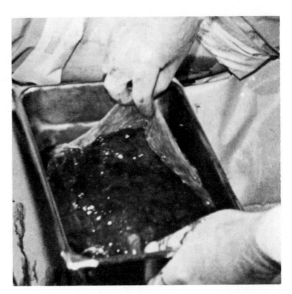

Figure 127.16

10. Observe the client for the separation of the placenta. There is usually a gush of blood before the expulsion of the placenta (Fig. 127-13). The fundus of the uterus rises in the abdomen when the placenta is in the vagina, and the cord lengthens (Fig. 127-14). Observe the placenta to see that it is intact and to ensure that no fragments have been retained (Figs. 127-15, 127-16). Observe the umbilical cord to see that there are two arteries and one vein.

CHARTING

Each hospital will have individual records for recording the progress of the labor and delivery. Make sure that the records are complete and that all information requested is provided. Record any deviations from normal.

DATE/TIME	OBSERVATIONS	SIGNATURE
9/18 1430	Vaginal examination performed after 2 hr of early labor. Cervical dilation approximately 2 cm. Effacement 75%. Small amount of pink discharge. Contractions q9min, approximately 20 sec. Membranes intact. FHT 138. Ambulating in hall with husband.	D. Perez RN

Discharge Planning Aspects

CLIENT AND FAMILY EDUCATION

1. If the client has had no prenatal instruction and has not had previous pregnancies, explain what will happen as clearly as time will permit. Tell the mother what to expect and how she can help herself. Explain to her spouse how he can provide help and support. If there is time, explain about breathing techniques. Offer reassurance and support.

2. Use the labor and delivery time to reinforce to the parents their new identify as a family unit, which now includes an additional member. Offer input that recognizes the infant as a member of the family. Allow the parents to listen to the FTH if possible. Encourage touch and sharing to make this a positive, family-centered experience.

3. If the mother will go home the same day that her baby is born, she will need additional information about caring for herself and her infant. In addition, she will be exhausted from the labor process and excited about the addition to her family. Teaching must be succinct and meaningful. Explain about possible complications. Tell her how to care for her baby. Offer as much of the information in written form as possible so that she will have it available for future reference.

REFERRALS

If the parents are concerned about family planning, they may be referred to local family planning clinics or counselors. If the client takes her baby home within the first 24 hours after delivery, she may benefit from a home visit by a visiting nurse association or home health agency in the next few days. If the parents are bewildered about caring for their new baby, they may be referred to parenting classes.

Evaluation

Quality Assurance

Documentation should follow the protocol set by the hospital. The forms and documents required by the state also must be completed. The forms should provide a progressive record of the labor process, including the time of arrival, status of the labor, and statement regarding prenatal instructions and care. The time and observations of rupture of the membranes should be noted. A progressive monitoring of the vital signs of the mother and the heart tones of the fetus should be reflected. Instructions given to the parents should be recorded. If electronic fetal monitoring is used, some means of historical preservation of all of the graphic record should be arranged. A record of the birth, including exact time and sex of infant, should be available. Monitoring during anesthesia should be reflected. Resuscitation efforts on the baby's behalf and Apgar scores should be reflected in the records. Careful monitoring of the mother for the first 1 to 2 hours after delivery must be in evidence. The chart also should show evidence that complications were recognized and actions were taken to prevent or reverse them, such as monitoring the fetal and maternal status during labor, checking the placenta, analysis of maternal and fetal blood, and inspection of the umbilical cord for proper number of vessels. Discharge instructions should be reflected with an assessment of the degree of understanding exhibited by the parents.

Infection Control

1. After the rupture of the membranes, the chance of infection is increased. The mother is usually kept in bed. All vaginal examinations are performed under strict sterile conditions.

2. Any equipment that comes in contact with the mother should be clean. If the equipment comes in contact with the birth canal, it should be sterile. Careful handwashing should be done before and after caring for the client in labor.

3. The delivery takes place under sterile conditions in the delivery suite. If family-centered birthing is done, the birth takes place in the birthing rooms. The equipment in the rooms is clean. Sterile equipment may be used for receiving and handling the baby. If sutures are required to repair the episiotomy or lacerations of the perineum, this is done using sterile technique. The emphasis is on involving the family in the birth; however, the prevention of cross-contamination of the mother and infant are still important considerations.

Technique Checklist

	YES	NO
Client and spouse had prenatal instructions regarding labor and delivery	_____	_____
Explanations offered	_____	_____
Records of		
Vaginal examinations	_____	_____
Rectal examinations	_____	_____
FHT	_____	_____
Maternal vital signs	_____	_____
Amniotomy	_____	_____
Contractions	_____	_____
Duration of labor _____		
To delivery room at _____		
Infant born at _____		
Father attended delivery	_____	_____
Delivered in		
Labor room _____		
Birthing room _____		
Delivery room _____		
Birthing chair _____		
Other _____		
Record of oxytocic drugs on chart	_____	_____
Placenta delivered at _____		
Intact	_____	_____
Antilactogenic hormone administered	_____	_____
Cord blood sample to laboratory	_____	_____
Umbilical cord inspected for proper		
Number of vessels	_____	_____
Vaginal flow	_____	_____
Apgar score		
1 min _____		
5 min _____		

128   Labor, Induction of

Overview

Definition

The process of starting labor by artificial means. In some situations, augmentation is used to intensify a labor that is progressing too slowly. Methods include intravenous administration of a dilute solution of an oxytocic agent or artificial rupture of the membranes (amniotomy).

Medical indications for induction of labor include primary uterine inertia, severe preeclampsia, prolonged pregnancy (>43 weeks), prolonged rupture of membranes, diabetes or severe iso-immunization, a fetus with a hemolytic disease, multigravidas who have a history of precipitate labor, and clients who must travel great distances to the hospital.

Rationale

Safeguard the mother and fetus.

Prevent complications which might interfere with the survival of the mother and/or the fetus.

Terminology

Cephalopelvic disproportion: The fetus' head is too large to fit safely through the natural birth canal because of the diameter of the pelvis.

Fetal heart rate patterns:

Normal: 120 to 160 beats/min

Bradycardia (fetal): under 100 beats/min

Tachycardia, marked (fetal): over 180 beats/min

Tachycardia, mild (fetal): 160 to 180 beats/min

Variability: the fluctuations that may occur that may range from 5 to 10 beats/min

Oxytocic agent: A drug that stimulates uterine contractions

Uterine inertia: The absence of uterine contractions during labor

Assessment

Pertinent Anatomy and Physiology

1. See Appendix I: *labor and delivery* (see also Technique No. 127, Labor and Delivery, Nursing Care During).

2. For a successful induction of labor, certain conditions are necessary. The cervix should be soft and at least partially effaced, or thinned. Some dilation of the cervix should be evidenced. The fetal head already should be settled into the pelvis.

3. Oxytocin is a hormone synthesized in the hypothalamus and transported to the pituitary, where it is released into the bloodstream. Natural oxytocin is released on stimulation of the nipples and dilation of the cervix and vagina. Intravenous oxytocin has a half-life of 3 minutes; therefore, blood levels drop quickly when the infusion is stopped.

Pathophysiological Concepts

1. Induction of labor is contraindicated in certain conditions. When spontaneous labor would be dangerous to the client and the fetus, as in cephalopelvic disproportion, induction is contraindicated. Women who have had previous cesarean births or bleeding during their pregnancy usually are not candidates for induction of labor. Women who are experiencing abnormal fetal presentation, overdistention of the uterus, or multiple pregnancies are not considered for induction of labor. There is increased risk of uterine rupture with an overlydistended uterus.

2. Oxytocin is a potentially dangerous medication that has been known to cause uterine rupture, hyperstimulation of the uterus, which causes hypoxia of the fetus, and abruptio placentae. To prevent these complications, the infusion must be administered carefully under controlled conditions.

Assessment of the Client

1. Assess the obstetric history of the client. Determine if she has had precipitate deliveries or any complications with delivering children previously. Assess for previous cesarean sections, noting reasons for them.

2. Assess the health status of the client. Determine if she has any chronic illnesses, such as diabetes, that might make her a candidate for induction. Determine the state of her present health. Assess vital signs for baseline measurements. Determine if she has had hypertensive problems during her pregnancy.

Plan

Nursing Objectives

Support the client throughout the procedure and ensuing labor and delivery.

Provide continuous monitoring of the fetal heart tones (FHT).

Provide information and reassurance to the client about what is happening and why.

Maintain close contact with family members.

Client Preparation

1. Explain the procedure to the client and her family. Provide enough information so that they will have a basic understanding of what will happen and the dynamics involved. Be available to answer any questions they may have.

2. Assist the client into a position of comfort. Provide pillows for positioning. Ask her to empty her bladder.

3. Prepare the client for manual rupture of the membranes, if this method of inducing labor will be used (see Technique No. 120, Amniotomy).

4. A baseline observation of fetal heart rate and uterine contractions should be made for 30 minutes before induction of labor. The method of preference is using an electronic fetal monitor with a uterine catheter to determine pressure. If this is unavailable, manual assessment of contractions may be done along with auscultation of FHT.

Equipment

Stethoscope and sphygmomanometer

Fetoscope or electronic fetal monitor

IV tray and fluids

Volume infusion pump

Watch (with second hand)

Sterile gloves for vaginal examination

Amniohook

Implementation and Interventions

Procedural Aspects

ACTION

1. Perform venipuncture with a catheter large enough to provide an adequate vehicle for administration of fluids (Fig. 128-1).

RATIONALE

The initial IV bag will be for hydration of the client. It usually will be continued after the oxytocic agent is discontinued.

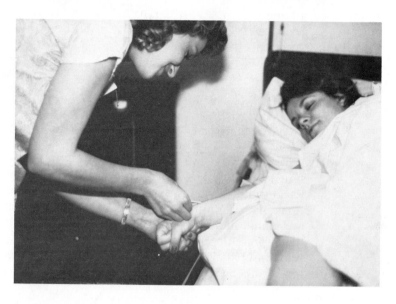

Figure 128.1

2. Prepare a second IV bag containing the oxytocic agent. The exact drug, dosage, and method of administration will be ordered. The second IV bag is then attached to the first by means of a piggyback infusion system. An infusion pump is applied to the oxytocic agent infusion to ensure the rate prescribed by the obstetric care provider. This rate is increased or decreased depending on the quantity and quality of the contractions. Rate modifications are prescribed by the care provider or by hospital policy.

The oxytocic agent must be well regulated to prevent overinfusion, a situation that could be catastrophic. The exact dosage and rate must be maintained at all times. Once the contractions are well under way, the infusion may be stopped to see if the labor will continue naturally.

3. Assess the fetal heart tones continually by electronic fetal monitoring during the oxytocin administration (Fig. 128-2). Any deviation in FHT or the appearance of contractions lasting more than 90 seconds indicates complications. The oxytocic agent should be stopped immediately until the situation has been resolved. An alternate solution, such as 5% dextrose in water, should be ready to infuse whenever the oxytocic agent must be stopped.

The FHT offer an excellent indication of the status of the fetus. Deviations may indicate fetal distress. Uterine contractions usually last from 30 to 60 seconds. Prolonged contractions may indicate that the dosage is too high or the infusion is running too rapidly.

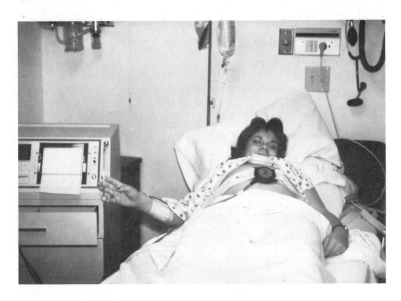

Figure 128.2

ACTION

4. Reassure the client as the contractions increase in frequency and duration. Monitor the client's blood pressure, pulse, and contractions. Observe the abdomen for tenderness or rigidity. Watch for vaginal bleeding.

Special Modifications

Slow progression of labor may occur. If the membranes have not yet ruptured, labor may be enhanced by changing the client's position frequently and encouraging her to walk. Relaxation techniques may also help. Assist the mother to take a warm shower, and provide a supportive, positive environment. Analgesic medications may help. Remind the client to empty her bladder at least every 2 hours. If these techniques do not promote the progress of the labor, administration of oxytocic drugs may be indicated. If the labor continues to be ineffective, cesarean section may be necessary.

RATIONALE

Reassurance and support may help the client to work with the contractions to make the labor progress smoothly. Abdominal tenderness and vaginal bleeding may indicate that the placenta has separated prematurely.

Labor may be slowed because of inappropriate use of analgesia, ineffective contractions, or inappropriate dilation of the cervix, which may not be ready for dilation. Other causes may be cephalopelvic disproportion or fetal malposition. Every effort should be made to allow the labor to progress naturally. A full bladder can inhibit labor and interfere with delivery.

Communicative Aspects

OBSERVATIONS

1. Watch for the danger signs that indicate that the oxytocic infusion should be discontinued and the physician notified. These include an increase or decrease in blood pressure with an increase or decrease in pulse, fetal hyperactivity, deviations in FHT, meconium-stained amniotic fluid, and prolonged contractions.

2. Observe for the desired response to the oxytocic drug. The desired response is initiation of moderate-to-strong contractions, lasting from 45 to 60 seconds and recurring every 2 to 3 minutes. The uterus should be relaxed in the interval between contractions.

3. Monitor the maternal pulse and blood pressure every 15 minutes after the initiation of oxytocin therapy. For comparison, a baseline value for each should be taken before the drug is started. This value is also a part of the assessment of the client's suitability for induction of labor.

4. Monitor the FHT continuously during the induction process. At the first sign of fetal distress, discontinue the oxytocin and evaluate fetal status carefully. Electronic fetal monitoring is the method of choice.

5. Monitor intake and output carefully on the client receiving oxytocin. This drug has a mild antidiuretic effect therefore fluid retention is possible.

6. Observe the infusion site to ensure that venous cannulation is maintained. It is important that the IV solution not infiltrate because absorption of the oxytocic agent from the tissue is difficult to control and assess. The IV catheter must remain patent. An infusion pump is used to ensure that the proper amount is administered over the desired period.

CHARTING

DATE/TIME	OBSERVATIONS	SIGNATURE
4/10 1630	Induction of labor started. Fetal monitor has been in place for 35 min. Baseline FHT 148. No contractions at this time. Cervix 2 cm dilation, 50% effaced. Membranes intact. Voided 250 ml clear urine. Has been ambulatory in hall for 2 hours. IV started with #18 ga Angiocath in right wrist. 1000 ml D5W infusing at keep-open rate. Oxytocin 10 units in 1000 cc D5W started to run at 5ml/min; infusion pump applied. T 98.2° F, P 78, R 20, B/P 120/72. Relaxed in bed, side-lying with pillows for support. No contractions.	M. Brown RN

Discharge Planning Aspects

CLIENT AND FAMILY EDUCATION

1. Explain to the client and her family why the induction is being done and how it will help the mother and baby. Explain induction of labor as being an adjunct to the natural birthing process. Answer any questions the family may have and reassure them about the procedure. Explain the danger signals to watch for, and enlist the assistance of the client and her family in reporting any untoward effects.

2. Tell the client how she can assist in progression of the labor if labor is slower than expected. Recommend comfort measures and other suggestions that may relax the client and allay any anxiety or tension. Tell her the reason for emptying her bladder every hour. Encourage her family to ambulate with the client. Demonstrate comfort measures such as backrubs and propping with pillows.

3. Prepare the family for the possibility of surgical intervention if the induction does not stimulate labor. Keep the information positive, stressing the safety of the mother and the fetus. Cesarean section can cause a variety of mixed emotions, not the least of which are fear and guilt. Keep the parents informed about the progress of the labor.

4. If an electronic fetal monitor is used, explain to the parents what information is being gathered and why. Allow them to be involved in the process and encourage them to associate the graphic tracings with the infant who will soon be part of their family.

Evaluation

Quality Assurance

Most hospitals require documentation of the need for induction of labor. Some require consultation and collaboration regarding the need for the procedure. Check each particular hospital's protocols to determine the documentation required. Documentation should include an assessment of the position, presentation, and status of the fetus. Dilation and consistency of the cervix before induction should be noted. The estimated gestational age and size of the fetus and expected date of confinement also should be reflected. Any tests for maturity should be reported on the chart. The process of induction should be recorded from the time of venipuncture or amniotomy through the birth. Any complications of induction should be noted, with notation about actions taken to reverse or report the problems.

Infection Control

1. Amniotomy is puncture of the sac in which for the past 9 months, the fetus has been protected from invasive organisms. Because the chance of infection is greatly enhanced after rupture of the membranes, the mother usually stays in bed. All vaginal procedures are performed using sterile technique.

2. Administration of oxytocic drugs is done intravenously using sterile technique. Any break in the skin is a potential entry point for microorganisms. A sterile dressing should be placed over the IV site. When the piggyback infusion containing the oxytocin is attached, the area of insertion must be aseptically prepared to reduce the chance of introducing microorganisms into the bloodstream.

3. Careful handwashing is done before and after any care given to obstetric clients.

Technique Checklist

	YES	NO
Procedure explained to client and spouse	_____	_____
Prenatal history available	_____	_____
Indication for induction or augmentation		
Preeclampsia	_____	_____
Primary uterine inertia	_____	_____
Prolonged pregnancy	_____	_____
Prolonged rupture of membranes	_____	_____
Hemolytic disease of fetus	_____	_____
Slow progression of labor	_____	_____
Other _____		
Type of induction		
Amniotomy	_____	_____
Administration of oxytocin	_____	_____
Baseline values obtained		
Fetal heart rate (30 min)	_____	_____
Maternal blood pressure	_____	_____
Maternal pulse	_____	_____
Progressive documentation of		
FHT	_____	_____
Maternal vital signs	_____	_____
Contractions	_____	_____
Dilation and effacement	_____	_____
Outcome of induction		
Successful labor and delivery	_____	_____
Cesarean section	_____	_____

Lochia, Observation of

Overview

Definition

Lochia is the discharge from the birth canal occurring after childbirth.

Rationale

Check the progress of postpartum healing and the involutionary process of the uterus.

Identify complications as early as possible.

Terminology

Decidua: The name given to the endometrium, or lining of the uterus, during pregnancy

Involution: The retrogression of the female reproductive organs to the normal, nonpregnant state

Assessment

Pertinent Anatomy and Physiology

1. Lochia is the natural discharge that follows the birth of a baby. Lochia rubra is the initial discharge occurring for the first 3 or 4 days after birth. It is a reddish color and consists of blood with a small amount of mucus, particles of decidua, and cellular debris that escape from the placental site. Lochia serosa is the discharge that appears about the 3rd or 4th day after birth and lasts for about 2 weeks. This drainage is reddish brown owing to the presence of exudate from the healing surfaces within the uterus and the breakdown of remaining debris. The discharge then turns into lochia alba at about the 14th day after birth. This discharge is marked by decreasing amounts of thinner, almost-colorless secretions. Lochia alba may persist for as long as 6 weeks after birth. Lochia provides evidence of how well the uterus is regenerating. Although the amount varies from client to client, the usual amount ranges around 200 ml to 300 ml total for the postpartum period. Mothers who have cesarean sections or who nurse their babies tend to have less lochia.

Pathophysiological Concepts

1. The presence of frank, fresh bleeding from the vagina is *not* normal. Neither is lochia containing large clots. Excessive lochia may indicate a relaxed uterus. Absence of lochia may indicate infection.

2. Foul-smelling lochia indicates complications. It may be due to infection or retention of clots. A retained sponge or packing also may cause unpleasant odors.

Assessment of the Client

1. Note the client's delivery date. Determine if the characteristics of the lochia are consistent with what would be expected for the length of time postpartum.

2. Assess the client's understanding of what lochia is and how it should progress during the postpartum period.

Plan

Nursing Objectives

Educate the client about the expected pattern of vaginal discharge after delivery and measures to take if unexpected patterns emerge.

Teach the client self-care of the perineum, episiotomy, and rectum.

Teach the proper technique of changing the perineal pad.

Assist the client to understand the need for frequent change of the perineal pad.

Recognize and report any signs of postpartum complications.

Client Preparation

1. Explain to the client about the vaginal discharge and the pattern it will assume.
2. The client usually will be most comfortable in the dorsal recumbent position when the lochia is checked. She should empty her bladder before the lochia is checked if the uterus will be massaged.

Equipment

Perineal pad
Washcloth

Implementation and Interventions

Procedural Aspects

ACTION	RATIONALE
1. Observe the lochia after delivery and at least every 15 minutes during the fourth stage of labor, that is, the initial hour after birth. Observe the amount and characteristics. The client should not saturate more than three perineal pads in a 15 min period. More discharge than this is considered abnormal and should be called to the attention of the obstetric care provider.	Excessive discharge during the initial hour after birth may indicate hemorrhage, a severe postpartum complication.
2. Remove the perineal pad to observe the lochia. If the client is unable to do so herself, cleanse the perineal area with a warm washcloth from front to back and apply a fresh perineal pad. Attach the pad to the belt in the front first, then in the back.	Application of a clean pad and cleansing the perineum is an excellent habit for the client to form while in the hospital. She should be taught to cleanse from front to back to avoid contamination from the rectal area.

Communicative Aspects

OBSERVATIONS

1. Observe the amount of lochia. Lochia should not be excessive. Saturation of more than three pads in 15 minutes is considered excessive. Lochia should not be nonexistent during the first 3 weeks postpartum, however. Absence of lochia may indicate infection or blockage of the cervix.
2. Observe the odor of the lochia. Lochia should not have an offensive odor. The characteristic odor is described as fleshy. Report any foul-smelling discharge.

3. Observe the characteristics of the lochia. There should not be large pieces of tissue in the lochia. This may be indicative of retained placental fragments and should be reported at once. Once the lochia has progressed from serosa to alba, it should not become dark again.

CHARTING

DATE/TIME	OBSERVATIONS	SIGNATURE
11/8 2100	Lochia rubra, saturating 1 pad every 2 to 3 hours, no clots. Perineal area cleaned and sterile pad reapplied. Need for cleansing from front to back explained. Expected changes in the lochia explained to client. Possible complications explained, with suggestions about when she should notify her physician about problems. B/P 118/66, P 20. Ambulatory in hall. To be discharged in the morning. ——————————————	M. Brown RN

Discharge Planning Aspects

CLIENT AND FAMILY EDUCATION

1. Explain the expected pattern of lochia to the client, as well as what to do if deviations from this pattern occur. She should understand the signs and symptoms of complications and should know how and to whom these should be reported. Explain the need for frequent changing of perineal pads using proper technique.

2. The amount of discharge tends to increase when the client becomes more active. When she gets out of bed for the first time after delivery, there may be a heavy discharge. She should be warned about this so that she will not think that something is wrong. She also should be told that the amount will increase when she is very active and conversely may be scant during inactive times, such as at night.

3. Alert the client to the hazards of using internal padding, such as tampons, to contain the lochia. This type of pad may cause trauma to the sensitive, healing tissue and may predispose to infection.

Evaluation

Quality Assurance

Documentation should contain periodic assessment of the appearance of the lochia. Explanations to the client about what to expect during the postpartum period regarding changes in the amount and color of the lochia should be reflected. The chart should contain evidence that the nurse knew possible complications and took measures to recognize, reverse, and report them.

Infection Control

1. Careful handwashing should precede and follow any care given to the postpartum client.

2. Cleansing the perineal area from front to back reduces the risk of contamination from the contaminated rectal area to the perineal area, which is considered clean. The perineal pad should not be applied to the back and pulled across the rectal area to be fastened in the front because of the possibility of contamination. It is fastened in the front first.

3. Moist, dark environments favor the colonization and proliferation of microorganisms. The pad should be changed frequently to prevent the growth of microorganisms. Advise the client to change the perineal pad every 4 hours, or more frequently, as needed.

Technique Checklist

	YES	NO
Process of lochia discharge explained to client	_____	_____
Client vaginal discharge checked q15min during initial hour after delivery	_____	_____
Periodic monitoring of amount and characteristics of lochia during hospitalization	_____	_____
Explanation of how to apply perineal pad	_____	_____
Client understands that lochia will change and decrease	_____	_____
Possible complications explained	_____	_____
Client understands when to notify her obstetric care provider	_____	_____

130   Perineal Light

Overview

Definition

Application of warmth to the perineal area with a heat lamp

Rationale

Provide localized warmth to promote the client's comfort.

Aid in the healing process of the episiotomy or laceration by keeping the perineal area dry and reducing edema.

Stimulate circulation to the perineal area to enhance the healing process.

Assessment

Pertinent Anatomy and Physiology

1. The area between the vagina and the anus is called the perineal body. It is composed of a mass of muscular and fibrous tissue that is capable of great stretching during childbirth.

2. An *episiotomy* is an incision made into the perineal body during birth to prevent uncontrolled laceration. The incision is made with blunt scissors. The episiotomy may be midline (directed straight back toward the anus), right mediolateral, or left mediolateral (Fig. 130-1).

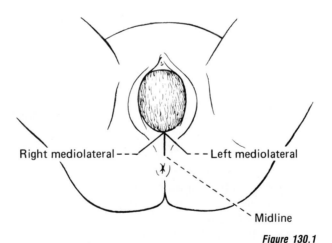

Right mediolateral ‑ ‑ ‑   ‑ ‑ Left mediolateral

Midline

Figure 130.1

Pathophysiological Concepts

Perineal laceration occurs when the perineal area is torn as it stretches to accommodate delivery of the baby. A first-degree laceration is one that does not involve muscle. Second-degree laceration involves the muscles of the perineal body but does not include the rectal sphincter. A third-degree laceration extends to include the rectal sphincter. A fourth-degree laceration extends into the rectum itself.

Assessment of the Client	1. Assess the extent of tissue involvement in the laceration or the episiotomy. Determine the state of healing and the condition of the perineal area.
	2. Assess the ability of the client to lie in the dorsal recumbent position with the knees bent. If there is a great deal of swelling, this position may be very uncomfortable.
	3. Assess the allergy history of the client if an anesthetizing spray is ordered for relief of local discomfort. These sprays may cause allergic reaction.

Plan

Nursing Objectives	Facilitate healing and comfort by the use of localized heat measures.
	Promote the safety of the client by proper placement and observation of the light during treatment.
	Prevent cross-contamination by thorough cleaning of the lights between client uses.
Client Preparation	1. Explain the procedure to the client. Be sure she understands why the light is used. She should know how the light will be positioned. Explain safety precautions.
	2. Cleanse the client's perineal area thoroughly before using the perineal light. Wash the area with a clean washcloth and warm water to remove any drainage, exudate, or anesthetizing spray.
	3. Allow the client to empty her bladder before beginning the procedure. A distended bladder may cause discomfort.
Equipment	Perineal light
	Padding if the light has stirrups
	Screen
	Perineal pad
	Medicated spray (if prescribed)

Implementation and Interventions

Procedural Aspects

ACTION	RATIONALE
1. Assist the client into a position of comfort flat on her back with her knees flexed. Place her heels on the bed or in the appropriate position on the perineal light base. If the perineal light has stirrups, place padding in the support areas. Assist the client to place her knees over the supports and to place her feet into the stirrups.	Pressure on the perineal area from tension on the sutures may add to the client's discomfort. Padding and correct positioning may relieve some of the tension.
2. If the client has an indwelling catheter, place a clean washcloth between it and the client's thigh to protect her from being burned.	Catheters can absorb and conduct heat.

ACTION

3. Place the heat lamp at a distance of 10 in to 12 in from the perineum (Fig. 130-2) with no larger than a 25-watt bulb. Check to see that the feet and legs are well away from the bulb. Adjust the light so that it shines directly onto the perineum. Allow a moment of adjustment so that the client can ascertain if the heat is too intense. If the client feels the lamp is too hot, move the lamp farther from the perineum or replace the bulb with one of smaller wattage. Observe the skin to see that it does not become discolored indicating that the lamp is too hot.

RATIONALE

Extreme care must be taken to avoid burning the client. The perineal area will be very sensitive from the stretching and bruising of the birth. Sensation may be impaired. Visualization of the skin along with the client's subjective comments about the light will help in assessing if the light is satisfactory.

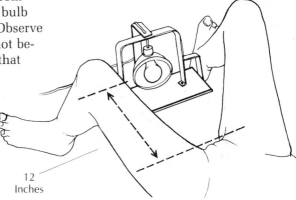

12
Inches

Figure 130.2

4. Place a sheet over the client and the lamp to provide privacy. Screen the client if further privacy is desired.

Attention to the client's privacy shows respect and consideration for her and promotes her self-image.

5. Leave the light on the client for 15 to 20 minutes or as prescribed by the obstetric care provider. If the client states that the light is too hot or her skin appears reddened, discontinue the treatment.

Local reaction to heat is vasodilation and increase in circulation. However, prolonged exposure to heat has the opposite effect and can cause tissue trauma and burns.

6. After the treatment, apply a clean perineal pad. Leave the client dry and comfortable.

Because lochia will continue for several weeks, the clean pad will absorb the lochia and promote feelings of comfort and well-being.

7. Clean and disinfect the equipment after each use. It should be cleaned with a germicidal solution and stored in a clean area.

Cross-transmission can occur if the equipment is not cleaned thoroughly between uses.

Communicative Aspects

OBSERVATIONS

1. Observe the episiotomy suture line for separation, discoloration, edema, bleeding, or purulent drainage and report their presence at once.

2. Observe the perineal area for signs that the light treatment may be too hot. If the area appears discolored or feels hot to touch, discontinue the treatment. If the client states that the lamp is too hot, discontinue it at once. The client should remain awake during the treatment so that she will be aware if the perineal area should become too warm.

3. Observe the client to see that she does not become overtired from the positioning.

CHARTING

DATE/TIME	OBSERVATIONS	SIGNATURE
5/12 1430	Perineal light applied for 15 min at a distance of 14 in. 25-watt bulb used. No signs of redness or statements of discomfort. Suture line intact and clean. No edema or discoloration noted. States that the light helps the tightness in the suture area.	M. Brown RN

Discharge Planning Aspects

CLIENT AND FAMILY EDUCATION

1. Explain to the client how the light works and what will be required of her. Be sure that she understands that the purpose of the light is to promote her comfort and to help the incision heal more quickly.

2. Use the time after perineal light treatment to explain the importance of proper cleansing of the perineal area for all women. Stress the importance of cleansing from front to back to avoid contamination with fecal material. If the client had a female baby or has female children, emphasize the importance of her teaching them also to cleanse from front to back.

Evaluation

Quality Assurance

Documentation should include a progressive summary of healing of the perineal area. Periodic observations should be made. Safety precautions taken to prevent injury to the client should be reflected. Explanations given to the client also should be noted.

Each hospital should have standard safety protocol regarding electrical equipment that provides for periodic checks of the safety and maintenance of this equipment. In addition, safety checks should provide that only bulbs of the proper wattage are available for heat equipment. A standard method of cleaning and disinfecting this type of equipment that meets or exceeds Centers for Disease Control standards should be adopted and communicated to the staff.

Infection Control

1. Thorough handwashing should precede and follow any treatments to obstetric clients.

2. Periodic cleansing of the perineum and changing of the perineal pad discourage the growth of microorganisms.

3. All equipment used consecutively for clients should be cleaned and disinfected thoroughly between uses.

Technique Checklist

	YES	NO
Procedure explained to client	_____	_____
Frequency of treatment _____		
Safety precautions		
Bulb watt _____		
Proximity to client _____ (in)		
Duration of each treatment _____ min		
Appearance of incision or laceration noted on chart at least daily	_____	_____
Complications prevented	_____	_____
Comfort measures explained to client for posthospital treatment	_____	_____

Postpartum Period Care

Overview

Definition

Care of the client from the birth of her infant until the reproductive system returns to its normal state. This period usually lasts from 6 to 8 weeks.

Rationale

Provide necessary care and support during the period required for return of the body to the natural, nonpregnant state. The postpartum period is a time of very rapid physiological change. In addition, psychological stress and exhaustion may arise as the client adjusts to her changing role and family needs.

Terminology

Mothering: Warm, tender behavior toward a child, the ability to love unconditionally

Puerperium: Postpartum, the six-week period after birth

Assessment

Pertinent Anatomy and Physiology

1. See Appendix I: *uterus, vagina.*
2. Involution is the process by which the female reproductive organs return to their normal, nonpregnant state. The most profound changes occur in the first 3 to 4 days after birth. After delivery, the uterus weighs about 2 lb (.9 kg) and is about the size of a grapefruit. The site of placental separation is marked by exposed vein endings that are constricted by the contraction of the uterine muscle. During the puerperium the uterus contracts and the depleted endometrium regenerates. Regeneration of the endometrium occurs in about 3 weeks except in the site of placental separation, which requires about 6 to 7 weeks to regenerate. Involution usually occurs more rapidly in primiparas and in breast-feeding mothers.
3. Lochia is the natural discharge that occurs after birth. It is initially red, changing to reddish brown and later to a whitish secretion after several weeks. Lochia also diminishes in amount throughout the duration of the puerperium. It may last as long as 6 weeks.
4. The cervix often is bruised after the strain of labor and delivery. It also may have small lacerations. The cervix reaches its normal state in about a month; however, it never returns to its prepregnancy state. After vaginal delivery, the cervix assumes a distinctive look. The external os remains slightly open and has lateral indentations where lacerations occurred during birth.
5. The vagina requires slightly longer to return to its natural state than the other reproductive organs. It has been greatly stretched during delivery. The rugae, or muscular folds, are generally discernible about 4 weeks after birth. The vaginal opening will remain slightly more stretched than it was before the pregnancy.
6. The external genitalia may be bruised and discolored after delivery. This area may remain sensitive for several weeks. If an episiotomy or laceration occurred during delivery, healing will probably proceed quickly; however, it may be 4 or 5 weeks before the muscle tone is restored.

7. During the early puerperium, the total volume of circulating blood remains high. It takes about a week for the blood volume to return to its prepregnant state. Iron supplements may be needed, especially if the woman is breast-feeding.

8. Breast development is accelerated during pregnancy. Colostrum, the thin, watery milk precursor, is present at birth. Actual milk production does not begin until about 2 days after birth, however. If the breasts are not emptied regularly, milk production decreases and eventually will stop in approximately 2 or 3 weeks. Antilactogenic drugs may be given after birth to suppress the production of milk.

9. Menstrual flow usually returns about 6 to 8 weeks after birth if the mother is not breast-feeding. Menstruation usually does not start while the mother is breast-feeding, although she may ovulate. Pregnancy is possible during the breast-feeding period.

Pathophysiological Concepts

1. Hemorrhage is a grave threat during the first hour after delivery (often called the fourth stage of labor). It usually results when the uterus fails to contract successfully, leaving the veins at the placental site open and bleeding. Contraction of the uterus causes constriction of the veins (see Technique No. 127, Labor and Delivery, Nursing Care During).

2. Puerperal infection is any bacterial infection that attacks the reproductive organs during labor and the postpartum period. Infection may develop from organisms already present in the woman's body or may be introduced during the labor and delivery processes. If not treated promptly and effectively, the infection may become systemic, resulting in septicemia.

3. Postpartum "blues" may occur in the first few weeks after delivery. This state usually involves feelings of slight to moderate depression and periods of weeping, over which the woman has no control. This generally passes without lasting effects. Postpartum depression, neuroses, or psychoses, on the other hand, interferes with the woman's ability to function. These conditions include anxiety states, phobias, obsessions, hypochondriasis, and severe depression. These clinical conditions require psychotherapy and possibly antidepressive medications for control.

Assessment of the Client

1. Assess the labor experience of the client to see if it met with her expectations. If she had a cesarean section, assess whether she had expected and was prepared for it.

2. Assess the physical parameters of the client, including vital signs and the presence of any chronic conditions that may or may not have been affected by the pregnancy.

3. Assess the client's emotional status, and her ability and readiness for self-care.

Plan

Nursing Objectives

Support and assist the client during the recovery phase.

Promote mother–infant bonding.

Teach self-care for an uncomplicated puerperium.

Assist the client in establishing priorities and making knowledgeable choices.

Provide information and referrals about methods of contraception, if the client desires.

Promote an understanding of infant growth and development.

Explain the physiological and psychological changes that are relevant to postpartum recovery.

Client Preparation

1. Make sure that the client has emerged safely from the uncertainty and danger of the fourth stage of labor. Measure vital signs to provide baseline values.

2. The puerperium may be facilitated by preparation during the prenatal period.

Equipment

See appropriate technique

Implementation and Interventions

Procedural Aspects

ACTION	*RATIONALE*
1. Ambulation usually is encouraged as soon as the mother has recovered fully from the anesthetic. Ask the client to call for assistance during her first attempts at ambulation after delivery. Allow her to sit on the side of the bed until feelings of faintness are gone. Encourage her to look straight ahead during ambulation. After she is stable, encourage the client to be out of bed frequently.	Activity stimulates the discharge of lochia. It also promotes feelings of well-being. Circulation, and bowel and bladder function, also are stimulated. Fainting and weakness are common following delivery. Progression to full ambulation should proceed at an individual rate.
2. Adequate rest is vital to the recuperative process. Explain to the family about the importance of rest and relief from tension and anxiety for the client. Provide a restful environment, spacing hospital procedures so that the client can rest adequately.	Labor and delivery is an exhausting process. Several hours of sleep are generally necessary after delivery. Adequate periods of uninterrupted sleep are important for the mother to feel rested.
3. Food and fluids usually are offered as soon as requested after delivery if the mother is not nauseated (Fig. 131-1). A well-rounded diet for the non-nursing mother would include the average number of calories for a person of her sex, build, and weight. The lactating client needs 700 additional calories each day, as well as vitamin supplements (see Technique No. 123, Breast-Feeding).	Most women are hungry after they recover from the immediate post-delivery exhaustion. Many have been without food for as long as 24 hours.

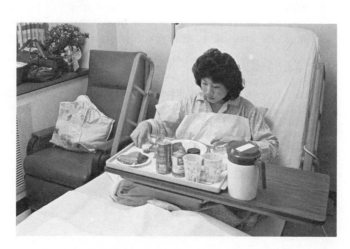

Figure 131.1

ACTION	RATIONALE
4. Postpartum exercises can be started on the first day. New exercises should be introduced gradually so that the mother will not become overly tired. Different hospitals, physicians, and midwives have various exercises that are recommended.	Exercise hastens the involution activities and promotes feelings of well-being. In addition, exercise promotes the physical fitness of the client.
5. Elimination may be sluggish after the birth. Constipation is a common problem. Encourage a well-balanced diet with fresh fruits and whole grains. Increasing fluid intake is also important. Suppositories or enemas may be prescribed unless the anal sphincter was torn or cut. In this case, elimination may be painful for a time. Administration of an analgesic may provide the relaxation that the client needs to have a bowel movement.	The release of abdominal pressure and the stretching and relaxation of the abdominal muscles contribute to bowel problems. In addition, discomfort and anxiety about stitches may promote constipation further.
6. Allow the mother to take a shower as soon as she is stable. Remain nearby during the first shower as the warm water may cause faintness. Tub baths generally are permitted 24 hours after delivery. Sitz baths in 2 in to 3 in of water may be prescribed after the first 24 hours to relieve the tenderness and discomfort and to promote healing of the perineum and episiotomy.	Bathing and attention to hygiene promote feelings of well-being and are positive to the client's self-image. For the first few days after birth, perspiration and body odor may be a problem as well. Showering and bathing provide a refreshing break.

Communicative Aspects

OBSERVATIONS

1. Observe the vital signs of the client throughout the postpartum hospitalization. Deviations may indicate complications and should be assessed carefully.

2. Observe the physical recovery from the pregnancy and delivery. Observe the lochia, perineum, breasts, and uterus (see the appropriate technique within this section).

3. Observe the interaction of the client and her infant. If she seems anxious or unsure, assist her and answer questions. Allow the client to express any feelings she may have, and respond in a nonjudgmental and accepting manner.

CHARTING

DATE/TIME	OBSERVATIONS	SIGNATURE
2/13 0915	Up to shower for first time. Stated that she was slightly dizzy and was assisted back to bed. B/P 118/74, P 72, R 22. After 20 min requested to go back to shower. Accompanied by nurse; no dizziness at this time. Showered and returned to bed without complications. Resting at this time. ——————	D. Perez RN

Discharge Planning Aspects

CLIENT AND FAMILY EDUCATION

1. Explain the involutionary process to the client. Be sure that she knows what to expect during the hospital and post-hospital periods. Explain about any restrictions on activity or diet, and answer any questions. If the teaching can be provided both orally and in written form, it may be more effective. When the client returns home and can reinforce previous teaching by reading it again, she may be more likely to remember and follow instructions. It is very important that the need for rest be stressed to the client. Many mothers find themselves with not only their prior responsibilities, but now with a new baby. In an attempt to meet all of these responsibilities, they may become overtired and strained. Stress the need for assistance during the initial post-hospital period; emphasize the importance of pacing and setting priorities.

2. Encourage the client to make and keep her follow-up appointment with her obstetric care provider. Continued follow-up care and supervision is important to the satisfactory recovery and prevention of complications. The first follow-up visit will probably be from 2 to 6 weeks after delivery.

3. Sexual activity will depend on the wishes of the couple and the extent of the obstetrical trauma. If the client had an episiotomy, healing may not be complete for about 4 weeks. Some discomfort may be noted. Lubrication of the vaginal walls may be inhibited for a short time. A water-soluble gel or contraceptive cream may be used.

4. Remind the client that some information should be maintained by her as an indication of the progress of her postpartum period. This information generally is to be brought with her when she comes for her follow-up visits and will provide an indication of her condition. Information will include noting when the lochia ceased, any vaginal discharges, weight gains or losses, breast changes, progress of lactation (how often and how long the baby nurses), and any bladder or bowel problems.

REFERRALS

A referral to a family planning counselor or clinic may ease the minds of the couple who are interested in spacing their children. Referral to an exercise class may help the client with her exercise program. Many local churches and colleges have community exercise programs. She should check with her obstetric care provider before undertaking a defined program of exercise to be certain that it is not too strenuous. Parenting services may be needed by the family who needs assistance in parenting skills.

Evaluation

Quality Assurance

Documentation during the postpartum period should stress monitoring of the client for early detection of deviation from what is expected during the postpartum period and emphasis on teaching the client self-care. Because the greatest portion of the postpartum recovery takes place out of the hospital, it is important that the client be prepared adequately for this period. Documentation should reflect what teaching was done and an assessment of the client's level of understanding and acceptance. Any deviations from the expected pattern should be documented, with a description of measures taken and results.

Infection Control

1. During the postpartum period, handwashing is very important. Stress to the client, by verbal instructions and by example, the importance of washing her hands before and after any care of herself or her baby.

2. The perineal area generally is considered clean rather than sterile. Washing with clean washcloths and soap are the method of cleansing. Stress the importance of cleansing from front to back to prevent contamination from the rectal area. Pads should be changed frequently to prevent colonization of microorganisms.

3. An early indication of infection is fever. The client should be encouraged to take her temperature daily and to report any elevations above 100°F.

4. Any foul-smelling discharge from the vagina or the suture area should be reported at once.

Technique Checklist

	YES	NO
Was the postpartum hospitalization without complications?	_____	_____

Number of days of postpartum hospitalization _____

Teaching of the client in the following areas

	ORAL	WRITTEN
Need for rest	_____	_____
Exercise plan	_____	_____
Diet	_____	_____
Lochia	_____	_____
Sexuality	_____	_____
Return of menses	_____	_____
Monitoring temperature	_____	_____
Breast care	_____	_____
Episiotomy care	_____	_____
Bowel care	_____	_____
Other _____		

_____

132   Postpartum Recovery Care

Overview

Definition

Procedures and observations of the new mother during the first 2 hours after delivery, referred to as the fourth stage of labor

Rationale

Assist the client to proceed through the fourth stage of labor with no complications.

Assist in alleviating the emotional and physical stress after delivery.

Provide support for the early mother–child relationship by means of early parental contact and interactions with the newborn.

Terminology

Postnatal: Occurring after birth, refers to the infant

Postpartum: After delivery or childbirth; refers to the mother

Puerperium: Synonymous with postpartum, the time from birth until physical and psychological recovery (approximately 6–8 weeks)

Assessment

Pertinent Anatomy and Physiology

See Appendix I: *labor and delivery.*

Pathophysiological Concepts

The danger during the immediate postpartum period is the failure of the uterus to continue contracting, allowing hemorrhage. With the expulsion of the fetus, the uterus begins involution. This change in the shape and size of the uterus causes the placenta to separate, and it is subsequently expelled. The change in shape and decreasing size of the uterus cause the loose vascular ends to be compressed, thus stemming the tendency to bleed. Relaxation of the uterine walls allows these open vessels to bleed freely, causing hemorrhage. Usually the muscular fundus will again contract, with firm, massaging pressure that stimulates the muscle fibers.

Assessment of the Client

1. Assess the labor and delivery process to see if this client is at risk for postpartum complications. If the client had an unusually long labor, a large baby, hydramnios, a multiple birth, induction of labor, or is a grand multipara (has had several previous births), she may be at risk for relaxation of the uterine muscles during the fourth stage of labor.

2. Assess the condition of the mother and the infant to determine if they may safely spend these first moments of the child's life together. This period has been shown to be critical to the mother–infant bonding process. If there are no contraindications, allow the parents to keep the infant in the recovery room with them (Fig. 132-1).

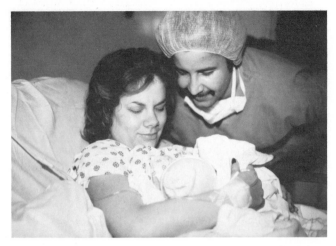

Figure 132.1

Plan

Nursing Objectives

Monitor the mother during the immediate postdelivery period to prevent complications.

Provide a family-centered post-delivery period.

Maintain complete records of the recovery period.

Client Preparation

1. Cleanse the vulva and perineum gently with warm, sterile water and apply a perineal pad.

2. Cleanse the upper portion of the body as needed. Dress the mother in a clean gown and cover her with a warm blanket.

3. Reposition the delivery table; gently lower both legs *simultaneously* from the stirrups.

4. If spinal anesthetic was used, tell the client that she will remain in the supine position for 8 to 12 hours, or as prescribed. Explain that this will help to prevent headache. Tell her to notify the nurse when she begins to regain feeling in her legs and feet.

5. Before moving the client onto the stretcher, check for the following:

   Lochia

   Change in blood pressure

   Fundus tone and location

   Bladder distension

   Color

   Respirations

Equipment

Sphygmomanometer and stethoscope

Suction capacity and catheter

IV equipment and supplies

Airways of various sizes

Perineal pads

Emesis basin

Oxygen capabilities with mask, cannula, or catheter

Recovery stretcher with side rails

Implementation and Interventions

Procedural Aspects

	ACTION	RATIONALE

ACTION

1. Provide an area that is quiet and restful for recovery from the birth. Keep the room dim and change the linens as needed to keep the client clean and comfortable. Change the perineal pad as needed and provide fluids if the client is not nauseated. Cover the mother with a warm blanket.

2. Check the client's vital signs on her admission to the recovery area and every 15 minutes thereafter for 1 hour. Check her fundus and massage if needed to express clots or maintain tone at least every 15 minutes. Note the amount of vaginal flow.

3. Check the client for bladder distension. If a blocking anesthetic was used, the client may be unaware that she needs to urinate. If the bladder becomes distended, straight catheterization may be needed.

4. Apply an ice pack to the episiotomy, if needed.

5. Administer analgesics as needed. Multiparas may experience afterpains.

6. Allow the client to verbalize her feelings during this period. She may be subject to a wide variety of emotions. Reassure her about the condition of her infant if the infant is not in the recovery room with her. Praise her for her efforts and assist in promoting the positive aspects of the birthing experience.

7. As soon as the mother's condition is stable, usually after 1 to 2 hours in recovery, she may be returned to her room. Before transfer, perform a thorough examination.

RATIONALE

The birthing process is very exhausting. The mother now needs rest and relaxation, as well as continual monitoring of physical condition. Chilling is a frequent reaction to loss of body mass, the muscular efforts of labor, perspiration, and exposure.

Constant monitoring of the client is the best defense against postpartal hemorrhage. Hemorrhage occurs when the contracted uterine muscle relaxes and allows the open ends of the blood vessels (where the placenta was attached) to bleed. Contraction of the uterus keeps these vessels constricted and prevents hemorrhage. If the uterus feels boggy, it may be full of clots and blood. Mild pressure will be sufficient to express these clots so that they will not interfere with the ability of the uterus to contract.

A distended bladder is uncomfortable. In addition, it may displace the uterus upward, causing distortion of the assessment of involution. A full bladder prevents the uterus from contracting and could cause increased bleeding.

Ice may relieve swelling and pain.

Afterpains are contractions of the uterus as it regresses to its nonpregnant state. They occur after every delivery, but successive pregnancies seem to make clients more aware of the discomfort.

The immediate postpartum period is a very critical time. The mother should be watched closely. Both she and her spouse should be allowed to verbalize their feelings. The nurse provides emotional support, reassurance, and physical surveillance during this period.

If hemorrhage has not occurred within the first hour after delivery, it is unlikely to occur at all. Proper communication promotes a smooth transition to the postpartum unit.

ACTION	RATIONALE
Check the fundus, the lochia, and the mother's vital signs. Check the episiotomy for hematoma and note the condition of the bladder. Complete the records and give an oral report to the receiving nurse.	

Special Modifications

If the client has had spinal anesthesia, monitor for the return of movement in the feet and legs. Ask the client to wiggle her toes each time her vital signs are checked. When movement begins to return, note the time on the client record.	Documentation of the return of function after spinal anesthesia is important for legal purposes. In addition, it is important to the overall assessment of the client's postpartal recovery.

Communicative Aspects

OBSERVATIONS

1. Observe the client for excessive blood loss during the first 2 hours after birth. Postpartum hemorrhage is most likely during this period. Indications of this may be rising pulse and respiratory rate accompanied by a lowered blood pressure. Observe the vital signs every 15 minutes for 1 hour, then every 30 minutes for 2 hours. Thereafter, the vital signs should be checked at least four times a day.

2. Observe the fundus during the recovery period. The fundus should be firm and rounded. If it is boggy or soft, massage until the muscle contracts. Mild massage may be used to express clots and drainage from the uterus; however, do not overmassage.

3. Hematoma of the episiotomy is indicated by severe, unrelievable pain, redness, and swelling of the perineal area. The hematoma may or may not be visible, but should be suspected if the client cannot get comfortable and continually changes positions seeking comfort.

4. Observe the color of the client's skin. Note the amount of lochia and signs of mental alertness on the mother's part.

5. Observe the interaction of the parents with their baby. Note the way in which they handle and relate to the baby. This may be important in later teaching.

CHARTING

Most hospitals have a special recovery record that allows quick, accurate, and comprehensive charting of the recovery room activities and measurements.

DATE	TIME	B/P	P	R	T(°F)	LOCHIA	FUNDUS	OBSERVATIONS NURSE
7/12	0930	118/72	76	18	99.2	Rubra/mod	UU	Holding infant
	0945	112/70	76	16		Rubra/mod	UU	
	1000	112/66	72	18		Rubra/mod	UU	Pad changed
	1015	110/70	78	18		Rubra/mod	2/U	Uterus displaced to right, bladder filling
	1030	110/70	80	18	99.0	Rubra/mod	3/U	Up to BR with assistance, voided 300 ml, pad changed
	1045	110/74	78	18		Rubra/mod	UU	
	1100	112/70	78	18		Rubra/mod	UU	Infant to nursery
	1115	110/68	72	16		Rubra/mod	UU	Episiotomy slightly swollen, no discoloration
	1130	114/70	78	18	99.8	Rubra/mod	UU	Pad changed, linen changed, uterus firm, transferred to unit 4C, full report given. States she understands about reporting passage of clots. C. Parker RN

Discharge Planning Aspects

CLIENT AND FAMILY EDUCATION

1. When the client is admitted to the recovery area, she will be both elated and exhausted. Provide a meaningful, family-oriented time by allowing the infant to be with the family in the recovery room if conditions permit. Explain to the client and her family that this period of time is one of monitoring to be sure that her body is returning to the nonpregnant state in the way that it should. Reassure the mother that she has done well during the labor and delivery process. Carry out the recovery room monitoring in an efficient and unobtrusive manner.

2. If the mother will be discharged after the recovery room period, she will need additional information about caring for herself and her infant. In addition, she will be exhausted from the labor process. Teaching must be brief, to the point, and meaningful. Offer as much of the information as possible in writing for future referral. Explain about possible complications, and clarify when she should call her obstetric care provider. Explain about feeding and caring for the infant. Answer questions as fully as possible. Referral to a home health nurse may enhance the security of the family who will remain in the hospital for a very short time.

Evaluation

Quality Assurance

Documentation should provide a clear, progressive picture of the immediate postpartum period. Forms will vary with each hospital. Data that should be monitored and charted are vital signs, condition of fundus, amount and appearance of lochia, condition of perineum, bladder distension, and any pertinent observations. Any complications should be noted as well as the outcomes. Time arriving and leaving recovery area should be noted. Any instructions given should be noted.

Infection Control

1. Careful handwashing should be done before and after any client contact.
2. Cleansing of the perineal area should be done with clean, warm cloths in the recovery room.
3. During the recovery phase, the pads that are placed on the client are sterile.

Technique Checklist

	YES	NO
Client to recovery room at _____		
Spouse or family accompanied client	_____	_____
Infant with client in recovery room	_____	_____
Vital signs		
Q15min for 1 hr	_____	_____
Q30min for 2 hr	_____	_____
Documentation of		
Vital signs	_____	_____
Condition of fundus	_____	_____
Vaginal flow	_____	_____
Condition of perineum	_____	_____
Bladder emptied _____ ml		
Uterus remained firm	_____	_____
Report of condition given to unit receiving client after recovery	_____	_____
Mother discharged after recovery period	_____	_____
Infant discharged	_____	_____
Conditions noted on discharge notes	_____	_____

133   Vulval and Perineal Care

Overview

Definition

Cleansing the vulva and perineal area during the postpartum period

Rationale

Prevent or reduce infection.

Provide a dry area for healing.

Observe the perineum.

Teach the client to care for her own personal hygiene and that of her female children properly.

Assessment

Pertinent Anatomy and Physiology

1. See Appendix I: *genitalia (female)*, *vagina*.
2. After the rigors of vaginal delivery, the mucosal surface of the vulval area may appear red for several weeks. The muscles of the pelvic floor may be torn and stretched. The perineum may be edematous and tender. Lacerations and bruising also may be present, especially in primiparas. The episiotomy and lacerations of the perineal area should heal within 4 to 6 weeks. Return of muscle tone is also expected in about 6 weeks.

Pathophysiological Concepts

Problems concerning the healing perineum may include infection. Infection may be caused by pathogenic organisms entering the area before, during, or after the birth process. Signs of infection or failure to heal are bloody drainage from the incision, failure of the incision to close properly, foul-smelling discharge, and an increase in pulse and temperature.

Assessment of the Client

1. Assess the stage of healing of the perineal area. Determine if the client is having pain or discomfort and the effectiveness of any prescribed comfort measures, such as medication and sitz baths.
2. Assess the ability of the client to assume the needed position for vulval and perineal care. If the client is experiencing pain, administration of an analgesic before administering the care may be advisable.
3. Assess the allergy history of the client if an anesthetic spray will be used to promote perineal and vulval comfort.

Plan

Nursing Objectives

Remove secretions and discharges from the vulva and perineal area.

Promote and monitor proper healing of the perineal area.

Reduce irritation and odor.

Prepare the area for local applications (e.g., dressings, heat, ice).

Provide comfort for the client.

Teach self-care and genital hygiene.

Record the condition of the area and the type and amount of discharge.

Client Preparation

1. Explain to the client what will occur during vulval and perineal care. Tell her the approximate schedule for this care, but emphasize that she may receive perineal care any time she feels uncomfortable, voids, or has a bowel movement. Explain that she will be able to care for herself as soon as she is ambulatory.

2. The client may be assisted to void before receiving perineal care because the dorsal recumbent position and cleansing of the perineal area may intensify the need to void if the bladder is full.

3. Remove the perineal pad before giving vulval and perineal care. Explain to the client that the pad is removed from front to back (i.e., the front is released and removed first and the back last). This prevents drawing the contaminated portion from the rectal area across the clean portion (the vulva). Dispose of the pad in a sack or bag.

Equipment

Cleansing solution or tap water and soap

Washcloths, cotton balls, or gauze sponges

Basin, pitcher or spray can

Bedpan

Perineal pad

Receptacle for soiled pad (bag or plastic sack)

Implementation and Interventions

Procedural Aspects

ACTION	*RATIONALE*
For the Client Who Cannot Get Out of Bed	
1. Generally, clean technique is considered satisfactory for reducing the spread of microorganisms. Handwashing should precede perineal care.	Pathogenic organisms may be transferred to susceptible surfaces by unclean or careless technique. All equipment used should be clean.
2. Assist the client into the dorsal recumbent position on the bedpan. Using soap and warm water on a washcloth, wash the perineal area gently and thoroughly with strokes from front to back. Use a different section of the washcloth for each stroke. Avoid the rectal area. Do not separate the labia during cleansing, and do not allow the rinse water to flow into the vagina (Fig. 133-1). Rinse the perineal area by pouring clean water over the area, letting it run into the bedpan, or by using a clean washcloth. All cleansing and rinsing should proceed from front to back.	Gravity may be used to catch the rinse water in the bedpan. Always use strokes from front to back to prevent contamination of the vulval area with organisms from the rectal area. Allowing cleansing or rinse water to seep into the vagina may predispose to infection.

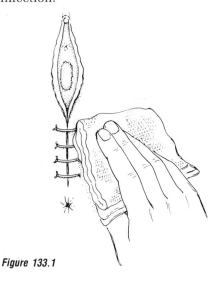

Figure 133.1

ACTION	RATIONALE
3. Dry the area gently with a clean cloth or towel.	Drying the area relieves irritation and promotes healing.
4. Assist the client to turn to Sims' position, that is, on her side with the uppermost leg flexed. Wash and dry the anal region.	Cleansing the anal region last promotes freshness while preventing the spread of microorganisms.
5. Apply a clean perineal pad. Attach the front first. Secure the pad firmly so that it does not move while it is being worn.	Care must be taken to prevent contamination of the vulval area with organisms from the rectal area.
6. Dispose of the soiled pad and any disposable equipment in a bag or sack. Clean the bedpan, basin or any other equipment used. Replace the equipment to its proper place.	Proper cleaning and disposal of equipment reduces odors and enhances the client's environment.

For the Client Who is Ambulatory

ACTION	RATIONALE
1. As soon as the postpartum client is ambulatory, she may do her own perineal and vulval care in the bathroom after each voiding and bowel movement. Explain to her that she should use a clean washcloth, making three strokes from front to back, and use a different portion of the washcloth for each stroke. She may use the spray bottle filled with tap water for cleansing. Provide an ample supply of washcloths in the bathroom. Place a linen hamper in the bathroom and a trash receptacle for disposal of washcloths and soiled perineal pads.	Self-care is important to the client's self-image and to successful transition to the home.
2. Other measures that may ease discomfort and tension in the perineal area are warm sitz baths or heat lamp (see Technique No. 130, Perineal Light). An inflated ring may be used when the client sits up to prevent pressure on the episiotomy. An ice pack, covered with a soft gauze material and applied over the perineal area, may decrease edema in the first 12 to 24 hours. Anesthetic sprays may decrease regional discomfort.	Comfort measures for the perineal area are aimed at decreasing the swelling and tension on the suture line. After 24 hours, one desired effect of treatment is increasing circulation to promote healing.

Special Modifications

1. If the client has an indwelling urinary catheter, clean all exudate from it with a washcloth and cleaning solution. Use strokes starting at the point of insertion and proceeding outward away from the body. Avoid tension on the catheter during cleaning. Use a different portion of the cloth for each stroke. Clean until all exudate is removed.

   The female urethra is short and vaginal discharge is a satisfactory medium for the growth of bacteria. Tension on the catheter may be traumatic to the tender vulva and perineal area.

2. If the client has had a cesarean section performed or has no lacerations or episiotomy, she should still have vulval and perineal care after each voiding and bowel movement.

   Encrustation of lochia provides an excellent medium for the proliferation of microorganisms.

Communicative Aspects

OBSERVATIONS

1. Observe the perineal area during vulval and perineal care for proper healing. After the mother begins her own self-care, observe the perineal area at least once daily to ensure that healing is progressing satisfactorily. Observe the episiotomy for edema, inflammation, separation, or the presence of a hematoma.

2. Observe the appearance of the lochia. Lochia during the first few days postpartum is red and has a fleshy odor. A foul odor indicates the presence of necrotic tissue or infection and should be reported at once. Some clots may be expressed from the uterus (see Technique No. 129, Lochia, Observation of).

CHARTING

DATE/TIME	OBSERVATIONS	SIGNATURE
7/18 0930	Vulval and perineal care given. Lochia reddish brown. Pad changed approximately q2hr. Vulva and perineum red and edematous. Episiotomy clean, intact, no signs of bleeding or discoloration. ————————————	D. Perez RN

Discharge Planning Aspects

CLIENT AND FAMILY EDUCATION

1. Explain to the client how to perform her own perineal and vulval care. This explanation may be done while the nurse is administering perineal care, during the immediate postpartum period.

2. Use this opportunity to teach the client that perineal pads should be put on and removed with consideration that the portion touching the rectal area should never be allowed to come in contact with the clean vulval area. The bowels normally harbor many kinds of bacteria. These bacteria in the bowel are harmless; however, if they are spread into the areas of open wounds or into the vaginal or urethral areas, they may cause serious infection. The pad should be fastened in the front and placed against the vulva. It should not be allowed to slide as it is being fastened in the back or during the time it is being worn. When removed, the pad should be taken from the vulva first and removed with a downward motion.

3. Explain the importance of cleansing from front to back after urinary and bowel elimination. This is particularly important in women because of the short length of the urethra and the proximity of the anus to the vaginal and urethral openings. If the client has had a female child, tell her that this is important when she changes the diaper and cleanses the baby's perineal area.

Evaluation

Quality Assurance

Documentation should reflect that the vulval and perineal care was given on a regular basis until the client can assume responsibility for her own care. The chart should show evidence that the client was instructed in proper technique and voiced an understanding of the principles of proper cleansing and preventing contamination. Any comfort measures should be noted with an assessment of their effectiveness. Periodic assessment of the status of healing of the perineal area should be made.

Infection Control

1. Perineal wounds and the buildup of dried lochia in the perineal region are conducive to the growth and proliferation of bacteria.
2. Vulval and perineal care is a clean procedure and should be preceded and followed by careful handwashing.
3. The importance of cleansing from front to back should be stressed both to the client and to the staff.

Technique Checklist

	YES	NO
Technique explained to the client	_____	_____
Handwashing explained and demonstrated each time care was rendered	_____	_____
Client instructions on vulval and perineal care		
Frequency	_____	_____
Method	_____	_____
Cleansing from front to back	_____	_____
Proper placement of perineal pad	_____	_____
Home care	_____	_____
Infection was prevented	_____	_____
Episiotomy or laceration healing without problem	_____	_____
Other comfort measures:		
Inflated ring	_____	_____
Sitz baths	_____	_____
Perineal light	_____	_____
Analgesics	_____	_____
Ice packs	_____	_____
Anesthetic spray	_____	_____

Vulval–Perineal Preparation

Overview

Definition
Removal of hair from the skin around the delivery area in preparation for birth of a baby

Rationale
Aid in the maintenance of a germ-free environment during delivery.

Provide optimal visualization during the delivery process.

Promote a cleaner environment for healing.

Terminology
Episiotomy: Incision of the vulval–perineal area to facilitate delivery and prevent uncontrolled laceration

Follicle, hair: A pouchlike depression in the skin in which a hair develops from the matrix at its base and grows to emerge from its opening on the body surface

Assessment

Pertinent Anatomy and Physiology
1. See Appendix I: *genitalia (female), skin, vagina.*
2. Hair is formed from germinal cells in the deep part of the hair follicle. A hair usually consists of a central core (medulla) surrounded by a cortex. The root of the hair is that part embedded in the follicle (usually slanting from the perpendicular), whereas the shaft projects above the surface of the skin. Two or more sebaceous glands are associated with each follicle. Hair is most prominent on the head, axillae, and pubic area of adults.

Pathophysiological Concepts
Hair around the pubic and perineal areas may harbor bacteria. However, there is growing evidence that shaving of the pubic and inner thigh hair is not effective in preventing infection and, in fact, may predispose to infection because of nicks and cuts resulting from the shaving process. Most obstetric-care providers have a preference as to how the preparation should be done.

Assessment of the Client
1. Assess the labor process to determine if the client is having contractions and, if so, their frequency and duration. It is usually preferable to shave the client before the labor progresses too far, to reduce the amount of discomfort.
2. Assess the ability of the client to lie in the dorsal recumbent position for the duration of the preparation procedure. If the client becomes hypotensive, periodic repositioning onto her side may be necessary during the preparation procedure.

Plan

Nursing Objectives
Remove the amount of hair specified in the prescribed type of preparation.

Protect the client by taking care not to scratch, scrape, or cut the skin during shaving.

Provide for the client's safety and comfort during the preparation.

Client Preparation

1. Explain the procedure to the client. Tell her why the preparation is being done.
2. Allow the client to empty her bladder before beginning the shaving preparation to promote comfort.

Equipment

Disposable prep kit
Germicidal soap
Antiseptic solution
Gauze sponges
Wash cloths
Lamp or adequate lighting
Warm water
Hip pad

Implementation and Interventions

Procedural Aspects

ACTION

1. Place a pad under the client's hips to protect the bed linen. Drape the client (Figs. 134-1, 134-2). Arrange adequate lighting.

RATIONALE

Adequate draping promotes the client's privacy and prevents chilling.

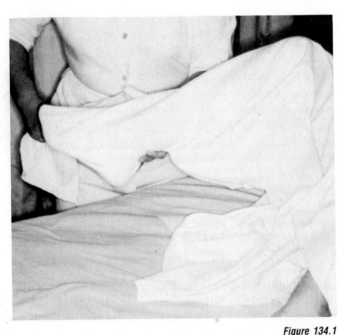

Figure 134.1

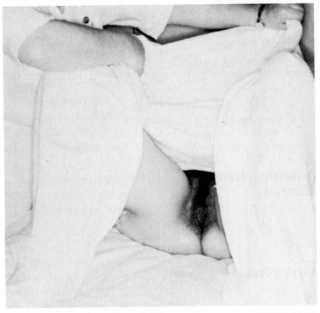

Figure 134.2

2. With the client in the dorsal recumbent position, knees flexed and separated, apply soap to the preparation area. Always work from front to back (Figs. 134-3, 134-4). Never reintroduce into the vaginal or perineal area a cloth that has come in contact with the anal region.

The rectal region harbors bacteria that are not harmful unless introduced into a susceptible area, such as the vagina or urethra.

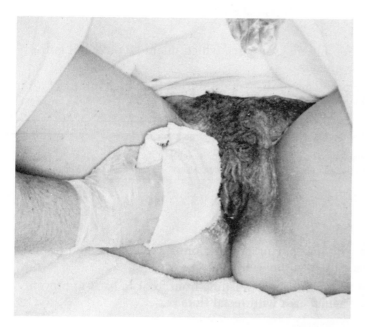

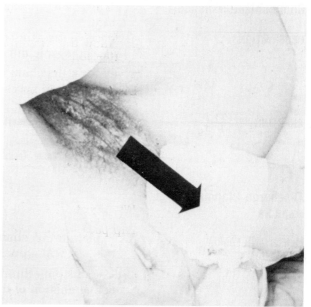

Figure 134.3

Figure 134.4

ACTION

3. Shave the prescribed area. Use short, downward strokes. Surrounding tissue may be held taut with a gauze pad in the other hand. Take care not to cut or nick the client, especially around the areas of moles, warts, or old scars. Shave the clean area first. Rinse this area with warm water or an antiseptic solution applied to a gauze sponge or cloth. Use a new sponge or cloth for each front-to-back stroke. Dry the area in the same manner. Turn the client to her side and ask her to flex the top leg. Shave the anal area and rinse. Once the razor has come in contact with the anal area, it is not reintroduced into the clean area around the perineum and vaginal canal.

Special Modifications

1. If the client experiences a contraction or faintness during the procedure, temporary repositioning to her side may be necessary.

2. For cesarean section, the entire abdomen and symphysis pubis is usually shaved and surgically prepared.

RATIONALE

Short strokes are less likely to cause accidental cuts or nicks in the skin. Moving from the clean area to the contaminated area helps prevent the spread of bacteria.

Hypotension due to compression of abdominal vessels may cause faintness. Repositioning usually reverses this problem.

The preparation for cesarean section is as for abdominal surgery.

Communicative Aspects

OBSERVATIONS

1. Observe the skin area for any nicks or cuts, which might be potential entries for pathogenic microorganisms.

2. Observe the client for problems or discomfort during the procedure. Reposition if necessary.

CHARTING

DATE/TIME	OBSERVATIONS	SIGNATURE
2/18 1300	Vulval–perineal prep from labia majora to anal region. No break in the skin integrity. Tolerated procedure without difficulty; no contractions. ————	D. Perez RN

Discharge Planning Aspects

CLIENT AND FAMILY EDUCATION

1. Explain to the client why the shaving preparation is being done. Tell her that the hair will grow back in about 6 weeks.

2. Use this opportunity to explain about washing from front to back to prevent contamination of the vaginal area with rectal flora.

Evaluation

Quality Assurance

Documentation should include the amount of skin area that was shaved. Any problems or complications, such as cutting the skin or discovery of previous breaks in the skin integrity should be noted. The client's response to the preparation should be noted. If contractions or hypotensive episodes interrupted the procedure, notation should include actions and outcomes.

Infection Control

1. Wash hands thoroughly before undertaking a shaving preparation of the client.

2. Always work from front to back. Never reintroduce any equipment into the vulval–perineal area once it has been in contact with the rectal region.

3. Report any breaks in the skin, which are potential entries for pathogens.

Technique Checklist

	YES	NO
Procedure explained to client	———	———
Type of preparation		
Pubic, perineal, vulval, and anal	———	———
Perineal, vulval, and anal	———	———
Abdominal	———	———
Other ———————		
Nicks and cuts of skin avoided	———	———
All movement from front to back	———	———
Tolerated procedure satisfactorily	———	———
Contractions	———	———
Hypotension	———	———

Unit Five

Techniques for Neonatal Clients

135   Admission to Newborn Nursery

Overview

Definition

The initial steps taken after birth and transport to the nursery to protect and safeguard the newborn in a controlled environment

Rationale

Prevent infection in the susceptible newborn.

Maintain constant temperature in the newborn.

Provide a basis for continuing evaluation by obtaining accurate baseline measurements.

Terminology

Ductus arteriosus: In fetal circulation, the vessel that connects the pulmonary artery to the aorta

Foramen ovale: In fetal circulation, the opening between the right and left atria of the heart

Ductus venosus: In fetal circulation, the vessel that connects the umbilical vein to the inferior vena cava

Vernix caseosa: The yellowish white, greasy, cheeselike substance that may cling to the newborn's skin after birth. It consists of secretions from sebaceous glands and epithelial cells. Its distribution over the body is variable, being heavier in the skin folds and between the labia of female infants.

Assessment

Pertinent Anatomy and Physiology

1. See Appendix I: *anus, bronchial tree, esophagus, heart, and skin.*
2. The neonate's respiratory system has been maintained by the placenta prior to birth. The abrupt change in environment necessitates quick reaction by the infant's system to take over the breathing and gaseous exchange, which are essential to extrauterine life. During the last few months of intrauterine life, the fetal lung contains a considerable amount of fluid. This fluid must be squeezed out of the air sacs so that normal respiration can begin. About one-third of the fluid is removed by the compression of the chest during the birth process. The remainder is absorbed by the pulmonary vessels. Infants with immature respiratory systems may have difficulty absorbing this fluid. The infant should begin to breathe normally about 1 minute after birth. The average respiratory rate is 40 to 44 breaths per minute without retraction or grunting. Infants are normally nasal breathers. Although the infant is somewhat cyanotic at birth, appearance of the lighter, pinker body color should occur within a few minutes.
3. At birth, the infant's circulatory system takes over when placental circulation stops. Blood ceases flowing through the umbilical vessels, and the fetal openings between the chambers of the heart and blood vessels (the ductus arteriosus, foramen ovale, and the ductus venosus) begin to close. Complete and permanent closure of the ductus arteriosus and foramen ovale usually occurs within the first 1 to 2 days after birth. The normal range of heart rate for the neonate is 120 to 180 beats per minute. The normal blood pressure is around 40 to 45 systolic and 20 to 25 diastolic.

4. The infant's body temperature may fall quickly at birth unless precautions against heat loss are taken. The infant uses shivering and metabolism to increase body temperature. Provision of a heated environment and reduction of the amount of physiologic stress the infant must manage help contribute to maintenance of adequate body temperature. The usual axillary temperature for the neonate should stabilize around 97°F (36.1°C).

5. An elevated bilirubin content in the neonate's blood causes a slight jaundiced appearance. This is called physiologic jaundice. It may increase during the first few days of life and generally disappears by the 14th day of life.

6. Initial stools of the neonate will be meconium, a black, sticky material. This may be preceded by expulsion of thick, grayish mucous. By the second to the fourth day, greenish brown to greenish yellow stools appear. They then change to yellowish semiformed (in breast-fed infants) or formed (in formula-fed infants) stools.

7. The umbilical cord begins to discolor and shrink soon after birth. Within a few days, the stump will dry up and turn black. After about 7 or 8 days, the stump sloughs off, leaving a granular area.

Pathophysiological Concepts

1. *Surfactant* is a substance lining the air sacs of the lungs. It reduces surface tension and keeps the sacs inflated by preventing their complete collapse during expiration. Immature infants or those who have suffered prenatal hypoxia may not manufacture surfactant. They then suffer from collapse of the air sacs, called respiratory distress syndrome. A hyaline membrane may form in the unexpanded air sacs, resulting in the infant being able to aerate only a small portion of the lung.

2. Shunting of small amounts of blood through the ductus arteriosus or the foramen ovale may occur when pressure variations occur within the neonate's heart. However, failure of these openings to close may lead to severe cardiac complications. Other congenital heart defects compromise the neonate. Cyanosis is the most common symptom of cardiac disease or problems.

3. Infants who become chilled must increase their metabolism, oxygen consumption and use of glucose. The side-effects are hypoglycemia, a state of acidosis, and inability to produce surfactant.

4. The head of the infant may be molded during delivery, giving it an elongated shape. This usually subsides in 1 to 2 days. *Caput succedaneum* is a swelling of the presenting portion of the cranium due to pressure during birth. The edema is usually absorbed in a few days. Swelling of the head due to accumulation of blood occurring after birth is called a cephalhematoma. It is usually due to birth trauma and may require several weeks to disappear.

5. The *fontanelles* are the areas located at the junction of the cranial sutures. Their size varies from wide open to almost closed. The size and tension of the fontanelles indicate the status of the infant. An increase in tension may indicate increased intracranial pressure or hydrocephalus. A decrease in the tension may indicate dehydration.

6. Failure of the infant to pass meconium during the first 24 hours of life may indicate an obstructed eliminatory system. The condition in which the lower bowel is not patent is called *imperforate anus*.

7. Continual regurgitation of oral liquids may indicate occlusion of the esophagus. Because of the possibility of aspiration, it is important to recognize this problem early and to withhold oral fluids until surgical repair can be done.

Assessment of the Client

The entire admission procedure is one of assessment of the newborn for ability to tolerate and adapt to extrauterine life. Assessment will be discussed under Procedural Aspects.

Plan

Nursing Objectives

Provide an environment in which the infant can satisfactorily recover from the trauma of birth.

Protect the infant from cross-contamination.

Ensure accurate identification of the infant.

Maintain a warm environment to conserve energy.

Provide careful observation of the newborn to detect abnormalities.

Promote the early establishment of the mother–child bond and the identification of the family unit.

Client Preparation

1. The infant should be properly identified in the delivery room. Identification should be attached to the infant's body in a manner that will prevent its becoming detached (Fig. 135-1). Identification may include foot-printing the infant and thumb-printing the mother.

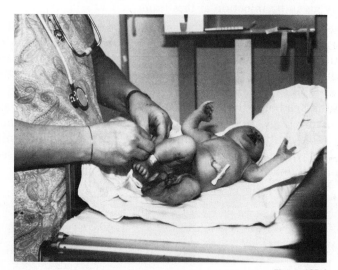 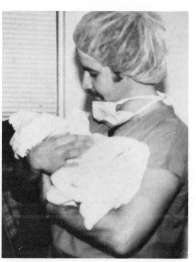

Figure 135.1   *Figure 135.2*

2. If the infant is stable, the parents should be allowed to meet and hold this new member of their family. The infant may remain with the mother in the recovery room. Some hospitals allow the father to carry the infant to the nursery (Fig. 135-2).

3. The infant is usually in stable condition before being transported to the nursery. The Apgar score (Technique 146) should have been completed in the delivery room. Adequate respiration should be established. Infants who are unstable are usually admitted to the neonatal intensive care unit (NICU) or are stabilized in the nursery and transported to the nearest NICU when possible.

Equipment

Balance scale with disposable covering

Tape measure

Rectal thermometer

Stethoscope

Controlled-environment warmer

Bulb syringe

Implementation and Interventions

Procedural Aspects

ACTION

1. Wash hands before and after handling each infant.

2. Assess the status of the infant upon admission to the nursery. If the infant is stable and is not experiencing respiratory distress, proceed with initial assessments. If the infant did not receive ophthalmic prophylaxis in the delivery room, it should be done now (see Technique No. 143, Eye Care, Initial). Vitamin K prophylaxis is usually given by injection at this time.

3. Weigh the infant upon admission to the nursery. Place the naked infant on a balanced scale covered with a cloth or paper covering (Fig. 135-3). Measure the circumference of the head and chest with a tape measure (Figs. 135-4, 135-5). Use extreme caution in handling the infant who may be wet and active and difficult to handle.

RATIONALE

Infants are extremely susceptible to infection because of the immaturity of their immune systems.

If the infant is in respiratory distress or is chilled, delay initial assessments until complications are reversed. Warming is necessary to conserve the infant's energy. Vitamin K is administered to augment the clotting mechanism, which is deficient at birth.

Loss of fluids will result in weight reduction. A loss of several grams is expected during the first few days of life. To evaluate this loss in distinguishing between normal and abnormal weight loss, an accurate initial weight measurement is essential. The paper or cloth lining of the scale will help prevent cross-infection of the infant.

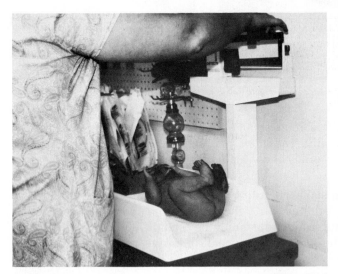

Figure 135.3

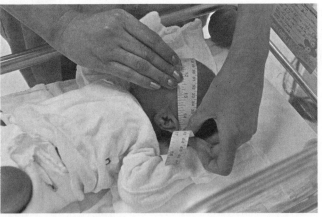

Figure 135.4

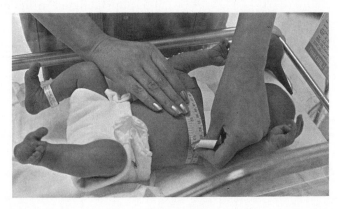

Figure 135.5

ACTION	*RATIONALE*
4. Assess the gestational age of the infant. There are a number of assessment tools that allow a systematic evaluation of physical and/or neurologic maturity of the infant.	It is possible to predict expected needs of the infant based on gestational age.
5. Measure the infant's vital signs. Auscultate the pulse apically for 30 seconds, preferably with the infant quiet. Count the respirations while the infant is quiet by observing the abdomen. Assess the infant for any grunting, chest retraction, or nasal flaring. Measure the initial temperature rectally. If any resistance is met, do not force the thermometer into the rectum. Measure the temperature by the axillary route and notify the physician. After the initial rectal measurement, axillary temperature measurements are generally taken unless otherwise stipulated by the pediatric care provider or hospital policy. Assess the infant's blood pressure by using a Doppler pressure-monitoring device. Measure the vital signs every 15 minutes for the first hour, then every 2 to 4 hours if the infant is stable and shows no signs of complications.	Vital signs are measured initially as an indicator of the neonate's condition and to provide baseline measurements for future comparisons. Since crying tends to elevate pulse and respiration rates, assessment during quiet, noncrying periods is preferred. Inability to pass the thermometer into the rectum may indicate imperforate anus. Forcing the thermometer might perforate the anus, causing grave complications. The chance of rectal perforation is also increased by repeated rectal temperature measurements.
6. Wipe the excess debris or materials from the infant's skin. Assess the infant for any abnormalities, bruises, or other trauma that may have occurred during the birth process. Take care to avoid chilling the infant.	After birth, the infant is frequently covered with dried blood and vernix caseosa. The infant is very susceptible to temperature changes and must be kept warm.
7. Check the clamp on the umbilical cord to ensure that it is tight and no leakage is occurring. Check the umbilical stump every 2 to 4 hours during the first 24 hours. Keep the cord area clean and dry to avoid infection (see Technique No. 140, Cord Care.)	The umbilical cord is clamped in the delivery room. Hemorrhage from the umbilical vessels is a possibility during the first 24 hours after birth. The moist, warm environment also makes the cord an ideal area for colonization of microorganisms.

ACTION	RATIONALE
8. Place the infant in a preheated, temperature-controlled environment. Check and chart the temperature every 4 hours while the infant is in this controlled environment. After stabilization of temperature, clothe the baby and place in an open crib. Clothing and coverings should provide warmth, but should not be constraining and confining. Place the infant in the side-lying position with the head slightly lower than the trunk. Keep a bulb syringe in the incubator or crib in case the infant requires nasal–oral suctioning (Fig. 135-6).	The infant requires several hours to stabilize the body's temperature-regulating mechanism. A controlled environment will help maintain body temperature until the infant is capable of self-regulation. The infant's nose, throat, and lungs have been filled with amniotic fluid before birth. The birth process and the initial breath clears most of the fluid. Using the principles of gravitational flow will help drain the remainder of the liquid. Suction may also help with removal of this fluid to prevent choking.

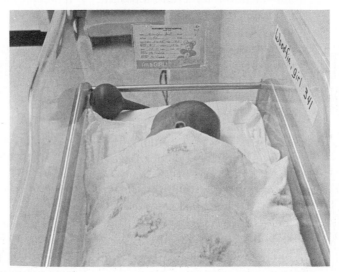

Figure 135.6

9. Allow the infant to rest during the first hours in the nursery.	The infant's primary need after birth is rest from the stress and rigors of the birth process.

Communicative Aspects

OBSERVATIONS

1. Observe the infant's activity, cry, and muscle tone. Periods of activity are expected to alternate with periods of sleep. If the infant has diminished reflexes or activity, abnormalities may be expected. Also, hypersensitivity to stimuli, shown by twitching, shaking, or an extremely high-pitched cry, may also indicate abnormalities.

2. Observe the color of the infant's skin. Initial pinkness with some cyanosis of the feet and hands is expected. Overall cyanosis, paleness, or pallor may indicate respiratory or circulatory problems. Observe for the yellowish tinge of jaundice.

3. Observe for indications that the infant is ready to eat. Observe for the first voiding and the first stool.

4. Observe the umbilical stump for hemorrhaging. Observe to see that the clamp is tight and remains in place.

5. Observe for any congenital abnormalities or for trauma that may have occurred during the birth process.

6. Infants who are at risk for hypoglycemia, such as those who have low birth weight or who had a difficult delivery, should be observed for decreased blood glucose levels.

CHARTING

DATE/TIME	OBSERVATIONS	SIGNATURE
3/14 0845	Admitted to newborn nursery after vaginal delivery at 0810. Carried to nursery by father. Male infant, weight 3,232 g; length 49.5 cm; head circum. 33 cm; chest 35.5 cm. T 97.4°F taken rectally with no difficulty. Apical pulse 128, R 40, blood pressure (Doppler) 45/24. Est. gestational age 40 weeks. No bruises or marks, slight redness over left eye. Slight elongation of head. Umbilical cord moist, no oozing or bleeding. Color pink except soles of feet and palms of hands. No stool and due to void. Credé's prophylaxis to eyes. Vitamin K 0.5 ml given IM. Placed in infant warmer. Report given to father and grandparents who are viewing baby at this time. ————————	N. Jones RN

Discharge Planning Aspects

CLIENT AND FAMILY EDUCATION

1. Allow the father and family members to witness the initial assessment if they wish. If the father is present at the assessment, demonstrate how to handle the baby carefully and confidently so that he will feel more comfortable with the infant. Provide a mechanism for the mother to know vital statistics of the infant as soon as possible. Mothers and families are generally very interested in weight and length, as well as in assurances that the infant is stable and healthy.

2. Provide the family with information about their infant during the observation period while the baby is stabilizing. They may be able to see the baby. Explain why warming the infant is necessary. When the infant is under a radiant warmer, clothing and diapers are generally not used. Seeing the infant without warm clothing may be disconcerting to the family who has been told that they may not hold their infant until warming is complete. Explain the principles behind radiant warmth, emphasizing that at this stage the clothing may inhibit warming. Tell them that when the infant is placed in an open crib, clothing and a diaper will be applied.

Evaluation

Quality Assurance

Documentation should include baseline vital signs and assessments. Evidence of frequent monitoring during the first hour (such as q 15 min) and consistent monitoring during subsequent time in the nursery (such as q 2–4 hr) should be evidenced. Any abnormalities should be noted and reporting should be documented along with follow-up activities and outcomes. Evidence of teaching and inclusion of the parents and family should be noted in the chart.

Infection Control

1. The immune system of the neonate is immature, making susceptibility to infection very great during this period. Careful handwashing should precede and follow care of each infant.

2. The area around the cord is usually cleansed with some type of bacteriostatic solution to prevent infection.

3. All equipment and materials that come in contact with the infant should be clean. Care must be taken not to cross-infect infants. All equipment used for subsequent infants should be cleaned and disinfected after use.

Technique Checklist   YES   NO

    Infant born at _____

      Infant received in nursery at _____

      Transported to nursery by _____

      Report of labor and delivery given   _____   _____

    Assessments made and recorded:

      Weight   _____   _____

      Length   _____   _____

      Head circumference   _____   _____

      Chest circumference   _____   _____

      Estimated gestational age _____ wks

      Vital signs

        Temperature _____

          Rectal _____

          Axilla _____

        Pulse _____

          Respirations _____

          Blood pressure _____

      Umbilical cord   _____   _____

      Ophthalmic prophylaxis   _____   _____

      Vitamin K prophylaxis   _____   _____

      Hypoglycemia testing   _____   _____

      Voiding   _____   _____

      Stool   _____   _____

    Parents informed of status of infant   _____   _____

    Complications or abnormalities noted _____

      Reported to physician   _____   _____

Bathing the Infant

Overview

Definition

The medium and method of cleansing the body of an infant

Rationale

Provide for cleanliness and comfort for the infant.
Cleanse the skin to remove microorganisms.
Permit observation of the child.

Terminology

Foreskin: The fold of skin over the glans penis in the male infant

Assessment

**Pertinent Anatomy
and Physiology**

See Appendix I: *skin.*

**Pathophysiological
Concepts**

Normal healthy skin has resident microorganisms that are not harmful. The skin is a natural barrier that protects underlying tissues from physical injury and bacterial invasion. In addition, it has a normal pH of 5 to 6, which is slightly acidic and is not supportive of microorganism growth. However, if a break occurs in the skin, pathogenic organisms are able to enter the blood stream, which is much more supportive to their growth. Mechanical cleansing of the skin and prevention of breaks in the skin surface will help prevent pathogenic invasion.

Assessment of the Client

1. Assess the physical condition of the infant in determining how much body surface to bathe. If the infant is very weak or debilitated, bathing may be confined to those areas that may be susceptible to colonization of microorganisms, such as the face and ears, the genitalia, and the rectum.
2. Assess the developmental level of the infant. If the child can sit up and there are no physical contraindications, allow the infant to sit in the tub or basin during the bath. *Never leave the infant unattended during the bath.*
3. Assess the knowledge level of the parents in soliciting their participation in the bath. If they are unfamiliar with proper safety precautions when bathing their infant, use the bath time to demonstrate. Assess the parent–child relationship. Determine if the parent is at ease with the child, amount of eye contact, and willingness of the parent to talk to the child.

Plan

Nursing Objectives

Promote proper hygiene and comfort of the child.
Observe the child's skin.
Assess the child's activity level, stage of development, and behavior.
Assess the child's physical condition.
Gain insight into the parent–child relationship.
Protect the integrity of the child's skin.

Client Preparation

1. Ensure that the bathing room is warm and drafts are eliminated.

2. Prepare all equipment within reach at the bedside. Fill the infant tub or basin half full of warm water, 43.3° to 46°C (110°–115°F).

3. Remove the child's clothing. Remove the pins from the diaper but leave it in place until the child is placed in the infant tub or until the genitalia are to be washed. Close the pins and place them out of the child's reach.

4. To many young infants, bath time is a very exciting and happy time. The medium of water is different from their normal world of hard and soft surfaces. This fact encourages experimentation and heightened activity. It is usually a good idea for the nurse to wear a covering over the uniform to protect against splashing.

Equipment

Linen for crib

Blanket

Diaper and infant clothing

Mild soap

Infant tub or basin

Implementation and Interventions

Procedural Aspects

ACTION

1. Place the infant in the tub supported by the nurse's hand. Keep hold of the infant during the entire procedure (Fig. 136-1). The infant may be bathed in the crib if placement in the tub is contraindicated by the presence of intravenous (IV) infusions, tubes, or dressings.

RATIONALE

Support and restraint by the nurse's hand provide an added safety measure to prevent falls and frightening the infant by accidental submersion.

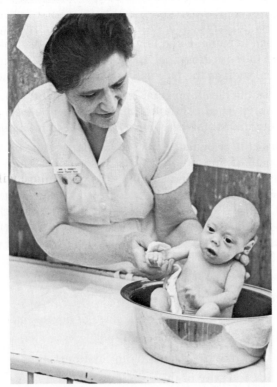

Figure 136.1

ACTION	**RATIONALE**
2. Using a clean, damp washcloth, wash the infant's eyes and face first. Using the corner of the cloth, gently wash one eye from the inner aspect outward to remove debris from the lid and skin around the eye. Using a different portion of the cloth, do the same for the other eye. Wash the face and external ears with warm water only. Lift the infant's chin and wash the neck reaching all creases.	The skin over and around the eyes is cleansed so that surface debris will not enter the eye itself, causing trauma and possibly contamination. The eye itself is not bathed because of its delicate and susceptible nature. To remove debris in the eye, sterile irrigation is necessary. Infants usually have short necks resulting in creases in which pathogenic microorganisms may colonize if these areas are not cleaned.
3. Using a very mild soap, wash the infant's hair and scalp. If the infant is in the tub, rinse the hair by reclining the infant in the tub supported by the nurse's hand. If the infant was not placed in the tub, the hair may be rinsed by holding the infant in the football hold and rinsing (see Technique 143, Bathing of Newborn, Initial).	Soap must be completely rinsed from the child's skin or it may serve as an irritant, causing itching and discomfort. Be certain that the infant is supported at all times to prevent falls and fright.
4. Lather and wash the infant's trunk, arms, and legs. Wash the genitalia. In the uncircumcised male infant, it is necessary to retract the foreskin over the penis each time the child is bathed to allow removal of the white, cheeselike exudate which forms there. After retracting the foreskin, allow water to run over the glans. Wash the rectal area last.	Wash the areas that are dirty. In the crawling infant, the hands, knees, and feet usually require additional attention. Cleansing of the glans penis must be done very gently. Since this area is very sensitive, do not rub it with a washcloth. Rinsing is usually sufficient to remove the exudate. Retraction of the foreskin also helps keep it stretched preventing later urinary problems. Microorganisms normally found in the rectal area may be pathogenic when transported to other areas of the body. For this reason, the rectum is bathed last.
5. Grasp the infant with a towel to ensure safe removal from the tub. Wrap the infant in a towel to prevent chilling. Dry the infant well and comb or brush the hair. Dress the infant and make the bed with fresh linen.	A squirming infant is sometimes difficult to hold. Being wet increases the problem because the infant is slippery. Using a towel as an extra safety feature will help prevent dropping the infant. Evaporation from the infant's wet skin may cause chilling. Drying quickly and thoroughly will prevent chilling and will increase comfort.

ACTION	RATIONALE
Special Modifications	
For the infant with an IV infusion, a cast, a dressing, or other areas that cannot be immersed in water, bring the tub of warm water to the bedside and bathe the infant lying in bed. A clean blanket may be placed under the infant to provide a clean environment and to promote warmth. Accessible areas should be bathed. It is particularly important to cleanse areas prone to colonization by microorganisms. The glans penis of the uncircumcised male infant may be cleansed by gently wiping it with a cotton ball.	Immobilized infants do not get dirty in the same fashion as they do when they are up and around. However, a bath is usually comforting and a welcome break from the enforced restriction on activities. In addition, restriction of movement may promote the growth of microorganisms in warm, moist areas.

Communicative Aspects

OBSERVATIONS

1. Observe the infant continuously during the bath to prevent accidents. Keep one hand on the infant to prevent accidental submersion, which is frightening to the infant.

2. Observe the skin for abnormalities such as rash and chafing. Observe for abnormalities of the joints, limbs, and other body surfaces.

3. Observe the infant's behavior during the bath. Determine if the infant seems to be in pain. Observe for indications of the infant's level of growth and development. Note the infant's sociability and physical range of motion.

4. Observe the infant's physical condition. Determine if the infant is well nourished. Observe any symptoms relating to the condition for which the infant has been hospitalized.

CHARTING

DATE/TIME	OBSERVATIONS	SIGNATURE
4/10 0930	Bathed with mild soap in infant tub in bathroom. Cool mist humidifier continuous in room. Playful during bath but did have two coughing episodes. Bilateral breath sounds still reveal moderate congestion. Returned to Croupette. Mother in attendance during bath. Safety measures stressed. Mother will bathe infant tomorrow with nurse observing.	C. Loo RN

Discharge Planning Aspects

CLIENT AND FAMILY EDUCATION

1. Stress to the parents the importance of preventing falls during bathing. Advise them never to leave their infant alone in the tub, even for one second. Explain to them that handling the wet infant with a dry towel will reduce the chance of dropping the infant.

2. Explain to the parents how to test the bath water to ensure that the infant is not burned. The water should feel warm to the inner aspect of the parent's wrist. Advise them never to add hot water to the tub with the infant in the tub. If the water gets too cool, they should remove the infant and add warmer water. The water should again be tested to ensure proper temperature before the infant is replaced into the tub.

3. Teach the parents the proper way to bathe a child, with emphasis on cleansing the contaminated areas last. Stress the necessity of cleansing from front to back when cleansing the genital area. If the male child is uncircumcised, the proper way to retract the foreskin and cleanse the glans penis should be taught.

4. Explain to the parents that there is a trend away from daily bathing of healthy infants. Daily bathing removes many of the natural oils that lubricate and protect the infant's delicate skin. Application of baby oils may cause dermatologic problems because of the presence of perfumes and other additives. It is often advisable to leave the natural oils alone to protect the infant. A current trend is to wash only the part of the baby that is soiled. If the infant soils a diaper, wash the genital and buttocks. If the infant gets food on both face and arms, wash the face and arms. It is no longer considered necessary to completely bathe the infant every day. When the child reaches the toddler stage, more frequent bathing may be necessary. But, again, stress that the infant or child should be bathed only when necessary.

Evaluation

Quality Assurance

Documentation of the child's bath is usually not made every day unless something extraordinary occurs or is observed. However, hospital policy should state the expected frequency of bathing, and deviations from this should be addressed in the chart. Any observations during bathing should be noted. Teaching of the parents and their observed understanding should be noted.

Infection Control

1. Cleanse the accumulated microorganisms from the skin to prevent colonization and proliferation into infection.
2. Label the infant's equipment, such as the bath basin, so that it will not be used for another client. If infant tubs or basins are used for consecutive clients, they must be cleaned and disinfected between each use.
3. Health-care personnel should engage in thorough handwashing before and after bathing the infant.
4. The skin is the natural protective barrier of the body. As long as the skin is intact, the chances of infections are minimized. Be careful not to scratch or otherwise traumatize the skin during bathing. Rings should be removed and long fingernails shortened.

Technique Checklist

	YES	NO
Explanation of procedure given to parents	_____	_____
Hands washed prior to starting bath	_____	_____
Type of bath		
In bed	_____	_____
In infant tub	_____	_____
Chilling avoided	_____	_____
Condition of skin noted	_____	_____
Constant attendance during bath	_____	_____
Bathed contaminated areas last	_____	_____
Teaching needs identified and addressed	_____	_____
Parents indicated understanding and acceptance of teaching	_____	_____

137 Bathing of Newborn, Initial

Overview

Definition   The initial cleansing of the remnants of birth from the infant's body

Rationale   Cleanse the infant.
Observe the infant for abnormalities.
Evaluate the infant's condition.

Terminology   ***Esophageal atresia:*** Occlusion or abnormal closure of the esophagus
Moro's reflex: A startle reflex, elicited by a sudden loud noise or jarring of the crib, in which the infant's arms extend outward with fingers spread, and then the hands are brought together.

Assessment

Pertinent Anatomy and Physiology
1. See Appendix I: *skin.*
2. The skin of the newborn is dark red or pinkish red. The hands and feet are often cyanotic for a few hours after birth. *Vernix caseosa,* a greasy, white, cheeselike material consists of an accumulation of secretions from the sebaceous glands. It covers the skin at birth. It may be present in a thin layer over the body; however, it is usually thicker in the folds and creases. It generally disappears after the first day.

Pathophysiological Concepts
The infant's temperature-regulating system is intact at birth. Because the infant does not usually shiver during the first hours after birth, chilling is combated by increased metabolism. This increase in metabolism depletes glucose and other energy sources and may cause acidosis and death if not reversed.

Assessment of the Client
1. Assess the temperature of the infant to determine if it has stabilized before undertaking the bath.
2. Assess the vital signs to determine if the infant is experiencing any complications that might indicate that the bath should be postponed.
3. Assess the infant's color to determine if adequate aeration of the lungs has occurred and to assess the adequacy of the circulatory system.
4. Assess the activity of the infant. Generally a period of activity is followed by a period of rest. Another period of activity then occurs about 2 hours after birth. After this time, the infant's condition has usually stabilized to the point that the bath may be safely done.

Plan

Nursing Objectives

Provide cleansing of the infant so that adequate visualization and assessment may be done.

Observe the infant for complications or problems.

Evaluate the infant's tolerance of activity and environment.

Enhance the family bond between the parents and the infant.

Client Preparation

1. The infant's initial bath is usually postponed until respiratory status is stabilized and body temperature has returned to approximately 98°F. This may take 3 to 4 hours.

2. The gross remnants of the birth process, such as blood on the head and face, will have been wiped away with dry cotton balls upon the infant's admission to the nursery.

3. Wrap the infant in a towel to prevent chilling during the bath.

Equipment

Cotton pads

Mild, nonmedicated soap

Warm, sterile water

Antiseptic, for cord care

Infant clothing

Implementation and Interventions

Procedural Aspects

ACTION	RATIONALE
1. Wash hands thoroughly before bathing the infant. Be sure that each infant has a separate crib for exclusive use.	The newborn has few defense mechanisms against unfavorable factors in the environment.
2. Use cotton sponges soaked with sterile water to remove blood from the face and head.	Soap should not be left on the infant's delicate skin because it may cause irritation.
3. Proceed with the bath, washing the eyes first. Wash from the inner canthus outward, using a clean cotton pad for each eye (Fig. 137-1). Wash the nose and ears, observing for abnormalities. Wash the hair with the mild soap and rinse thoroughly (Fig. 137-2). Hold the infant in the "football hold," that is, under the arm and balanced on the nurse's hip with the head supported by the nurse's hand (Fig. 137-3). Wash the feet if footprint identification was done. Remove meconium from the perianal area with a front to back motion. A mild, nonmedicated soap may be used. Rinse the washed areas thoroughly.	Take care not to contaminate the infant. Prevention of infection is critical at this stage. Because the infant is likely to be active, a firm hold is essential to prevent dropping. Supporting the head prevents strain on the infant's neck muscles.

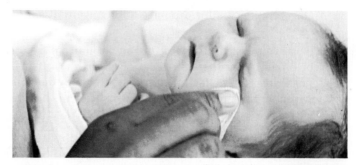

Figure 137.1

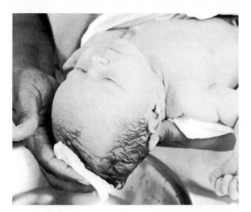

Figure 137.2

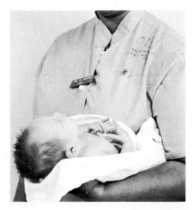

Figure 137.3

ACTION	RATIONALE
4. Cleanse around the cord area with a cotton ball and antiseptic. Dry the area but do not cover it.	Because the cord provides a direct entrance into the infant's circulatory system, it must be kept clean until it closes.
5. Do not wash the vernix from the rest of the infant's skin unless it is grossly soiled.	The American Academy of Pediatrics has stated that evidence indicates that the vernix caseosa may serve a protective function and no evidence indicates that it is harmful to the infant. Therefore, it is not washed from the infant's skin.
6. Leave the infant in a side-lying position.	Lying on the side facilitates drainage of mucus and helps prevent aspiration and choking.

Communicative Aspects

OBSERVATIONS

1. Observe the color of the infant. If color is cyanotic or pale, notify the physician. Physiologic jaundice may give a yellowish tinge to the skin. This should be reported to the physician.

2. Observe the eyes for hemorrhage or capillary rupture. Note edema of the eyelids or neuromuscular problems indicated by random movements of downward displacement of the eyes (setting-sun sign). Also note the presence of tearing, which usually does not occur until several months of age.

3. Observe the nasal area for drainage, cleft lip, and septal defects. Observe the appearance of mucus in the mouth, which might indicate esophageal atresia. Observe the palate for abnormalities.

4. Observe the ears for drainage and congenital abnormalities, such as low-set ears.

5. Observe the head for molding and abnormal lumps, which may indicate fluid or blood under the skin because of birth trauma. Observe the anterior and posterior fontanelles for depression or bulging. Observe the facial appearance and note the presence of forceps marks and birthmarks.

6. Note the presence of swollen glands and nodes in the neck area.

7. Observe the chest for retracting and for any trauma that may have occurred during the birth process.

8. Observe the fingers and toes for congenital absence or extra digits. Observe for tremors. Note the presence of club feet and asymmetry.

9. Observe the trunk for abdominal distension, hernia, spina bifida, meningocele and masses. Note the condition of the cord. Observe for oozing or bleeding.

10. Observe the genitalia for vaginal discharge (normal) and proximation or flaring of the labia majora. Observe the presence of the testes in the scrotum. Note the presence of meconium and/or urine, which indicates that voiding and stool elimination have occurred.

11. Observe the general degree of infant's alertness. Note the presence of reflexes, such as the Moro's reflex. Observe the activity level and muscle tone of the infant. Note the cry; a high shrill cry may indicate complications.

CHARTING

Notations about voiding, stool, or any other pertinent observations should be appropriately charted.

DATE/TIME	OBSERVATIONS	SIGNATURE
1/7 0900	Admission bath given. Small bruise, approx. 2 cm diameter on left shoulder. Alert and crying. Moro reflex apparent. Fontanelles soft. Lusty cry, no retractions. Small amount of meconium stool. Cord moist with no oozing or bleeding, cleaned with antiseptic. Face, head, and perianal areas cleaned with sponges and warm water. Reasons for bath and limitations of the area bathed explained to parents who state their understanding. With parents at this time. —————————————————————	 C. Loo RN

Discharge Planning Aspects

CLIENT AND FAMILY EDUCATION

1. Explain to the parents what the vernix caseosa is and why it is not removed. Emphasize its lubricant quality and explain that it will be absorbed or rubbed off by clothing in a day or two.

2. Tell the family that the intent of the initial bath is to improve the comfort and appearance of the baby. It also affords an opportunity for the nurse to inspect and observe the infant. Explain that the baby will be kept clean and dry in the nursery. Encourage the parents to participate in the infant's care as soon as possible.

Evaluation

Quality Assurance

Documentation should include any abnormalities observed during the bath. Notation of reporting of abnormalities and action taken should also be made. Extent of the bath and explanations to the parents should also be included.

Infection Control

1. The infant's defense system is immature, and infection is a constant threat. Use sterile or clean equipment in bathing the infant.

2. Careful handwashing should precede and follow any care rendered to infants. Jewelry should not be worn because it may harbor microorganisms. A surgical scrub may be done when the nurse reports for duty to ensure the removal of as many microorganisms as possible. This scrub does not take the place of handwashing between infants.

Technique Checklist

	YES	NO
Procedure explained to parents	_____	_____
Observations noted on chart	_____	_____

Bath included

    Head _____

    Face _____

    Perianal region _____

    Other _____

Complications or abnormalities

_____

_____

138   Bundling the Infant

Overview

Definition

The process of encasing the infant in a blanket

Rationale

Provide security for the infant.
Maintain adequate warmth.
Facilitate safer and easier handling of the infant.

Assessment

Assessment of the Client

1. Assess the infant's temperature before removal from the heated crib environment. The temperature should be stabilized above 97°F before the infant is removed and wrapped in a blanket.
2. Assess the infant's respiratory status. If excessive mucus is present, the infant must be observed carefully and suctioned as needed.

Plan

Nursing Objectives

Maintain security without constricting movement.
Facilitate aeration of lungs by keeping the infant's airway patent.

Client Preparation

1. Check the infant to ensure that the diaper and clothing are dry before bundling. Be sure that pins and other closures are secured.
2. Examine the infant for normal breathing and movement before wrapping.

Equipment

Blanket

Implementation and Interventions

Procedural Aspects

ACTION	RATIONALE
1. Lay the blanket on a flat surface. Place the infant supine in the middle of the blanket. Bring the left side of the blanket across the front of the infant (Fig. 138-1). Bring the bottom of the blanket up and tuck it inside the overlapping portion (Fig. 138-2). Bring the right side across and tuck it under the infant's body (Fig. 138-3). Make the blanket tight enough to give a sense of security, but not too constricting or confining. The infant should be able to move both arms and legs while in the blanket (Fig. 138-4). If the infant is to be placed	The fetus is accustomed to a warm, stable, confining environment. After birth, the temperature fluctuations and vastness of the surroundings may have an unsettling effect on the newborn infant. Being closely wrapped in a warm blanket may provide a sense of security.

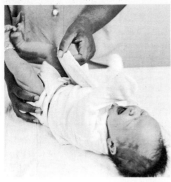

Figure 138.1

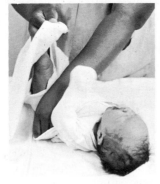

Figure 138.2

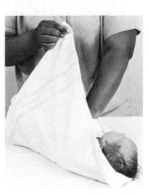

Figure 138.3

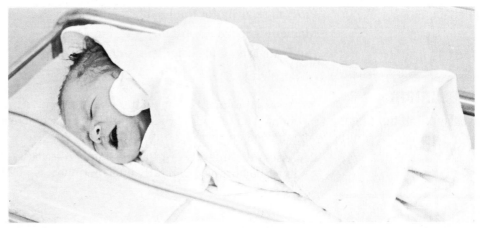

Figure 138.4

ACTION	RATIONALE
on the right side, the right side of the blanket is brought across first.	
2. Place the infant in the side-lying position. A rolled diaper may be placed against the infant's back for support.	The side-lying position facilitates the drainage of mucus.

Communicative Aspects

OBSERVATIONS

1. Observe the infant's color and respiratory rate to be sure that breathing is not inhibited by drainage in the throat or by the constriction of the blanket.

2. Observe the blanket to see that it does not become too loose because of infant's activity.

CHARTING

DATE/TIME	OBSERVATIONS	SIGNATURE
3/15 0845	Apical pulse 110, Resp 36. Suctioned with bulb syringe. Bundled and turned to right side.	C. Loo RN
0915	Sleeping quietly, no cyanosis or choking.	C. Loo RN

Discharge Planning Aspects

CLIENT AND FAMILY EDUCATION

Teach the parents the bundling technique. Emphasize the need to avoid too much constriction of movements. Explain why the infant is placed in the side-lying position and proper use of the bulb syringe if suctioning will be done at home.

Evaluation

Quality Assurance

Documentation should include notation of safety precautions when the infant is bundled (i.e., respiratory rate, color, any problems). It is usually not necessary to document every occasion of bundling the infant. Generally, documentation occurs when the bundling is done following another technique or problem.

Infection Control

1. Careful handwashing should precede and follow care of each infant
2. Blankets and other linen should be for the exclusive use of a single infant. No linen should be shared in the nursery. If the blanket comes in contact with the floor or other contaminated surface, it should be discarded and a clean one used.

Technique Checklist

	YES	NO
Bundling technique explained to parents	_____	_____
Adequate respiratory status maintained	_____	_____

139 Circumcision Care

Overview

Definition

Treatments and considerations given to the care of the infant male genitalia after surgical excision of the prepuce (foreskin) of the penis

Rationale

Prevent infection.

Minimize the infant's discomfort.

Facilitate cleansing of the penis.

Promote proper male hygiene.

Fulfill a religious or cultural ritual.

Terminology

Phimosis: Stenosis or narrowing of the preputial orifice so that the foreskin cannot be pushed back over the glans penis

Prepuce: Foreskin or fold of skin over the glans penis

Assessment

Pertinent Anatomy and Physiology

1. See Appendix I: *genitalia (male).*
2. At birth, the male infant's scrotum may be edematous. This condition usually resolves in several days. Normally, both of the testes have descended into the scrotal sac in the term infant. The prepuce of the penis usually does not separate from the glans until the child is several months old.
3. Circumcision involves removal of the prepuce partially or totally from the glans of the infant.

Pathophysiological Concepts

1. Undescended testicles, also called *cryptorchidism,* results from failure of one or both testicles to descend from the intra-abdominal cavity through the inguinal canal. This usually occurs during the 8th or 9th month of gestation. Uncorrected bilateral cryptorchidism leads to sterility and may predispose the client to the development of testicular cancer. The testicles atrophy, probably because of the body-cavity temperature higher than that to which testes in the scrotum are exposed.
2. *Smegma* is a cheeselike material that collects under the foreskin. When bacteria is present, irritation results.

Assessment of the Client

1. Assess the condition of the male genitalia. Note the presence of undescended testes or scrotal edema.
2. Assess the bleeding and clotting time of the infant before the circumcision is done. If the clotting time is extended, notify the primary-care provider.
3. Assess the condition of the circumcision. Determine if the area is bleeding or appears abnormal.

Plan

Nursing Objectives Assist the practitioner in the circumcision procedure as needed.

Prevent infection of the circumcision site.

Observe for bleeding.

Promote healing by keeping the area clean and dry.

Allay the parents' anxiety about the procedure and aftercare.

Client Preparation

1. Be sure that the parents know why the procedure is done and exactly what will happen. The American Academy of Pediatrics has stated that there are no actual medical indications for circumcision during the neonatal period. They affirm the rights of the parents to know this and to be allowed to make a truly informed consent. This is the physician's responsibility. However, the nurse has the responsibility to answer questions honestly and to be sure that the parents understand what is happening to their infant.

2. Feedings may be withheld for 1 hour prior to circumcision, since the infant may regurgitate during the procedure.

3. Circumcision is considered a surgical procedure. The written consent of one or both parents is required before it can be done. Consult the hospital policy manual or the laws of the state to determine what kind of consent is required.

Equipment Adequate lighting

Preparation solution

Circumcision board

Dressing, such as a petrolatum gauze (if ordered)

Circumcision set containing surgical equipment for circumcision (a disposable clamp may be used)

Implementation and Interventions

Procedural Aspects

ACTION	RATIONALE
1. Set up the circumcision area before bringing in the infant. Place the circumcision board (Fig. 139-1) on the surface. Pad the board to promote comfort and place the infant on the board. Secure him with the restraining straps (Fig. 139-2). Do not leave the infant unattended. If the procedure is delayed, place the infant back in the crib until ready.	Since the infant is sensitive to extremes in temperature, he should not be exposed to the room environment any longer than necessary. The procedure should proceed efficiently. When unavoidable delays occur, removing the infant back to his crib ensures his safety and warmth.
2. Cleanse the penis and surrounding area with a disinfectant. Assist the practitioner during the procedure. After the clamp is removed, apply the prescribed dressing. Observe the circumcision for several minutes to ensure that clotting is taking place before applying the dressing.	A clamp generally is used to control the bleeding by placing pressure on the excised surfaces. Once the clamp is removed, a dressing may be used to control bleeding or to absorb oozing. Cleansing the area with a disinfectant reduces the number of microorganisms and helps prevent infection.

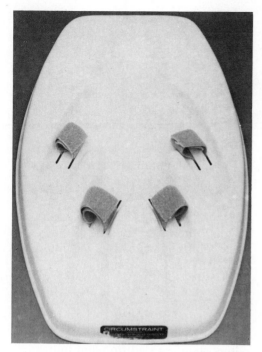

Figure 139.1

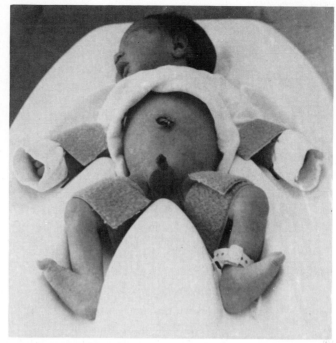

Figure 139.2

ACTION	*RATIONALE*
3. Apply a loose diaper over the circumcised area. Dress and bundle the infant before returning him to the crib. Cuddle the infant for a few minutes before placing him in his bed. Unless contraindicated, allow his mother to hold and cuddle him after the procedure. The infant may be fed if he is hungry.	The infant may cry during the procedure because of the discomfort or the restraint. However, this usually ceases after the procedure is completed. Allowing the mother to hold and comfort her child will reassure her about his condition and will contribute to mother–infant bonding.
4. Observe the infant for 12 hours for any signs of bleeding at the circumcision site. Position the infant on his side. If bleeding should occur, place a sterile 4 × 4 gauze pad over the circumcised area and apply gentle pressure until the bleeding stops or the physician performs surgical repair.	Bleeding is a possible complication of circumcision. Side-lying promotes drainage of mucus and prevents pressure on the circumcision site from the diaper and bed linens.
5. Report excessive bleeding to the physician. Some oozing or slight bleeding is expected; however, continuous frank bleeding is a severe complication and must be reported.	If the infant's clotting time is prolonged, bleeding may occur to an extent that places the infant in a compromised state. Bleeding must be controlled.

ACTION	*RATIONALE*
6. The dressing and diaper may stick to the raw area. To prevent trauma and pain, use sterile water to soak the dressing and diaper free during diaper changes. If the dressing is a tight, pressure-type dressing, it is not removed for several days. However, if the dressing is loose, it is usually removed with each diaper change. Petrolatum gauze may be applied.	Once the clot has started to form, trauma or abrasion to the area may dislodge the clot and cause pain and bleeding. If the clot adheres to the diaper or dressing, soaking it may prevent trauma to the delicate tissues caused by pulling the diaper free. Medicated gauze may prevent irritation of the circumcised area.
7. Change the infant's diaper as soon as possible after he voids.	Voiding may cause a burning sensation. Prolonged exposure to the acidic urine may cause discomfort to the circumcision area.

Special Modifications

Jewish Circumcision

Assemble the equipment. The circumcision is usually done in a specialized area, not in the nursery. Place the restraining board at the left side of the circumcision setup. Dress the infant as requested. Place a small amount of wine on gauze in a nipple and place it on a sterile towel. Assist the infant's godfather into a sterile gown and show him where and how to scrub his hands. Assist in restraining the infant. Offer him water or wine from the nipple during the circumcision. Assist as requested. During the procedure, the rabbi will pour a small amount of wine in a sterile medicine glass and offer it to the baby with a sterile spoon during the ceremony. Apply petrolatum gauze to the circumcision after completion. Return the clothes to the infant's mother if he is to remain in the hospital. Jewish circumcision is usually done on the 8th day of the child's life unless he is ill.

Jewish circumcision is based on long-standing tradition and follows prescribed laws and rituals. The nurse usually will be asked to participate if assistance is needed.

Communicative Aspects

OBSERVATIONS

1. Observe the circumcision site very closely for the first 2 hours to detect bleeding tendency. The circumcision should be checked frequently during the first 12 hours to ensure that proper clotting has taken place.

2. Observe the circumcision for signs of proper healing, (i.e., closure of wound, patency of urinary meatus, absence of infection). It is normal for a yellowish exudate to form over the glans after the first 24 hours. This should not be removed. It will disappear in several days.

CHARTING

DATE/TIME	OBSERVATIONS	SIGNATURE
5/7 1100	Procedure explained to parents. They state that their other son had this done and they are familiar with the procedure. Feedings withheld for past hour. Circumcision done in nursery treatment room. Strapped to circumcision board. Nurse in attendance at all times. Apical pulse 126, Resp 26, T 98.2 F. Petrolatum gauze applied to circumcised area. Slight oozing of serous fluid, but no frank bleeding. Taken to mother for feeding. Checked q 5 min for 15 min, then q 15 min for 2 hours. No signs of bleeding. Normal healing and possible complications explained to mother. Took breast-feeding without problems. Asleep on left side in nursery at this time. ————————	N. Jones RN

Discharge Planning Aspects

CLIENT AND FAMILY EDUCATION

1. Explain to the parents what will happen during circumcision. Explain that the infant may feel discomfort each time he urinates after the procedure. This will probably occur for several days. Tell the parents that they will have to take some precautions about how they handle the infant for a few days so that pressure is not placed on the circumcision, causing discomfort.

2. Tell the parents how to care of the circumcision after discharge from the hospital. Explain that the area should be washed with warm, soapy water. Advise them not to try to disinfect the area with antiseptics or astringents, such as alcohol, because this is extremely painful and irritating to the infant. Adequate cleansing will be possible with warm water and a mild soap. The area should be rinsed and a clean diaper reapplied. If a medicated gauze is recommended, show the parents how to apply it.

3. Explain possible complications to the parents. Tell them to report excessive bleeding, foul odor, or failure of the circumcision to heal in 7 to 10 days.

Evaluation

Quality Assurance

Documentation should include any information or teaching to the parents. Preparations for the procedure should be documented. The infant's vital signs should be recorded prior to the procedure to serve as a baseline should complications arise. Any problems during the procedure should be recorded. The presence of dressings should be reflected. Evidence that the nurse was aware of the possibility of bleeding should appear in the record, with precautions taken. Follow-up care and evidence of safe and consistent monitoring of the circumcised area should be reflected. Reassurance and attention to the needs and anxieties of the parents should also be reflected. Discharge instructions should be documented.

Infection Control

1. Careful handwashing should be done before and after handling any infant. It is especially important to wash hands carefully when changing the diaper of the newly circumcised infant.

2. If dressings are applied, they should be sterile. Sterile technique is used to provide direct care to the circumcision.

3. Diapers should be changed as soon as possible after soiling. The warm, moist environment is ideal for the growth of microorganisms that might infect the circumcision.

4. The parents should be cautioned to watch for infection after discharge from the hospital. They should be told that discoloration, redness and swelling, or a foul odor are all indications that the circumcision may be infected; they should report these to their health-care provider.

Technique Checklist

	YES	NO
Procedure explained to parents		
By nurse	_____	_____
By physician	_____	_____
Other _____		
Circumcision done on _____ (date)		
Consent signed	_____	_____
Feedings withheld for _____ hour(s)		
Vital signs checked before circumcision	_____	_____
Clotting progressed satisfactorily	_____	_____
Circumcised area monitored frequently	_____	_____
Complications _____		
_____		
Possible complications explained to parents	_____	_____
Parents understand how to care for circumcision at home	_____	_____
Demonstrated competence	_____	_____

140 Cord Care

Overview

Definition

Care of the remaining umbilical stump on a newborn infant

Rationale

Ligate and seal the cord to prevent hemorrhage and infection.
Keep the cord clean and dry.

Terminology

Clamp: A mechanical device for the compression of blood vessels

Ligature: A binding tie of thread or wire

Wharton's jelly: A gelatinous substance in the umbilical cord

Assessment

Pertinent Anatomy and Physiology

1. The *umbilical cord* extends from the fetus to the placenta. It provides a means to transport nutrients from the mother to the fetus. It also provides a means to transport waste from the fetus to the mother for elimination. At term, the cord is smooth and gray, measuring approximately 50 cm to 55 cm in length and 2 cm in diameter. The cord contains no pain receptors. The cord normally contains two arteries, which return deoxygenated blood to the placenta, and one larger vein, which transports oxygenated blood to the fetus. These vessels may be longer than the cord and tend to coil up in the umbilical cord, giving it a lumpy appearance. These vessels are supported by a gelatinous substance called Wharton's jelly, which lubricates and cushions them, preventing tight coiling or kinking that might interfere with the fetal circulation.

2. At birth, the cord is cut and ligated close to the infant's abdominal wall. The purpose is to prevent oozing or bleeding. The cord will dry up and fall off in about 5 to 8 days.

Pathophysiological Concepts

The number of vessels in the cord is important because in at least 1% of neonates, a two-vesseled cord (one umbilical vein and one umbilical artery) will be noted. Various anomalies are present in at least 10% of these infants. This condition is more common in multiple pregnancies.

Assessment of the Client

1. Assess the cord of the infant at birth to ensure the presence of two arteries and one vein.

2. Assess the amount of Wharton's jelly present in the cord. If the amount is excessive, greater care in observing the cord is necessary. After birth, the Wharton's jelly dries up. If there is a large amount, the ligature on the cord may become loose when the jelly dries up, causing shrinking of the cord.

3. Assess the parents' knowledge level and experience to determine how much teaching is appropriate.

Plan

Nursing Objectives   Observe the attachment of the umbilical cord for indication of anomalies.
Prevent infection and hemorrhage.
Facilitate the natural sloughing of the cord.
Alleviate the parent's anxiety about the cord.

Client Preparation   Remove the infant's shirt and diaper before giving cord care.

Equipment   60% or 70% Alcohol or prescribed antiseptic solution
Antibiotic ointments and medications, if ordered
Cotton balls or gauze pads

Implementation and Interventions

Procedural Aspects

ACTION

1. Check the clamp for satisfactory placement and closure. The tie, clamp, or band should be tightly secured (Fig. 140-1).

RATIONALE

The umbilical cord provides access to the infant's vascular system. Failure to seal the cord completely could result in hemorrhage.

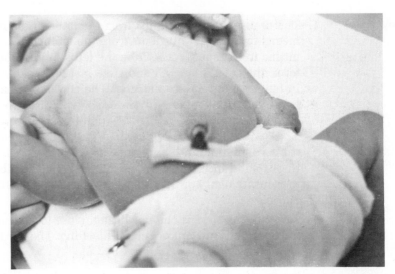

Figure 140.1

2. Keep the cord dry and exposed to the air. Clean the cord and surrounding area with alcohol or the prescribed solution on a cotton ball or gauze pad (Fig. 140-2). Clean from the base of the umbilical stump outward in a circular motion. Lift the cord out of the way to facilitate cleansing.

A moist, warm environment is a breeding ground for bacteria. Daily removal of as many bacteria as possible reduces the chances of infection.

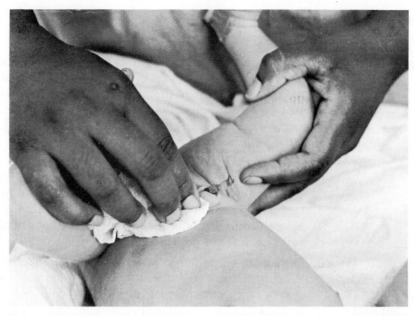

Figure 140.2

ACTION

RATIONALE

Special Modifications

If exchange transfusion may be needed, the umbilical stump is left longer than usual and must be kept moist and intact. Apply sterile gauze soaked in saline solution, which is held in place by a loose-fitting binder. After the exchange transfusion is complete, the cord may be kept moist in case a second transfusion is needed (see Technique No. 100, Exchange Transfusion, Assisting In).

In the case of Rh incompatibility, the infant may suffer from a condition called erythroblastosis fetalis. In this condition, the blood is exchanged for an equal amount of compatible blood. The mechanism for this exchange is a catheter inserted into the umbilical vein.

Communicative Aspects

OBSERVATIONS

1. Check the tie or clamp on the umbilical cord every 15 minutes for the first few hours, until it is fairly certain that the cord will not hemorrhage. As the Wharton's jelly dries up, the cord may tend to shrink slightly. As this happens, the previously secure ligature may become loose and allow oozing or flow of blood. The cord should then be observed each time the diaper is changed for satisfactory progressive healing. Watch for signs of oozing, seeping, or bleeding.

2. Observe the cord for redness, foul odor, moisture, or discharge from the umbilical stump, which may indicate infection.

CHARTING

DATE/TIME	OBSERVATIONS	SIGNATURE
8/19 0815	Umbilical stump cleansed with 60% alcohol and exposed to the air for 10 min. clamp intact and no signs of oozing or infection. Diaper applied below umbilical level. Mother observed procedure and will demonstrate it before going home tomorrow.	J. Morgan RN

Discharge Planning Aspects

CLIENT AND FAMILY EDUCATION

1. Explain to the parents why the cord area must be kept clean and the technique involved. Tell them that alcohol will facilitate drying and will discourage infection. Explain the procedure for applying diapers so that the cord area is left exposed. Allow them to demonstrate their understanding and competency. This will allow assessment of their skill and will bolster their self-confidence.

2. Tell the family that the cord will fall off naturally when the baby is 5 to 8 days old. Caution them against trying to detach it before it falls off by itself. Tell them that separation might be accompanied by slight bleeding but that this should be only slight and should stop quickly. It will take several days before the naval has healed completely. They should observe the area to be sure that infection does not occur.

3. Emphasize to the family that the infant should not be bathed in a tub until the cord has successfully separated and the naval area has healed. Explain that this will help prevent infection.

4. Ask the parents to report to their pediatric care provider any bleeding, redness, discharge, or odor around the stump. If the stump does not fall off in 7 to 8 days, they should notify their care provider.

Evaluation

Quality Assurance

Documentation should include an assessment of the condition of the cord and stage of healing. If problems are present, the person to whom they were reported should be noted. Teaching of the parents should be noted, with assessment of their understanding and competence in performing the procedure.

Infection Control

1. Careful handwashing should precede care of the infant.

2. Asepsis must be maintained until healing of the cord is complete. Bacteria can cause an infection, which can extend to the peritoneum, liver, and even into the blood.

3. The infant's diaper should not cover the umbilical cord, since the warm wet environment may predispose the infant to colonization by bacteria.

4. Tub bathing of the infant is generally discouraged until the cord has dropped off and the naval area has completely healed.

Technique Checklist

	YES	NO
Technique explained to parents	———	———
Physiology of cord explained	———	———
Cord observed q 15 min for ——— hr		
Cord cleansed daily with ———		
Cord care demonstrated to parents	———	———
Return demonstration	———	———
Complications		
Hemorrhage	———	———
Premature release of ligature	———	———
Infection	———	———
Umbilical catheter for infusion	———	———

141   Diapering

Overview

Definition

Protecting and covering the external genitalia by means of an absorbent material drawn up between the legs and fastened at the waist

Rationale

Remove irritants on the infant's skin and provide a dry environment.
Assess the adequacy of elimination.
Provide care for irritated buttocks or genitalia.
Provide an opportunity for mother–infant interaction.

Assessment

Pertinent Anatomy and Physiology

See Appendix I: *genitalia (female)*, *genitalia (male)*, *skin*.

Pathophysiological Concepts

Diaper rash is a skin reaction that occurs when the skin comes in contact with the acidic urine. In fair-skinned infants, it may occur even with the most conscientious care.

Assessment of the Client

1. Assess the condition of the infant's skin. Assess the presence of diaper rash or problems with the external genitalia.
2. Assess the understanding and experience of the parents in changing diapers.

Plan

Nursing Objectives

Make a neat, serviceable diaper.
Prevent skin reactions.
Keep the infant as dry and comfortable as possible.
Maintain a safe, therapeutic environment.
Provide the infant with auditory, visual, and tactile stimulation.

Client Preparation

Place the infant on a flat, safe surface for diaper change.

Equipment

Cloth or disposable diaper
Two large diaper pins (for cloth diaper)
Receptacle for soiled diapers
Medication, if prescribed
Washcloth, warm water, and towel

Implementation and Interventions

Procedural Aspects

ACTION

1. Wash hands thoroughly. Gather equipment and place within reach. Place the infant on a flat surface and do not leave unattended. Remove the soiled diaper and dispose of it in the designated receptacle. Close each pin as soon as it is removed and place each well out of the infant's reach. Lubricate diaper pins, if necessary, by sticking them into a bar of soap.

2. Wash the genitalia first, then the buttocks, with warm water. Dry the area thoroughly. In females, wash from the front to the back to avoid contamination of the vulva with waste material from the anus. Male infants should also be washed from the front to the back, especially while the circumcision is healing. Apply medications as prescribed.

3. If a disposable diaper is used, place it on the infant and fasten the adhesive tabs. Check to see that it is not too tight or too loose. The diaper should be checked frequently to ensure that the infant's skin is not in contact with the urine for extended periods.

4. Fold the cloth diaper so that it will fit the infant. The two most common methods of folding are the kite-fold and the rectangular-fold (see Client Education section of this procedure). Place the diaper under the infant and draw it between the infant's legs (Fig. 141-1).

RATIONALE

Having the equipment in reach eliminates the temptation to leave the infant to go and get something forgotten. Since the infant can move so suddenly, the risk of falls is great if he or she is left unattended even for 1 second.

The rectal area contains resident flora that are not dangerous to the infant. However, when these flora are transmitted to another part of the body, they can cause infection. The rectum is always washed last.

Although many disposable diapers are said to keep the infant dry, it is possible for the skin to be in contact with urine. The disposable diaper should be changed as soon as it is soiled, just as is the cloth diaper.

The bulk of the diaper should be near the genitalia so that it will absorb the urine and feces. However, too much bulk is uncomfortable and confining.

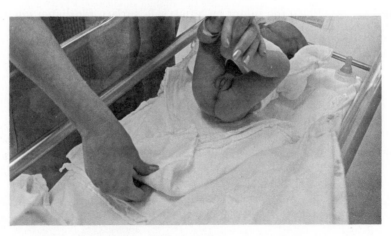

Figure 141.1

ACTION

5. Secure the diaper at each side by inserting a pin horizontally through both the front and the back sections. Place two fingers between the diaper thicknesses and the infant's skin to prevent sticking the baby with the pin. Direct the pin away from the infant's abdomen (Fig. 141-2).

RATIONALE

The pins used to secure the diaper must be closed securely. In case one should accidentally come open, it should be pointing away from the abdomen to prevent trauma. Keeping the nurse's fingers between the diaper and the infant allows better guidance of the pin and prevents sticking the infant.

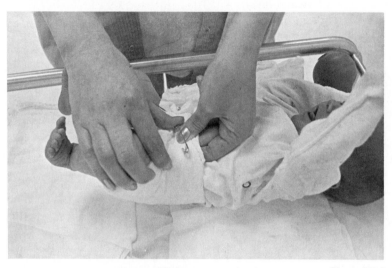

Figure 141.2

6. Leave the infant in a clean and comfortable environment. Place the soiled linen in the proper receptacle.

Soiled linen can offer a medium for bacterial growth and should be kept away from the infant.

Special Modifications

If the infant is very small, regular cloth or commercial diapers may be too large. The diapers may be tucked or folded to fit. Experiment to find the best fold that will produce the desired effects.

Extra folding can produce a proper fit and increase comfort.

Communicative Aspects

OBSERVATIONS

1. Observe the infant frequently to determine if the diaper is soiled. The diaper should be changed whenever it is soiled.
2. Observe the infant for signs of diaper rash. If the condition is serious, medicated creams or ointments may be prescribed.

CHARTING

Most hospitals have forms for the numerical charting of the number of diaper changes for each infant, as well as a description of the feces (i.e., meconium, yellow liquid, yellow formed, etc.). Anything inconsistent with what would normally be expected should be charted in the nurses' progress notes and reported to the proper person.

Discharge Planning Aspects

CLIENT AND FAMILY EDUCATION

1. Demonstrate to the parents how to fold the diaper. The two methods are as follows:

   Kite-fold diaper (Fig. 141-3)—Open or fold the diaper into a large square. Fold in corner A on dotted line E-D. Fold in corner C on dotted line F-D, making a point at D. Fold corner B down to adjust to desired hip size. Fold D upward to desired width. Place the base of the triangle under the infant's buttocks at waist level. Draw the folded point, D, between the infant's legs, up over the abdomen, and fasten it to the two back corners with pins at the waist level.

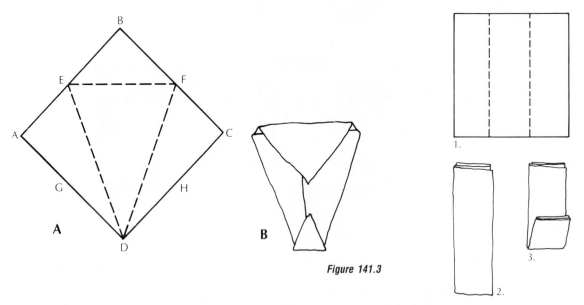

Figure 141.3

Figure 141.4

Rectangular-fold diaper (Fig. 141-4)—Place a square diaper on a flat surface. Fold it into thirds, lengthwise. Fold up the bottom third to the midway portion of the diaper to form extra thickness. Place one half of the folded diaper under the buttocks; draw up the remainder between the legs and over the abdomen. Pin securely at both sides. Because of the pattern of urine flow, females may require the extra thickness over the posterior area and males may require extra thickness over the anterior area.

2. Explain to the parents the need for frequent diaper changes and thorough cleansing of the infant's genitalia and buttocks. Emphasize the need to wash from front to back to prevent contamination from the rectal area. Tell the parents that the area is dried well to prevent irritation of the skin and to discourage growth of microorganisms, which flourish in a warm, moist environment.

3. Tell the parents that the use of plastic pants is discouraged because they tend to retain heat and encourage urine stagnation and bacterial growth. Cloth diapers should be washed separately with a mild detergent. Rinsing the diapers twice will help ensure that all of the soap is removed and may reduce skin irritation.

4. Emphasize the importance of safety factors in changing the infant's diaper. Tell the parents to close the pins as soon as they are removed from the diaper and to place them out of the child's reach. Caution them about the need to remain in constant attendance to prevent falls when the infant is on a flat surface.

Evaluation

Quality Assurance

Documentation should include an accurate count of the number of diaper changes. The presence of urine and/or feces should be noted. The color and texture of the fecal material should be noted. If any untoward findings occur, these should be noted in the nurses' progress notes, along with documentation of who was notified, actions taken, and outcomes. If the infant is ill or is having intake and output monitored, the diapers may be weighed to assess the amount of urine being excreted.

Infection Control

1. Careful handwashing is essential before and after changing the infant's diaper. It is important to emphasize to the parents that they should wash their hands before and after changing the infant's diaper.

2. Prolonged exposure of the delicate skin to stagnant urine may lead to skin breakdown. This may predispose the infant to infections. Stress to the parents the importance of changing the diapers frequently and keeping the infant clean and dry.

3. Soiled diapers may provide a satisfactory medium for the growth and proliferation of microorganisms. The diapers should be stored in a special receptacle and should be laundered frequently.

Technique Checklist

	YES	NO
Diaper changes documented in chart	_____	_____
Explanations to parents about:		
Need for frequent diaper change	_____	_____
Diaper-folding techniques	_____	_____
Importance of cleansing from front to back	_____	_____
Need for proper handwashing	_____	_____
Prevention of diaper rash	_____	_____
Safety factors	_____	_____

142   Exchange Transfusion, Assisting with

Overview

Definition

Replacement of the circulating blood of the neonate by withdrawing blood and injecting the blood of the donor in equal parts. The process is continued until about 70% to 80% of the newborn's blood has been replaced, approximately 500 ml.

Rationale

Reverse the complications of sepsis in the neonate.

Remove some of the antibodies causing hemolysis of red blood cells in the infant's circulation.

Decrease the amount of toxic products in the infant's circulation.

Decrease serum bilirubin levels.

Prevent kernicterus in the infant.

Elevate a low hemoglobin level.

Terminology

Antibodies: Proteins that are produced in the body in response to invasion by a foreign agent, known as an antigen, and that react specifically with it. In hemolytic diseases of the newborn due to Rh incompatibility, antibodies pass through the placenta and produce agglutination of the infant's red blood cells.

Antigen: A foreign substance in the body that stimulates the production of antibodies

Communicable: Transmissible from person to person, either directly or indirectly

Hemolysis: A process in hemolytic conditions of the newborn in which incompatibility causes red cells to clump together

Kernicterus: A condition of the newborn in which there is brain damage associated with high levels of bilirubin in the blood

Sepsis: A pathologic state resulting from the presence of microorganisms or their poisonous products in the bloodstream

Assessment

Pertinent Anatomy and Physiology

1. The *Rh factor* is a protein substance that is called an antigen and is found on the surface of red blood cells. Those persons who possess the factor are referred to as Rh positive (D) and those lacking it are Rh negative (d). Blood type is inherited.

2. The major blood groups are A, B, AB, and O. Each type has antigens that may be incompatible with the antigens of any of the other groups.

Pathophysiological Concepts	1. A common indication for exchange transfusion is the removal of pathologic microorganisms from an infant who is considered septic. A frequent cause of sepsis in the neonate is group B hemolytic streptococcus, which is contracted during passage through the birth canal. Infants with sepsis have a tendency to bleed. Exchange transfusion not only serves to remove the pathogens from the infant's circulation, but also provides fresh antibodies and additional clotting factors.
	2. The circulatory systems of the fetus and mother are completely separated. However, a break in the placental barrier may allow some of the fetal cells to escape into the maternal circulation. This may take place during delivery or after an abortion. These fetal cells stimulate the formation of antibodies in the mother's circulation. During subsequent pregnancies, the antibody formation is enhanced and may pose a danger to the infant when the maternal antibodies enter the fetal circulation and begin to hemolyze the baby's red blood cells. The rapid destruction of red blood cells causes bilirubin to spill into the amniotic fluid. The baby attempts to compensate for this destruction of red blood cells by replacing those lost with immature red cells, called erythroblasts. The baby may develop anemia, which may result in fetal death in utero.
	3. One indication for the need for exchange transfusion is ABO incompatibility. This involves a newborn with type O blood and a mother with type A or B. The clinical manifestations are similar to those of Rh incompatibility, jaundice, enlarged liver, and enlarged spleen.
Assessment of the Client	1. Note the blood types of the infant and the mother. Problems may be expected when the mother is Rh negative and the infant is Rh positive.
	2. Assess the maternal history to determine if there is a likelihood that she may become sensitized. This sensitization may occur from a previous pregnancy that lasted beyond 8 weeks' gestation or from previous blood transfusions.
	3. Assess the infant for yellow-stained vernix or cord, which may indicate bilirubin problems. Edema and ascites may also be present.
	4. Assess the placenta for enlargement. In hemolytic disease, the placenta may weigh proportionally more than in the healthy newborn.
	5. Assess the infant for a tendency to bleed. Note during heel stick if the blood takes an unusually long time to clot.

Plan

Nursing Objectives	Prevent sepsis or infection by maintaining sterile technique.
	Report and record desired and undesired effects of the transfusion.
	Recognize the signs and symptoms of a blood reaction.
	Prevent system overload from excessive infusion, causing shock and cardiac failure.
	Monitor the infant's condition and record the procedure.
	Observe and record systematically the venous pressure of the infant during the exchange.
	Prevent hemorrhage by attention to bleeding and clotting factors.
Client Preparation	1. Give the parents a clear, concise explanation of the need for the exchange transfusion.
	2. Do not feed the infant for several hours before the procedure to ensure an empty stomach. If the infant has already eaten, the stomach contents may be aspirated through a nasogastric tube to reduce the chance of regurgitation and aspiration.

3. Immobilize the infant with light restraints on a circumcision board. The usual site of infusion is the umbilical vein. Other possible sites are the jugular or femoral vessels. Use a radiant heat cradle to keep the infant's temperature within the thermoneutral zone. Measure the infant's vital signs to provide baseline parameters against which to measure subsequent readings.

4. Apply cardiac and respiratory monitors before starting. If monitor equipment is not available, a stethoscope may be placed over the apex of the infant's heart to provide continued auscultation of the heart rate. Apply blood pressure monitoring equipment for continual pressure monitoring throughout the technique.

5. Resuscitation equipment, such as oxygen, ventilatory assistance devices, masks, airways, endotracheal intubation equipment, adaptors, suction, and emergency medications should be readily available.

Equipment

Sterile disposable exchange transfusion tray

Venisection cut-down tray

Fresh donor's blood, which must not be more than 5 days old (2 units are usually available in case 1 is contaminated)

Blood warmer or a warm water bath for warming blood (100°F)

Skin disinfectant solution and applicators

Sterile gown, gloves, drapes, caps, and masks

Transfusion record

Cardiorespiratory monitor

Medications, such as calcium gluconate, sodium bicarbonate, and 50% glucose solution

Radiant warmer

Implementation and Interventions

Procedural Aspects

ACTION	RATIONALE
1. Check the donor card carefully for age, type, and Rh, and to ensure that the donor blood is free of sickle cell trait. Be sure, also, that the donor unit has a hematocrit of at least 50 and a pH over 7.2.	It is essential to give the right blood to the right client. If the hematocrit is below 50, the infant may become anemic. If the pH is below 7.2, the infant may become acidotic.
2. Assist in setting up the blood and the transfusion equipment. Run the tubing from the blood through the warming mechanism. Prepare the skin site with disinfectant. Sterile drapes are applied. The transfuser and anyone directly assisting will wear caps, gowns, and masks.	Warming the blood before it reaches the infant helps prevent cold stress and vasospasm. It also allows the blood to flow more freely by decreasing the viscosity. Sterility and disinfection help prevent cross-contamination.
3. Record the initial central venous pressure once the catheter has been placed. The transfuser then begins the exchange procedure.	The pressure is checked during the procedure. A change from 10 cm to 12 cm pressure is an indication that fluid overload may be occurring and status must be reassessed. The initial pressure reading provides a baseline for future measurements.

ACTION	*RATIONALE*
4. The transfuser will exchange equal amounts of blood while maintaining a venous pressure of 10 cm to 12 cm. If this pressure is increased during the procedure, the exchange will be stopped. The transfusion may be continued with a deficit of blood volume, since 10 ml to 20 ml of blood may be removed and sent to the laboratory for testing.	Heart failure can occur from fluid overload. An indication of fluid overload is increased venous pressure.
5. Record the time the exchange transfusion began. With each successive withdrawal of infant's blood and injection of donor blood, note the time, amount in and out, and cumulative amounts in and out. The total time for exchange transfusion is usually about 1 hour, although it may vary greatly.	Accurate records of amounts in and out are important to assess infant response and need for further transfusion.
6. After 100 ml of blood have been exchanged, calcium gluconate may be given to stabilize the cardiac rhythm. Monitor the infant's vital signs, including blood pressure.	Stabilization of cardiac rhythm reduces the chance of cardiac arrest. Calcium preparations are given to overcome the danger of tetany, which may result from the depletion of calcium by the large amount of sodium citrate in the donor blood.
7. At the end of the transfusion, protamine sulfate may be given to counteract the effects of the heparinized blood that was infused.	The heparinized blood can affect the infant's coagulation ability for 4 to 6 hours after exchange.
8. After the transfusion is completed, the transfuser may either remove the catheter or leave it in the vessel with an intravenous infusion or plug attached. If the catheter is left in place, be sure that adequate restraints are applied to ensure that the child will not pull it out. The catheter should be secured with a sterile dressing and tape. If the catheter is removed, place a small compression bandage over the area. Observe for bleeding.	Observe the infant to prevent hemorrhage from the transfusion site.

Communicative Aspects

OBSERVATIONS

1. During the exchange, constantly monitor the cardiac rate, skin color, color of withdrawn blood, and the infant's respirations. Monitor the vital signs during the transfusion. It is imperative to monitor continuously the blood pressure, either by an external pressure monitoring apparatus or by monitoring the venous pressure. Blood pressure fluctuations are usually the first indicator of infant distress.

2. Observe the transfusion site for hemorrhage. After the transfusion is completed, observe the site every hour for 4 hours and then every 4 hours for 24 hours.

3. Observe the infant for signs of transfusion complications, such as heart failure, hypocalcemia, hyperkalemia, and sepsis. Indications include cardiac arrythmias and convulsions. Blood reactions are manifested by skin rashes, fever, and possibly seizures.

CHARTING

Charting should include complete and accurate documentation of the procedure and the amounts of blood infused and removed. Nursing progress notes should include the following:

Verification of checking blood

Baseline vital signs and venous pressure

Time the exchange transfusion began

Time, amounts in and out, and cumulative totals of amounts

Blood pressure, heart and respiratory rates during transfusion

Medications administered, amount, time, and result

Follow-up observations

Pertinent information about the procedure

Information given to parents

EXCHANGE TRANSFUSION RECORD

Infant _____ Boy Doe _____   Birth weight __3.1 kg__

Exchange time started __08:30__   Exchange time completed _____09:15_____

TIME	OUT		IN					
	AMT	TOTAL	AMT	TOTAL	B/P	P&R	MEDS	OBSER
0830	20	20	20	20	45/25	150–54		
0834	20	40	20	40	40/25			
0837	20	60	20	60	40/25			
0845	20	80	20	80	45//22	156–54		

Discharge Planning Aspects

CLIENT AND FAMILY EDUCATION

1. Explain the procedure to the parents. Be sure that they understand the physiology of the blood and the reason why the exchange transfusion is needed.

2. Tell the family about signs to watch for after the exchange transfusion. The infant will be observed in the nursery for at least 24 hours. However, the parents need to know what is happening and to feel that they have a part to play in the infant's progress.

Evaluation

Quality Assurance

Documentation should include the signs and symptoms that prompted the need for exchange transfusion. The entire exchange procedure should be progressively documented on the chart. The total amount infused and removed should be noted. Any observations before, during, and after the procedure should be noted in the chart. The progress notes should reflect that the nurse knew what the possible complications were and took steps to avoid or reverse them. The teaching of the parents should be noted. Disposition of the infusion catheter should be reflected. Any complications and their reporting and outcomes should be noted.

Infection Control

1. Exchange transfusion provides direct access to the circulatory system of the newborn. Since the newborn has very few defense mechanisms, every precaution must be taken to prevent cross-contamination of the infant. Careful handwashing is essential. Sterile technique is maintained during the procedure.

2. The transfusion site should be cleansed with a disinfectant before beginning. The site is covered with a sterile dressing after the transfusion is completed, whether or not the catheter is removed.

Technique Checklist

	YES	NO
Procedure explained to parents	_____	_____
Reason for exchange transfusion _____		
Time exchange started _____		
Documentation of amounts infused and removed	_____	_____
Time exchange ended _____		
Observation after infusion		
Q1hr for 4 hr	_____	_____
Q4hr for 24 hr	_____	_____
Sterility maintained during transfusion	_____	_____

143   Eye Care, Initial

Overview

Definition
The instillation of prophylactic agents into the eyes of the newborn infant

Rationale
Protect the infant from developing ophthalmia neonatorum.
Comply with state laws.

Terminology
Conjunctiva: The delicate membrane that lines the eyelids and covers the exposed surfaces of the sclera

Credé's method: Prophylactic eye treatment named for the Viennese physician who introduced it in 1881

Prophylaxis: Preventive treatment

Assessment

Pertinent Anatomy and Physiology
See Appendix I: *eye, labor and delivery.*

Pathophysiological Concepts
Ophthalmia neonatorum is the term used to refer to any hyperacute purulent conjunctivitis occurring during the first 10 days of life. It is usually contracted during the birth process from infected vaginal discharge of the mother.

Assessment of the Client
1. Assess the condition of the newborn to ensure that adequate respirations have been established and the infant is stable.
2. Assess the mother's condition. If she is able, the infant may spend the first hour after birth with her. The National Society to Prevent Blindness has stated that a delay of 1 hour after birth before administration of eye prophylaxis is not harmful to the infant. This has proven to be a very important time in the mother–infant bonding process.

Plan

Nursing Objectives
Administer the eye prophylaxis within 1 hour after birth.
Prevent ophthalmic problems for the newborn.
Promote mother–infant bonding.

Client Preparation
1. With a sterile cotton ball and a small amount of sterile water, gently wipe the eyes of the neonate to remove blood, vernix, and other debris before administering the prophylactic solution or ointment. Wipe from the inner toward the outer corner of the eye.
2. Position the infant in the supine position on a stable, flat surface.

Equipment	Sterile cotton balls and sterile water
	Medication (erythromycin [0.5%] ophthalmic ointment or drops in single-use tubes or ampules, or tetracycline [1%] ophthalmic ointment or drops in single-use tubes or ampules, or less frequently used is 1% silver nitrate ampule)
	Sterile pin

Implementation and Interventions

Procedural Aspects

ACTION	RATIONALE
1. *Ophthalmic drops:* Puncture the end of the medication ampule with a sterile pin. Gently open the infant's eyelids. Instill 2 drops on the conjunctival sac (Fig. 143-1). Allow the solution to run across the entire conjunctiva. Carefully manipulate the eyelids to ensure that the medication spreads throughout the entire surface. Puncture the other ampule and instill 2 drops into the other eye in the same manner.	The agent must reach all parts of the conjunctival surface to be effective.

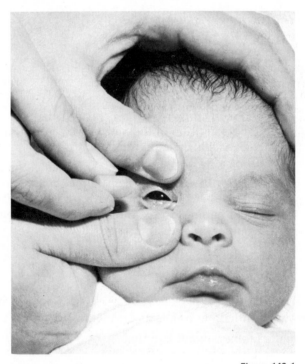

Figure 143.1

ACTION	RATIONALE
2. *Ophthalmic ointments* (erythromycin or tetracycline): Gently open the infant's eyelids and place a thin line of ointment along the inner aspect of the lower lid. Carefully manipulate the eye in order to spread the agent to all parts of the conjunctival surface. *Do not touch the eye with the tip of the tube.* Repeat the procedure in the other eye, using the same tube of medication.	The agent must reach all parts of the conjunctivae. Touching the eye with the tube may cause trauma to the delicate eye lining.
3. After 1 minute, gently wipe the excess medication from the eyelids and surrounding skin with sterile water. *Do not irrigate the eyes.*	Irrigation may reduce the effectiveness of the medication.

Communicative Aspects

OBSERVATIONS

1. Observe the medication to ensure that it spreads over the entire conjunctival sac.

2. Observe the eye to see that the medication and secretions that flow from the eyes after instillation are wiped from the infant's skin.

3. It is possible for the infant to exhibit an allergic reaction to the medication. Observe the infant for signs of allergic reaction for several hours after instillation.

CHARTING

DATE/TIME	OBSERVATIONS	SIGNATURE
7/19 1430	0.5% erythromycin ointment instilled in each eye. Excess medication cleansed from around the eye. Technique explained to parents who gave permission. Infant with mother in recovery room for 45 minutes before receiving eye treatment.	N. Jones RN

Discharge Planning Aspects

CLIENT AND FAMILY EDUCATION

The family should understand the need for and laws regarding the instillation of eye drops for prophylaxis in the newborn.

Evaluation

Quality Assurance

Documentation should include written verification that the infant received prophylactic treatment. The type of medication should be noted, along with the amount placed in each eye. Follow-up treatment should be noted. Explanations to the parents should be noted. Any untoward effects or complications should be reflected in the chart.

Infection Control

1. Wash hands carefully before doing eye treatments.

2. Do not touch the medication tube to the eye of the infant.

Technique Checklist

	YES	NO
Procedure explained to parents	———	———
Medication instilled in each eye	———	———

Erythromycin ———

Tetracycline ———

Silver nitrate ———

Baby born at ——— (time)

Eye prophylaxis at ——— (time)

	YES	NO
Precautions taken to spread medication over entire conjunctival sac	———	———

144   Feeding the Infant

Overview

Definition

Nourishing the newborn by artificial means (*i.e.*, by means other than breast-feeding)

Rationale

Provide the nourishment required for normal growth.

Provide the infant with a feeling of love and security.

Offer an opportunity to enhance the mother–child bond.

Assessment

Pertinent Anatomy and Physiology

1. See Appendix I: *esophagus, intestine (large), intestine (small), and mouth.*

2. The stomach and small intestine of the newborn infant are mature enough to utilize the substances in human milk. Salivary, gastric, pancreatic, and intestinal digestion become increasingly able to deal with more complex foods as they are introduced into the infant's diet. Before the age of 3 months, the infant is unable to digest fat in the stomach. Because the fats in commercial formulas is almost the same as that in human milk, these fats are digested. Fat from other sources is not digested. Human milk protein is digested almost completely in the intestinal tract. After the age of 4 months, the salivary glands assist in the breakdown of starches. Pepsin and hydrochloride in the stomach also aid in digestion of milk and other substances.

3. The sucking and swallowing reflexes are present at birth. Feeding time meets the infant's need for closeness and tactile stimulation. After the second month, the infant begins to equate mother with food. Feeding schedules vary; the newborn usually eats about 5 times a day and should soon sleep through the night. After the age of 3 months, the infant will be able to swallow with less tongue protrusion. The infant at this age will recognize the bottle as a source of food and will not readily accept a cup.

Pathophysiological Concepts

1. *Esophageal atresia* is the abnormal closure of the esophagus. It may be associated with *tracheoesophageal fistual,* an opening between the esophagus and the trachea. The result is aspiration of ingested liquids into the trachea and respiratory tract. These infants tend to drool excessively and choke, cough, and become cyanotic during feedings. If the atresia is not accompanied by tracheoesophageal fistula, the ingested food is not tolerated and is regurgitated. The infant is not fed orally, and surgical correction is needed.

2. Propping the bottle with the infant lying down is a dangerous practice because of the possible physiologic consequences. The nipple may block the air passage, or the infant may regurgitate and aspirate formula. This can result in lung infection or death. Infants who are propped in the horizontal position have a higher incidence of otitis media, since the eustachian tube orifice opens during swallowing, and mucus from the nose can drain into the duct and occlude it.

Assessment of the Client

1. Assess the infant's ability to take oral food soon after birth. The infant may be given sterile water to ensure patency of the esophagus. If the infant becomes choked or cyanotic, withhold feeding until the physician has been notified. A small nasogastric tube may be threaded into the stomach to ensure esophageal patency.

2. Assess the structure of the infant's mouth. Determine the presence of cleft palate or other physical abnormalities that might interfere with sucking.

Plan

Nursing Objectives

Ensure that the infant is receiving enough nourishment.

Instruct the mother in proper feeding technique.

Evaluate the infant's tolerance of the formula.

Client Preparation

1. Be sure that the infant is clean and dry before beginning the feeding period. Feeding time should be a comfortable and satisfying experience for both the mother and the infant.

2. Water or other liquids should not be given for an hour before feeding time so that the infant will be ready to eat.

Equipment

Bottle of formula (see Technique No. 145, Formula Preparation in the Home).

Implementation and Interventions

Procedural Aspects

ACTION	RATIONALE
1. Assist the mother to wash her hands before feeding the baby. Provide her with a comfortable chair, preferably one with arms.	Microorganisms are spread by direct contact. Since the infant's immune system is immature, every effort should be made to prevent the spread of microorganisms. A position of comfort facilitates a positive feeding experience.
2. Show the mother how to hold the infant snugly in the crook of one arm. The bottle is held with the other hand (Fig. 144-1). The infant's head should be on a higher plane than the rest of the body.	Holding the infant promotes a feeling of trust and security. If the head is higher than the rest of the body, there is less chance of choking because gravity can be used to facilitate swallowing.
3. Gently insert the nipple along the infant's tongue. The opening in the nipple should be large enough for the feeding to flow smoothly, but should not be so large that excessive formula fills the infant's mouth. If the opening is too small, aggressive but unproductive sucking efforts will result. The bottle should be held at an angle so that the nipple is always filled with formula.	The infant's sucking efforts should result in adequate feeding. Too much formula may cause choking, and too little will result in tiring. If the nipple becomes filled with air, the air will be sucked and swallowed by the infant, resulting in gastric discomfort.

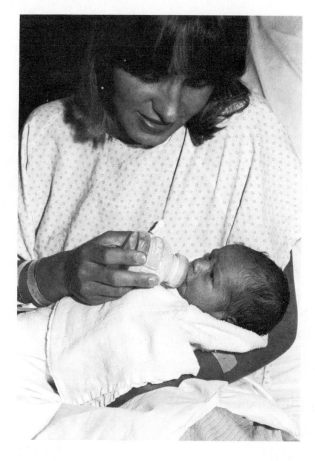

Figure 144.1

ACTION	*RATIONALE*
4. Feed the infant slowly. Allow an opportunity for the removal of swallowed air during the feeding by removing the bottle from the infant's mouth. Place the infant against either shoulder (Fig. 144-2) and gently pat the middle and upper back. The infant may also be placed in a sitting position with the head supported (Fig. 144-3) or lying prone with the head supported to facilitate breathing (Fig. 144-4). Gentle patting or stroking of the infant's back will facilitate removal of swallowed air. This technique, called "burping" or "bubbling" may be done at the beginning of the feeding, after 1 ounce of formula has been taken, and after the feeding is completed.	Air trapped in the gastrointestinal (GI) tract can cause cramping and discomfort. Slight pressure on the infant's stomach and gentle patting or stroking of the back will aid in the removal of the swallowed air. Since the neck muscles are immature, the head should be supported.

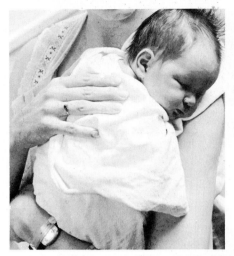

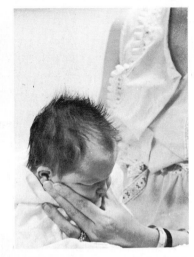

Figure 144.2   *Figure 144.3*

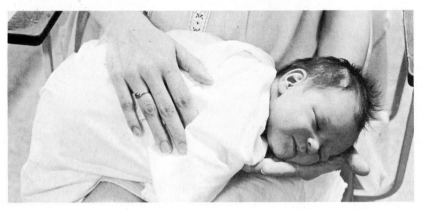

Figure 144.4

ACTION	RATIONALE
5. Be careful not to overfeed the infant. The formula should be at room temperature or slightly warmer. Ready-to-feed formulas at room temperature do not require warming. Refrigerated formulas should be warmed in a pan of water. The formula should feel warm to the touch when dropped onto the inner aspect of the mother's arm. After feeding, allow the infant to rest quietly.	Overfeeding causes abdominal discomfort and regurgitation. Cold formula may cause abdominal cramping. Allowing the infant to rest after feeding minimizes the danger of overtiring and regurgitating.

Communicative Aspects

OBSERVATIONS

1. Observe the infant's tolerance of the feeding. Observe to see that the formula is not being ingested too quickly or too slowly. Rate may be altered by changing the size of the hole in the nipple.

2. Observe the amount of formula taken. Observe the amount, appearance, and frequency of regurgitation.

3. Observe the mother's technique of feeding and handling her baby. Demonstrate methods for assisting the baby to remove swallowed air. Observe the eye contact and closeness between the mother and the baby.

CHARTING

Most hospital records provide a means for recording each feeding, which includes the time, type of formula, amount, and any regurgitation. Any problems, such as frequent regurgitation or choking should be documented in the nurses' progress notes.

Discharge Planning Aspects

CLIENT AND FAMILY EDUCATION

1. Emphasize to the parents the importance of holding the infant for *every* feeding. The primary developmental task of the infant is the development of trust. The closeness of the parent who is feeding the infant and the tactile stimulation all promote feelings of trust and enhance the parent–infant relationship. Discourage the practice of propping the bottle.

2. Demonstrate the methods of feeding the infant and how to assist the infant in removing swallowed air. Allow the mother to return the demonstration until she feels comfortable feeding her infant.

3. Teach the mother about care of bottles and formula preparation. Tell her how to ensure that the formula is ready to feed to her infant. Explain safeguards for storage and preparation of formula (see Technique 145, Formula Preparation in the Home).

Evaluation

Quality Assurance

Documentation should include some notation about explanations given to the parents in feeding techniques and an assessment of their understanding and ability. A progressive record of the amount and frequency of feedings should be reflected. Any problems with the formula should be noted.

Infection Control

1. Careful handwashing is essential before and after feeding the infant. In addition, hands should be washed before preparing the feeding or handling the feeding equipment.

2. Every effort should be made to keep the nipple free from contamination after introducing it into the baby's mouth. During periods when the infant is being held for removal of swallowed air, the bottle should be set upright and the cap replaced. The cap should be set top side down during the feeding so that the portion that fits over the nipple remains free from direct contact with contaminants.

3. Unused formula is an excellent breeding ground for bacteria. After each feeding, the unused portion should be discarded.

Technique Checklist

	YES	NO
Technique for feeding demonstrated	_____	_____
Return demonstration	_____	_____
Feedings taken without problems	_____	_____
Regurgitation _____		
Cramping _____		
Choking _____		
Cyanosis _____		
Documentation of amount and frequency of feedings	_____	_____
Techniques for assisting the infant to remove swallowed air demonstrated	_____	_____
Infant weight maintained within safe limits	_____	_____

145   Formula Preparation in the Home

Overview

Definition

The process for mixing and storing the infant feedings; this technique is usually taught to the mother in anticipation of discharge from the hospital. Formula is a mixture for feeding the infant. Types of formula include the following:

Prepared, ready-to-use formulas, available in cans and bottles

Powdered or concentrated formulas, which are mixed with water

Formula prepared by mixing evaporated milk, dextrose, and water

Rationale

Teach the mother how to prepare feedings safely and confidently.

Provide adequate nutrition for the infant.

Prevent infection or contamination due to poor technique.

Terminology

Aseptic method: Formula preparation in which the bottles, nipples, nipple caps, and equipment for making the formula are sterilized before the formula is prepared

Sterile: Free from germs, bacteria, and other microorganisms

Terminal method: Formula preparation in which the formula is prepared and poured into bottles that are then sterilized

Assessment

1. Assess the sucking and swallowing reflexes of the infant. Note the amount and type of formula taken in relation to nutritional needs after discharge.

2. Assess the mother's ability to understand and follow directions to determine which type of education efforts will be most effective. Assess the need for home health nurse visits.

3. Assess the home environment in relation to teaching. Ask the mother about the availability of hot and cold running water, sewage arrangements, cleanliness of drinking warer, availability of refrigeration, and cooking heat arrangements.

Plan

Nursing Objectives

Teach the mother a method of formula preparation that takes her individual needs and abilities into account.

Equipment

Commercially prepared formulas: liquid concentrate, powder or ready-to-feed (Fig. 145-1)

Can opener

Bottles (Fig. 145-2)

Nipples, caps, and collars

Brush

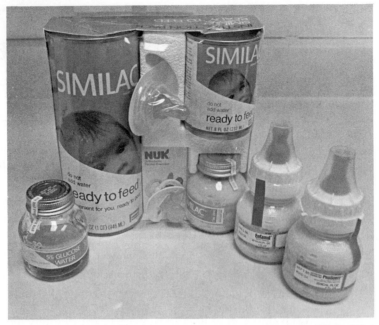

Figure 145.1

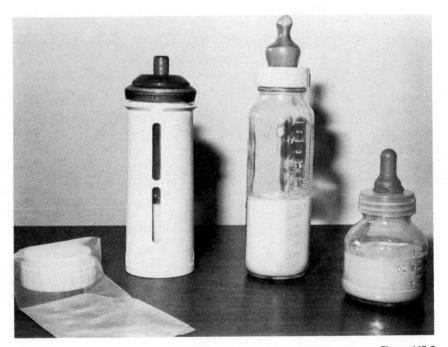

Figure 145.2

Implementation and Interventions

Procedural Aspects

ACTION

1. Formula preparation should always be preceded by thorough hand-washing. The area for preparation should be clean and free from contaminants.

2. Encourage the mother to follow the formula manufacturer's directions. Although many packages still contain the directions for sterilizing the water before diluting powdered or concentrated formula, this is not recommended unless the sanitation conditions in the home leave some question as to the safety of the drinking water for the newborn. In these cases, sterile water should be used. Under normal circumstances, the formula may be diluted with tap water. The physician will usually prescribe the type of formula to be used.

3. Milk solids can coat the sides of the bottle during heating of the formula. If the bottles are not cleaned immediately after use, this film will adhere to the sides of the bottle and may result in contaminated formula. To prevent this, the bottle, nipple, and cap should be rinsed immediately after use and left to soak until washed with warm soapy water.

4. Bottles, nipples, caps, and collars should be washed with warm, soapy water and rinsed well in hot water. A brush may be used to remove milk solids. This should be done in a clean basin or in the dishwasher with no other dishes. Water should be forced through the nipple to ensure that the nipple opening is cleaned.

RATIONALE

Microorganisms may contaminate the feeding by direct contact with unclean hands or surfaces.

Sterilization of tap water may decrease the normal fluoride content and should be avoided unless there is a chance that the water is contaminated.

Contamination with heat-resistant organisms may cause digestive problems for the infant as these microorganisms are transmitted through the contaminated formula. Removal of the milk film discourages the proliferation of heat-resistant microorganisms.

Soapy water and thorough rinsing is usually adequate to prevent cross-contamination of the infant. Pathogens may grow in the confined area of the nipple opening unless it is cleaned consistently.

ACTION	*RATIONALE*
5. Proper storage and disposal of unused portions is very important. Unused portions of cans of prepared formula may be covered and stored in the refrigerator for 24 hours. Opened containers of powder may be covered and stored in a cool, dry place. Unused portions of feedings should be discarded. If several bottles of formula are prepared at one time, they should be stored in the refrigerator until ready to be used.	Microorganisms can grow and proliferate in opened cans and containers. Refrigeration retards the growth of microorganisms.
6. Formula should be at room temperature for feeding. The ready-to-feed bottle does not require refrigeration and may be fed as soon as it is opened. Reconstituted formulas may be prepared with water at room temperature and may be fed at once. Refrigerated feedings should be warmed to room temperature by placing them in boiling water for a few minutes.	The infant usually prefers feedings that are of a consistent nature. As the infant grows older, formula directly from the refrigerator may be accepted. Refrigerated formula should be heated to room temperature instead of letting it warm by standing, since microorganisms can grow during the time it takes for the milk to warm up.

Special Modifications

If the sanitary conditions seem to indicate the need for further cleanliness measures, instruct the mother on further precautions to prevent contamination of formula. She may be instructed to boil the bottles, rings, and caps for 15 minutes. The nipples should be boiled for 5 minutes. The formula should be prepared with sterile water and added to the bottles which are refrigerated at once. Assess the mother's motivation and the environmental situation. Recommend formula preparation techniques that seem most likely to be carried out and that will benefit the infant most.	The principles of cross-contamination should be explained to the mother. If she understands why precautions are taken, she may be more willing to carry out prescribed procedures. Obviously, it seems futile to design elaborate sterilization methods if the mother has no motivation or ability to carry them out. The instructions should take a common sense approach to the best method that is most likely to be followed. A home-health referral may be an alternative to ensuring that the formula preparation is the best possible one for this family.

Communicative Aspects

OBSERVATIONS

1. Observe the mother feeding her infant. Observe for proper positioning of the infant, with the head higher than the body. Also observe for closeness and mother–infant interaction.

2. Observe the mother during return demonstrations to assess her understanding of the principles of cross-contamination and what is clean and what is contaminated.

CHARTING

Charting should include any instructions given to the parents and serve as assessment of their understanding and acceptance.

DATE/TIME	OBSERVATIONS	SIGNATURE
7/18 1800	Formula preparation instructions given to mother and father in anticipation of discharge home tomorrow. Neither parent could offer an explanation of what was clean and what was contaminated during the preparation procedure. Both also stated they did not understand why the infant could not just drink milk like the other children in their apartment building. One week supply of ready-to-feed formula given to family. Will demonstrate preparation and feeding again tomorrow. Physician notified of parents' statement. Community Health Nurse referral made today. CH nurse will come to meet family this afternoon and will make daily visits or as needed. ————————	C. Loo RN

Discharge Planning Aspects

CLIENT AND FAMILY EDUCATION

1. Be sure that the family understands the method of formula preparation and the safety precautions involved. Answer any questions and anticipate any problems based on the environmental assessment. Demonstrate techniques if needed and ask the mother to return the demonstration. Explain the principles of cross-contamination and caution the mother about proper handwashing before preparing the formula or feeding the infant.

2. Emphasize the importance of proper dilution of formulas. Formulas that are prepared with too much diluent may compromise the nutrition of the infant who is not receiving the required amount of nutrients. Underdilution may cause an increase in the renal solute, with ensuing dehydration.

3. Referral to a visiting health nurse may be needed to assess adequately the environmental problems involved in formula preparation at home.

Evaluation

Quality Assurance

Documentation should include instructions given to the parents with an assessment of their understanding. If problems were encountered or are anticipated, referrals should be noted. Assessment of return demonstrations may also be indicated. The chart should reflect that nursing staff took environmental considerations into account when giving formula-preparation instructions. Other considerations might include motivation, financial factors, availability of assistance, and previous experience.

Infection Control

1. The goal of formula preparation instructions and procedures is to prevent contamination of the milk and subsequent contamination and infection of the infant. Eliminating the opportunity for direct contact with contaminants helps prevent contamination. Careful handwashing and adequate cleansing of the preparation surface are important.

2. Once the formula is prepared, it should be refrigerated to prevent or reduce the growth of microorganisms. Formula that has been at room temperature for a significant amount of time (30 minutes–1 hour) should be discarded.

Technique Checklist

	YES	NO
Formula preparation technique explained	_____	_____
Parents exhibited an understanding of:		
Preparation technique	_____	_____
Prevention of contamination	_____	_____
Storage of formula	_____	_____
Amount to feed infant	_____	_____
Feeding technique	_____	_____
Environmental assessment done	_____	_____
Anticipated problems addressed	_____	_____
Referral made _____		

146 Neonatal Assessment, Initial (Apgar Scoring)

Overview

Definition

Evaluation of the newborn infant's condition at birth

Rationale

Provide an objective assessment based on accepted criteria at critical intervals in the infant's first hours of life.

Engage in efficient assessment of the neonate's adjustment to extrauterine life and identification of potential problems.

Terminology

Apgar scoring: A method for making a clinical evaluation of the newborn's condition 1 minute and 5 minutes after birth

Apnea: Cessation of breathing

Anoxia: Deficiency of oxygen

Asphyxia: Anoxia and carbon dioxide retention resulting from failure of respiration

Hypoxia: Inadequate oxygen content in inspired air

Resuscitation: The restoration of life or consciousness in one apparently dead, which includes measures such as assisted ventilation and external heart massage

Assessment

Pertinent Anatomy and Physiology

1. See Appendix I: *heart, lungs, skeletal muscles.*

2. The heart rate of the newborn may be observed as pulsations of the umbilical cord at its attachment to the abdomen or by auscultation. At birth, the circulatory system undergoes drastic changes. Blood ceases to flow through the umbilical vessels and the placenta. Fetal openings in the heart and vessels, the ductus arteriosus, the foramen ovale, and the ductus venosus, begin their closure process, which may take several days to complete. This incomplete closure may be responsible for transient heart murmurs heard in newborns. Normal heart rate in the newborn is in the range of 120 to 180 beats per minute.

3. The respiratory system must function immediately after birth. Gaseous exchange has taken place previously through the placenta. Pulmonary ventilation must begin immediately after birth. If the lungs are not structurally developed to a sufficient degree, adequate aeration is impaired. The lungs have not usually developed sufficiently to support life until after the 26th week of gestational life.

4. The newborn's skin is dark red or pinkish red shortly after birth, becoming pinker in a week or 2. Pallor and pale lips and mucous membranes are not normal. The hands and feet may be slightly cyanotic for an hour to 2 after birth until peripheral circulation has had time to improve. The skin of the neonate is best observed in sunlight.

5. The infant is born with certain reflexes that may signify normal development. The presence or absence and the quality of these reflexes provide indications of the adequacy of the nervous system.

6. The newborn generally has a very good muscle tone. The extremities are usually found in a state of flexion with strong resistance to antagonistic movement. The premature infant generally has less muscle tone than the full-term newborn.

Pathophysiological Concepts

1. A heart rate below 100 beats per minute may indicate asphyxia. Resuscitation may be imminent. The infant with depressed cardiac rate cannot adequately oxygenate the blood and may develop circulatory problems very quickly.

2. Persistent blueness of the hands and feet may indicate inadequate oxygenation due to pulmonary problems, heart disease, or birth trauma. When insufficient oxygen is available in peripheral circulation, the skin may take on a bluish or darkened appearance.

3. Poor muscle tone may indicate a disturbance of the pH of the blood and tissues. This is usually related to asphyxiation.

4. Reflexes are spontaneous actions in response to neural stimulation. Absence or depression of reflexes may indicate neurologic disturbances.

5. Limpness or flaccidity at birth may indicate that the infant is suffering from shock or neurologic injury. These symptoms may also be induced by prenatal narcotic administration to the mother.

Assessment of the Client

Since this technique deals with assessment of the infant, assessment will be considered in the Procedural Aspects section.

Plan

Nursing Objectives

Evaluate the infant's condition at birth by assessing the five vital indicators of status: heart rate, respiration effort, muscle tone, reflexes, and color.

Identify any abnormalities and implement immediate treatment as indicated.

Client Preparation

1. The infant is assessed from the moment of birth by someone who observed the birth and remains in constant attendance with the infant during the first moments of life. Assessments are generally done with the infant's clothing removed so that full visualization may be accomplished. Natural daylight provides the best lighting for assessment of the neonate.

2. While doing the assessment, keep the infant in a well-lit, warm environment free from drafts. Keep the air passages cleared. Gentle patting or massaging may serve as a stimulus to circulation.

Equipment

Stethoscope
Rating form

Implementation and Interventions

Procedural Aspects

ACTION	RATIONALE
1. Perform the Apgar scoring method 1 minute after birth without regard to the delivery of the placenta. Each sign is evaluated according to the degree in which it is present. Each sign is ranked 0, 1, or 2. One score is given to each of the signs, and these scores are added together. The possible ranking of the infant is between 0 and 10, with 10 being the highest. A total score of 0 to 3 represents severe distress; 4 to 6 indicates fair condition; 7 to 10 indicates good condition.	The Apgar Scoring System was developed by Dr. Virginia Apgar in 1952. It provides a consistent method of assessing and reporting the condition of the newborn infant.
2. Repeat the Apgar scoring 5 minutes after birth.	After 5 minutes, the infant's respiratory status and circulatory system should have stabilized. The Apgar score at this time should present a fairly accurate assessment of the infant's ability to adjust to extrauterine life.
3. Interpret the Apgar score according to the Apgar Rating Scale (Chart 146-1). A score of 0 to 3 indicates that resuscitation is needed immediately. With a score of 4 to 6, the air passages should be cleared; oxygen may be administered by mask with the flow not to exceed 2 liters per minute. With a score of 7 to 10, the infant may need only supportive care to ensure a patent airway and provide additional heat, and continued observation.	The Apgar score will given an indication of the amount of assistance required for the infant to survive. It will also alert the practitioner to the possibility of congenital problems.

CHART 146-1 Apgar Rating Scale

SIGN	0	1	2
Heart rate	Absent	Slow (below 100 beats/min)	Over 100 beats/min
Respiratory effort	Absent	Slow, irregular	Good, crying
Muscle tone	Limp, flaccid	Some flexion of extremities	Active motion
Reflex			
1. Response to slap on foot or	No response	Weak cry or grimace	Vigorous cry
2. Response to catheter in nostril	No response	Grimace	Cough or sneeze
Color	Blue, pale	Body pink; extremities blue	Completely pink

ACTION	*RATIONALE*
4. After completing the Apgar scoring, continue to evaluate the infant. After the cord is cut and before the final clamp is placed on the cord, examine the cord surface closely for the correct number of vessels—two arteries and one vein. Examine the head and body for abnormalities. Check the fontanelles for bulging. Auscultate the chest to indicate the position of the heart, the rate and rhythm of the apical pulse, and air flow into the lungs. Note the presence of jaundice. Palpate the abdomen for enlargement of the liver, spleen, or kidneys. Observe the shoulders for fracture. Place a finger on the clavicle and move it. As soon as the infant is stable, perform eye care (see Technique No. 143, Eye Care, Initial). The infant will receive a full examination upon transfer to the nursery (see Technique 135, Admission to the Newborn Nursery).	The presence of only one artery in the umbilical cord may indicate severe congenital anomalies. Other abnormalities found upon initial assessment may provide vital information for use in later assessments and monitoring.

Communicative Aspects

OBSERVATIONS

1. The heart reate is the most important sign in Apgar scoring. Auscultate the rate with a stethoscope or observe the pulsation of the umbilical cord where it attaches to the abdomen. Determine the rate. Listen for murmurs that may be present in the normal newborn for several days.

2. Respiratory effort is the second most important sign. Observe to see that respirations are well established 1 minute after birth. Respirations should be rapid and regular. Observe for rate and quality.

3. Observe the quality of the infant's muscle tone by ability to keep extremities flexed, even when antagonistic force is gently applied. Observe for natural flexion of extremities. The infant will usually attempt to assume the prenatal posture, which is usually one of flexion of the entire body, or "folded into a position of comfort."

4. Reflex irritability should be acute when the infant is awake. Some reflexes are diminished during sleep. Observe the reflex action of the infant.

5. When the infant's condition has stabilized, observe for the following:

   Eyes: Abnormalities such as cataracts

   Nose: Passageway, appearance of septum

   Ears: Location of pinna, presence of skin tags

   Mouth: Cleft lip and/or palate, facial muscles

   Neck: Masses

   Anus: Imperforate

   Extremities: Number of fingers and toes, birth defects such as clubbing or webbing, birth marks

   Genitalia: Hernia, hydrocele, undescended testicles

Abdomen: Umbilical hernia

Gross Reflexes:

Moro's—startle reflex

Grasp—grasping object when placed in hand

Tonic neck—head turned to one side with arm and leg on same side extended

Rooting—head turns to side when cheek is touched

Sucking—sucking on hand, fingers, anything near mouth

Swallowing—swallows after sucking and obtaining fluids

CHARTING

Charting is usually done on an Apgar Scoring Scale, where the score may be calculated and recorded. The Apgar score is usually recorded on the birth record, the nursery record, and wherever else recommended according to hospital policy.

Discharge Planning Aspects

CLIENT AND FAMILY EDUCATION

The family should know the infant's Apgar score and should understand what it means. Explain that a low Apgar score may only mean that the infant adjusted slightly more slowly to extrauterine life and may not indicate permanent damage.

Evaluation

Quality Assurance

Documentation should include an assessment of the Apgar Score at 1 and 5 minutes.

Infection Control

1. Sterile gown and gloves are usually used to handle the infant during the first moments of life. Surgical scrub handwashing should precede donning the sterile garb.

2. Be sure that equipment used for consecutive infants is adequately cleaned between infants to prevent cross-contamination.

Technique Checklist

	YES	NO
Apgar score at 1 min _____		
Apgar score at 5 min _____		
Apgar scoring explained to parents	_____	_____
Evaluation of infant before transfer to nursery	_____	_____

147 Phenylketonuria (PKU) Screening

Overview

Definition

Testing the blood of the newborn for the disease phenylketonuria, or PKU (Chart 147-1)

CHART 147-1 Diagnostic Tests for PKU

TEST	PROCEDURE	COMMENTS
Gutherie test	A few drops of blood are taken from the heel, placed on a filter, and sent to the laboratory for assessment.	Used in wide-scale screening. Positive if the level of phenylalanine is above 8 mg/100 ml.
La Du-Michael method	5 ml of blood is taken; serum is separated and tested.	Level above 8 mg/100 ml indicates PKU.
Dinitrophenylhydrazine test (DNPH)	1 ml urine is collected. An equal amount of DNPH solution is added.	Immediate reaction of pale yellow-orange is negative. Change to opaque bright yellow is positive.
Phenistix test	Test stick is pressed against a wet diaper and compared with chart.	This test is not accurate unless the infant is about 6 wk old.
Diaper test	10% ferric chloride is dropped onto a freshly wet diaper.	A green spot is positive. This test indicates the possibility of PKU. It is not used until the infant is about 6 wks old.

Rationale

Identify the presence of PKU as early as possible.

Implement immediate treatment to prevent mental retardation.

Identify those families who would benefit from future genetic counseling.

Terminology

Metabolism: The sum of all the physical and chemical processes by which living organized substance is produced and maintained; also, the transformation by which energy is made available for the use of the organism

Phenylalanine: An essential amino acid found in animal and vegetable protein

Assessment

Pertinent Anatomy and Physiology

The amino acid, phenylalanine, is essential to metabolism. A certain level is necessary for the satisfactory functioning of the body. The ingested excess must be degraded to prevent accumulation in the tissues.

Pathophysiological Concepts

PKU is a genetic disease that results in a defect in the metabolism of the amino acid phenylalanine. The problem develops because of a deficiency of the enzyme phenylalanine hydroxylase. The infant with PKU is unable to convert phenylalanine to tyrosine. Phenylalanine not incorporated into body tissue accumulates in the body. If the condition is not treated, mental retardation and brain damage can result. The accumulation of phenylalanine eventually spills over into the urine. In PKU, the amount of phenylalanine present in the tissues must be kept at the amount necessary for metabolism; this is accomplished by dietary control. In an infant with PKU, the serum phenylalanine level rises rapidly after birth as the infant begins milk feedings.

Assessment of the Client

1. Assess the dietary intake of the infant prior to testing for PKU. Assess the infant for feeding problems or vomiting before the test, which might render a false-negative result. The infant must have ingested a significant amount of protein for 2 or 3 days before the test.

2. Assess the parents' understanding level if the infant is to be brought back at a later time to have the PKU testing done. Assess the chance of compliance and offer instructions and counseling in a positive manner to gain compliance with treatment prescriptions.

Plan

Nursing Objectives

Arrange for the testing in an expeditious manner to ensure early detection, accurate results, and appropriate treatment.

Refer families for genetic or nutrition counseling if indicated.

Provide emotional support.

Client Preparation

1. Be sure that the infant has taken satisfactory quantities of milk feedings for several days prior to the test.

2. Explain the procedure to the parents and obtain their permission. Many states require PKU testing by law. Consult the hospital policy manual to determine what type of consent is required.

Equipment

Antiseptic and cotton balls

Disposable blood lancet

Filter paper

Implementation and Interventions

Procedural Aspects

ACTION

1. *Guthrie test:* Place the infant prone on a flat surface and make the heel accessible. Cleanse the heel with an antiseptic solution (Fig. 147-1). Stick the heel with a sterile lancet (Fig. 147-2) and collect the blood on the filter paper. The circles on the filter paper must be completely filled with blood.

RATIONALE

The heel is cleaned to prevent contamination of the specimen. The vascular heel of the infant is an excellent location for blood specimen collection when small amounts are needed.

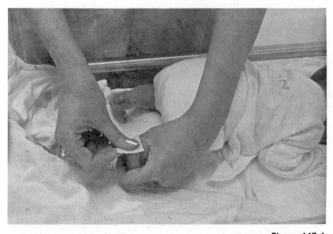

Figure 147.1

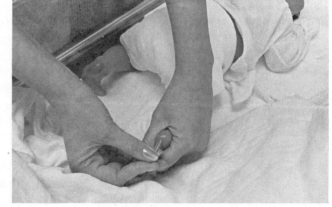

Figure 147.2

ACTION	*RATIONALE*
2. If one of the other tests is done, assist with collecting the blood or urine specimen. Be sure that the test is done correctly and report the results.	Various tests have age limitations. The urine testing is usually not done until the infant is 6 weeks old.
3. Arrange for a follow-up test, which is usually done if the first test is negative.	If the test is negative, a second test may be ordered to ensure that the first reading was not a false-negative due to inadequate ingestion of milk.

Communicative Aspects

OBSERVATIONS

1. Clinical features of PKU usually follow a pattern. The newborn appears normal and characteristically has blond hair, blue eyes, and fair skin. After a period of time, the infant will fail to grow. Symptoms such as vomiting and skin rashes may appear. By the age of 6 months, signs of mental retardation may be seen. The child may have a "musty" odor. Hyperactivity and unpredictable, erratic behavior may also be seen. The child usually appears very immature and dependent, with poor interpersonal-relations skills.

2. Observe the infant after collecting the blood specimen to ensure that clotting takes place and bleeding is prevented.

3. Women with PKU should be identified because maternal phenylalanine is absorbed by the placenta. Pregnant women with PKU should resume their PKU diet before and during pregnancy.

CHARTING

DATE/TIME	OBSERVATIONS	SIGNATURE
4/10 1530	Rt. heel stick for PKU testing. Specimen on filter paper sent to laboratory. Small amount of bleeding after heel stick. Mother instructed about why test was done. Gave permission and expressed interest in results. ———————	N. Jone RN

Discharge Planning Aspects

CLIENT AND FAMILY EDUCATION

1. Inform the parents about the nature of PKU. Emphasize that it is controllable if found early enough. Stress the importance of screening the child. Determine if the screening is mandated by law. If so, inform the parents of actions that they must take to be in compliance with the laws of the state. Since the child must have been on feedings for several days before the test is done, it is possible that the mother will have to bring the infant back to the clinic or hospital for testing after discharge. This is especially true if the mother and infant were discharged early. Emphasize the importance of keeping the follow-up appointment to have the PKU testing done.

2. If the child is found to have PKU, the parents will require a great deal of teaching, support, and counseling. Explain the need for early and continued treatment. The treatment of PKU is dietary. After diagnosis has been confirmed, the diet is planned to limit the ingestion of phenylalanine to 10 mg to 20 mg/kg/24 hours. The normal intake is more than 100 mg/kg/24 hours. This reduction will lower blood levels of phenylalanine to 2 mg to 6 mg/100 ml. Food lists are available for families to follow. Lofenalac, a commercially prepared formula from which 95% of the phenylalanine has been removed, is used for PKU babies. It contains protein in the form of casein hydrolysate and amino acids and provides the essential minerals, vitamins, fats, and carbohydrates. Low-protein strained foods are generally introduced later. The adequacy of the diet will be monitored by blood and urine testing at frequent intervals as the infant grows. Frequent monitoring is essential to ensure that

enough phenylalanine is being ingested to meet metabolic demands but not enough to cause neural disorders.

3. Emphasize to the parents of PKU children that damage to the central nervous system can be minimal if the diet is started before the age of 3 months. The duration of the diet is controversial. Some recommend that the diet be continued through adolescence.

4. PKU requires long-term treatment. Referral to a clinic or public health department may allow the mother to feel supported and confident about caring for her special child.

Evaluation

Quality Assurance

Documentation should contain written evidence that the PKU test was performed. Observation for untoward effects of the testing should be noted. If the test was not done, the reason should be stated, such as "dismissed same day as birth; infant to be returned to clinic for PKU testing on Friday, 3/15." Documentation should include any instructions or teaching of the parents. An assessment of the parents' likelihood of returning for follow-up testing or care should be noted. If there is reasonable doubt that the parents will return the child for PKU testing, a referral to a visiting nurse association to collect the sample may be made. Other arrangements may be made according to the laws of the state and the policy of the city and hospital.

Infection Control

1. Careful handwashing should precede and follow handling any infant.

2. Cleansing the heel with a disinfectant reduces the change of introducing pathogenic microorganisms into the infant's system.

Technique Checklist

	YES	NO
PKU testing _____		
PKU testing not done	_____	_____
Reason documented in chart	_____	_____
Follow-up appointment given	_____	_____
Parents understand need to keep appointment	_____	_____
PKU suspected or confirmed	_____	_____
Explanation given to parents	_____	_____
Dietary counseling given	_____	_____
Follow-up care arranged	_____	_____
Genetic counseling recommended to parents	_____	_____

148   Phototherapy

Overview

Definition

The use of intense fluorescent light for treating neonatal hyperbilirubinemia

Rationale

Reduce the serum bilirubin in a full-term or premature neonate.

Terminology

Bilirubin: The yellowish or orange-colored pigment in the bile that is carried to the liver by the blood; produced from the degradation of the hemoglobin of the red blood cells

Hyperbilirubinemia: Excessive bilirubin in the blood

Jaundice: A condition due to the deposition of bile pigment in the blood, causing yellowness of the skin, eyes, mucous membranes, and body fluids

Kernicterus: Abnormally high levels of unconjugated bilirubin, which, unless reversed, result in brain damage and death

Assessment

Pertinent Anatomy and Physiology

Bilirubin is a breakdown product of hemoglobin that is released when red blood cells die and their membranes rupture. Two main forms of metabolism of bilirubin occur in the body: *conjugaton,* which takes place in the liver, and *photodecomposition,* which takes place in the skin under the influence of light. The bilirubin resulting from the breakdown of hemoglobin is unconjugated. Because it is fat-soluble, not water-soluble, it cannot be excreted by the kidneys. Bilirubin is conjugated by the process of being bound to albumin, which transports it to the liver, where it is converted into conjugated bilirubin. This type of bilirubin is water-soluble and is excreted through the bile ducts.

Pathophysiological Concepts

Photodecomposition of bilirubin takes place in the skin under the stimulus of blue light and is not dependent on enzyme action. The amount of bilirubin decomposed depends on the area of skin exposed to light, the wave length and intensity of the light, and the length of exposure. If the natural or artificial methods of disposal of bilirubin are insufficient, the bilirubin level rises progressively, and the infant becomes increasingly jaundiced as the bilirubin passes from the blood into the skin and other tissues, such as the brain. Brain cells do not tolerate the presence of the bilirubin, and cell death may occur.

Assessment of the Client

1. Assess the amount of jaundice of the infant by looking at the nailbeds and the sclera (whites of the eyes). A yellowish tinge to the skin is often evident.
2. Assess the parents' level of understanding of the jaundice, the use of phototherapy, and the implications of the therapy. Assess the parents' level of anxiety.
3. Assess the amount of milk the infant has received prior to initial appearance of the jaundice. Determine if the infant is breast-fed or bottle-fed. Assess the age of the infant and any family history of jaundice in other children.

Plan

Nursing Objectives

Follow safety measures before, during, and after the use of phototherapy.

Meet the needs of the infant for oxygenation, hydration, safety, and warmth.

Observe carefully for adverse reactions.

Offer an explanation and reassurance to the parents about the need for and expected outcomes of phototherapy.

Client Preparation

1. Protect the infant's eyes by placing an eye protector over them.
2. Be sure that the safety shield is in place under the lamp to protect the infant from the danger of broken glass, dust, and overexposure to ultraviolet radiation.
3. Label the enclosed crib or controlled environment crib with the infant's name.
4. Protect the genitals from the ultraviolet light by covering them with a surgical face mask.

Equipment

Phototherapy light (such as the Bili-lite, which operates from a 110 V a.c. supply with a three-wire ground cord and plug)

Eye covers, in the newborn or premature size

Open or enclosed crib

Implementation and Interventions

Procedural Aspects

ACTION	RATIONALE
1. Undress the infant and place the infant in an enclosed or open crib with warmer capabilities.	The infant is undressed to maximize the amount of surface exposed to the light. Since the infant cannot be covered with a blanket, some type of external warming capability is necessary.
2. Be sure that eye and genital covers are in the proper position (Fig. 148-1). They must be on at all times when the baby is under the light. However, remove the eye covers every 3 or 4 hours at the times the baby is fed so that the eyes may be exposed to the air. The genital cover will be removed and changed when soiled.	The covers protect the delicate tissue of the eye, which is susceptible to damage from the light. However, eye infection may result if the eyes are covered continuously. In addition, the child needs the visual stimulation available during periodic removal of the covers.
3. Place the phototherapy source (such as the Bili-lite) over the top of the crib at close range, approximately 18 inches from the mattress level. Do not place the light directly on top of the enclosed crib. Leave the light in place for the time specified by the physician.	The light should be close enough to provide the infant with the benefits of phototherapy but should not present safety hazards. The duration of phototherapy usually is determined by measuring the serum bilirubin.

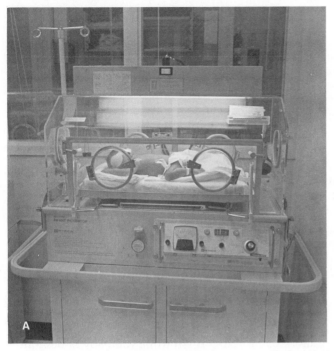

Figure 148.1A

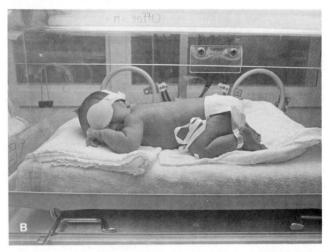

Figure 148.1B

ACTION	*RATIONALE*
4. Turn the infant over periodically to prevent pressure on any part of the body. Bathe the infant daily while under the light.	Movement and turning of the infant are not contraindicated by the phototherapy. Excretion of some of the waste products of hemoglobin breakdown through the skin makes the daily bath very important.

Communicative Aspects

OBSERVATIONS

1. Observe the degree of jaundice and note the progression or regression during phototherapy. Note particularly the sclera, nailbeds, gums, and skin. Jaundice progresses in a cephalocaudal direction; the further down the body the jaundice is found, the higher the bilirubin level.

2. All infants undergoing phototherapy must be observed for immediate untoward effects of phototherapy, which include loose, green stools, increased water loss through the skin, hyperthermia, and increased metabolic rate.

3. If the plastic shield is not in place, the ultraviolet light may cause a skin rash. Observe for proper positioning of the shield each time the baby is placed in the crib.

4. Flammable material should not be placed on the light hood. Observe to see that diapers and other materials are not placed there.

5. Monitor the body temperature of the infant. Hyperthermia is a side effect of phototherapy. Hypothermia may result if the infant is in an open crib without an external warming source.

6. Because of the water loss through the skin, monitor the state of hydration, body weight, and the specific gravity of the urine at least once a day.

CHARTING	DATE/TIME	OBSERVATIONS	SIGNATURE
	5/25 0900	Bili-lite applied because of increasing yellowish tinge to skin. Eyes and genitals covered, diaper and clothing removed. Complete explanation of reasons for phototherapy and expected results given to parents. Both are very upset at this time. Explanation will be repeated this afternoon after mother feeds baby.	C. Day RN

Discharge Planning Aspects

CLIENT AND FAMILY EDUCATION

1. Explain why the phototherapy is necessary and what the expected effects are. Tell the family that the infant will not be harmed by the therapy, but that failure to use this form of therapy can cause dire consequences. Explain the mechanism of kernicterus if the parents seem able and willing to understand. Explain why the infant must be undressed and why the eyes and genitals are covered. The idea of the baby lying with no clothes may be disturbing to the parents. Explain that the crib is warm and that the baby is safe and comfortable.

2. Demonstrate how to hold and feed the baby. Reassure the parents that being under the light will not alter the baby's appetite or need to be held and cuddled. The parents may feel more comfortable if handling the baby is demonstrated.

Evaluation

Quality Assurance

Document the time the baby was placed under phototherapy and safety precautions taken, such as placement of the light and application of eye and genital covers. Laboratory values that support the need for phototherapy should be a part of the child's permanent chart. Explanations to the parents and their reaction should be noted. Daily monitoring of the extent of jaundice and attention to adequate intake and output should be reflected.

Each hospital should have a standardized method of ensuring the safety and efficiency of electrical equipment, such as the phototherapy lights. Documentation of routine maintenance should be evidenced by log sheets or tags on equipment.

Infection Control

1. Periodic removal of the eye coverings is necessary to prevent the colonization of microorganisms in the dark, moist environment provided by their placement over the eyes. Clean debris from the child's eyes with a soft, moist cloth, moving from the inner to the outer corner of the eye.

2. Wash hands thoroughly between clients in the nursery to prevent cross-contamination.

3. Bathe the infant as often as needed to prevent infection and discomfort. The loss of fluid and particles through the skin may require frequent cleansing of the infant's skin.

4. All equipment used for consecutive clients must be cleaned between uses. This is particularly vital for infants whose natural immunity is immature, thus rendering them particularly susceptible to disease. Terminal disinfection according to the hospital routine should be done on all equipment that will be used by consecutive newborns.

Technique Checklist

	YES	NO
Reasons for phototherapy explained to parents	_____	_____
Initial bilirubin level _____		
Final bilirubin level _____		
Protective devices applied when under light		
Eye pads	_____	_____
Genital covering	_____	_____
Eye coverings removed q _____ hr	_____	_____
Eyes cleansed q _____ hr		
Duration of phototherapy _____		
Documentation of intake and output assessment on chart	_____	_____
Complications or side-effects		
Loose, green stools	_____	_____
Dehydration	_____	_____
Hyperthermia	_____	_____
Hypothermia	_____	_____
Physical parameters monitored		
Daily weight	_____	_____
Temperature q _____ hr		
Specific gravity of urine q _____ hr	_____	_____
Apical heart rate	_____	_____

149 Resuscitation of the Newborn

Overview

Definition

Implementation of efforts to initiate or restore life or consciousness to a newborn

Rationale

Establish normal respiration in the depressed neonate in an expedient manner. Avoid the complications of continued anoxia.

Terminology

Apnea, apneic: Without respirations

Asphyxia: Decreased oxygen and/or increased carbon dioxide in the system

Fourth stage of labor: The 2 hours after delivery of the placenta, when the mother's reproductive organs begin returning to the nonpregnant state

Premature: Infants born before 37 weeks' gestation

Third stage of labor: From birth of the baby to delivery of the placenta

Assessment

Pertinent Anatomy and Physiology

1. Appendix I: *lungs, trachea.*
2. Prior to birth, the infant has been aerated by gaseous exchange through the placenta. The fetal lung is filled with fluid. Most of this fluid is compressed from the lungs during the rigors of the birth process. The remainder is absorbed by the body within an hour after birth.
3. Adequate maturation of the lungs is necessary for successful functioning of the respiratory system. Pulmonary ventilation and circulation are critical to the survival of the infant in extrauterine life.

Pathophysiological Concepts

The infant who does not breathe at birth will have compromised blood gas values. The PO_2 will decrease, reflecting a decreased oxygen concentration in the blood. The PCO_2 will reflect a rise in the accumulation of carbon dioxide in the blood. The pH of the blood and tissues will fall, indicating an acidic condition. The abnormal condition of the blood will have cardiovascular effects, resulting in a decrease in the rate and eventual cessation of the heartbeat.

Assessment of the Client

1. Infants with an Apgar score of 0 to 3 will probably need vigorous resuscitation (see Technique No. 146, Neonatal Assessment, Initial). An Apgar score of 4 to 6 indicates that the infant is moderately depressed and should be observed carefully and assessed frequently for resuscitation needs.
2. Assess the airway to be sure it is clear before instituting resuscitation efforts. Suctioning with a bulb syringe may clear the airway adequately. Assess the status of the infant's tongue to ensure that it is not obstructing the airway. If it is, pull the infant's chin forward and upward in a position of slight hyperextension.

Plan

Nursing Objectives

Provide oxygen and decrease the amount of carbon dioxide in the bloodstream.

Expand and maintain the integrity of the lungs.

Maintain adequate circulation.

Maintain the infant in a warm environment.

Observe the infant for early signs of fetal distress, such as bradycardia or prolonged apneic periods.

Allay the anxiety of the parents.

Avoid complications from resuscitation efforts.

Client Preparation

Client preparation is not indicated. The resuscitation technique may be initiated upon the birth of a distressed infant. At every delivery, working resuscitation equipment should be ready in case it is needed. Although many infants may be identified as being at risk before birth, it is not always possible to predict when resuscitation will be indicated. For that reason, equipment should be ready for use in every delivery.

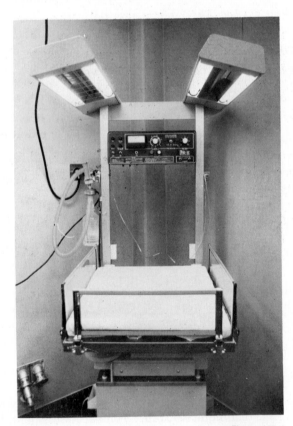

Figure 149.1

Equipment

Heated open crib accessible to the nurse (Fig. 149-1).

Bulb syringe for suctioning

Resuscitation bag equipped with a pressure manometer and various sizes of masks and endotracheal adapters

Pharyngeal airways or endotracheal tray (see Technique 98, Endotracheal Intubation)

Umbilical catheterization tray with fluid

Blood pressure monitoring equipment

Stethoscope

Suction catheters (sizes 5 F–10 F) and aspiration syringe or aspiration catheter

Emergency drugs, syringes, and needles

Antiseptic cleansing solution and tape

Implementation and Interventions

Procedural Aspects

ACTION

1. Hold the infant's head in a position slightly lower than the trunk and turned to the side. Clear the oral pharynx by suctioning with a small-bulb syringe. Gently rubbing the infant's back, towel drying the skin, or gentle suction will usually initiate respiration.

2. If the infant has not started spontaneous breathing within 1 minute after birth, start resuscitation. Clamp and tie the cord. Auscultate the heartbeat to determine sufficiency. If the cardiac rate falls below 80 beats/minute, oxygenation of the lungs is urgent.

3. Ensure the patency of the airway. Nasopharyngeal suctioning may be sufficient to clear the airway and allow spontaneous respiration. If the infant fails to breathe spontaneously, administer 100% oxygen by a bag or mask at the rate of 30 to 40 breaths per minute. Be sure that the mask forms a seal over the infant's nose and mouth. The first breath may be more vigourous than those needed for subsequent respirations. This initial breath may stimulate breathing. Subsequent breaths should be gauged by the rise and fall of the infant's chest, usually around 20 to 40 cm/water pressure.

RATIONALE

Fluid arises from the alveolar cells of the lungs and must be drained by gravitational pull into the trachea so that it can be suctioned or removed by coughing of the infant. Vigorous stimulation of the newborn, such as slapping on the back or buttocks may endanger the infant and should be avoided.

In just a few minutes, the pH level can fall to a level that is incompatible with life. When the cord is clamped, the infant is no longer receiving gaseous exchange with the placenta. Self aeration is essential. Bradycardia or muffled heart sounds can also indicate the need for assisted oxygenation.

The airway may contain meconium, fluids, or mucus, which inhibit the act of respiration. A high concentration of oxygen for a short period is not believed to be harmful to the infant. The wet lining of the lungs adhere to each other and may be parted by the initial inflation, thus instituting respiration.

ACTION

RATIONALE

4. Failure to adequately aerate the lungs may result in cardiac suppression. If the heart rate remains very low or ceases, external cardiac massage may be indicated. Use the two thumbs at midsternum level. Place the fingertips under the infant's axillae, wrapping around to the back (Fig. 149-2). Compress the infant's sternum with the thumbs at a rate of 100 compressions per minute. Discontinue compressions every 30 seconds for a brief time to check for spontaneous heartbeat. Check frequently for the presence of peripheral pulses. Another method of cardiac compression is by using two fingers on the infant's sternum (Fig. 149-3). The infant is placed in a supine position. Once the heart begins to beat spontaneously, cardiac massage may be stopped.

Compression of the lower third of the sternum may cause liver damage. A compression rate of 100 per minute with an assisted ventilation rate of 30 per minute will render a 3:1 ratio. External massage is usually indicated if the heart rate is less than 50 beats per minute after 30 seconds of ventilation.

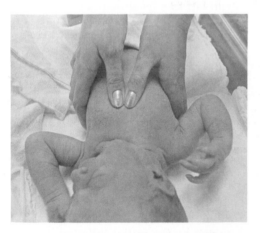

Figure 149.2

Figure 149.3

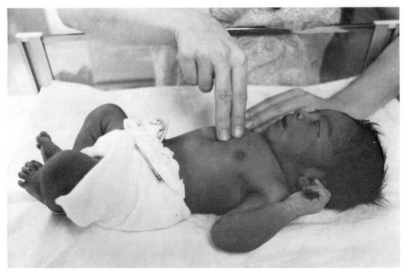

5. If initial resuscitation efforts fail to revive the infant, fluid and electrolyte therapy may be indicated. Prepare umbilical catheterization equipment and emergency drugs.

6. Be sure that the infant is kept warm during the resuscitation effort.

Acidosis may be reversed by the administration of drugs such as sodium bicarbonate. Epinephrine and/or narcotic antagonists may also help revive the infant.

This is a critical period in the life of the infant. Warmth is essential. Cooling the infant induces increased metabolic demands to maintain body temperature, resulting in metabolic acidosis in addition to respiratory acidosis.

ACTION	RATIONALE
7. Offer support and information to the mother and father. Keep them informed of their infant's progress and help allay their apprehension.	The mother will be in the third or fourth stage of labor when resuscitation techniques are being carried out. She will need physical and emotional support.

Communicative Aspects

OBSERVATIONS

1. Observe for adequate aeration of the infant's lungs during resuscitation, indicated by the rise and fall of the infant's chest. The sound of the air entering the lungs must also be auscultated. Observe for cardiac sufficiency by auscultation of the heart and palpation of the peripheral pulses. Also, note the infant's color and initiation of spontaneous movement.

2. Careful observation is essential during the postresuscitation period. During this critical time, complications from prolonged asphyxia may manifest themselves. The heart rate should be monitored continuously by a cardiac monitor. Observe for bradycardia, which may be due to hypoxia, and tachycardia which may indicate that acidosis has not been corrected. Symptoms such as cyanosis, grunting, and nasal flaring indicate that the infant is having difficulty with adequate respiration. Renal complications are also possible. Anuria, oliguria, hematuria, and proteinuria may occur because of renal damage during the oxygen deprivation period. Gastrointestinal (GI) symptoms include abdominal distension, blood in the stool, and delayed stomach emptying. Hypoxic damage to the brain may cause seizures.

CHARTING

DATE/TIME	OBSERVATIONS	SIGNATURE
10/19 0800	Resuscitated in the delivery room. Apgar 1 at birth, no spontaneous respirations, no movement, color pale, heart rate inaudible. Intubation accomplished with 3.5 endotracheal tube and O_2 administered after suctioning. Weak cry response attempted with spontaneous respirations in 45 sec. Respirations still poor quality. Umbilical catheter inserted by Dr. K. 100 ml D_5W running keep open at this time. Pulse is 112, clearly audible. Five-min Apgar is 6. Taken to Neonatal ICU in warmer. Parents reassured about baby's condition and got to see him as he was taken to nursery. Father accompanied baby to nursery.	C. Loo RN

Discharge Planning Aspects

CLIENT AND FAMILY EDUCATION

1. The parents need a great deal of support during this time. They will seek and deserve to have information about their infant's condition. Honesty is the best approach when dealing with a highly emotional situation such as infant resuscitation. Building false hope should be avoided; however, caring and truthful support are never inappropriate.

2. If long-term effects of asphyxia are expected, the parents should be told about possible symptoms and appropriate actions. Referrals to a neonatal intensive care center may be made if the infant cannot be stabilized adequately.

Evaluation

Quality Assurance

Documentation should contain a progressive record of what occurred during the resuscitation. The Apgar scores should be noted. The symptoms that prompted resuscitation should be documented. Any ancillary procedures, such as endotracheal intubation, should be noted in the chart. The outcome of the resuscitation effort should be reflected with follow-up observations or transfer notes. Any medications or intravenous solutions administered should be noted on the appropriate portion of the chart.

Infection Control

1. Equipment used for resuscitation of the newborn should be sterile and ready to use whenever needed. After use, the equipment should be cleaned, disinfected, and sterilized for the next use.

2. The nurse(s) and other health-care personnel responsible for the infant during delivery should engage in a sterile surgical scrub prior to delivery of the baby. Sterile gown and gloves may be worn to protect the infant from cross-contamination.

Technique Checklist

	YES	NO
Time of birth _____		
Apgar 1 min _____		
Apgar 5 min _____		
Time resuscitation began _____		
Suctioned with bulb syringe	_____	_____
Suctioned with catheter	_____	_____
Endotracheal intubation	_____	_____
Tube size _____		
Cardiac massage	_____	_____
Umbilical catheterization	_____	_____
Drugs administered _____		
_____		
Solutions _____		
Infant kept warm during procedure	_____	_____
Parents kept informed of infant's progress	_____	_____
Infant placed on respirator	_____	_____
Time of spontaneous respiration _____		
Time infant pronounced dead _____		

150 Weighing the Newborn

Overview

Definition

Obtaining the infant's daily weight

Rationale

Provide a basis for future evaluation.

Determine the infant's progress.

Compare to accepted norms for assessment.

Terminology

Kilogram (kg): A unit mass in the metric system; 1000 grams (g), or 2.2. pounds avoirdupois

Pound (lb): A unit of mass in the avoirdupois system, containing 16 ounces (oz); equivalent to 453.592 g

Assessment

Pertinent Anatomy and Physiology

It is normal for infants to lose weight during the first few days of life. This is due to a low fluid intake and loss of excess fluid in the body during adjustment to the extrauterine environment. The weight normally stabilizes by the 3rd or 4th day and then begins to increase. Appoximately half of all full-term babies weigh between 3000 g and 3500 g (6½ lb–7½ lb).

Pathophysiological Concepts

Premature or ill infants lose weight over a longer period of time and regain the weight more slowly than healthy infants. A great deal of the metabolic activity of the ill infant is used in restoration of homeostasis. The premature infant is attempting to survive with many immature organs and systems. Nutrients are being used for maturation of systems; formation of fat and muscle does not begin until the infant is physiologically able to spare the nutrients for these processes.

Assessment of the Client

Assess the status of the infant to ensure stability and adequate warmth. If the infant is unstable or chilled, delay weighing until it can safely be carried out without compromising the infant.

Plan

Nursing Objectives

Weigh the infant accurately and record the weight daily.

Notify the physician of major discrepancies in weight.

Involve the parents in the infant's care by keeping them informed of the daily weights.

Client Preparation

Remove all of the infant's clothing for weighing.

Equipment

Balance scale with tray

Disposable coverings for tray

Implementation and Interventions

Procedural Aspects

ACTION	RATIONALE
1. Place a clean disposable pad over the scale tray. Set the scale balance on 0.	A pad will help prevent cross-contamination of the infant.
2. Place the unclothed infant on the scale tray. *Never leave the infant unattended on the scale tray.* Use one hand to set the balance. Keep the other hand about 1 inch above the infant but not touching the infant's body (Fig. 150-1).	Keeping a hand over the infant will prevent falls but will not alter the actual weight of the infant.

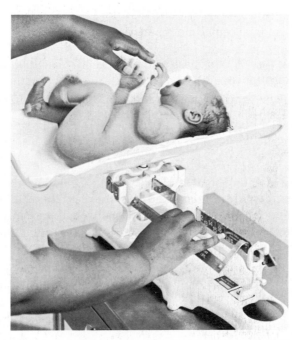

Figure 150.1

ACTION	RATIONALE
3. After weighing, dress the infant and return to the crib or warmer. Chart the weight.	To maintain temperature, the infant is dressed and wrapped when in bed. If a radiant warmer is used, it provides a thermoneutral environment.
4. Weigh at approximately the same time each day.	Daily weights at the same time provide a more accurate measurement.

Communicative Aspects

OBSERVATIONS

1. Observe the child during the weighing procedure to ensure safety.
2. Observe the weight of the child. Great fluctuations in weight must be accounted for (i.e., loss of 10% or more of the birth weight).

CHARTING

Accurate recording of weight should be charted each day, or as prescribed.

NAME	DATE 1/3	DATE 1/4	DATE 1/5
Baby Boy Doe	3.3 kg	3.0 kg	3.1 kg

Discharge Planning Aspects

CLIENT AND FAMILY EDUCATION

1. Reassure the parents that an initial weight loss of several ounces is to be expected. Keep the parents informed of daily weights.

2. Show the parents how to weigh their infant safely at home. Stress safety factors in weighing the infant. Explain that the infant may be slippery when unclothed and a firm grip on the infant is necessary. Stress that they must never leave the infant unattended on the scale.

Evaluation

Quality Assurance

Documentation should include the initial weight and all subsequent weights. Any large discrepancies should be noted in the nurses' progress notes with an assessment of possible causes and follow-up actions. Hospital policy should provide a mechanism for ensuring that every newborn is weighed at least one time each day.

Infection Control

1. Careful handwashing should precede and follow handling of any infant.

2. Equipment used for consecutive infants should be cleaned between uses or covered to prevent cross-contamination. Cover the scale with a disposable towel before placing the infant on it.

Technique Checklist

	YES	NO
Initial weight _____		
Family notified of initial weight	_____	_____
Subsequent weights documented	_____	_____
Parents informed of daily weights	_____	_____
Parents instructed about home weights	_____	_____
Weight of infant upon discharge	_____	_____

Appendix I   Synopsis of Normal Anatomy and Physiology

The following anatomy and physiology concepts are intended as a brief review to provide a background for understanding various aspects of each technique. In the body of the technique, referrals will be made to the portions of this section that are relevant. The items are arranged in alphabetical order for easy reference. Anatomical and physiological information pertinent to only one technique are found in that technique.

***Anus, anal canal* (Fig. A1):** The anal canal is the terminal portion of the large intestine. It is the opening to the outside of the body. Powerful sphincter muscles guard the anal opening. Relaxation of the sphincter muscles is a voluntary action.

***Biliary system* (Fig. A1):** Bile is a greenish yellow fluid that is formed in the liver and is important to digestion because it aids in the emulsification of fats and facilitates the absorption of fats and fat-soluble vitamins. The chief bile-transporting duct from the liver is the common hepatic duct. It joins the cystic duct from the gallbladder to form the common bile duct. The common bile duct descends behind the pancreas, where it usually joins the pancreatic duct, forming a single dilated tube that opens into the duodenum. The bile and pancreatic juice thus is transported into the duodenum to aid in digestion.

***Bladder* (Fig. A2):** The urinary bladder is a thick-walled, muscular sac that lies behind the pubis. It serves as a reservoir for urine and is emptied periodically. The mucous membrane lining of the bladder is present in folds (rugae) that disappear as the bladder distends with urine.

Blood: The chief function of the blood is to maintain normal cell function by the constant exchange of nutrients and wastes with the cells. Arterial blood is bright scarlet; venous blood is a very dark red. The constituents of whole blood are water, dissolved solids, erythrocytes (red blood cells), leukocytes (white blood cells) and thrombocytes (blood platelets). The viscosity of blood is about four times as great as that of water. Normally, the blood not only fills the vascular system but also distends it slightly. The sudden loss of large quantities of blood causes a reduction in volume and pressure and may interfere with the collection of an adequate specimen.

Clotting of the blood is a normal defense mechanism that guards against the possibility of hemorrhage. Clotting begins with a spasm of the vessel, which reduces blood flow. A platelet plug is then formed as the platelets circulating in the bloodstream adhere to the wound and form a sticky aggregate. The unstable platelet plug becomes cemented in place with fibrin strands. Coagulation takes place as the fibrin clot prevents loss of any more blood. The clot gradually begins to retract, drawing together the sides of the wound. As the clot gradually dissolves, it is replaced with scar tissue. Several factors are essential for proper sequential formation of a clot. Absence or interference with any of these factors results in abnormal clotting. Chemical agents may be used to prevent blood specimens from clotting.

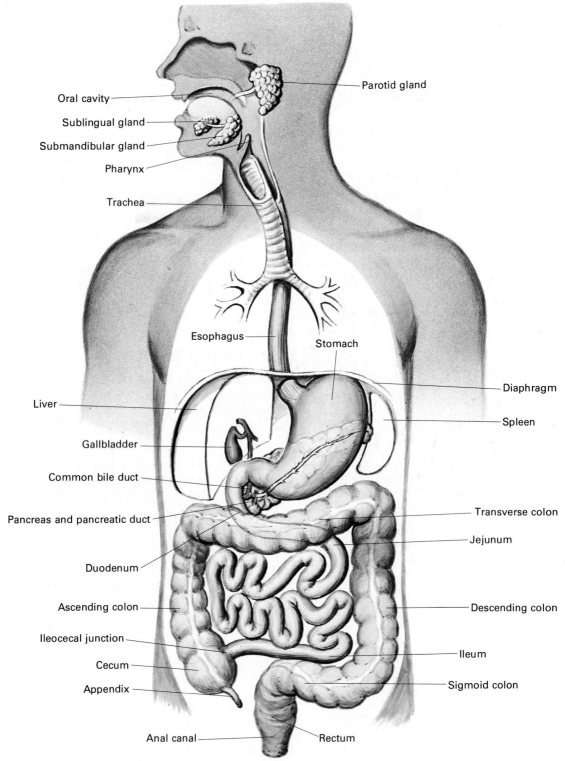

Oral cavity

Sublingual gland

Submandibular gland

Pharynx

Trachea

Esophagus

Stomach

Liver

Gallbladder

Common bile duct

Pancreas and pancreatic duct

Duodenum

Ascending colon

Ileocecal junction

Cecum

Appendix

Anal canal

Parotid gland

Diaphragm

Spleen

Transverse colon

Jejunum

Descending colon

Ileum

Sigmoid colon

Rectum

Figure A1.
The digestive system.

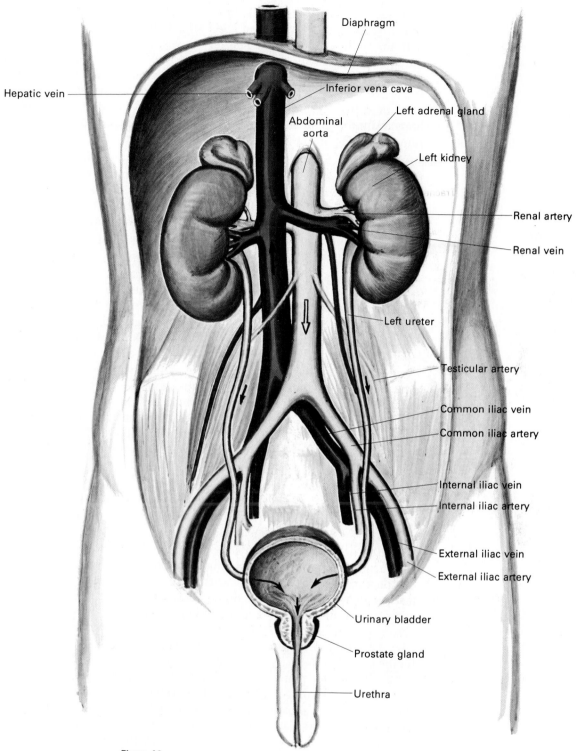

Figure A2.
Overview of the urinary system, with major blood vessels.

Blood vessels: Blood is transported throughout the body by arteries (from the heart), veins (to the heart), and capillaries (where major gaseous exchange with the tissues occurs). The shorter the vessel and the greater its diameter, the lower the resistance to flow. Long, narrow vessels offer more resistance. Arterial pressure is determined by the cardiac output and the peripheral resistance. Arterial pressure is highest in the aorta because it is closest to the heart muscle itself; it is lower as the blood flows away from the heart and branches into the smaller arteries and arterioles. Veins normally follow the same course as do the arteries.

Bone marrow: Bone marrow is one type of blood-forming tissue that is confined to the cavities of the bones. In the marrow are vast numbers of unattached blood cells in various stages of development. If demand for red blood cells exceeds supply, the bone marrow will release premature cells, the presence of which in the blood is indicative of pathology. Platelets, important in blood coagulation, are fragments of larger cells found in the red bone marrow.

Bone repair: The bones most frequently broken are the long bones of the arms and legs and the bones of the pelvis (Fig. A3). Bone repair is carried out in three stages: 1) formation of a procallus, 2) development of a fibrocartilaginous callus, and 3) conversion of the fibrocartilaginous callus to bone. During the initial stage, there is bleeding into the surrounding tissues and between the bone fragments, with development of a blood clot. The granular procallus develops at the site of the clot. In about 5 days, the bone-building cells, or *osteoblasts*, enter the area and form the callus, which within the next few days will serve to immobilize the fragments of the fracture. This tissue differentiates to form the various layers of the bone. Calcium salts then are laid down, and the callus is replaced with osseous material, which eventually is remodeled so that the bone returns to its original state. The most common types of fractures are the simple, compound, comminuted, and greenstick (Fig. A4).

Brain (Fig. A5): The average adult brain weighs about 3 lbs. Brain size is not normally indicative of intelligence. The brain attains its full size by age 18 to 20. The cerebrum, the largest part of the brain, contains the neural mechanism necessary for discrimination and correlation of sensory impulses and recollection of past experiences. The advanced cerebrum is what sets humans apart from animals. Other functions of the cerebrum are motor skills, speech, complex intellectual activities, sensory reception, hearing, sight, smell and taste, memory, learning, and sleep. The midbrain contains centers for posture and orientation in space. The medulla oblongata contains centers for cardiac, vasomotor, and respiratory control. The cerebellum serves primarily for the coordination of muscular activity. The outer covering of the brain is formed by the cranial bones. The meninges or coverings of the brain are the dura mater and the pia mater, which are separated by the arachnoid layer. The cerebrospinal fluid is a clear, colorless watery fluid that fills the ventricles of the brain and the subarachnoid spaces around the brain and the spinal cord. Twelve paris of cranial nerves originate in the undersurface of the brain and pass through the base of the brain on the way to their destination.

Breast (Fig. A6): The female breasts are located on either side of the sternum, extending to the axilla and downward to the area of the second to the sixth rib. The size varies. Each breast is composed of lobes that function in the production and delivery of milk during lactation. The nipple is a projection located slightly below the center of each breast. It contains perforations that allow the milk to be excreted from the breast. The pigmented area around the nipple is called the areola.

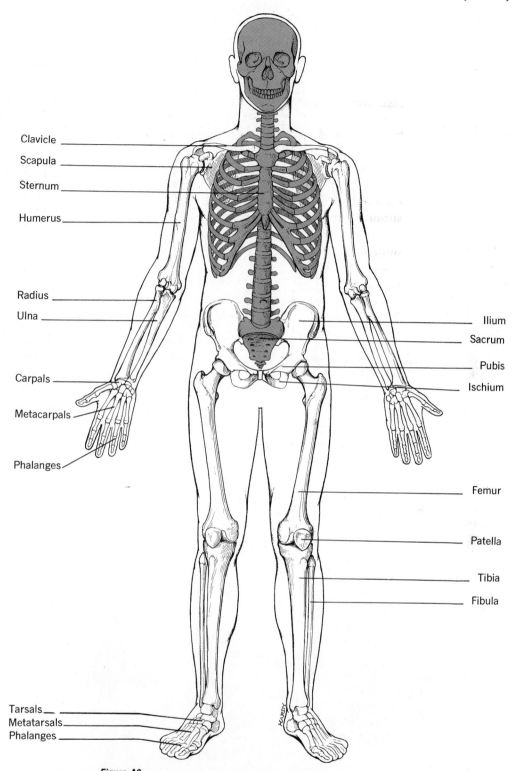

Figure A3.
The skeleton. Bones of the head and the trunk that form the axial skeleton are shaded, and those of the extremities forming the appendicular skeleton are not shaded.

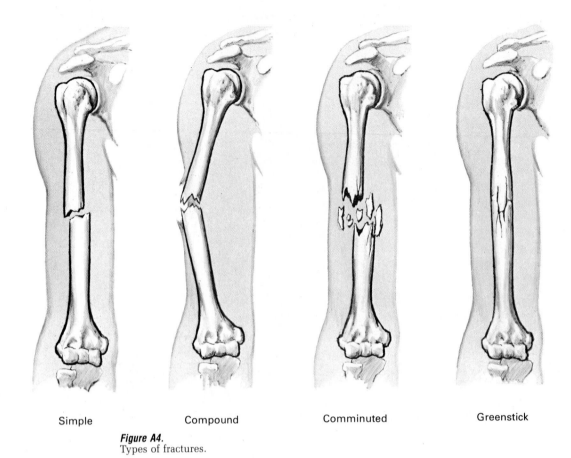

Simple   Compound   Comminuted   Greenstick

Figure A4.
Types of fractures.

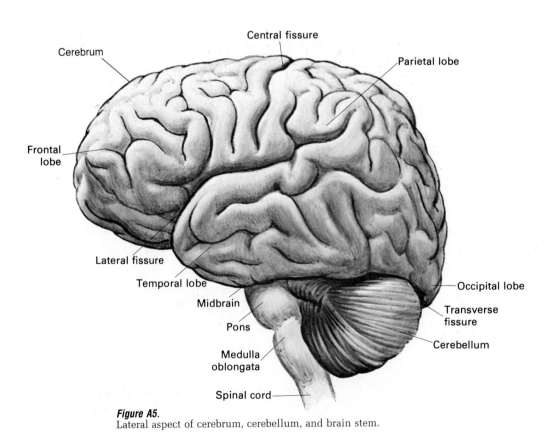

Figure A5.
Lateral aspect of cerebrum, cerebellum, and brain stem.

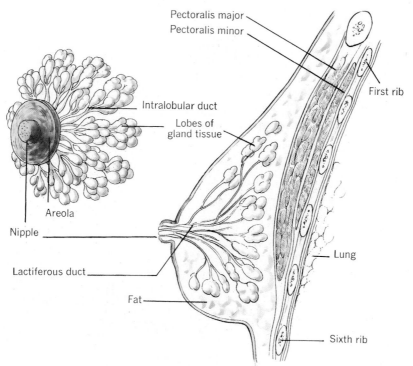

Figure A6.
Glandular tissue and ducts of the mammary gland.

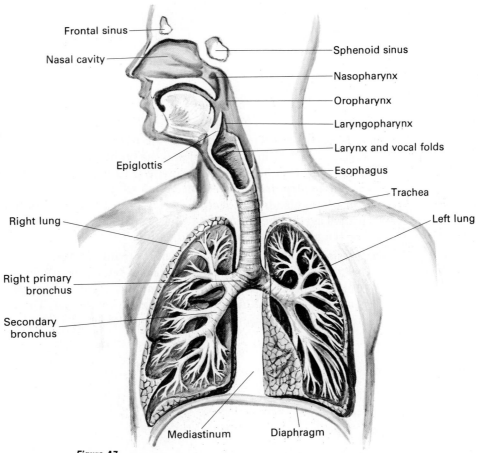

Figure A7.
The respiratory system.

***Bronchial tree* (Fig. *A7*):** The bronchial tree consists of the bronchi and their extensions into the lungs. The trachea divides into the right and left primary bronchi. The right primary bronchus is more nearly vertical, shorter, and wider than the left because of the displacement on the left side by the heart. The primary bronchi branch into secondary bronchi as they enter the lung, three on the right and two on the left. These then branch into smaller tubes called bronchioles. The respiratory tract is lined with mucous membranes. Fluid is essential to the production of the watery mucus that is normally present.

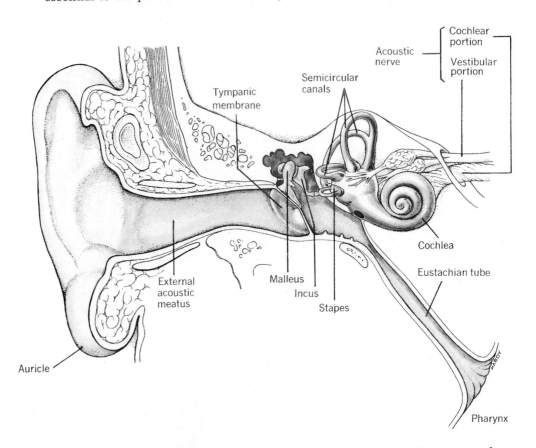

Figure A8.
Diagram of the ear, showing the external, middle, and internal subdivisions.

***Ear, external* (Fig. *A8*):** The external portion of the ear receives sound waves and consists of the pinna (auricle) and the auditory canal. The auditory canal extends inward, forward, and downward from the pinna to the tympanic membrane (eardrum), a distance of about 4 cm (1½ in). The auditory canal is lined with glands that secrete a brown earwax, cerumen, that serves as a protective agent. The external auditory canal should be pink and smooth, and the tympanic membrane should be intact.

***Ear, internal* (Fig. *A8*):** The middle ear, or tympanic cavity, is a tiny, irregular cavity in the temporal bone, the lateral wall of which is formed mainly by the tympanic membrane (eardrum). The tympanic membrane is attached so that it vibrates with all audible sound waves entering the ear. The middle ear communicates with the nasopharynx and the mastoid air cells of the temporal bone.

Esophagus (**Fig. A1**): The esophagus is a muscular, collapsible tube about 25 cm (10 in) long lying behind the trachea. It begins at the pharynx and ends as it enters the stomach. Passage of food through the esophagus is not under voluntary control. The muscles exhibit wavelike contractions that propel the food through the digestive tube into the stomach. Mucus is the only secretion in the esophagus that serves to reduce friction so that the food will slide easily through the tube.

Eye, external (**Fig. A9**): The orbit is the cavity that surrounds and protects the eye, the body's receptor for vision. The eyeball consists of three layers, or coats, that surround the transparent internal structures. The fibrous coat consists of the sclera and the cornea. The sclera is the white of the eye, and the cornea is a transparent tissue that refracts light rays and allows them to enter the eyeball, where they finally reach the retina. The vascular coat is heavily pigmented and contains many of the blood vessels that nourish the eye. The iris is suspended between the cornea and lens and is responsible for eye color. It also regulates the amount of light entering the eye by causing the pupil to constrict in bright light and to dilate in dim light. The third coat is the retina, which is the innermost layer of the eyeball. Posteriorly the retina is continuous with the optic nerve.

Eye, internal (**Fig. A9**): The fundus of the eye is the portion that is seen on ophthalmoscopic examination, namely, the retina, with several distinctive landmarks. Near the center of the retina is a small, yellowish spot called the macula. The center of the macula, called the fovea centralis, is the area of most acute vision. A short distance to the nasal side of the fovea centralis is a pale disk. This area is called the optic disk and is the point of optic nerve attachment. Various blood vessels may be seen branching from the central artery, which enters the eyeball in the center of the optic disk.

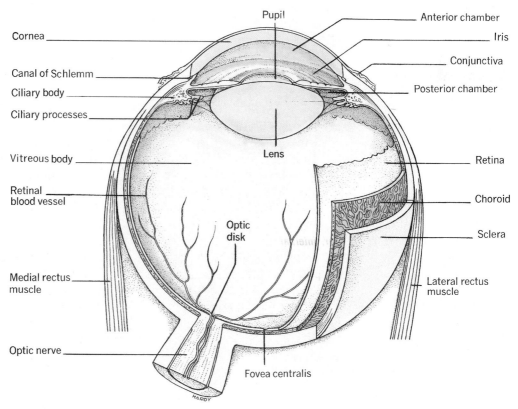

Figure A9.
Transverse section of the eyeball.

Foot: The foot serves to support the weight of the body and provides a strong lever for the muscles of the calf in walking and leaping. The curves of the foot, the longitudinal arch (from the heel to the toe) and the transverse arch (crosswise in the foot), are maintained by powerful ligaments, muscles, and tendons that hold the bones in proper alignment. The bones of the ankle are the dorsal ends of the fibula and tibia. The bones of the foot are the tarsal bones, the metatarsals, and the phalanges, which are the bones of the toes (Fig. *A*3). In the foot, upward movement at the ankle joint is called dorsal flexion and downward movement at the ankle joint is called plantar flexion (extension). Turning the sole of the foot inward is called inversion and turning it outward is called eversion.

Gallbladder (Fig. *A*1): The gallbladder is a muscular, membranous sac about the size and shape of a small pear. It is located on the undersurface of the liver. The function of the gallbladder is to store and concentrate bile. When food enters the duodenum, a hormone is released that stimulates the gallbladder to contract and empty the bile contents into the duodenum when it is needed.

Genitalia, female (Fig. *A*10): The female genitalia consists of the mons pubis, labia majora, labia minora, clitoris, and vestibule. The mons pubis, also called the mons veneris, is a rounded pad of fat in front of the symphysis pubis. The labia majora are two folds of skin extending backward from the mons pubis toward the anus. The labia minora are two smaller folds of skin situated between the labia majora. There are no sweat glands located within the labia minora. The clitoris is a small structure composed of erectile tissue lying at the anterior junction of the labia minora. The vestibule is the cleft between the labia minora into which open the vagina and urethra. Bartholin's glands are located on either side of this area. The perineal body is the area between the vagina and anus.

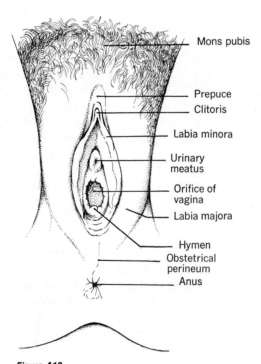

Figure A10.
External genitalia of female.

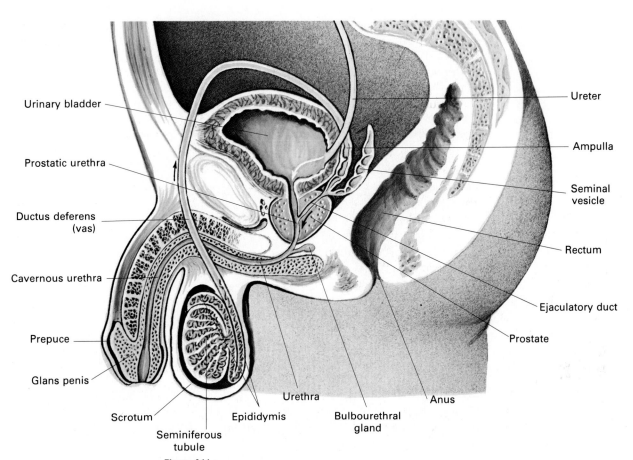

Urinary bladder

Prostatic urethra

Ductus deferens (vas)

Cavernous urethra

Prepuce

Glans penis

Scrotum

Seminiferous tubule

Epididymis

Urethra

Bulbourethral gland

Anus

Prostate

Ejaculatory duct

Rectum

Seminal vesicle

Ampulla

Ureter

Figure A11.
The male reproductive system. Arrows indicate course of spermatozoa through the duct system from epididymis to urethra.

***Genitourinary system, male* (Fig. *A*11):** The male genitourinary system has two basic functions: urine elimination, and reproduction. This system consists of a pair of gonads, the testes, a system of excretory ducts, and accessory organs. The testes are suspended outside the body between the thighs in a pouch called the scrotum. Within each testis are the coiled seminiferous tubules concerned with the production of sperm. Sperm are transported to the urethra by means of a series of tubes. The last tube, the ejaculatory duct, enters the urethra near the prostate gland. The penis is an external organ composed of erectile tissue. The urethra proceeds through the penis to open to the outside of the body. The distal end, the glans penis, is covered with a fold of skin called the prepuce, or foreskin, which is removed during the surgical procedure called circumcision.

***Heart* (Fig. *A*12):** The heart is a hollow, muscular organ located in the space between the lungs in the thoracic cavity. About two thirds of the heart lies to the left of the midline. The heart is composed of four chambers that are separated by valves. Blood is pumped from the right side of the heart into the lungs for aeration. It is received from the lungs into the left side of the heart, which then pumps the blood out into the body. The heart is slightly larger than a clenched fist.

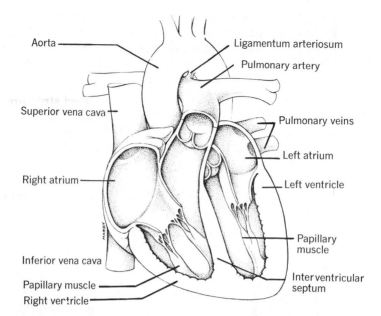

Aorta

Ligamentum arteriosum

Pulmonary artery

Superior vena cava

Pulmonary veins

Left atrium

Left ventricle

Right atrium

Papillary
muscle

Inferior vena cava

Interventricular
septum

Papillary muscle

Right ventricle

Figure A12.
Interior of the heart. Arrows
indicate the direction of blood
flow.

One cardiac cycle means one complete heartbeat, consisting of contraction
(systole) and relaxation (diastole) of the heart muscle. The heartbeat is initiated by the pacemaker cells of the sinoatrial (SA) node. The impulse from the
SA node filters through the muscle mass of both atria, causing them to contract simultaneously. When the impulse reaches the atrioventricular (AV)
node, there is a slight delay before it progresses through the ventricles, causing simultaneous contraction of these lower chambers as well. The slight
delay allows atrial systole to complete. Every beat of the heart is accompanied by an electrical charge. Electrolytes in the body fluids and tissues act as
conductors to the skin surface. The conduction system controls the rhythm
and the pumping action of the heart.

Intestine, large (Fig. A1): The large intestine is about 2.5 meters (4½ ft–5 ft) in
length and about 6 cm (2½ in) in diameter. It is divided into four sections:
the cecum, the colon, the rectum and the anal canal. The appendix arises
from the cecum about 2.5 cm. (1 in) below the ileocecal valve. The colon is
divided into several sections: the ascending colon, which travels up the right
side of the lower abdomen; the transverse colon, which runs across the body
below the level of the umbilicus; and the descending colon, which extends
downward along the left side of the abdomen. Activity in the large intestine
is limited to mechanical evacuation of the contents, which is facilitated by
the secretion of mucus. Bacterial activity also takes place. No enzymes are
secreted in the large intestine.

Intestine, small (Fig. A1): The small intestine is the portion of the alimentary canal
or digestive system in which the greatest amount of digestion and absorption
takes place. It is a coiled tube extending from the stomach to the large intestine. It is approximately 7 meters (23 ft) in length and 4 cm (1½ in) in diameter. The small intestine is composed of three sections: the duodenum,
jejunum, and ileum. The duodenum is the shortest, widest, and most firmly
attached portion of the small intestine, composing the first 25 cm (10 in). It is
shaped in the form of the letter C, and the head of the pancreas lies in the
hollow that it forms. The jejunum forms the next portion of the small intestine and extends to the portion called the ileum. The ileum is the terminal
end of the small intestine, which joins the large intestine at a right angle.

Mechanical activity in the small intestine involves contractions, which serve to mix the digestive juices with the contents as well as to bring the contents in contact with the intestinal wall so that portions can be absorbed for use by the body. Peristalsis, which is the wavelike contraction that propels contents through the small intestine, also occurs.

***Kidneys* (Fig. *A3*):** The kidneys are two bean-shaped structures located in the back of the abdominal cavity. Filtration is a kidney function whereby fluids and small particles are removed from the blood. Normally about 125 ml of fluid is filtered each minute. Only about 1 ml of this is excreted as urine. The average output is about 1440 ml/day. The kidneys perform both excretory and endocrine functions. While excreting wastes, kidneys selectively reabsorb those materials that are needed to maintain a stable internal environment.

Labor and delivery: At the end of pregnancy, a state which lasts about 40 weeks, the uterus begins wavelike contractions that will build in intensity to expel the fetus from the intrauterine environment. The onset of labor usually is heralded by certain signs. These signs of impending labor include lightening (a feeling of respiratory relief as the pregnant uterus drops into the pelvis, releasing some of the pressure on the diaphragm), false contractions (called Braxton–Hicks contractions), changes in the cervix, show (pink-tinged mucus discharge from the vagina), and rupture of the membranes. The first stage of labor consists of dilation of the cervix. Intermittent, regular contractions that become stronger and closer together are responsible for forcing the fetus down the birth canal and into the extrauterine world. With each contraction, the fluid-filled amniotic sac is pushed against the cervix. This wedgelike action serves to efface (obliterate) the cervical canal and dilate the cervix in preparation for birth (Figs. *A*13, *A*14). Usually the amniotic sac ruptures spontaneously during this process and the fluid escapes through the vagina. When dilation of the cervix is complete, the second stage of labor begins. This stage features delivery of the infant through the cervical canal and vagina (Fig. *A*15).

The second stage of labor is termed the stage of expulsion. The forces for expelling the fetus from the maternal body are the involuntary contractions of the uterus and voluntary abdominal muscle contractions. As the fetus proceeds down the birth canal and the presenting part enters the vagina, the perineum begins the bulge. Crowning refers to the emergence of the fetal head through the vaginal opening. Birth follows very quickly. The infant usually emerges head first with typical turning to accomodate passage of the shoulders and torso through the birth canal. The infant may emerge feet first, a situation called breech birth; however, this type of birth may be accompanied by complications and close observation is necessary. Following the birth of the infant, there is usually a gush of retained amniotic fluid and perhaps a small amount of blood. The third stage of labor is the delivery of the placenta. The placenta separates from the uterine wall and is delivered through the vaginal canal. The uterus contracts after delivery of the infant. The placenta is not contractile tissue and actually peels off of the uterine wall as the uterus changes shape and becomes smaller. The uterus continues to decrease in size after birth, a process called involution, causing closure of the open blood vessels at the placental site. The fourth stage of labor involves the first two hours after birth, during which the uterus must remain contracted to prevent bleeding from the placental site. Involution progresses during this stage.

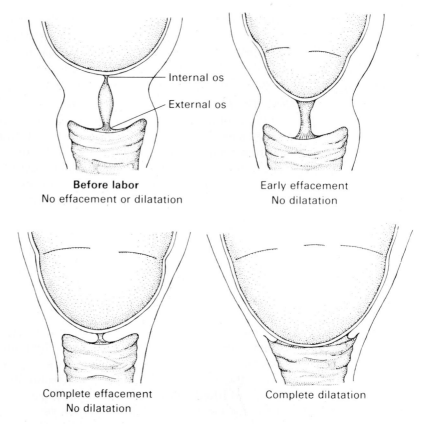

Internal os

External os

Before labor
No effacement or dilatation

Early effacement
No dilatation

Complete effacement
No dilatation

Complete dilatation

Figure A13.
Stages in cervical effacement and dilatation.

FIG. 11-4. *Cervical dilatation in centimeters (actual size).*

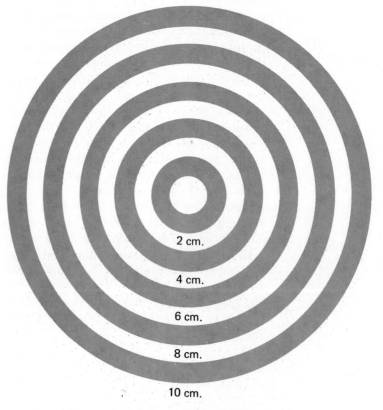

2 cm.

4 cm.

6 cm.

8 cm.

10 cm.

Figure A14.
Cervical dilatation in centimeters (actual size).

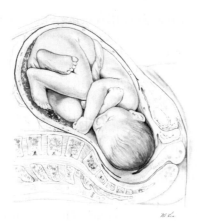

Normal flexion during descent in left occiput anterior position.

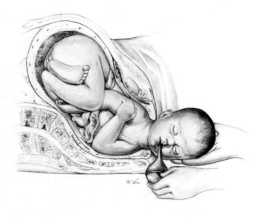

External rotation of the head produces internal rotation of the body.

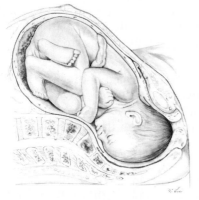

Internal rotation to occiput anterior position.

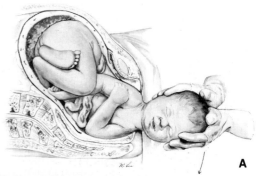

Delivery of the anterior shoulder, (A) and delivery of the posterior shoulder (B) are followed by delivery of the body.

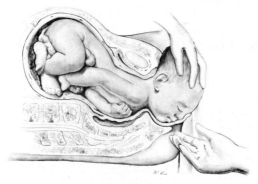

Birth of the head by extension.

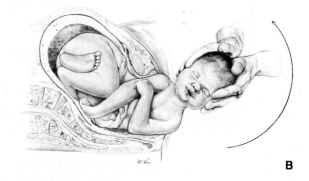

Figure A15.
Progression of the infant through the birth canal.

Lungs (Fig. **A7**): The lungs are two cone-shaped organs that occupy the thoracic cavity. The right lung is shorter and broader owing to the presence of the heart. Each lung is covered by a transparent, two-layered membrane called the pleura. The two layers form the visceral pleura, which adheres to the lung surface, and the parietal pleura, which lines the inner surface of the chest wall. The two layers are separated by a potential space. The pleural layers glide across each other because of the effect of a thin film of serous fluid. The lungs house a branching tree of respiratory tubes that grow progressively smaller and through which air enters and exits. The smallest portion of the bronchial network is that of the alveoli, in which the gaseous exchange between lungs and blood takes place by diffusion.

Mouth: The mouth is the first portion of the digestive tract. Its boundaries include the teeth, hard and soft palates, and the tongue. The roof of the mouth is formed by the bony/hard palate anteriorly and the soft palate posteriorly. The soft palate is drawn upward during the act of swallowing to close the nasopharynx and prevent food from entering the nasal cavities. The tongue is an accessory organ important in chewing, swallowing, and speaking. As the food is chewed, it is broken down into small particles and is mixed with saliva before being pushed through the pharnyx into the esophagus.

Ovaries (Fig. **A16**): The ovaries are small, almond-shaped bodies located on either side of the uterus. The end of each ovary is in contact with the free end of the fallopian tube into the uterus. The oocyte is formed in and released from the ovary into the tube. If it encounters sperm in the fallopian tube, fertilization may occur.

Pregnancy: Pregnancy begins with fertilization of a mature ovum by a spermatozoon. This fertilization takes place in the distal third of the uterine tube. The fertilized ovum, called a zygote, begins immediate division as it travels along the uterine tube toward the uterus. It reaches the uterus in about 3 or 4 days in the form of a fluid-filled ball called a blastocyst. Here it adheres to and later implants into the uterine lining, the endometrium. Following implantation, small fingerlike cords of cells, called villi, penetrate into the surrounding uterine tissue. This becomes the maternal side of the placenta. A fetal membrane, called the amnion, surrounds the growing embryo by the body stalk, which later becomes the umbilical cord. The umbilical cord contains two umbilical arteries and one umbilical vein, which convey fetal blood to and from the placenta to nourish the growing fetus and remove wastes. The placenta provides for respiration, nutrition, and excretion needs of the fetus. Oxygen and nutrients from the mother diffuse from the maternal circulation through the walls of the villi into the fetal bloodstream. Waste is removed by the same process. The placenta maintains the growing embryo and fetus until birth. The periods of intrauterine life are:

Preembryonic period: From the moment of fertilization to about two weeks later

Embryonic period: From the beginning of the third week to the end of the eighth week, when placental circulation is well established

Fetal period: From the beginning of the ninth week until birth

Rectum (Fig. **A1**): The rectum extends from the sigmoid colon to the anal canal and is about 13 cm (5 in) long. Fecal material passes into the rectum just before defecation. Stretching of the rectum arouses the desire to defecate.

Sigmoid colon (Fig. **A1**): The sigmoid colon extends from the descending colon at the level of the pelvic brim to the rectum. The sigmoid is filled with feces because of the action of the large intestine, which pushes its contents into the sigmoid colon.

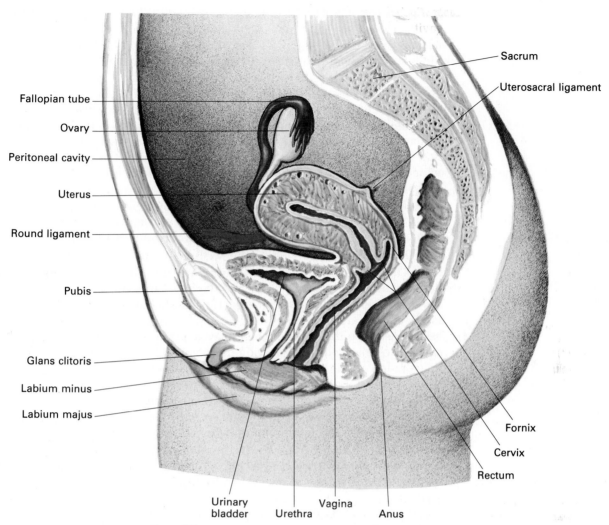

Figure A16.
Female reproductive organs, as seen in sagittal section.

Skeletal muscles: The skeletal muscles are voluntary muscles under the control of the conscious will. Muscle tone refers to a normal state of tension that is common to all healthy muscle. It involves a sustained mild contraction that gives the muscle firmness but does not produce movement. Skeletal muscles move the bones around the joints by contracting and relaxing so that locomotion can take place. Muscles are designated *flexors* when they decrease the angle between the bones and *extensors* when they increase the angle between the bones. Muscle tissue is able to produce movement of the internal and external body parts. Muscle tissue has the properties of excitability and contractility. Excitability is the capacity to respond to a change in the environment; contractility is the action potential of the muscle. The human body functions best in the vertical position. The lungs function optimally when the diaphragm is allowed to contract down into the abdominal cavity. Lying flat in bed allows the viscera to place abnormal pressure on the heart and respiratory apparatus. Physical exertion and mobility stimulate circulation, increase metabolism, and facilitate normal body functions. The chief muscles involved in ambulation are those of the legs and thighs. The normal walking pace for adults is 70 to 100 steps per minute. Elderly people generally have a slower pace.

Skeletal system (Fig. *A*3): The skeletal system forms the strong supporting framework for the body and protects soft tissues and organs. Bones are composed of an organic matrix, calcium salts, and bone cells. The organic matrix provides the framework and strength for the bones. The calcium salts form about 70% of the bone, filling the matrix and adding strength. Bone cells work in a constant state of equilibrium to maintain bone growth and strength. Abnormal stress on the bone results in structural problems, however. Bones are classified on the basis of their shape. The four classes are the long bones, containing a strong tube of compact bone with a hollow space in the center that is filled with marrow; the short bones, located in the wrist and ankle, which are cubical in shape; the flat bones, which are thin and composed of two plates of compact bone surrounding a layer of spongy bone; and the irregular bones, appearing in various shapes throughout the body. With the exception of the joints, bones are completely covered with a dense fibrous membrane called the periosteum. Periosteum is important in the early growth of bones as well as in the nourishment of bone tissue.

Skin (Fig. *A*17): The skin is the body's first line of defense. It provides a protective barrier, covering the entire surface of the body. It is composed of two layers, the dermis and epidermis. The epidermis is the outermost layer. The deeper layers of cells are continually undergoing mitosis, with some of the cells being pushed to the outside where they die from lack of nourishment. These cells provide a protective function on the outside of the skin by preventing dehydration of the lower layers. The blood supply to the skin is important in regulation of temperature and nourishment of the tissue cells. The skin has normal resident microorganisms that are not harmful.

The cutaneous glands continually secrete substances onto the skin. The sebaceous glands are found almost everywhere on the surface of the body, except the palms of the hands and the soles of the feet. They produce an oily secretion called sebum that prevents hair from becoming dry and brittle and that forms an oily layer on the skin surface, keeping it soft and helping to waterproof it.

Sweat glands are of two types: apocrine and eccrine. Apocrine sweat glands are confined primarily to the axilla, areola of the breasts, and the anogenital area. The milky, sticky secretions of these glands are decomposed by the action of bacteria normally found on the skin. This decomposition gives rise to the distinctive odor of sweat. The eccrine glands are distributed all over the body. Their excretory function is primarily responsible for the loss of body heat by evaporation.

Stomach (Fig. *A*1): The stomach is a distensible, saclike organ at the end of the esophagus that receives swallowed food, secretes gastric juice, and serves as an organ of digestion. When the stomach is empty, the mucous membrane lining is seen as folds (rugae). These folds gradually smooth out and disappear as the stomach becomes distended with food. Gastric juice is the highly acid secretion produced by glands in the mucosa of the stomach that aids in the chemical breakdown of food.

Teeth: The teeth are accessory organs of the digestive tube. Each person has two sets of teeth, the first (deciduous teeth) are lost during childhood to be replaced by permanent teeth. Permanent teeth are intended to last for life. The roots of the teeth fit into sockets in the mandible and the maxillae. The teeth are used for chewing the food, or mastication. This action grinds it into small particles and mixes it with saliva.

Trachea (Fig. *A*18): The trachea, or windpipe, is a flexible, tubular structure that extends from the larynx downward through the midline of the neck into the thorax (Fig. *A*7). It is about 11 cm (4½ in) in length and lies in front of the esophagus. The U-shaped cartilage that form the trachea have their open side next to the esophagus so that when a large bolus of food is swallowed, slight encroachment on the back of the trachea is allowed.

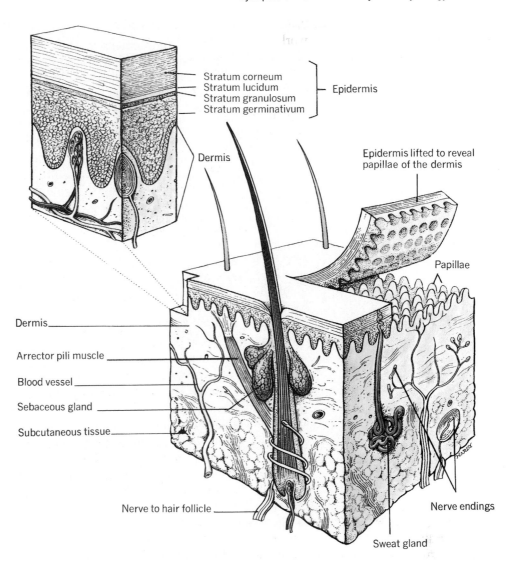

Stratum corneum
Stratum lucidum
Stratum granulosum
Stratum germinativum
— Epidermis

Dermis

Epidermis lifted to reveal papillae of the dermis

Papillae

Dermis

Arrector pili muscle

Blood vessel

Sebaceous gland

Subcutaneous tissue

Nerve endings

Nerve to hair follicle

Sweat gland

Figure A17.
Three-dimensional view of the skin.

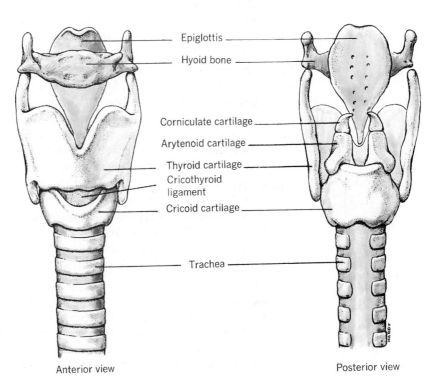

Epiglottis

Hyoid bone

Corniculate cartilage

Arytenoid cartilage

Thyroid cartilage

Cricothyroid ligament

Cricoid cartilage

Trachea

Figure A18.
The laryngeal cartilages.

Anterior view

Posterior view

***Ureters* (Fig. *A2*):** The ureters are tubes about 30 cm (12 in) long that transport urine from the kidneys to the bladder. There is no valve at the ureteral opening into the kidney pelvis; however, as the urine pressure in the bladder begins to rise, the flexible ends of the ureters are compressed against their supports in the bladder wall. This prevents backflow of urine.

***Urethra* (Figs. *A2*, *A16*):** The urethra is the tube that conveys urine from the bladder to the exterior. The female urethra is 2.5 cm to 3.5 cm (1 in–1½ in) in length. As it curves downward from the bladder, it is united firmly with the anterior wall of the vagina. An external sphincter surrounds the orifice and enables one to control the escape of urine voluntarily. The male urethra consists of three portions: the prostatic portion is about 2.5 cm (1 in) long and extends from the urinary bladder to the pelvic floor. During its course, it is surrounded completely by the prostate gland. The membranous portion and the cavernous portion, which is in the penis, constitute the remainder of the male urethra.

Urination: Urination (micturition) refers to emptying of the urinary bladder. When about 250 ml of urine has accumulated in the bladder, receptors transmit an impulse that stimulates a desire to empty the bladder. Although emptying of the bladder is reflex in nature, it is initiated by an effort of the will and a voluntary removal of restraint.

***Uterus* (Fig. *A16*):** The uterus is a hollow, thick-walled, muscular organ, the lower portion of which connects with the vagina. Along both distal edges of the upper border are the openings of the fallopian tubes. The upper portion is called the body, or fundus, and the lower portion is called the cervix. The uterus is suspended by heavy muscles and ligaments. The upper portion of the uterus is free, movable, and rests on the upper surface of the bladder; therefore, when the bladder is full, the uterus may be tilted backward. The uterus is capable of great expansion during pregnancy to accommodate the fetus. The function of the uterus is to contain the fetus during pregnancy and expel the fetus and placenta during the birth process.

***Vagina* (Fig. *A16*):** The vagina is a muscular tube about 9 cm (3½ in) long lying between the bladder and the urethra anteriorly and the rectum posteriorly. It proceeds downward from the uterus to the outside of the body. The upper end is attached to the cervix. The surface of the vagina is a series of folds (rugae). It serves as an excretory duct of the uterus and provides a depository for sperm during sexual intercourse.

***Vertebral column* (Fig. *A19*):** The vertebral column, or backbone, of the adult consists of 26 separate bony segments arranged in a series to form a strong, flexible pillar. Ligaments help to hold the segments in the proper position. There are seven cervical vertebrae (in the neck), twelve thoracic vertebrae (in the thorax), five lumbar vertebrae (in the small of the back), five fused vertebrae forming the sacrum (in the lower back), and one coccyx, or tailbone. An intervertebral disk composed of cartilaginous material serves as a buffer between each of the vertebrae. The vertebral column provides the strength and rigidity necessary to support the head, trunk, and upper extremities. The normal curves of the column provide some of the resilience and spring essential for walking and jumping. In addition, the vertebral column surrounds and protects the spinal cord and the origins of the the spinal nerves.

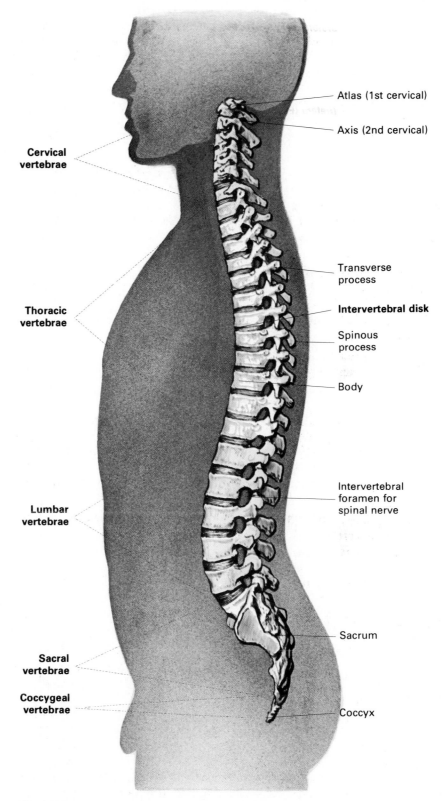

Cervical vertebrae

Atlas (1st cervical)

Axis (2nd cervical)

Thoracic vertebrae

Transverse process

Intervertebral disk

Spinous process

Body

Lumbar vertebrae

Intervertebral foramen for spinal nerve

Sacral vertebrae

Sacrum

Coccygeal vertebrae

Coccyx

Figure A19.
Lateral aspect of the vertebral column.

Appendix II   Charting Abbreviations

Rules Governing Initials and Abbreviations for Charting

1. Abbreviations should be used consistently. Imaginative abbreviations that are meaningful to only a few have no place on the client's record.
2. Abbreviations and initials should not be used in portions of the chart that are likely to be used for legal purposes.
3. If there is any possibility that the abbreviation or initial will be misinterpreted, the word should be spelled out.

Acceptable Initials and Abbreviations for Charting

General Terms

abd	abdomen
ac	before meals
AC	alternating current
accom	accommodation
ACTH	adrenocorticotropic hormone
ad	to, up to
ADH	antidiuretic hormone
ad. lib.	as desired
adm	admission
AFB	acid-fast bacillus
AK	above knee
alb	albumin
alk	alkaline
AM	morning
amb	ambulate
amp	ampule
amt	amount
anes	anesthesia, anesthetic
ant	anterior
AP	anteroposterior
APC	aspirin, phenacetin, caffeine
approx	approximately
ARM	artificial rupture of membranes (amniotic)
ASA	acetylsalicylic acid (aspirin)
ASHD	arteriosclerotic heart disease
AV node	atrioventricular node
ax	axillary
BBB	bundle branch block
BCG	bacillus Calmette–Guérin (vaccine for tuberculosis)
b.i.d.	twice a day
bisp	bispinous or interspinous diameter (pelvic measurement)
BK	below knee
BM	bowel movement
BMR	basal metabolic rate
BP	blood pressure

BPH	benign prostatic hyperplasia
BRP	bathroom privileges
C	centigrade
c̄	with
C_1, C_2 (etc)	first cervical vertebra, second vertebra (etc)
Ca	calcium
CA	cancer, carcinoma
cap	capsule
cath	catheter, catheterized
cc	cubic centimeter
CCU	coronary care unit
CHF	congestive heart failure
CHO or carbo	carbohydrate
Cl	chloride
cm	centimeter
CNS	central nervous system
CO_2	carbon dioxide
COPD	chronic obstructive pulmonary disease
comp	compound
conc	concentrate, concentrated
cont	continued, continuous
CPD	cephalopelvic disproportion
CPR	cardiopulmonary resuscitation
C&S	culture and sensitivity
CS	cesarean section
CSF	cerebrospinal fluid
CVA	cerebrovascular accident
CVP	central venous pressure
cysto	cystoscope, cystoscopy
CZI	crystalline zinc insulin
DC	discontinue; direct current
DC	diagonal conjugate (pelvic measurement)
D&C	dilatation and curettage
diab	diabetic
diag	diagnosis
diam	diameter
dil	dilute, diluted
disc	discontinue
dl	deciliter
DNS	Director of Nursing Service
DOA	dead on arrival
Dr.	doctor
dr	dram
DTs	delirium tremens
D/W	distilled water
Dx	diagnosis
EDC	expected date of confinement
EENT	eye, ear, nose and throat
elix	elixir
EOM	extraocular movement
epith	epithelial
ER	emergency room
et	and
et al	and others
etc	and so on
exam	examination

exp lap	exploratory laparotomy
expir	expiration, expiratory
ext	extract, external
F	Fahrenheit
F cath	Foley catheter
F.H.	family history
FHS	fetal heart sound
FHT	fetal heart tones
fl, fld	fluid
FOC	frontal–occipital circumference
fract	fracture
ft	feet
G in W *or* glyc. in W	glycerin in water
gal	gallon
GB	gallbladder
GC	gonorrhea
GI	gastrointestinal
g	gram
gr	grain
Grav I, grav II *(etc)*	primigravida, secundigravida (etc)
gt	drop
GU	genitourinary
gyn	gynecology
H *or* (H)	hypodermic
h	hour
H et H *or* H&H	hemoglobin and hematocrit
H&P	history and physical
Hb *or* Hgb	hemoglobin
HC	head circumference
HCG	human chorionic gonadotropic hormone
HCl	hydrochloric acid
Hct	hematocrit
Hg	mercury
H_2O	water
H_2O_2	hydrogen peroxide
HOB	head of bed
hosp	hospital
hr	hour
hs	hour of sleep; bedtime
ht	height
hx	history
I	iodine
ICU	intensive care unit
I&D	incision and drainage
ID	intradermal
IICU	infant intensive care unit
IM	intramuscular
inspir	inspiration, inspiratory
inter	between
I&O	intake and output
IOP	intraocular pressure
IPPB	intermittent positive-pressure breathing
IQ	intelligence quotient
irrig	irrigation, irrigated
iss	one and one-half

IT	inhalation therapy, intertuberous (pelvic measurement)
IV	intravenous
K	potassium
Kg	kilogram
$KMnO_4$	potassium permanganate
L	liter
L *or* lt	left
L_1, L_2, L_3 *(etc)*	first lumbar vertebra, second lumbar vertebra, third lumbar vertebra (etc)
lab	laboratory
lap	laparotomy
lat	lateral
lb	pound
LE	lupus erythematosus
lg	large
LH	luteinizing hormone
liq	liquid
LLL	left lower lobe (lung)
LMP	last menstrual period
LP	lumbar puncture
LR	lactated Ringer's (IV solution)
LUL	left upper lobe (lung)
L&W	living and well
M	male, thousand
m	minim; meter
max	maximum
mcg (*or* μg)	microgram
med	medicine
mEq	milliequivalent
mEq/L	millequivalents per liter
Mg	magnesium
mg, mgm	milligram
MI	myocradial infarction
mid	middle
min	minute, minimum
ml	milliliter
mm	millimeter
Mn	manganese
mo	month
MS	morphine sulfate, multiple sclerosis
N	normal, nitrogen
Na	sodium
NB	newborn
neg	negative
neuro	neurology, neurologic
NICU	neonatal intensive care unit
no	number
noct	nocturnal (night)
non. rep.	do not repeat
NPO	nothing by mouth
NS	neurosurgery
N/S	normal saline
N&V	nausea and vomiting
'o'	orally
O_2	oxygen

O₂ cap	oxygen capacity
O₂ sat	oxygen saturation
obs *or* OB	obstetrics
O.C.	obstetrical conjugate (pelvic measurment)
occ	occasional
occ. th.	occupational therapy
o.d.	daily
OD	right eye, overdose
OFC	occipital–frontal circumference
oint	ointment
op	operation
ophth	ophthalmology
opt	optimal
OR	operating room
ortho	orthopedic
OS	left eye
OT	occupational therapy
oto	otology
OU	both eyes
oz	ounce
P	pulse
p̄	after or post
PA	posteroanterior
palp	palpable
Pap	Papanicolaou smear test
PAR	postanesthesia recovery
Para I, Para II *(etc)*	primipara, secundipara (etc)
paracent	paracentesis
Path	pathology, pathological
pc	after meals
PE	physical education
ped	pediatrics
PEEP	positive end expiratory pressure
percuss. & ausc.	percussion and auscultation
PERLA	pupils equal and reactive to light and accommodation
PIH	pregnancy-induced–hypertension (toxemia)
PKU	phenylketonuria
pH	hydrogen concentration
P.I.	present illness
PID	pelvic inflammatory disease
P.M.	afternoon
PMP	previous menstrual period
PNP	pediatric nurse practitioner
PO	phone order
p.o.	per os (by mouth)
poplit	popliteal
pos	positive
postop	postoperative
prep	preparation
preop	preoperative
PRN	whenever necessary
prog	prognosis
prot	protein
psych	psychiatric, psychiatry
pt	pint
PT	physical therapy
pulv	powder

PVC	premature ventricular contraction
PVD	peripheral vascular disease
PZI	protamine zinc insulin
q	every
q.i.d.	four times a day
qh	every hour
q2hr, q3hr *(etc)*	every 2 hours, every 3 hours (etc)
q.o.d.	every other day
q.n.	every night
q.n.s.	quanity not sufficient
q.s.	quantity sufficient
qt	quart
quant	quantity, quantitative
R	rectal, respirations; right
resp	respiratory, respiration
req	request, requisition
RHF	right heart failure
RLL	right lower lobe (lung)
RLQ	right lower quadrant (abdomen)
RML	right middle lobe (lung)
ROM	range of motion
rt	right
rt'd	returned
RUL	right upper lobe (lung)
RUQ	right upper quadrant
Rx	therapy, treatment
s̄	without
SAD	sugar and acetone determination
SA node	sinoatrial node
SC	subcutaneous
SCIV	subclavian intravenous
S.H.	social history
sig	write or label
sm	small
SMR	submucous resection
sod. bicarb.	sodium bicarbonate
sol	solution
SOS	may be repeated once if urgently required
spec	specimen
sp. fl.	spinal fluid
sp. gr.	specific gravity
s. s. enema	soap suds enema
Staph	Streptococcus
stat	immediately, once only
stillb	stillbirth
Strep	Steptococcus
subcu	subcutaneous
subling	sublingual (under the tongue)
supp	suppository
surg	surgery, surgical
sympt	symptom
syr	syrup
Sx	symptoms
T	temperature
T&A	tonsillectomy and adenoidectomy

tab	tablet
TAT	tetanus antitoxin
Tb	tubercle bacillus
TB	tuberculosis
tbsp	tablespoon
temp	temperature
t.i.d.	three times a day
tinct	tincture
TL	tubal ligation
TLC	total lung capacity, tender loving care
TLV	total lung volume
TPR	temperature, pulse, respiration
tr	tincture
trach	tracheostomy
tsp	teaspoon
TUR	transurethral resection
U	unit
UA	urinalysis
ung	ointment
URI	upper respiratory infection
UTI	urinary tract infection
urol	urology, urologic
vag	vaginal
VC	vital capacity
VD	venereal disease
VI	volume index
vit	vitamin
vit. cap.	vital capacity
VO	verbal orders
vol	volume
VS	vital signs
WBC	white blood cells
wd	well-developed
wn	well-nourished
wt	weight

X-ray Abbreviations

AP	anteroposterior
AP & Lat	anteroposterior and lateral
^{198}Au	radioactive gold
Ba enema	barium enema
Ba swallow	barium swallow
CAT	computerized axial tomography
Co	cobalt
ECG (EKG)	electrocardiogram
echo	echo encephalogram
EEG	electroencephalogram
EMG	electromyograph, electromyogram
GB series	gallbladder series
GI series	gastrointestinal series
^{131}I	radioactive iodine
IV cholangiogram	intravenous cholangiogram
IVP	intravenous pyelogram
KUB	kidney, ureters, bladder

MFT	muscle function test
UGI	upper gastrointestinal series

Laboratory Abbreviations

acid p'tase	acid phosphatase
AFB	acid fast bacillus
AG	albumin–globulin ratio
alk	alkaline
alk p'tase	alkaline phosphatase
ANA	antinuclear antibody (test for lupus erythematosus)
ASO or ASTO	antistreptolysin
baso	basophile
bili	bilirubin
bl. cult.	blood culture
Bl. time	bleeding time
Br	bromide
BSP	bromosulphalein
BUN	blood urea nitrogen
C	carbon
Ca	calcium
CBC	complete blood count
ceph. floc.	cephalin flocculation test
chol	cholesterol
chol. est.	cholesterol ester
CI	color index
Cl	chloride
CPK	creatine phosphokinase
CO_2	carbon dioxide
coag. time	coagulation time
creat	creatinine
CRPA	C-reactive protein antiserum
diff	differential count
eos	eosinophils
FBS	fasting blood sugar
Fe	iron
fib	fibrinogen
glob	globulin
gluc	glucose
g %	grams per hundred milliliters of serum or blood
Hct	hematocrit
Hgb or Hb	hemoglobin
h.p.f.	per high-powered field (used only in describing urine sediments)
I	iodine
ict. ind.	icterus index
LDH	lactic dehydrogenase
LE cell	lupus erythematosus cell
lymph	lymphocytes
MCH	mean corpuscular hemoglobin
MCV	mean corpuscular volume
mg %	milligrams per hundred milliliters of serum or blood
mono	monocytes

NH$_3$N	ammonia nitrogen
NPN	nonprotein nitrogen
PBI	protein-bound iodine
pCO$_2$	partial pressure of carbon dioxide
pH	hydrogen concentration
PKU	phenylketonuria
PO$_4$	inorganic phosphorus
polys	polymorphonuclear leukocytes
pro. time	prothrombin time
PSP	phenolsulfonphthalein
RBC	red blood count
sed. rate	sedimentation rate
SGOT	serum glutamic oxaloacetic transaminase
SGPT	serum glutamic pyruvic transaminase
SMAC	sequential multiple analyzer with computer
SMA-12	sequential multiple analysis of 12 chemistry constituents
STS	serologic test for syphilis
T$_3$ test	triiodothyronine test
T$_4$ test	a test for thyroxine
TGR	thromboplastin generation time
TPI	*Treponema pallidum* immobilization test
UA	urinalysis
VDRL	flocculation test for venereal disease
WBC	white blood count
Zn	zinc

Commonly Used Symbols

$>$	greater than
$<$	less than
$=$	equal to
♀	female
♂	male
@	at
&	and
#	pound or number
ℨ	dram
℥	ounce
$\times$	times
i	one time
ii	two times
iii	three times
iv	four times
v	five times
vi	six times
vii	seven times
viii	eight times
ix	nine times
x	ten times

Appendix III   Commonly Used Conversion Techniques for Calculation of Drug Dosages

1. To convert from one form of measurement to another, the basic equivalents are

   60 mg = 1 gr (grain)
     1 mg = 1/60 gr
   0.06 g = 1 gr
       1 g = 15 gr
      30 g = 1 oz
   1 ml* = 15 m (minims)
    30 ml = 1 fluid oz

2. Commonly used conversions may be summarized as follows:
   a. *Grams to grains:* multiply the number of grams by 15.
   b. *Grains to grams:* divide the number of grains by 15.
   c. *Milligrams to grains:* divide the number of milligrams by 60.
   d. *Grains to milligrams:* multiply the number of grains by 60.
   e. *Grams to ounces:* divide the number of grams by 30.
   f. *Ounces to grams:* multiply the number of ounces by 30.
   g. *Fluid ounces to milliliters:* multiply the number of fluid ounces by 30.
   h. *Milliliters to fluid ounces:* divide the number of milliliters by 30.
   i. *Milliliters to minims:* multiply the number of milliliters by 15.
   j. *Minims to milliliters:* divide the number of minims by 15.

3. Weight and liquid measures: Always try to visualize the quantity with which you are concerned.
   a. 1 minim (m) is about the size of a drop of water.
   b. 1 grain (gr) is approximately the weight of a drop of water.
   c. 1 fluid dram is approximately a teaspoonful.
   d. 1 teaspoonful of water weighs about 1 dram (dr).
   e. 1 ounce (oz) almost fills a medicine cup.

4. Tables of approximate equivalents
   Weights

| APOTHECARY UNITS | | METRIC UNITS | | HOUSEHOLD |
WEIGHT	LIQUID	WEIGHT	LIQUID	UNITS
1 gr	1 m	0.06 g	0.01 ml (or cc)	1 drop
15 gr	15 m	1 g	1 ml	15 drops
1 dr (or 60 gr)	1 fluid dr (or 60 m)	4 g	4 ml	1 t (or 60 drops)
1 oz	1 fluid oz	30 g	30 ml	2 T
1 lb	12 oz	360 g	360 ml	2 teacupsful
	1 pt	500 g	500 ml	2 glassesful
	1 qt	1 kg	1 liter or 1,000 ml	4 glassesful
	1 gal	4 kg	4 liter or 4,000 ml	16 glassesful

* milliliter (ml) is considered equivalent to 1 cubic centimeter (cc).

METRIC	APOTHECARY
30 g	1 oz (480 gr)
4 g	1 dr (60 gr)
1 g	15 gr
0.6 g (600 mg)	10 gr
0.32 g (300 mg)	5 gr
0.1 g (100 mg)	1½ gr
0.06 g (60 mg)	1 gr
0.05 g (50 mg)	¾ gr
0.04 g (40 mg)	⅔ gr
0.03 g (30 mg)	½ gr
0.02 g (20 mg)	⅓ gr
0.015 g (15 mg)	¼ gr
0.012 g (12 mg)	⅕ gr
0.01 g (10 mg)	⅙ gr
0.008 g (8 mg)	⅛ gr
0.0064 g (6 mg)	1/10 gr
0.005 g (5 mg)	1/12 gr
0.004 g (4 mg)	1/15 gr
0.003 g (3 mg)	1/20 gr
0.002 g (2 mg)	1/30 gr
0.0015 g (1.5 mg)	1/40 gr
0.0012 g (1.2 mg)	1/50 gr
0.001 g (1 mg)	1/60 gr
0.0008 g (0.8 mg)	1/80 gr
0.0006 g (0.6 mg)	1/100 gr
0.0005 g (0.5 mg)	1/120 gr
0.0004 g (0.4 mg)	1/150 gr
0.0003 g (0.3 mg)	1/200 gr
0.00025 g (0.25 mg)	1/250 gr
0.0002 g (0.2 mg)	1/300 gr

Volume

METRIC	APOTHECARY
30 ml (or cc)	1 fluid oz (490 m)
10 ml	2½ fluid dr
4 ml	1 fluid dr (60 m)
1 ml	15 m
0.6 ml	10 m
0.3 ml	5 m
0.06 ml	1 m
500 ml	1 pt
1,000 ml (1 liter)	1 qt

References and Suggested Readings

Bates B: A Guide to Physical Examination, 3rd ed. Philadelphia, JB Lippincott, 1983

Beland I, Passos J: Clinical Nursing: Pathophysiological and Psychosocial Approaches, 4th ed. New York, Macmillan, 1981

Bobak I, Jensen M: Essentials of Maternity Nursing. St. Louis, CV Mosby, 1984

Broadribb V: Introductory Pediatric Nursing, 3rd ed. Philadelphia, JB Lippincott, 1983

Brunner L, Suddarth D: Textbook of Medical–Surgical Nursing, 5th ed. Philadelphia, JB Lippincott, 1984

Burrell Z, Burrell L: Critical Care, 4th ed. St. Louis, CV Mosby, 1982

Carpenito L: Nursing Diagnosis: Application to Clinical Practice. Philadelphia, JB Lippincott, 1984

Chaffe E, Lytle I: Basic Physiology and Anatomy, 4th ed. Philadelphia, JB Lippincott, 1980

Chow M et al: Handbook of Pediatric Primary Care, 2nd ed. New York, John Wiley & Sons, 1984

Creighton H: Law Every Nurse Should Know, 4th ed. Philadelphia, WB Saunders, 1981

Fiesta J: The Law and Liability: A Guide for Nurses. New York, John Wiley & Sons, 1983

Garner J, Simmons B: Guideline for Isolation Precautions in Hospitals. Atlanta, GA, Centers for Disease Control, 1983

Hamilton A: Critical Care Nursing Skills. New York, Appleton–Century–Crofts, 1981

Hamilton P: Basic Maternity Nursing, 5th ed. St. Louis, CV Mosby, 1984

Hammond B, Lee G: Quick Reference to Emergency Nursing. Philadelphia, JB Lippincott, 1984

Hawkins J, Higgins L: Maternity and Gynecological Nursing: Women's Health Care. Philadelphia, JB Lippincott, 1981

Howe J: Nursing Care of Adolescents. New York, McGraw-Hill, 1980

Johnson B et al: Standards for Critical Care. St. Louis, CV Mosby, 1981

Kozier G, Erb G: Techniques in Clinical Nursing: A Comprehensive Approach. Menlo Park, CA, Addison–Wesley, 1982

Lewis L: Fundamental Skills in Patient Care, 3rd ed. Philadelphia, JB Lippincott, 1984

Lippincott Manual of Nursing Practice, 3rd ed. Philadelphia, JB Lippincott, 1982

Mason M, Bates G: Basic Medical–Surgical Nursing, 5th ed. New York, Macmillan, 1984

McConnell E, Zimmerman M: Care of Patients with Urologic Problems. Philadephia, JB Lippincott, 1983

Metheny N, Snively W: Nurses' Handbook of Fluid Balance, 4th ed. Philadelphia, JB Lippincott, 1983

NAACOG Standards for Obstetric, Gynecologic, and Neonatal Nursing, 2nd ed. Washington, DC, The Nurses' Association of the American College of Obstetricians and Gynecologists, 1981

Phipps W et al: Medical Surgical Nursing. St. Louis, CV Mosby, 1983

Pikl B (ed): Massachusetts General Hospital Manual of Pediatric Nursing Practice. Boston, Little, Brown & Co, 1981

Phillips C: Family-centered Maternity/Newborn Care: A Basic Text. St. Louis, CV Mosby, 1980

Porth C: Pathophysiology: Concepts of Altered Health States, Philadelphia, JB Lippincott, 1982

Reeder S, Mastroianni L, Martin L: Maternity Nursing, 15th ed. Philadelphia, JB Lippincott, 1983

Russo R, Gurruraaj V: Practical Points in Pediatrics, 3rd ed. Garden City, NY, Medical Examination Publishing Company, 1981

Sana J, Judge R: Physical Assessment Skills for Nursing Practice, 2nd ed. Boston, Little, Brown, & Co, 1982

Smith M et al: Child and Family: Concepts of Nursing Practice. New York, McGraw–Hill, 1982

Smith S, Duell D: Nursing Skills and Evaluation: A Nursing Process Approach. Los Altos, CA, National Nursing Review, 1982

Sporin E, Walton M, Cady C: The Children's Hospital of Philadelphia Manual of Pediatric Nursing Policies, Procedures, and Personnel. Oradel, NJ, Medical Economics Books, 1984

Thomas C (ed): Taber's Cyclopedic Medical Dictionary, 14th ed. Philadelphia, FA Davis, 1981

Vestal K (ed): Pediatric Critical Care Nursing. New York, John Wiley & Sons, 1981

Whaley L, Wong D: Essentials of Pediatric Nursing. St. Louis, CV Mosby, 1982

Whitson B, McFarlane J: The Pediatric Nursing Skills Manual. New York, John Wiley & Sons, 1980

Wieczorek R, Natapoff J: A Conceptual Approach to the Nursing of Children: Health Care from Birth through Adolescence. Philadelphia, JB Lippincott, 1981

Index